Anatomy & Physiology for Health Professions

An Interactive Journey

Bruce J. Colbert
Director of Allied Health
University of Pittsburgh at Johnstown

Jeff Ankney
Director of Clinical Education
University of Pittsburgh at Johnstown

Karen T. Lee
Associate Professor of Biology
University of Pittsburgh at Johnstown

PEARSON
Prentice Hall
Upper Saddle River, New Jersey 07458

Library of Congress Cataloging-in-Publication Data
Colbert, Bruce J.
Anatomy and physiology for health professionals : an interactive journey / Bruce J. Colbert, Jeff Ankney, Karen T. Lee
p. ; cm.
ISBN 0-13-151268-4
1. Human anatomy. 2. Physiology. I. Ankney, Jeff. II. Lee, Karen T. III. Title.
[DNLM: 1. Anatomy. 2. Physiological Processes. QS 4 C684a 2006]
QM23.2.C64 2006
612—dc22
2005027594

Publisher: Julie Levin Alexander
Assistant to Publisher: Regina Bruno
Executive Editor: Mark Cohen
Associate Editor: Melissa Kerian
Development Editor: Jill Rembetski, Triple SSS Press Media Development
Media Editor: John J. Jordan
Director of Production and Manufacturing: Bruce Johnson
Managing Production Editor: Patrick Walsh
Production Liaison: Christina Zingone
Production Editor: Patty Donovan, Pine Tree Composition
Manufacturing Manager: Ilene Sanford
Manufacturing Buyer: Pat Brown
Art Director/Cover Designer: Cheryl Asherman
Interior Design: Wanda España
Medical Illustrators: Barb Cousins/Hutchinson Studio and Imagineering Media Services Inc.
Director of Marketing: Karen Allman
Senior Marketing Manager: Harper Coles
Manager of Media Production: Amy Peltier
Media Project Manager: Stephen Hartner
New Media Production: Hector Grillone, Anne Lukens, Jody Small, and Kate Stillings, Pearson Video Production Services, Red Frog, Inc.
Composition: Pine Tree Composition, Inc.
Printer/Binder: Banta Book Group
Cover Printer: Phoenix Color Corp.

Image Credits
Stamp with postal marks: Sharon Swanson/Getty Images, Inc.–Illustration Works
Anatomy of Shoulder Injury: Russell Thurston/Getty Images, Inc.–Photodisc
Compass: Dana Mardaga/Images.com

Notice:
The authors and the publisher of this volume have taken care that the information and technical recommendations contained herein are based on research and expert consultation, and are accurate and compatible with the standards generally accepted at the time of publication. Nevertheless, as new information becomes available, changes in clinical and technical practices become necessary. The reader is advised to carefully consult manufacturers' instructions and information material for all supplies and equipment before use, and to consult with a health care professional as necessary. This advice is especially important when using new supplies or equipment for clinical purposes. The authors and publisher disclaim all responsibility for any liability, loss, injury, or damage incurred as a consequence, directly or indirectly, of the use and application of any of the contents of this volume.

Pearson Education LTD.
Pearson Education Singapore, Pte. Ltd
Pearson Education, Canada, Ltd
Pearson Education–Japan
Pearson Education Australia PTY, Limited
Pearson Education North Asia Ltd
Pearson Educación de Mexico, S.A. de C.V.
Pearson Education Malaysia, Pte. Ltd
Pearson Education, Inc. Upper Saddle River, New Jersey

PEARSON
Prentice Hall

10 9 8 7 6 5 4 3
ISBN 0-13-151268-4

DEDICATIONS

To all the future health care professionals learning Anatomy and Physiology. May your chosen professions be as personally rewarding as ours have been.

—*Your Travel Guides*
Bruce, Jeff, and Karen

To those closest to me, who share this wonderful journey through life: my wife Patty, my sons Joshua and Jeremy, my Mom, and my brothers and sister. And to Jen and Kristi Jan, who, through my sons, have become part of this family. Finally, to the memory of my Dad, who taught me the importance of education.

—*Bruce*

To the most wonderful family a person could ever wish for, and a better one than I probably deserve: Patty, Zack, Emily, Sara, Mom, and Dad, and, of course, Rusty. And to my past teachers and professors; here's proof that underachievers sometimes do hit their stride!

—*Jeff*

I dedicate this book to my family who have always supported me, no matter where life has taken me; not only my "real" family; my late father, Ed, my mother Pat, brother Eddie, sister-in-law Sheila, and assorted aunts, uncles, and cousins, who really had no choice but to be part of my life, but also those members of my extended family who have inexplicably chosen to be part of my life, giving me the gift of their friendship. I couldn't have done it without them.

—*Karen*

CONTENTS

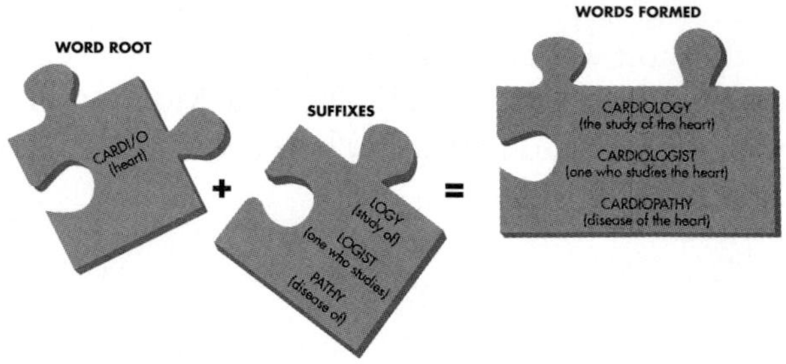

WORD ROOT
CARDI/O (heart)
+
SUFFIXES
LOGY (study of)
LOGIST (one who studies)
PATHY (disease of)
=
WORDS FORMED
CARDIOLOGY (the study of the heart)
CARDIOLOGIST (one who studies the heart)
CARDIOPATHY (disease of the heart)

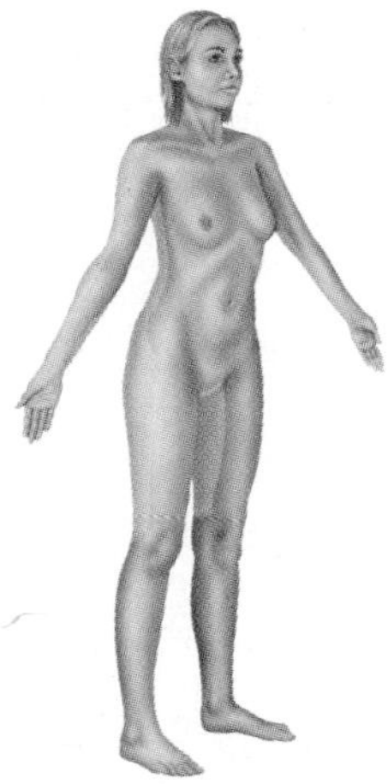

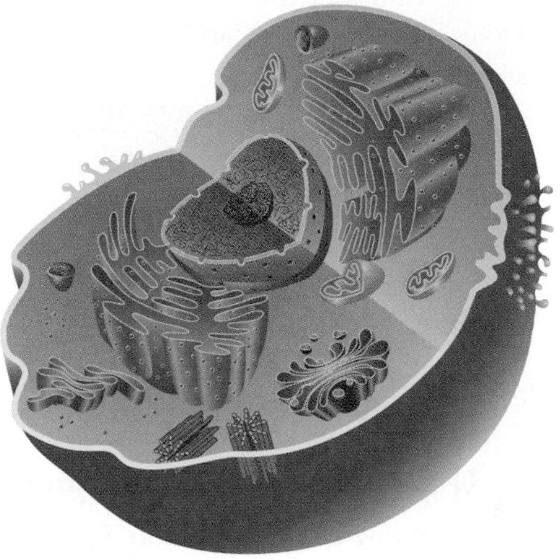

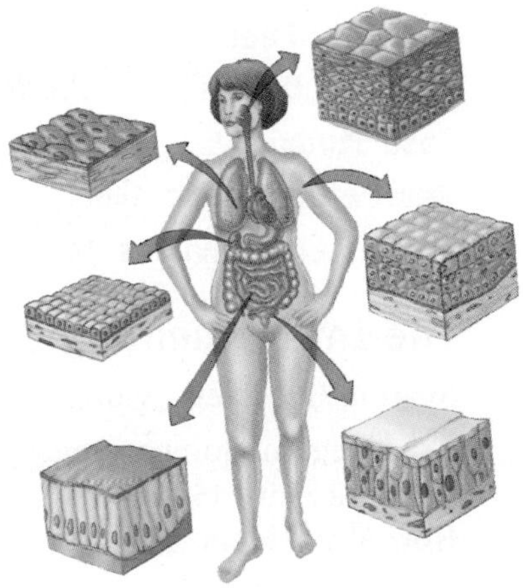

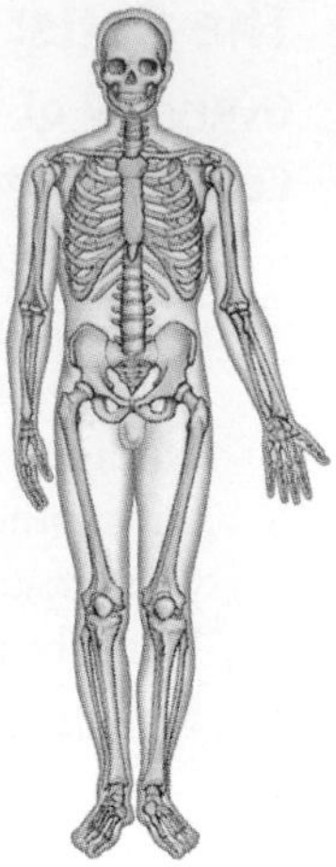

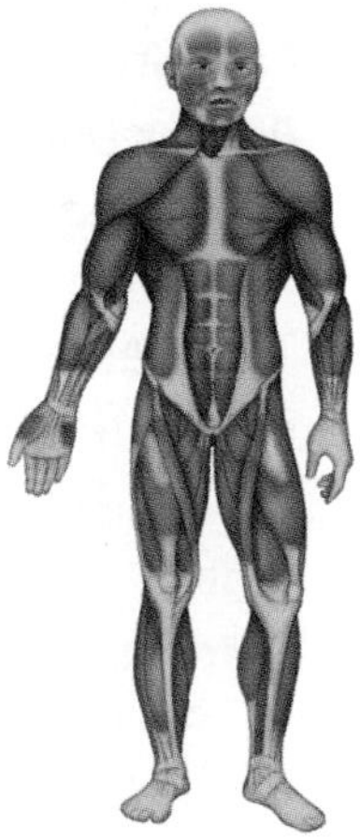

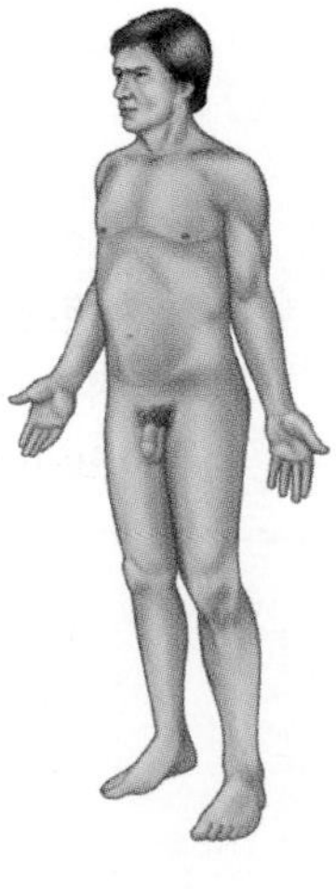

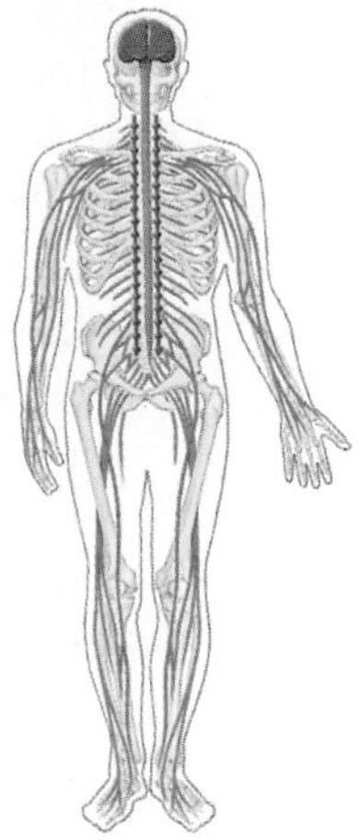

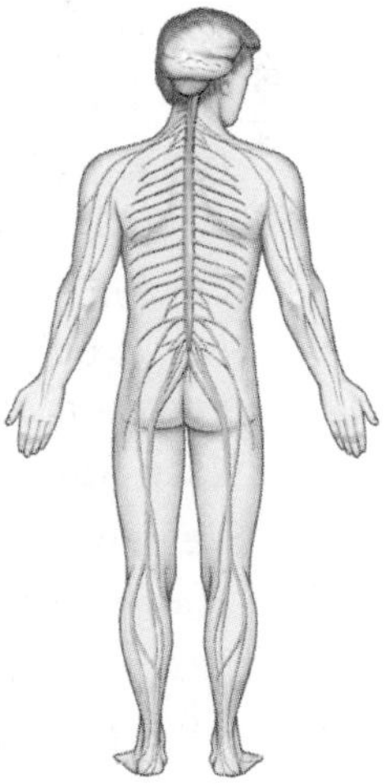

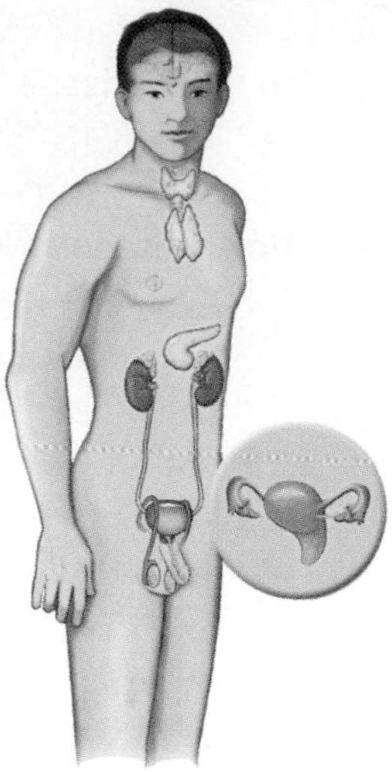

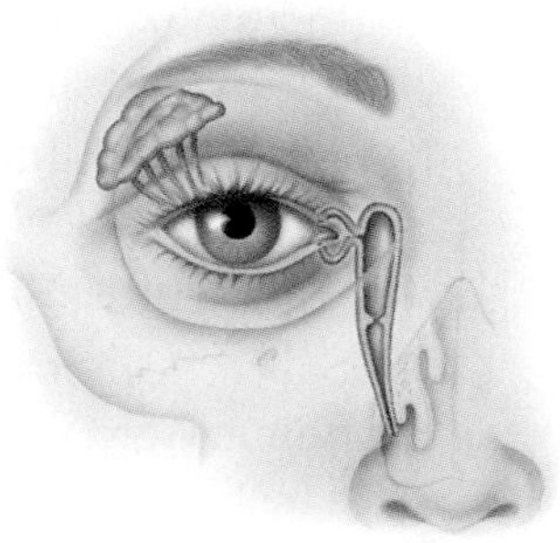

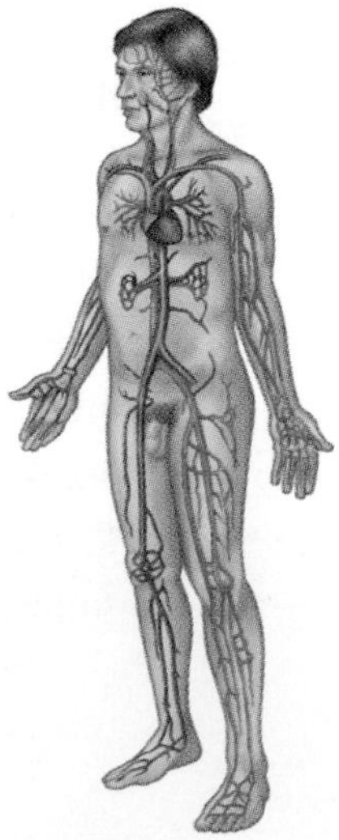

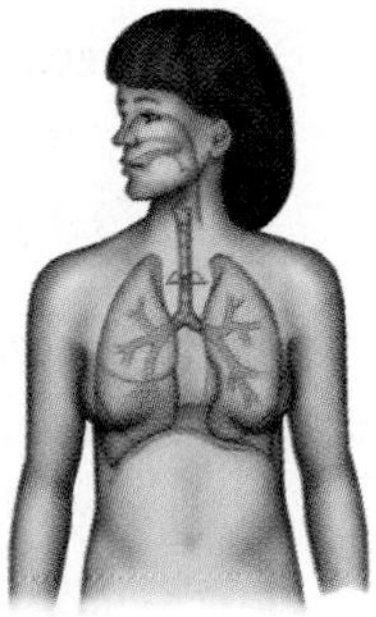

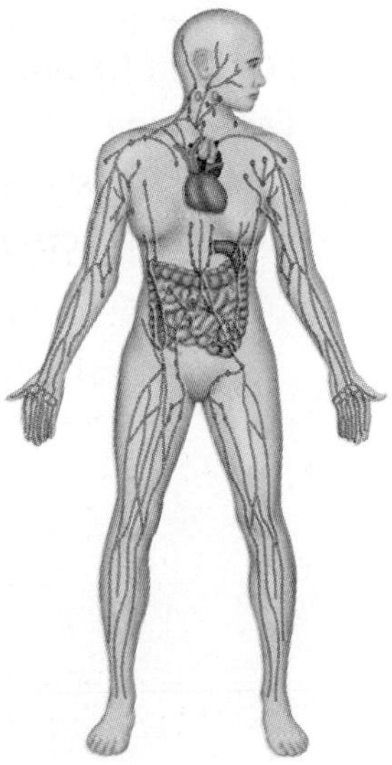

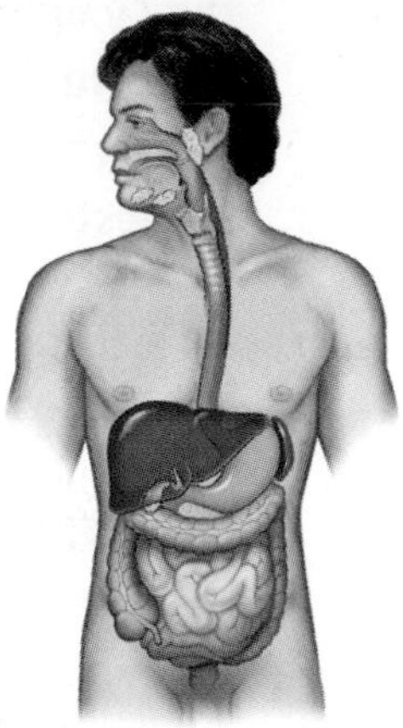

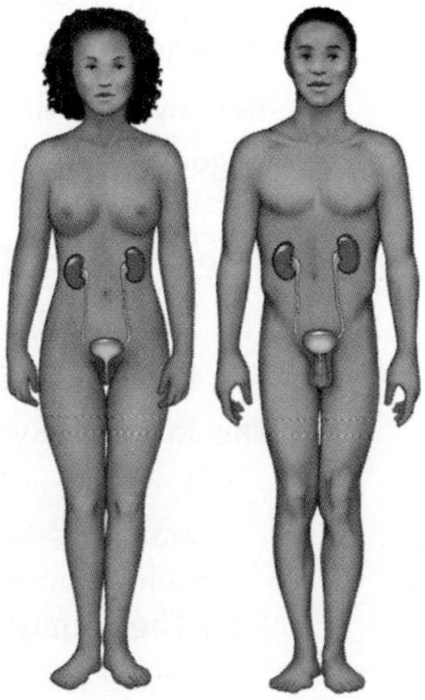

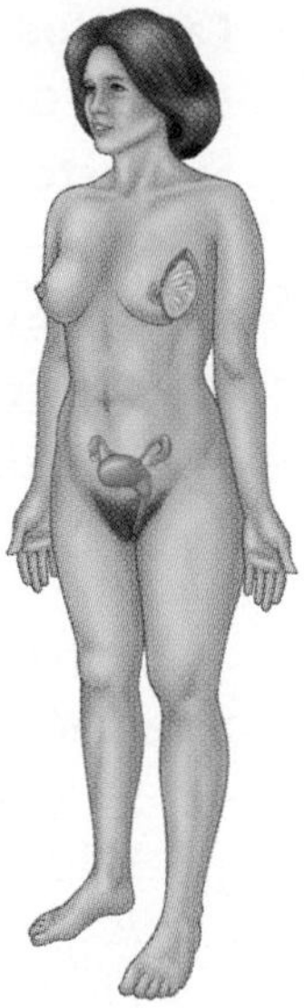

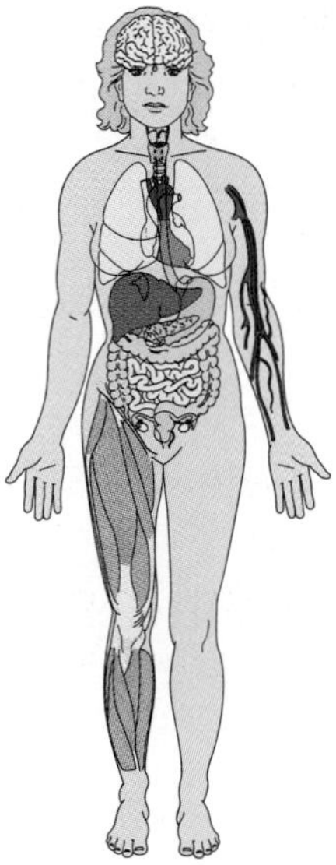

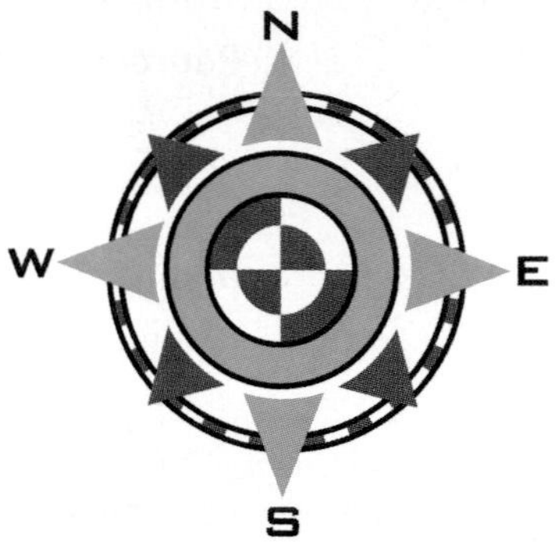
N
W
E
S

ABOUT THE AUTHORS

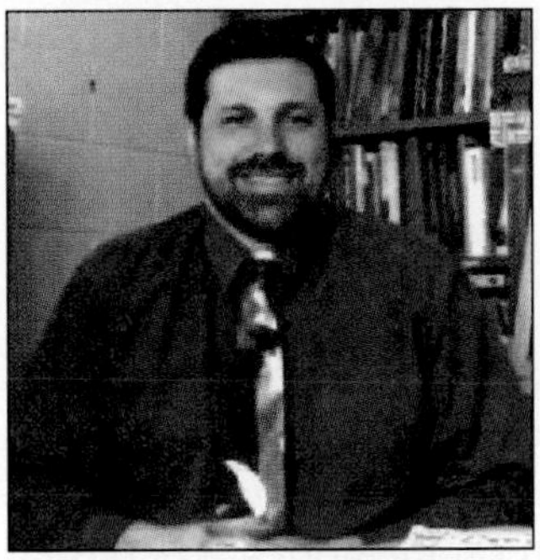

Bruce Colbert is the Director of the Allied Health Department at the University of Pittsburgh at Johnstown. He holds a Master's in Health Education and Administration, has authored four books, written several articles, and given over 175 invited lectures and workshops at both the regional and national level. Many of his workshops provide teacher training involving techniques to make the health sciences engaging and relevant to today's students. In addition, he does workshops on developing effective critical and creative thinking, stress and time management, and study skills. He is an avid basketball player, even after three knee surgeries, which may indicate he has some learning difficulties.

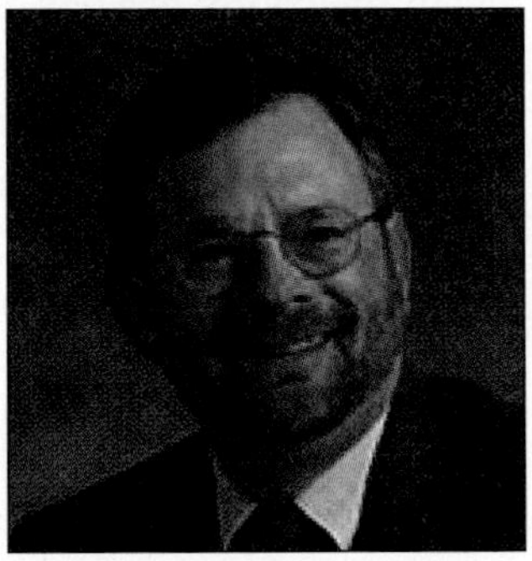

Jeff Ankney is the Director of Clinical Education for the University of Pittsburgh at Johnstown Respiratory Care program where he is responsible for the development and evaluation of hospital clinical sites. In the past, Jeff has served as a public school teacher, Assistant Director of Cardiopulmonary Services, Program Coordinator of Pulmonary Rehabilitation, and a member of hospital utilization review and hospital policy committees. He is a consultant on hospital management and pulmonary rehabilitation concerns. Jeff was also the recipient of the American Cancer Society Public Education Award. He is a pretty fair fly fisherman and wing shot, although his springer spaniel, Rusty, would probably disagree.

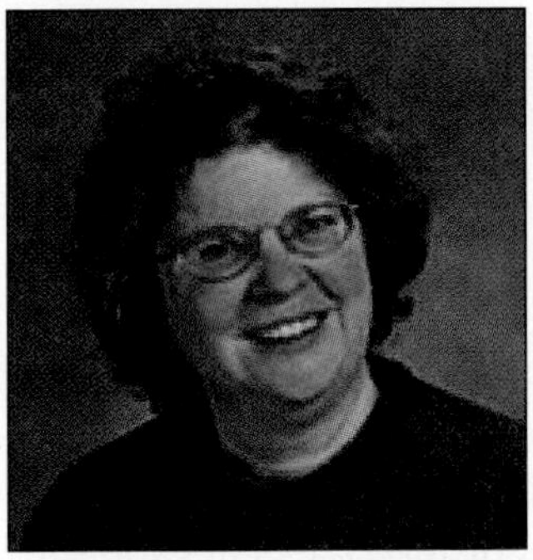

Karen Lee is an Associate Professor in the Biology Department at the University of Pittsburgh at Johnstown, where she teaches all the anatomy courses, including Anatomy and Physiology for Nursing and Allied Health students. She presents regularly at scientific conferences and has published several articles on crustacean physiology and behavior. An active member of the Council on Undergraduate Research, she is also the chair of the University of Pittsburgh at Johnstown's annual undergraduate symposium. For the last fifteen years she has sung bass in women's barbershop choruses and quartets and more recently has been harmonizing with any singer or guitar player who will let her near the microphone.

PREFACE

We have made every effort to put together an Anatomy and Physiology book that students would actually enjoy reading. This book is supplemented with a CD and dedicated website that reinforces the concepts and allows for a visual and interactive learning experience.

Anatomy and Physiology is a critical academic course you must master to succeed in the health professions. ***Anatomy and Physiology for Health Professionals: An Interactive Journey,*** along with the accompanying *Study Success Companion*, integrated CD, and website, are written in a manner that will enhance learning of the material versus mass memorization of facts. Too often students adopt the strategy of memorizing massive amounts of information and simply storing it in their short-term memories. Then they literally spew this information during their exams, which may allow them to *survive* the course. However, memorization alone does not help learners internalize the material and make the lasting connections that will help them *thrive* as a health care practitioner.

In the course of a day as a health professional, you will be exposed to a variety of diseases involving all parts of the body and, therefore, must truly learn the workings and interrelatedness of all the body systems and functions. Imagine someone saying to you, as a loved one has a cardiac arrest, "Sorry, I memorized CPR six months ago but now I forget what to do." We think you get the picture.

So what have we done to facilitate learning the material? First, we have placed study skills and stress management tips in a *Study Success Companion* in the back of your book to help you along your journey through this class and beyond. Second, we have strived to make anatomy and physiology "come alive" by using an engaging writing style to make it seem as if we are sitting next to you talking about the concepts. We hope you consider us assistants to the most important guide through this journey: your teacher.

Humor, where appropriate, and analogies to compare the human body to everyday things to which you can relate, has been interwoven throughout the text. Finally, we have added special features in a unique fashion tailored to the visual learning styles and relevant learning that today's students require.

We have worked hard and sincerely hope these features will help make studying Anatomy and Physiology a positive experience. Have a safe and happy journey!

ACKNOWLEDGMENTS

To Jill Rembetski who acted as our guide through the development and completion of this textbook. To all those at Prentice Hall who were so helpful and friendly in this monumental process. A special thanks goes to Mark Cohen for his enthusiastic belief and support in the vision and execution of this unique project. Thank you to a great group of reviewers who helped shape this project with their thoughtful insights. Finally, special thanks to Jan Snyder and Jamie Kusher for putting up with two quirky authors and helping in so many ways.

CONTRIBUTORS

Instructor's Manual

Debra S. McKinney, RN, BSN
Practical Nursing Program Director
TESST College of Technology
Alexandria, Virginia

Test Bank

Nina Beaman, MS, RNC, CMA
Program Area Coordinator
Allied Health
Bryant and Stratton College
Richmond, Virginia

Joy Harden, RN, BSN, CNOR, MBA
Former Director of Health Services Education
Virginia College
Mobile, Alabama

PowerPoint Lecture

Debra S. McKinney, RN, BSN
Practical Nursing Program Director
TESST College of Technology
Alexandria, Virginia

Companion Website

Margaret N. Anfinsen, RN, MSN
Associate Program Manager
Allied Health Studies
Southwest Florida College
Fort Myers, Florida

Minda Brown, RMA
Instructor
Medical Assisting
Pima Medical Institute
Colorado Springs, Colorado

Student CD-ROM

Margaret N. Anfinsen, RN, MSN
Associate Program Manager
Allied Health Studies
Southwest Florida College
Fort Myers, Florida

Joy Harden, RN, BSN, CNOR, MBA
Former Director of Health Services Education
Virginia College
Mobile, Alabama

Mary Warren-Oliver, BA
Clinical Coordinator
Medical Assisting
Gibbs College
Vienna, Virginia

Workbook

Nadine Forbes, M.S.
Research Associate
Department of Comparative Medicine
Johns Hopkins University
Baltimore, Maryland

Classroom Response System

Joel Scott, LMT
Consultant
Massage Therapy
Blue Cliff Career College
Mobile, Alabama

REVIEWERS

Margaret N. Anfinsen, RN, MSN
Associate Program Manager
Allied Health Studies
Southwest Florida College
Fort Myers, Florida

Nina Beaman, MS RNC CMA
Program Area Coordinator
Allied Health
Bryant and Stratton College
Richmond, Virginia

Dorothea Best, RN, BA, BSHS
Medical Program Director
McCann School of Business and Technology
Scranton, Pennsylvania

Jeanine Brice, RN, MSN
Assistant Professor
Nursing
Pasco-Hernando Community College
New Port Richey, Florida

Minda Brown, RMA
Instructor
Medical Assisting
Pima Medical Institute
Colorado Springs, Colorado

Carmen Carpenter, RN, BSN, CMA, MS
Chair
Allied Health Science and Medical Assisting
South University
West Palm Beach, Florida

Stephanie Cox, BA, LPN
Program Director
Allied Health
York Technical Institute
Lancaster, Pennsylvania

Susan DeGirolamo, RMA, NCPT, NCICS
Medical Program Director
CHI Institute, Southampton Campus
Southampton, Pennsylvania

Kathie Folsom, MS, BSN, RN
Chair
Health Occupations
Skagit Valley College
Oak Harbor, Washington

Nadine Forbes, M.S.
Research Associate
Department of Comparative Medicine
Johns Hopkins University School of Medicine
Baltimore, Maryland

Shirley Jelmo, CMA
Faculty Coordinator & Instructor
Medical Assisting
Pima Medical Institute
Colorado Springs, Colorado

Dee Ann Kerr, BA, MA
Campus Director
Minnesota School of Business
Waite Park, Minnesota

Jennifer A. Leach, BS
Department of Allied Health
Lehigh Valley College
Center Valley, Pennsylvania

Stacey Long, BS
Instructor, Massage Therapy
Miami Jacobs Career College
Dayton, Ohio

Janet M. Bohachef Martin, B.A., M.Ed.
Assistant Professor/Director
Medical Laboratory Technology
Amarillo College
Amarillo, Texas

Andrew E. Muniz, OT, BBA, MBA
Allied Health Sciences
Baker College
Auburn Hills, Michigan

Ruth Ann O'Brien, MHA
Director of Allied Health
Medical Assisting
Miami-Jacobs Career College
Dayton, Ohio

Eddie Rhodes, Jr., MEd., MT(AMT),CPT(ASPT)
Phlebotomy Instructor
West Georgia Technical College
LaGrange, Georgia

Sharon Romine, RN, BSN, MSN
Department of Nursing
Bessemer State Technical College
Bessemer, Alabama

Mary K. Sargent, MS
Assistant Professor of Biology
Ivy Tech State College
Valparaiso, Indiana

Jaqueline T. Smith, AAS, CPhT
Instructor
National College of Business and Technology
Bluefield, Virginia

Barbara Snyder, CMA
Program Director
Medical Department
Thompson Institute
Harrisburg, Pennsylvania

Irma Villarreal, MS
Professor
Health Information
DeVry University
Irving, Texas
and
Medical Assisting Program
Everest College
Dallas, Texas

Joyce A. Wilson, RN, BA
Instructor
Vocational Nursing
South Plains College
Levelland, Texas

SPECIAL FEATURES DIRECTORY LISTING

Chapter 1

In-Text Features

CD Interactive Exercises

Video on Medical Specialties, 1-1
Video on Vital Signs, 1-2
Interactive Games and Puzzles, 1-3

Companion Web site

Professional Profiles:

- Medical Assisting
- Medical Records and Health Information Technician
- Medical Transcriptionist

Related Internet Links
Additional Review Questions

Chapter 2

In-Text Features

CD Interactive Exercises

Additional Video Information on Body Positions, 2-1
Videos on Ultrasound, MRIs and Other Diagnostic Imaging, 2-2
Interactive Drag-and-Drop Exercise to Reinforce Body Cavities, 2-3
Interactive Drag-and-Drop Exercise to Reinforce Anterior and Posterior Body Regions, 2-4
Interactive Games and Puzzles, 2-5

Companion Web site

Professional Profiles

- Radiologic Technology
- Surgical Technology

Related Internet Links
Additional Review Questions

Chapter 3

In-Text Features

CD Interactive Exercises

Companion Web site

Chapter 4

In-Text Features

CD Interactive Exercises

Companion Web site

Chapter 5

In-Text Features

CD Interactive Exercises

Companion Web site

Chapter 6

In-Text Features

CD Interactive Exercises

Companion Web site

Chapter 7

In-Text Features

CD Interactive Exercises

Companion Web site

Chapter 8

In-Text Features

CD Interactive Exercises

Companion Web site

Chapter 9

In-Text Features

CD Interactive Exercises

Positron Emission Tomography (PET) Scan of the Brain, 9-1
Drag-and-Drop Exercise: Brainstem and Arachnoid Space, 9-2
Video on Parkinson's Disease, 9-3
Videos of Absence Seizures, Alzheimer's Disease, Autism, Bipolar Disorder, Dissociative Identity Disorder, Epilepsy, Obsessive-Compulsive Disorder, Complex Partial Seizures, Schizophrenia, Generalized Tonic-Clonic Seizure, and Panic Attacks, 9-4
Interactive Games and Puzzles, 9-5

Companion Web site

Professional Profile
- Pharmacy

Related Internet Links
Additional Review Questions

Chapter 10

In-Text Features

CD Interactive Exercises

Animation and Video Spotlighting the Pathology of Diabetes, 10-1
Interactive Games and Puzzles, 10-2

Companion Web site

Professional Profiles:
- Phlebotomy
- Dietician

Related Internet Links
Additional Review Questions

Chapter 11

In-Text Features

CD Interactive Exercises

Video on Opthalamic Medications and Their Delivery, 11-1
Interactive Drag-and-Drop Exercise of the Eye Structures and 3-D Animation of the Eye, 11-2
Video on Tympanic Membrane Thermometer Measurements, 11-3
Animation of the Workings of the Middle Ear, Adolescent Ear and Child's Ear, 11-4

Companion Web site

Professional Profiles:

- Ophthalmology and Opticians
- Audiologist

Related Internet Links
Additional Review Questions

Chapter 12

In-Text Features

CD Interactive Exercises

Companion Web site

Professional Profiles:

- Cardiovascular Technology

Related Internet Links
Additional Review Questions

Chapter 13

In-Text Features

CD Interactive Exercises

Animation on Gas Exchange, 13-1
3-D Animation of the Respiratory System and an Interactive Drag-and-Drop Labeling Exercise, 13-2
Videos on Various Oxygen Delivery Devices and Respiratory Treatments, 13-3
Interactive Drag-and-Drop Labeling Exercise Concerning the Alveolar Area, 13-4
Interactive Exercise on Labeling the Muscles of Ventilation, 13-5
Animations and Videos on COPD, Asthma, ARDS, Allergic Rhinitis, Apnea and Tuberculosis, 13-6
Interactive Games and Puzzles, 13-7

Companion Web site

Professional Profiles
- Respiratory Therapist
- Perfusionist

Related Internet Links
Additional Review Questions

Chapter 14

In-Text Features

CD Interactive Exercises

Video on Lymphatic Drainage Massage Therapy, 14-1
3-D Illustration of the Lymphatic System, 14-2
Interactive Drag-and-Drop Exercise of the Lymphatic System, 14-3
Pathology Spotlight on Skin Cancer, 14-4
Video on Proper Hand Washing Technique, 14-5
Animation of T Cell Destruction by HIV, 14-6
Pathology Spotlight on Leukemia, 14-7
Animation of the Treatment of Severe Allergic Reactions with an EpiPen, and Allergic Rhinitis, 14-8
Interactive Games and Puzzles, 14-9

Companion Web site

Professional Profiles
- Nuclear Medicine
- Pharmacy

Related Internet Links
Additional Review Questions

Chapter 15

In-Text Features

CD Interactive Exercises

3-D Animation of the Digestive System, 15-1
Animation of GERD, 15-2
Interactive Drag-and-Drop Labeling of the Digestive System, 15-3
Interactive Drag-and-Drop Exercise of the Intestinal Wall, 15-4
Videos on Anorexia and Bulimia, Eating Disorders and Diabetes, 15-5
Interactive Games and Puzzles, 15-6

Companion Web site

Professional Profile
- Medical Profession: Dietician
- Dental Assistants and Hygienists

Related Internet Links
Additional Review Questions

Chapter 16

In-Text Features

CD Interactive Exercises

3-D Animation of the Urinary System, 16-1
Interactive Labeling Exercise for the Kidney, 16-2
Animation of Renal Blood Flow, 16-3
Animation of Hypovolemic Shock, 16-4
Video of Ultrasound Procedure, 16-5
Drag-and-Drop Exercise on Labeling the Urinary Bladder, 16-6
Videos on Renal Failure and Kidney Stones, 16-7
Interactive Games and Puzzles, 16-8

Companion Web site

Professional Profile
- Ultra Sound Technician

Related Internet Links
Additional Review Questions

Chapter 17

In-Text Features

CD Interactive Exercises

Companion Web site

Professional Profiles
- Doula or Midwife

Related Internet Links
Additional Review Questions

Chapter 18

In-Text Features

CD Interactive Exercises

Companion Web site

Study Success Companion

In-Text Features

A User's Guide to the Features of This Book

We have designed this textbook to be fun, interesting, and rich in features to aid your understanding of this challenging topic. Here is a quick guide to what makes this text different from others. We hope that the special highlights of this book enhance your learning experience as the journey of your health care career unfolds.

SPECIAL FEATURES MAKE LEARNING FUN

Medical Terminology Guides

While this is not a medical terminology book, understanding and pronouncing medical words is critical to your success. You will find proper pronunciations and word part analysis in the margins where key terms are introduced. Audio pronunciation of terms is contained on both your CD as well as the student website at www.prenhall.com/colbert.

> **scope** *instrument to examine*
> **microscopic anatomy**
> *(MY kroh scop ic ah NAH tom ee)*
> **micro** = *small*
> **macroscopic anatomy**
> *(MAK roh scop ic ah NAH tom ee)*
> **macro or gross** = *large*
>
> **cyto** = *cells*
> **histo** = *tissues*
> **ology** = *the study of*

> *Clinical Application*
>
> **DO YOU KNOW YOUR LEFT FROM YOUR RIGHT?**
>
> By now, it should be clear that a precise, standardized language with directional terms is needed to study anatomy and physiology and apply it in a health care setting. Something as simple as left and right can become critical. For example, suppose you are a surgical technologist and are ordered to put a tag around a patient's right leg to designate it as the leg to be amputated in an upcoming surgery. If you approach the patient from the bottom of the bed and place the tag on the leg on YOUR right side, you have erroneously placed it on the patient's left leg, and this could have disastrous results. The take-home message is that left and right *always* refer to the patient's left and right, *not yours.*

Clinical Applications

These highlight boxes show the relevance of what you are learning and how that knowledge is needed in clinical practice. This feature includes topics such as aging, major diagnostic studies, and therapeutics.

p. 27

Applied Sciences

Instead of having a separate non-integrated chemistry or physics chapter, the sciences are presented in context.

> *Applied Science*
>
> **A USEFUL APPLICATION OF A DEADLY TOXIN**
>
> Botulism is a potentially deadly disease caused by food poisoning with the *Clostridium botulinum* bacteria. Science has found a way to utilize the poison generated by this bacteria for medical and cosmetic treatment. Small amounts of botulinus toxin are injected into facial muscles to stop previously untreatable facial twitching. The toxin basically paralyzes the muscles. The same toxin is used to treat wrinkles without the use of surgery and is known as Botox injections.

p. 143

Amazing Body Facts

These are "that's awesome" kinds of facts to give an appreciation of just how wonderful the human design is. For example, nerve impulses can travel at speeds of up to 426 feet per SECOND!

Amazing Body Facts

MAGNETOTAXIS: SOME BACTERIA RESPOND TO MAGNETIC FIELDS

Believe it or not, some bacteria can sense and respond to a magnetic field. These types of bacteria are sensitive to Earth's magnetic field and orient themselves to this force! This ability to move in response to magnetic forces is called *magnetotaxis.* This discovery was made by Richard Blakemore as he observed bacteria living in sulfide-rich mud from a lake. As he changed the position of the mud, the bacteria would reorient themselves to Earths's magnetic field. Upon further examination, Blakemore determined that these bacteria possessed particles of iron oxide, a magnetic metal compound that is stored in a cell structure called *magnetosome.*

p. 61

Learning Hints

We present helpful hints to facilitate learning difficult concepts. These may sometimes be amusing stories or other learning aids.

Learning Hint

MNEMONIC DEVICES

A mnemonic device is a tool used to help you memorize long lists. It can be very useful in anatomy. To make a mnemonic device, take the first letter of each part of the list you are trying to memorize and make it into a sentence. For example, the five great lakes in order from west to east are Superior, Michigan, Huron, Erie, and Ontario. The mnemonic device used to remember the right order is **S**am **M**ade **H**arry **E**at **O**nions, much easier to remember than the lakes themselves. An example for the cranial nerves is this one: **O**n **O**ld **O**lympus **T**owering **T**ops **A** **F**inn **V**ith **G**erman **V**alked **A**nd **H**opped.

p. 205

Test Your Knowledge

After a concept is fully developed within a chapter, a "Test Your Knowledge" section will insure you understand what was just covered before moving on and running the risk of getting really lost on your journey.

TEST YOUR KNOWLEDGE 5-3

Answer the following:

1. What is the difference between the axial skeleton and the appendicular skeleton?
2. Which of the following bones is considered to be part of the axial skeleton?
   a. humerus
   b. patella
   c. femur
   d. sternum
3. The number of vertebra in the thoracic region is
   a. 5
   b. 7
   c. 12
   d. 120
4. Describe the difference between flexion and extension.

p. 117

Snapshots from the Journey

This is a concise review summary of key points covered within each chapter.

Snapshots from the Journey

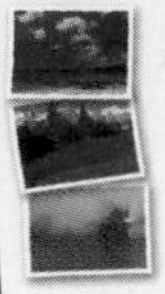

- The body can assume many different positions, and to standardize the study of anatomy, scientists often reference the anatomical position. In the anatomical position, the person stands with face and toes forward, hands at sides, and palms facing forward. Other positions, such as the prone, supine, and Fowler positions, are used in health care for assessment and treatments.
- The body can be divided by the use of planes into different sections. For example, the transverse, or horizontal plane divides the body into superior and inferior sections. The median, or midsagittal, plane divides the body into equal right and left halves, and the frontal, or coronal, plane divides the body into anterior and posterior sections.
- Directional terms, such as internal and external, proximal and distal, superficial and deep, central and peripheral, help us to navigate the body.
- It is important to always remember that directions such as right and left are referenced from the *patient's* perspective and NOT yours.
- The body has several cavities that house anatomical structures (mainly organs). For example, the cranial cavity houses the brain, the thoracic cavity houses the heart and lungs, the abdominopelvic cavity houses the digestive and reproductive organs, and the spinal cavity houses (guess what) the spinal cord.
- The body has many specific regions. For example, the umbilical region is found around your naval, or belly button, and the femoral region is located in the upper inner thigh area.
- The directional terms, anatomical landmarks, body regions, and body cavities are all important to know so that health care professionals can communicate in specific terms that leave no room for confusion.

p. 38

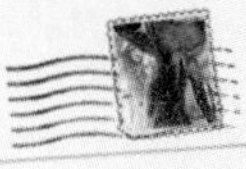

Case Study

A 40-year-old male patient presents with complaints of tinnitus and vertigo. He complains that his hearing is getting progressively worse and he is having dizzy spells and nausea.

Describe the patient's complaints in your own words.

What possible disease is present?

What part of the ear is affected and why?

p. 264

Case Studies

A case study pulls together many of the points discussed within the chapter to show the inter-relatedness of what you are learning. The case study is followed by end-of-chapter review questions to test your overall knowledge.

ANCILLARIES GUIDE YOUR JOURNEY

Study Success Companion

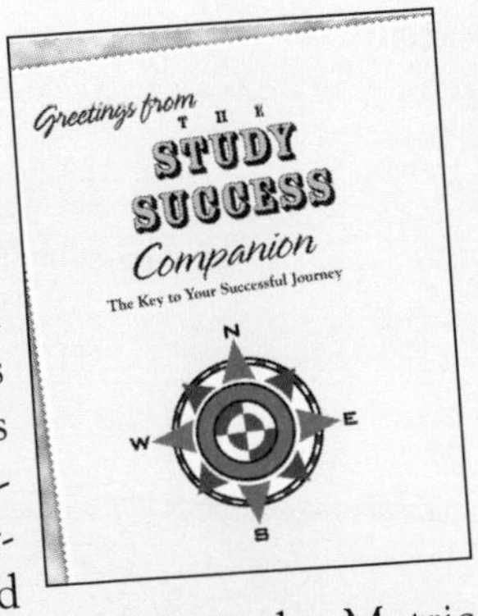

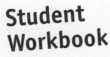

Your Study Success Companion will help you establish a good foundation for your trip. This appendix includes study skills and stress management techniques to help you as you journey through Anatomy and Physiology. It also contains topics such as the Metric System in case you do not have this background and need a self taught mini-refresher.

Student Workbook

This supplemental workbook contains even more practice and reinforcement opportunities and helps you prepare for quizzes and exams.

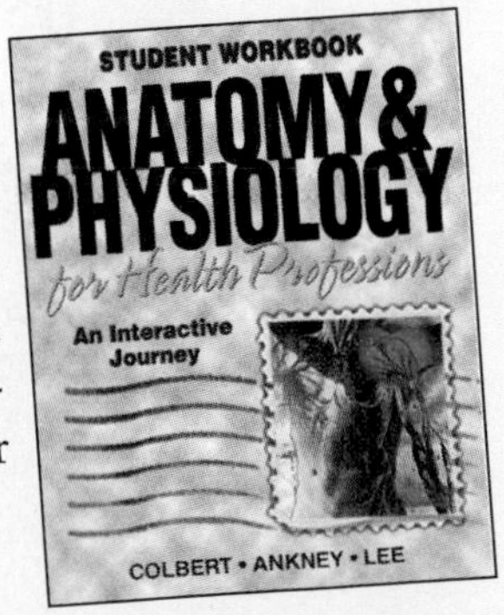

INTEGRATED MULTIMEDIA BRINGS CONCEPTS ALIVE

CD-ROM Interactive Exercises

At the completion of selected sections we prompt readers to visit the CD-ROM to view animated or video presentations of what is described in the book as well as interactive exercises. The CD-ROM contains:

- Animations and short videos
- Interactive games and puzzles
- Audio pronunciation glossary

6-4 With physical activity and the daily stress of life, muscles often become sore and fatigued. Massaging techniques help to stimulate blood flow and relax tense muscles. To understand more about various massage techniques, please go to your CD-ROM to view videos showing several different methods of massage.

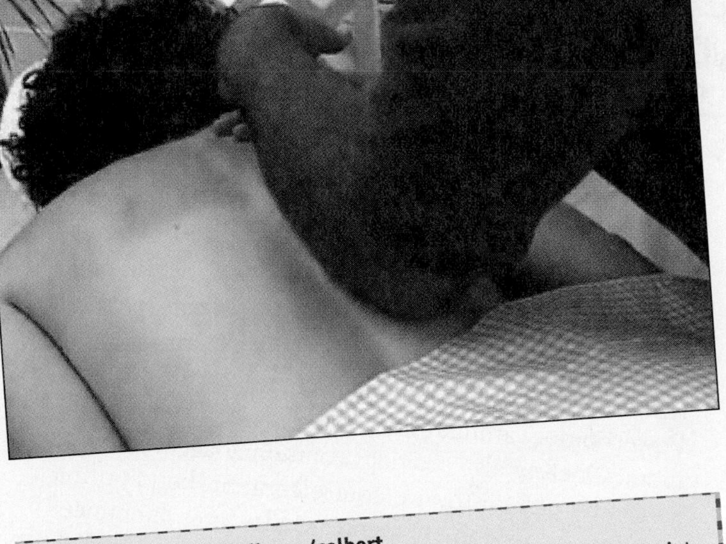

Companion Website

Located at **www.prenhall.com/colbert** the companion website complements the textbook and CD-ROM. The features include:

- A variety of healthcare career video profiles and corresponding internet links for each chapter
- Quizzes in multiple question formats that offer immediate scoring and feedback.
- Audio glossary in which key terms are pronounced.
- Drug Updates for the drugs discussed in each chapter.
- Links to updates on news items related to healthcare from ***The New York Times.***
- Related web links (i.e. American Heart Association)
- **Syllabus Manager™.** Faculty adopting this textbook have free access to the online Syllabus Manager. It offers a host of features that facilitate the students' use of the Companion Website, and allows faculty to post syllabi and course information online. For more information or a demonstration of please visit **www.prenhall.com/demo**, click Companion Web Sites then Syllabus Manager Tour.

www.prenhall.com/colbert
Not only do the skeletal muscles facilitate movement but, integrated with the nervous system, they provide support for posture while standing or sitting. Promoting balance and posture, along with proper muscle function, is one of the responsibilities of physical therapists. Physical therapists perform many therapies, such as range of motion (ROM) exercises, to ensure full muscle movement. Occupational therapists assist patients in utilizing and adapting their muscle function to perform activities of daily living and improving their quality of life. Massage therapists work directly on the muscles to aid in their relaxation and optimal functioning. To learn more about these professions, please go to the Web site for this chapter.

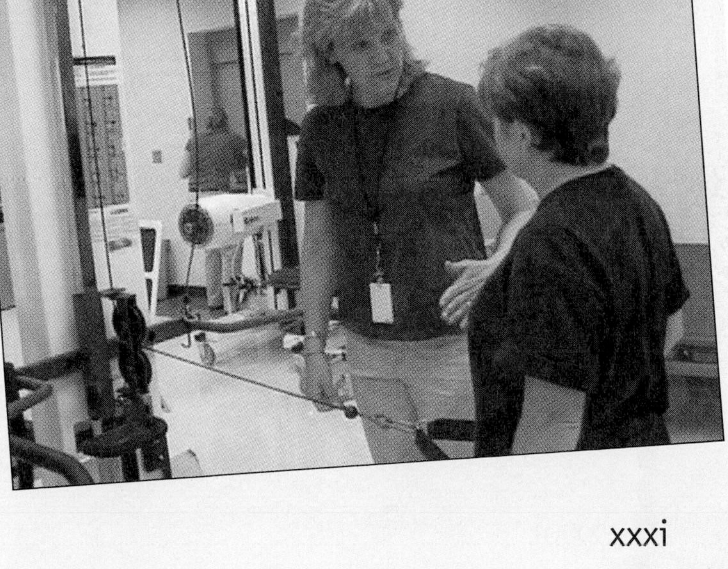

TEACHING ANCILLARIES BRING OUT THE BEST IN INSTRUCTORS

This text offers a rich array of ancillary materials to benefit instructors and help infuse a spark in the classroom. The full complement of supplemental teaching materials is available to all qualified instructors from your Prentice Hall Health sales representative.

Online Course Management Systems

Instructors wishing to facilitate on-line courses will be able to access OneKey, an integrated on-line resource that brings a wide array of resources together in one convenient place for both students and faculty. OneKey features everything you and your students need for out-of-class work, conveniently organized to match your syllabus. OneKey's online course management solution features interactive modules, text and image PowerPoints, animations, videos, case studies, and more. OneKey also provides course management tools so faculty can customize course content, build online tests, create assignments, enter grades, post announcements, and communicate with students. OneKey content is available in Blackboard, WebCT, and the nationally hosted version CourseCompass platform. Please contact your Prentice Hall Health sales representative for a demonstration or go online to www.prenhall.com/onekey.

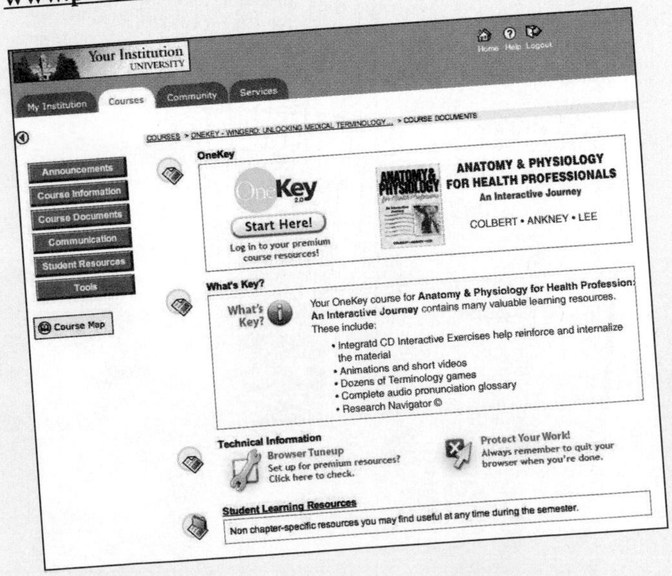

Instructor's Resource Manual

This manual contains a wealth of material to help faculty plan and manage the anatomy and physiology course. It includes many teaching tips, individual and team activities and games, ethical dilemmas, outlines, learning objectives, a wealth of extra "Did You Know" teaching pearls, answers to the chapter review activities, and a complete 900 question test bank. The IRM also guides faculty how to assign and use the text-specific Companion Website, www.prenhall.com/colbert, and the CD-ROM that accompany the textbook.

Instructor's Resource CD-ROM

Packaged along with the Instructor's Resource Manual, this cross-platform CD-ROM provides many resources in an electronic format. First, the CD-ROM includes the complete 900 question test bank that allows instructors to generate customized exams and quizzes. Second, it includes a comprehensive, turn-key lecture package in PowerPoint format. The lectures contain discussion points along with embedded color images from the textbook as well as bonus illustrations, animations, and videos to help infuse an extra spark into classroom experience. Instructors may use this presentation system as it is provided, or they may opt to customize it for their specific needs.

A COMMITMENT TO ACCURACY

It is vital that the content of this book and all ancillary resources be completely accurate, matching the need for precision in today's healthcare environment. In order to attain the highest level of accuracy possible throughout this educational program, we put an extensive development process into place. No fewer than a dozen content experts have read each page of chapter for accuracy, including all test questions, the website, the student CD-ROM, and all other ancillary resources.

While our intent is for all books to be error-free, it is possible for some mistakes to get through our system. Prentice Hall takes this issue seriously and therefore welcomes any and all feedback that you can provide along the lines of helping us enhance the accuracy of this book. If you identify any errors that need to be corrected in a subsequent printing, please send them to: Prentice Hall Health Editorial; Health Professions Corrections; 1 Lake St.; Upper Saddle River, NJ, 07458.

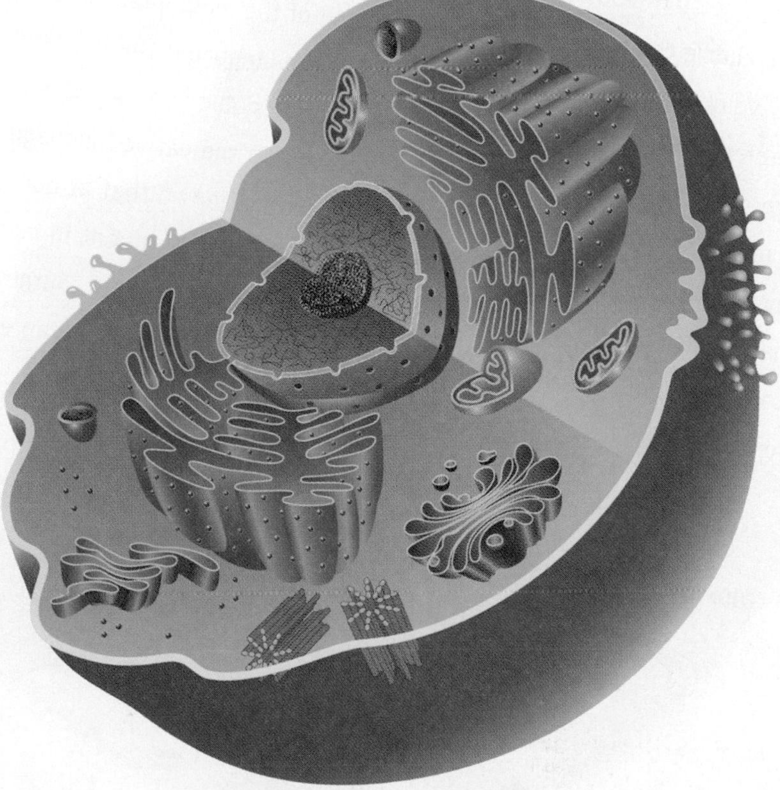

Greetings from ANATOMY & PHYSIOLOGY

Learning the Language

Imagine getting ready to travel to a foreign country where we do not speak the language. To maximize the success of our journey, one of the most important preparatory steps is to develop a basic understanding of the native language. The key language upon which health professions and the study of anatomy and physiology are based is medical terminology. Therefore, this chapter lays the foundation of learning the native language (medical terminology) of medicine. Future chapters build on this foundation so that at our journey's end, we not only will understand anatomy and physiology, but will be fluent in medical terminology. This chapter also assists in understanding the road signs along our journey. The special features to enhance our journey are presented by identifiable icons, and an explanation of each feature is given in the user's guide.

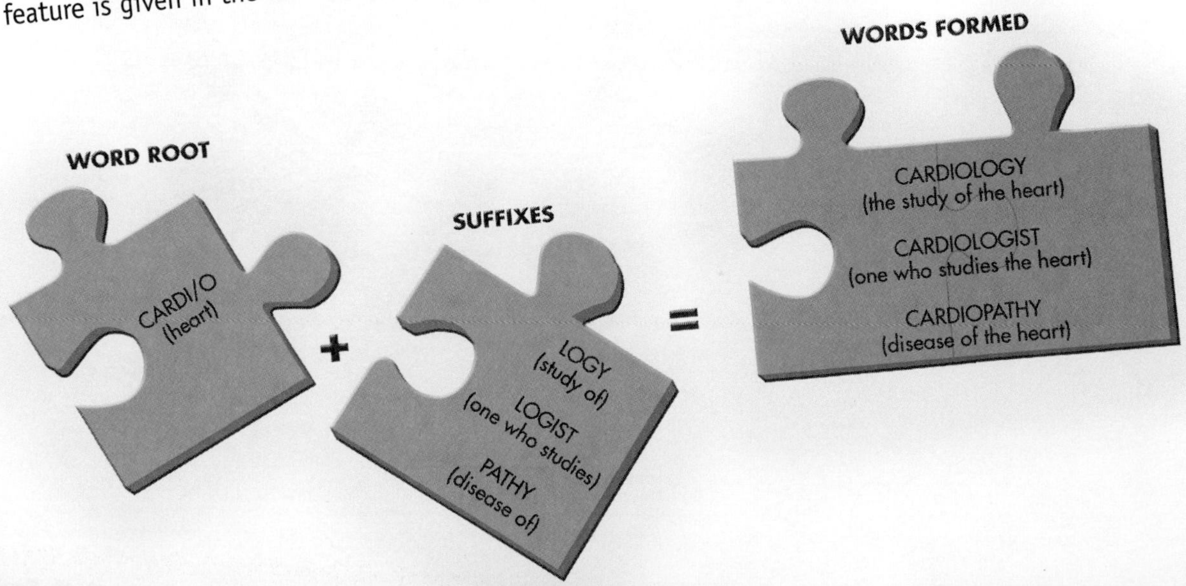

Chapter 1

LEARNING OBJECTIVES

At the end of your journey through this chapter, you will be able to:

- Understand the term *anatomy and physiology* and its various related areas
- Relate the importance and purpose of medical terminology to anatomy and physiology
- Construct and define medical terms using word roots, prefixes, suffixes
- Explain the concept and importance of homeostasis
- Contrast the metabolic processes of anabolism and catabolism

MULTIMEDIA APPLICATIONS

CD-ROM Interactive Exercises

- Video on medical specialties, 1-1
- Short videos on vital Signs, 1-2
- Interactive puzzles and games with medical terminology, 1-3

www.prenhall.com/colbert

- Professional Profiles:
  - Medical Assisting
  - Medical Records and Health Information Technician
  - Medical Transcriptionist
- Related Internet Links
- Additional Review Questions

Pronunciation Guide

Correct pronunciation is important in any journey so that you and others are completely understood. Here is a "see and say" Pronunciation Guide for the more difficult terms to pronounce in this chapter.

anabolism (ah NA bow lizm)
anatomy (ah NA tom ee)
catabolism (ka TA bow lizm)
diagnosis (dye ahg NOH siss)
etiology (ee tee ALL oh jee)
homeostasis (hoh mee oh STAY siss)
macroscopic anatomy (MAK roh scop ic ah NA tom ee)
microscopic anatomy (MY kroh scop ic ah NA tom ee)
metabolism (me TA bow lizm)
pathology (path ALL oh jee)
physiology (fiz ee ALL oh jee)
prognosis (prog NOH siss)
syndrome (SIN drohm)

WHAT IS ANATOMY AND PHYSIOLOGY?

You're probably so accustomed to hearing the words anatomy and physiology used together that you may not have given much thought to what each one means and how they differ. They each have unique meanings. Let's take a closer look.

Anatomy

anatomy *(ah NAH tom ee)*

Anatomy is the study of the internal and external *structures* of plants, animals, or for our focus, the human body. The human body is an amazing and complex structure that can perform an almost limitless number of tasks. To truly understand how something works, it is important to know how it is put together. Leonardo da Vinci, in the 1400s, correctly drew the human skeleton and could be considered one of the earliest anatomists (one who studies anatomy). The word anatomy is from the Greek language and literally means "to cut apart," which is exactly what you must do to see how something is put together. For example, the study of the arrangement of the bones that comprise the human skeleton, which is the anatomical framework for our bodies, is considered anatomy.

scope *instrument to examine*

microscopic anatomy *(MY kroh scop ic ah NAH tom ee)*
micro = *small*

macroscopic anatomy *(MAK roh scop ic ah NAH tom ee)*
macro or gross = *large*

cyto = *cells*
histo = *tissues*
ology = *the study of*

Just as we can subdivide biology into more specific concentrations, such as cell biology, plant biology, and animal biology, we can also broadly divide anatomy into **microscopic anatomy** and **macroscopic** anatomy, sometimes called **gross anatomy.** Microscopic anatomy is the study of structures that can be seen and examined only with magnification aids such as a microscope. The study of cellular structure (cytology) and tissue samples (histology) are examples of microscopic anatomy.

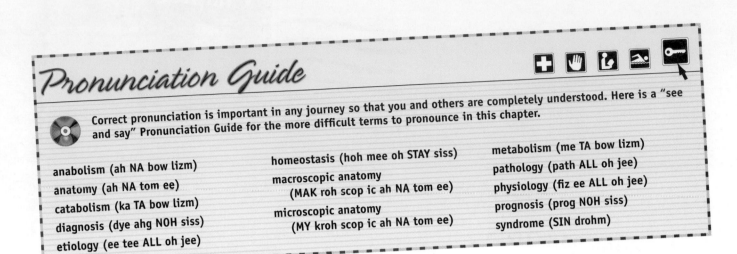

Gross anatomy represents the study of the structures visible to the unaided or naked eye. For example, the study of the various bones that make up the human body is gross anatomy. Viewing an X-ray of the arm to determine the type and location of a broken bone is considered an examination of gross anatomy.

Physiology

physiology *(fiz ee ALL oh jee)*
physio = *relationship to nature*
logy = *study of*

Physiology focuses on the *function* and vital processes of the various structures making up the human body. These physiologic processes include muscle contraction, our sense of smell and sight, how we breathe, and the list goes on. We will focus on each of these processes in their respective chapters. Physiology is closely related to anatomy because it is the study of how an anatomical structure such as a cell or bone actually functions. Physiology deals with all the vital processes of life and is more complex and, therefore, has many subspecialties. Human physiology, animal physiology, cellular physiology, and neurophysiology are just some of the specific branches of physiology.

Putting It All Together

In summary, anatomy focuses on *structure* and how something is put together, whereas physiology is the study of how those different structures work together to make the body function as a whole. For example, anatomy would be the study of the structure of the red blood cells (RBCs), and physiology would be the study of how the RBCs carry vital oxygen throughout our body. Figure 1–1 ■ shows deformed RBCs (sickle shaped) that are present in the dis-

> *Learning Hint*
>
> **USING THE MARGINS OF THIS BOOK**
>
> Notice that the margin notes present a breakdown of the medical terms discussed in the text. Sometimes you may already know the term and may not need to refer to the margin note, but it is always there to help reinforce the word. On occasion, you may even see a short little story on the word origin where it is of interest or helps to further explain the term.

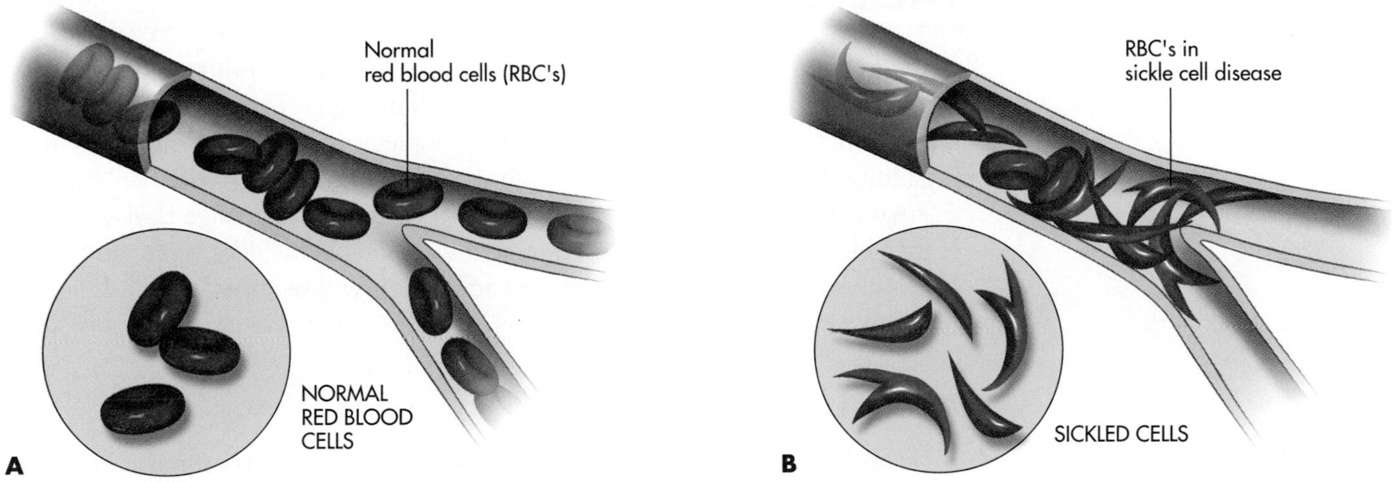

FIGURE ■ 1–1

A. Normal red blood cells (RBCs) are flexible and donut shaped and move with ease through blood vessels. **B.** The anatomical distortion of the *structure* of RBCs in sickle cell anemia affects its normal *function* to carry oxygen. In addition, the sickle cells lose their ability to bend and pass through the small blood vessels, thereby causing blockages to blood flow.

ease sickle cell anemia. Because of the anatomical deformity, the physiological process of effectively carrying oxygen is adversely affected.

You will notice on your journey that the design of a structure is often related to its function. For example, the type of joint located between bones is dictated by the functions of those bones: hinge joints are located at the knees where back and forth bending movement is required, while a ball and socket joint of the hip provides for a greater range of motion.

Therefore, it makes sense to combine these two sciences into anatomy and physiology (A&P). Human anatomy and physiology forms the foundation for all medical practice. Anything that upsets the normal structure or functioning can be called disease, and the study of disease is **pathology.** Another synonymous term for pathology is pathophysiology.

pathology *(path ALL oh jee)*
patho = *disease; disease literally means not (dis) at ease*

TEST YOUR KNOWLEDGE 1-1

Indicate whether the following examples are gross anatomy or microscopic anatomy by putting a G or M in the space provided.

1. ______________ viewing an X-ray to determine the type of bone break
2. ______________ classifying a tumor to be cancerous by cell type
3. ______________ viewing bacteria to determine what disease is present
4. ______________ examining the chest for any obvious deformities
5. ______________ a histotechnologist and cytotechnologist primarily study this type of anatomy

THE LANGUAGE

Even if you're traveling to another city within your home country, you will most likely need to learn a few things about the language its citizens speak. For example, think of the many different names people use to identify a sandwich made on a long skinny roll. Your "sub" might be someone else's "grinder" or "hoagie."

Anatomy and physiology also has its own unique language that you must learn before you can converse comfortably. Some words, like *heart, lungs,* and *blood pressure,* are already familiar to you. Others will seem strange and foreign. Let's take a closer look.

Medical Terminology

As stated earlier, the language of anatomy and physiology is primarily based on medical terminology. Understanding medical terminology may seem like an overwhelming task because, on the surface, there appears to be SO many terms. In reality, there are only a relatively few root terms, prefixes, and suffixes, but they can be put together in a host of ways to form numerous terms.

Each medical term has a basic structure upon which to build, and this is called the word root. For example, *cardi* is the word root for terms pertaining to the heart. Rarely is the word root used alone. Instead, it is combined with prefixes and suffixes that can change its meaning. Prefixes come before the word root, while suffixes come after the word root. The suffix **ology** means "study of," and therefore, we can combine cardi and ology to form **cardiology,** which is the study of the heart. The prefix *tachy* means "fast" and can be placed in front of the word root to form **tachycardia,** which means a fast heart rate. Figure 1–2 ■ shows the components of a medical term.

Often you will be given a combining form, which is the word root and a connecting vowel (usually o), to make it easier to pronounce and combine with pos-

Learning Hint

COMBINING AND FORMING MEDICAL TERMS

If a suffix begins with a vowel, drop the vowel in the combining form. For example, the combining form for stomach is gastr/o, and if we add the suffix for inflammation, *itis,* the medical term becomes *gastritis.*

cardi = *heart*
logy = *study of*
tachy = *fast*
ologist = *one who studies*

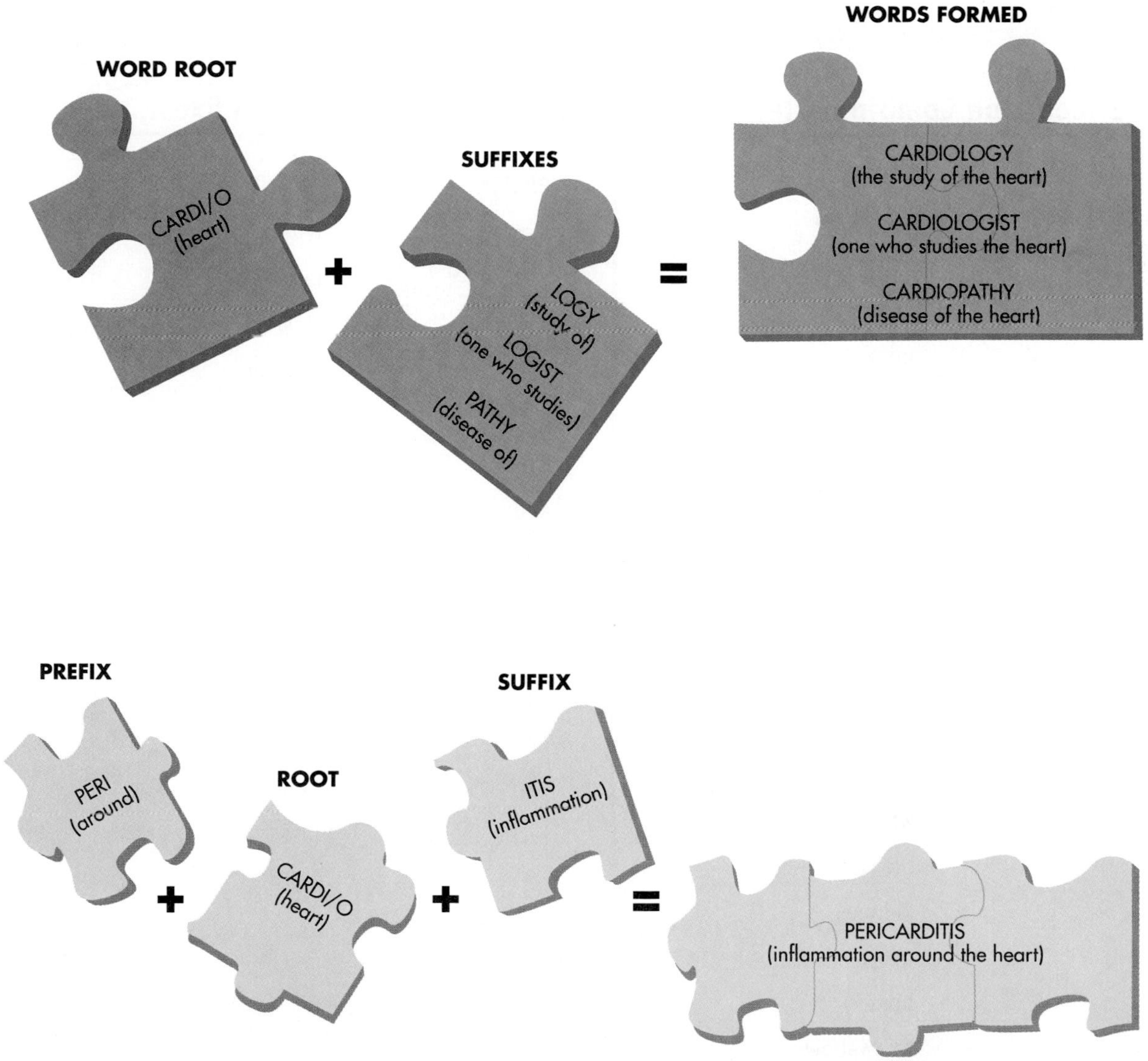

FIGURE ■ 1–2

How prefixes and suffixes can be combined with a word root to form many medical terms.

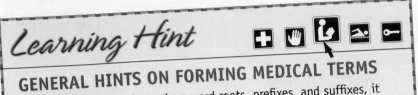

Learning Hint

GENERAL HINTS ON FORMING MEDICAL TERMS

While you can learn the various word roots, prefixes, and suffixes, it gets confusing trying to put them correctly together. In most instances, the medical definition indicates the last part of the term first, especially when suffixes are used. For example, an inflammation of the stomach is gastritis, not itisgastro, and one who studies the stomach is a gastrologist, not an ologistgastro. When using prefixes, you usually put the parts together in the order you say the definition. For example, slow heart rate is bradycardia, not cardiabrady. As with general rules, there are exceptions, but with practice it will become familiar to you.

sible suffixes. For example, the combining form for heart is cardi/o. Listed in Table 1–1 are some common combining forms to get you started.

Now let's add some common prefixes that can be placed before the word roots to alter their meaning (see Table 1–2).

Finally, let's add some common suffixes (Table 1–3) and then see what kinds of words we can form with just these few parts.

Using tables 1–1, 1–2, and 1–3, look at all the terms you can make from just the one word root, cardi/o. Cardiology is the study of the heart, and a cardiologist

TABLE 1–1 Common Combining Terms

WORD ROOT/ COMBINING FORM	MEANING
abdomin/o	abdomen
angi/o	vessel
arthr/o	joint
cardi/o	heart
cyan/o	blue
cyt/o	cell
derm/o	skin
erythr/o	red
gastr/o	stomach
glyc/o	sugar
hepat/o	liver
hist/o	tissue
leuk/o	white
mamm/o	breast
nephr/o	kidney
neur/o	nerve
oste/o	bone
phag/o	to swallow
path/o	disease
rhin/o	nose

TABLE 1–2 Common Prefixes

PREFIX	MEANING
a or an	without
acro	extremities
brady	slow
dia	through
dys	difficult
electro	electric
endo	within
epi	upon or over
hyper	above normal
hypo	below normal
macro	large
micro	small
peri	around
tachy	fast

is one who studies the heart. Bradycardia is a slow heart rate, tachycardia is a fast heart rate, and an electrocardiogram is an electrical recording of the heart. If your heart were enlarged due to inflammation (carditis), you would have cardiomegaly, which would mean you have heart disease (cardiopathy). The Tin Man from *The Wizard of Oz* thought he had no heart (acardia), but realized that he had a heart all the time.

Note

Most of the medical terms are derived from the Greek and Latin languages because much of the science of medicine originated in Greek and Latin cultures. When we refer to Latin, we mean the ancient society that lived in the Mediterranean region, and not in Latin America.

TABLE 1–3 Common Suffixes

SUFFIX	MEANING
algia	pain
cyte	cell
ectomy	surgical removal of
gram	the actual recorded record
graphy	the process of recording
ist	one who specializes
itis	inflammation of
logist	one who studies
logy	study of
sis	disease or condition of
otomy	cutting into
ostomy	surgically forming an opening
megaly	enlargement of
pathy	disease
phobia	fear of
plasty	surgical repair
penia	decrease or lack of
scope	instrument to view or examine

Abbreviations

Abbreviations are used extensively in the medical profession. They are useful in simplifying long, complicated terms for disease, diagnostic procedures, and therapies that require extensive documentation. For now, review Table 1–4 for some common abbreviations you may have heard in a health care setting or on television.

Of course you will learn many more terms and abbreviations as we explore the upcoming chapters and become fluent in conversational medical language. This will help you to avoid using lay terms (common, everyday terms) to describe medical and anatomical concepts. Now you know that the correct term for "getting a nose job" is **rhinoplasty.**

rhinoplasty *(RYE noh plass tee)*
rhino = *nose*
plasty = *surgical repair*

TABLE 1–4 Common Medical Abbreviations

ABBREVIATIONS	MEANING
A&P	anatomy and physiology
BP	blood pressure
CPR	cardiopulmonary resuscitation
GI	gastrointestinal
ICU	intensive care unit
NPO	Latin *nil per os,* which means "nothing by mouth"
SOB	shortness of breath
STAT	Latin *statim,* which means "immediately"
ER/ED	emergency room/emergency department

Note: ER was popularized by the television show of the same name. However, in actuality it is really a whole department and not just a room, so most prefer the abbreviation ED which stands for Emergency Department.

TEST YOUR KNOWLEDGE 1-2

Define the medical terms:

1. acrocyanosis
2. gastritis
3. rhinoplasty
4. bradycardia
5. mammogram
6. cytomegaly

Give the correct medical term:

7. inflammation of the kidneys
8. removal of the stomach
9. enlarged heart
10. disease of the bones
11. one who studies the nerves

www.prenhall.com/colbert
The professionals who work in medical assisting must become very familiar with medical terminology in their workplace. Other professionals who deal extensively with the medical charts and records of patients must also master this language. Examples of these professions are medical coders, medical transcriptionists, and health information technicians. If you want to learn more about these professions, please go to the website to view videos and read their professional profiles.

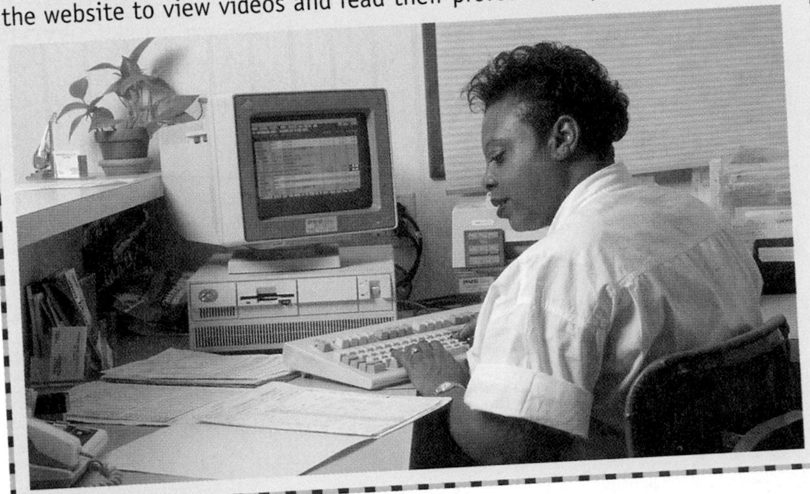

The Metric System

Whereas medical terminology represents the written and spoken language for understanding anatomy and physiology, the metric system is the "mathematical language" of anatomy and physiology. For example, blood pressure is in millimeters of mercury (mm Hg), and organ size is usually measured in centimeters (cm). Medications and fluids are given in milliliters (ml) or cubic centimeters (cc), and weight is often measured in kilograms (kg). What exactly does it mean when you are taught that normal cardiac output is 6 liters per minute? You can now see why you must be familiar with the metric system in order to truly understand anatomy and physiology and medicine. While the metric system may seem complicated if you are not familiar with it, it really isn't if you have a basic understanding of math.

There are two major systems of measurement in our world today. The United States Customary System (USCS) is used in the United States and Myanmar (formerly Burma) and the International System of Units (SI) is used everywhere else, and especially in health care. The SI system is also known as the international or **metric system** and is based on the power of 10. The metric system is also the system used by drug manufacturers.

The USCS system is based on the British Imperial System and uses several different designations for the basic units of length, weight, and volume. We commonly call this the **English system.** For example, in the English system, volumes can be expressed as ounces, pints, quarts, gallons, pecks, bushels, or cubic feet. Distance can be expressed in inches, feet, yards, and miles. Weights are measured in ounces, pounds, and tons. This may be the system you are most familiar with, but it is not the system of choice used throughout the world and within the medical profession because the English system has no common base and is therefore very cumbersome to use. It is difficult to know the relationship between each unit of

1-1 Medical Specialties
There are numerous medical specialties (ologists), and just by going to the Yellow Pages of the phone book, you can see firsthand the vast array that exists—from anesthesiologists to urologists. Each of these specialty terms is covered in its respective chapter, but if you're so excited and can't wait to know more, go to the CD to view a video on medical specialties and learn a few more word roots along the way.

measure because they are not based in an orderly fashion according to the powers of 10 as in the metric system. For example, how many pecks are in a gallon? Just what is a peck? How many inches are in a mile? These all require extensive calculations and memorization of certain equivalent values, whereas in the metric system, you simply move the decimal point the appropriate power of 10.

This has been a brief overview of the two types of measurement systems that you will encounter in your everyday activities as a health care professional. If you want to learn more about the metric system, please refer to your student *Study Success Companion* at the end of this text, where a simplified explanation is given on how to easily use the metric system in the health care setting.

THE LANGUAGE OF DISEASE

This chapter is about planning for a smooth trip by learning the language. However, even with the most careful planning, things can still go wrong. Things such as flat tires, airport delays, and loss of money or credit cards can ruin a trip. Similarly, problems can happen to the human body. Ideally, the body works to make things function smoothly and in balance. Sometimes things happen to alter those functions. Eating habits, smoking, inherited traits, trauma, environmental factors, and even aging can alter the body's balance and lead to **disease.** Disease, simply put, is a condition in which the body fails to function normally.

disease *(dih ZEEZ)*
dis = *not; literally, disease means "not at ease"*

While this is an A&P course that focuses on *normal* function and structure, it is often helpful to reinforce the concepts with some elaboration of what can go wrong. Therefore, at the end of each system chapter, a *brief* discussion on some of the major diseases associated with that system is provided. An even further in-depth discussion is contained on the CD-ROM as optional material. For example, a future physical therapist or massage therapist may want to spend more time exploring in-depth disease information on the muscular system; a dental hygienist may wish to learn more about the function of teeth in the digestive system, and a radiologic technologist may focus on the skeletal system. For now, a brief discussion on some of the unique language of disease is needed to lay the foundation for future discussions.

Note

The word gnosis is Greek for knowledge. Dia means through or complete, and therefore diagnosis literally means "know through or completely." Pro is a prefix meaning before or in front of, and prognosis literally means the foreknowledge or predicting of the outcome of a disease.

diagnose *(dye ahg NOHS)*
etiology *(ee tee ALL oh jee)*
prognosis *(prog NOH siss)*

Signs and Symptoms of Disease

Think back to a time when you were sick. You may have had a fever, cough, nausea, dizziness, joint aches, or a generalized weakness. These are examples of what we call **signs** and **symptoms** of disease. While the terms signs and symptoms are often used interchangeably, each has its own specific definition. Signs are more definitive, objective, obvious indicators of an illness. Fever, or monitoring the change in the size or color of a mole are good examples of signs. **Vital signs** are common, measurable indicators that help us to assess the health of our patients. Vital signs are the signs vital to life and include pulse (heart rate), blood pressure, body temperature, and respiratory rate. The vital sign standard

1-2 Go to the CD-ROM to learn more about pulse sites and to view short videos on the proper way to take vital signs.

values can change according to the patient's age and sex.

Symptoms, on the other hand, are more subjective and more difficult to measure consistently. A perfect example of a symptom is pain. Tolerance to pain varies among individuals, so an equal amount of pain (as in a headache) applied to a number of people could be perceived as a light, moderate, or intense level of pain depending on each individual's perception. In spite of the fact that symptoms are hard to measure, they are still very important in the diagnosis of disease. Sometimes a disease exhibits a set group of signs and symptoms that may occur at about the same time. This specific grouping of signs and symptoms is known as a **syndrome.** Signs, symptoms, and syndromes are further explained throughout the rest of our textbook as they relate to the anatomy and physiology of the various body systems.

Discovering as many signs and symptoms as possible can help to **diagnose** a disease. A diagnosis is an identification of a disease determined by studying the patient's signs, symptoms, history, and results of diagnostic tests. Getting the medical history can help in determining the **etiology,** or cause, of the disease. The **prognosis** is the prediction of the outcome of a disease. Hopefully, your *prognosis* for doing well in this anatomy and physiology course is excellent.

Clinical Application

THE VITAL SIGN OF PULSE

The pulse is commonly taken by applying slight finger pressure over the radial artery located in each wrist (on the thumb side) and counting the number of beats in a 60-second period (please see Figure 1-3 ■). The normal heart rate for an adult is 60 to 100 beats per minute, child rate is approximately 70 to 120, and a newborn's rate is 90 to 170 beats per minute. If an adult has a heart rate of 165 beats per minute, what medical term would you use to describe that condition?

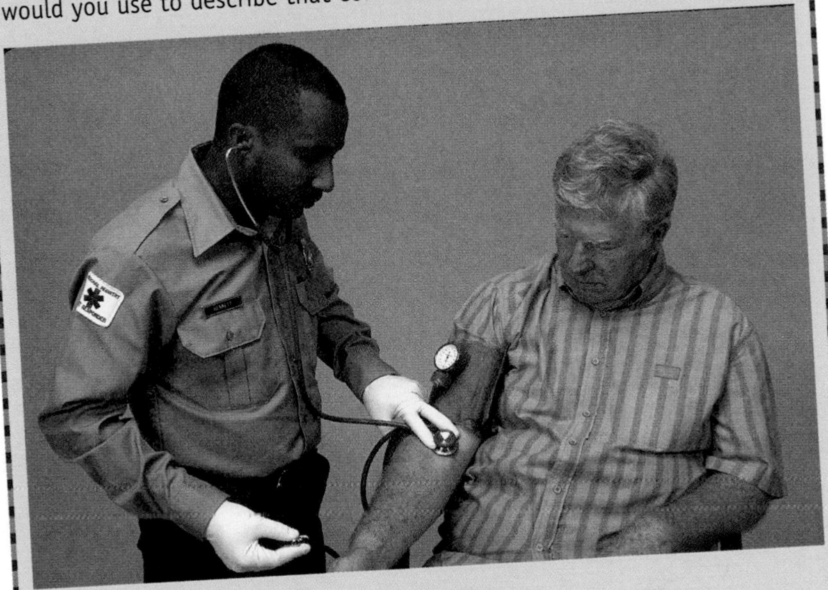

FIGURE ■ 1-3

Taking a pulse is vital to the proper measurement of blood pressure.

TEST YOUR KNOWLEDGE 1-3

Answer the following questions:

1. Check which of the following are vital signs:

_______________ a. pulse

_______________ b. pain

_______________ c. blood pressure

_______________ d. age

_______________ e. indigestion

_______________ f. respiratory rate

_______________ g. body temperature

2. Which of the following is the medical term for the cause of a disease?
   a. prognosis
   b. diagnosis
   c. etiology
   d. syndrome

3. Which of the following is the medical term for the outcome of a disease?
   a. prognosis
   b. diagnosis
   c. etiology
   d. syndrome

ANATOMY AND PHYSIOLOGY CONCEPTS YOU WILL ENCOUNTER ON YOUR JOURNEY

In this section, we take a closer look at some additional concepts related to the study of anatomy and physiology that you will learn more about as you journey through the chapters in this text.

Metabolism

metabolism *(me TA bow lizm)*

If you travel to other countries, you will see many different cultures and customs. Even though each culture is unique, they all share certain similarities. The same can be said in anatomy and physiology. We all share certain functions that are vital to survival. All humans, for example, need food in order to produce complex chemical reactions necessary for growth, reproduction, movement, and so on. **Metabolism** refers to all of the chemical operations going on within our bodies. Metabolism requires various nutrients or fuel to function and produces waste products much like a car consumes gas for power and produces waste, or exhaust. Metabolism, for now, can be thought of as "all the life-sustaining reactions within the body."

Clinical Application

METABOLIC SYNDROME, OR SYNDROME X

There is a disturbing new syndrome affecting nearly one quarter of the United States adult population. Known as Metabolic Syndrome, or Syndrome X, a patient with this syndrome exhibits three of the following five common conditions: high blood sugar levels (hyperglycemia), high blood pressure (hypertension), abdominal obesity, high triglycerides (a lipid substance in the blood), and low blood level of HDL (which is a good form of blood cholesterol). Individuals who exhibit this syndrome are at an increased risk for a form of diabetes, heart attacks, and/or strokes. This is essentially a syndrome that is created as a result of poor diet and lack of exercise.

Metabolism is further subdivided into two opposite processes. **Anabolism** is the process by which simpler compounds are *built up* and used to manufacture materials for growth, repair, and reproduction, such as the assembly of amino acids to form proteins. This is the *building* phase of metabolism. **Catabolism** is the process by which complex substances are *broken down* into simpler substances. For example, the breakdown of food into simpler chemical building blocks for energy use is a catabolic process. An abnormal and extreme example of catabolism is a starvation victim whose body "feeds upon itself," actually consuming the body's own tissues.

anabolism *(ah NA bow lizm)*
ana = *up, as in build up*
catabolism *(ka TA bow lizm)*
cata = *down, as in tear down*

Homeostasis

For the body to remain alive, it must constantly monitor both its internal and external environment and make the appropriate adjustments. In order for cells to thrive, they must be maintained in an environment that provides a proper temperature range, balanced oxygen levels, and adequate nutrients. Heart rate and blood pressure must also be monitored and maintained within a certain range or setpoint for optimal functioning depending upon the body activity. **Homeostasis** is the physiologic process that monitors and maintains a stable internal environment or equilibrium. Survival depends upon the body's ability to maintain homeostasis. Homeostatic regulation refers to the adjustments made in the human organism to maintain this stable internal environment.

homeostasis *(hoh mee oh STAY siss)*
homeo = *unchanging*
stasis = *standing still; as you will soon see, stasis is not an accurate term because homeostasis is actually a dynamic state of equilibrium*

The thermostat in your house functions like a homeostatic mechanism. A temperature is set and then maintained by a sensor that monitors the internal environmental temperature and either heats the house if the sensor registers too cold or cools the house if the sensor registers too hot. There is a continuous feedback loop from the sensor to the thermostat to determine what action is needed. Because the feedback loop opposes the stimulus (cools down if too hot, heats up if too cold), it is referred to as a **negative feedback loop.**

The body also relies on negative feedback loops that continually sense the internal and external environment and the body makes adjustments to maintain homeostasis (see Figure 1–4 ■). The hypothalamus in the brain represents the body's thermostatic control. If the hypothalamus senses a very cold environment, it opposes this cold stimulus (negative feedback loop) and performs physiologic processes to gain heat within the body to maintain an internal temperature near 98.6°F. The body begins to shiver, and this increased muscular activity generates heat. In addition, since most heat loss is through peripheral areas (head, arms, and legs), the body decreases the size of the peripheral blood vessels (vasoconstriction), causing the blood to be deeper from the skin surface where the heat would be lost to the cold environment. This keeps the blood closer to the core of the body where it is warmer. Of course, we can assist the body by wearing a heavy coat and hat which would remove much of the stress of the cold environment or simply get out of the cold to a warmer environment.

Conversely, if you are in the desert and the temperature is 120 degrees F,

Amazing Body Facts

BIZARRE SIGNS AND SYMPTOMS!

Here are some strange signs and symptoms that have been indications of diseases. To keep lawyers from making a ton of money on this book, please note that there are other signs, symptoms, and tests to determine specific diseases. Please do not use this list of oddities as a sole diagnostic tool! Void where prohibited, you must be 18 years of age to play, cannot be used with other coupons, and all other restrictions apply.

1. Generalized itching skin can be an indication of Hodgkins disease.
2. Sweating at night may indicate tuberculosis.
3. A desire to eat clay or starchy paste may indicate an iron deficiency in the body.
4. Breath that smells like fruity flavored chewing gum may be an indication of diabetes.
5. A magenta colored tongue is indicative of a riboflavin deficiency.
6. A patient with profound kidney disease often doesn't have moons (cuticles) on his or her fingernails.
7. A hairy tongue may mean that a patient's normal mouth flora has died from improper use of antibiotics.
8. Spoon-shaped fingernails may point to an iron deficiency in the body.
9. Brown linear streaks on the fingernails of fair-skinned people may indicate melanoma (skin cancer).

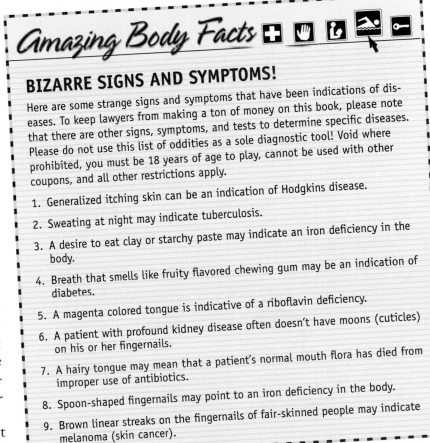

the body senses this as too hot and stimulates physiologic processes to cool you down. These processes include sweating (evaporation is a cooling process) and enlarging the peripheral vessels (peripheral vasodilation) in order to dissipate the body heat into the external environment. In health care practice, if a patient presents with a very high temperature, he or she may need to be rapidly cooled with ice packs or baths to reduce their temperature toward the normal range. Much of health care practice is just that—assisting the body through therapy and treatments in returning it to homeostasis.

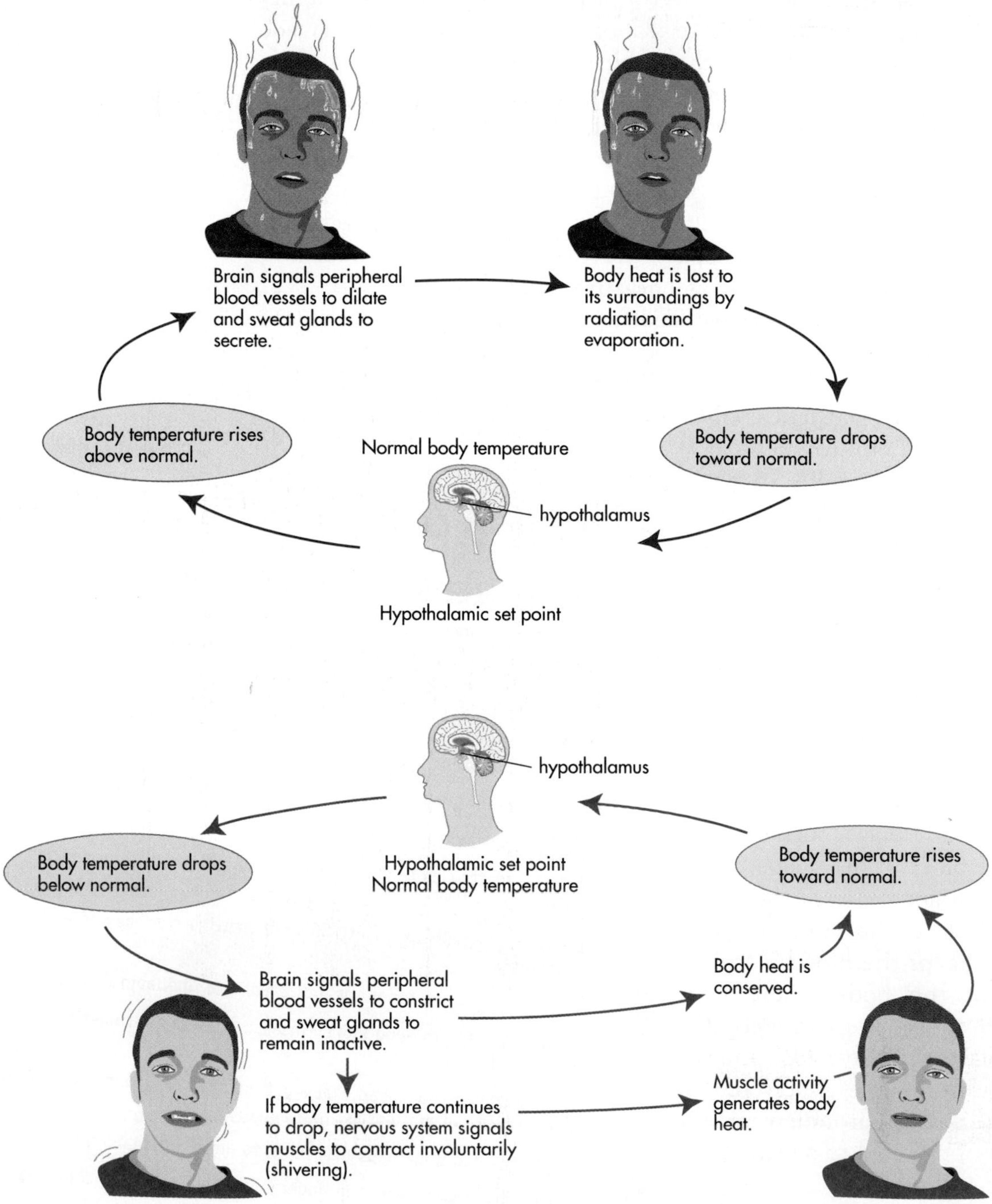

FIGURE ■ 1–4

The homeostatic control of normal body temperature (37°C or 98.6°F).

Your body is also capable of **positive feedback,** which increases the magnitude of a change. This process is also known as a vicious cycle. Positive feedback is not a way to regulate your body, because it increases a change away from the ideal setpoint. Often, positive feedback is harmful if the vicious cycle cannot be broken, but sometimes positive feedback is necessary for a process to run to completion.

A good example of necessary positive feedback is the continued contraction of the uterus during childbirth. When a baby is ready to be born, a signal, not well understood at this time, tells the hypothalamus to release the hormone oxytocin from the posterior pituitary. Oxytocin increases the intensity of uterine contractions. As the uterus contracts, the pressure inside the uterus caused by the baby moving down the birth canal increases the signal to the hypothalamus. More oxytocin is released, and the uterus contracts harder. Pressure gets higher inside the uterus, the hypothalamus is signaled to release more oxytocin, and the uterus contracts yet harder. This cycle of ever-increasing uterine contractions due to ever-increasing release of oxytocin from the hypothalamus continues until the pressure inside the uterus decreases—that is, until the baby is born.

Clinical Application

"BREAKING" A FEVER

It is believed that most fevers are the body's way of making an inhospitable environment for a pathogen to survive. Why is it when someone begins sweating after a prolonged fever (increase in body temperature), the fever is said to be "breaking?" A fever sets the hypothalamus to a higher setpoint temperature. The body increases metabolism to generate more heat to reach this now higher set temperature. Once whatever is causing the fever is gone, the hypothalamus set temperature is turned back down to the true normal. The body must now rapidly get rid of the excess heat by the cooling process of evaporation through sweating.

SUMMARY

Snapshots from the Journey

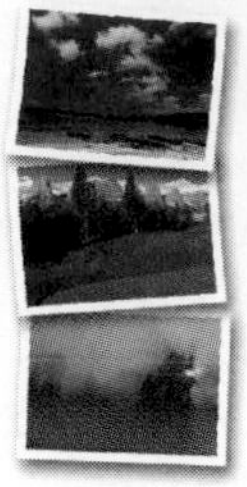

- Anatomy is the study of the actual internal and external structures of the body, and physiology is the study of how these structures normally function. Pathology is the study of the disease processes by which abnormal structures and abnormal body functions can occur.
- Medical terminology is the language of medicine and combines word roots, prefixes, and suffixes to construct numerous medical terms to describe conditions, locations, diagnostic tools, and so on.
- The metric system is the mathematical language of medicine based on the powers of 10. If you require more practice with this system, please go to your student Study Companion Guide at the end of this text for a simplified review.
- Metabolism refers to all of the chemical operations going on within the body and can be broken down into two opposite processes. The building phase of metabolism is anabolism, in which simpler compounds are *built up* and used to manufacture materials for growth, reproduction, and repairs. The tearing down phase is catabolism, in which complex substances are *broken down* into simpler substances, such as food broken down for energy use.
- The body tries to maintain a balanced or stable environment called homeostasis. It must constantly monitor the environment and make changes to maintain this balance. It often accomplishes homeostasis through negative feedback loops.

Case Study

A 66-year-old Asian male involved in a vehicular accident is taken to the ICU with SOB and abdominal pain. He has acrocyanosis, tachycardia, and a past medical history of cardiopathy. He weighs 150 pounds and is 5 feet 6 inches tall. His chest X-ray shows an enlarged heart. His facial injuries will require future rhinoplastic surgery. An electrocardiogram and lower GI series is ordered.

a. Where exactly in the hospital was the patient taken?

b. Describe the patient's color, heart rate, and breathing.

c. What is the medical term for what the X-ray showed?

d. What future facial surgery will he need?

REVIEW QUESTIONS

Multiple Choice

1. Which of the following is an example of microscopic anatomy?
   a. viewing an X-ray
   b. examining the shape of an organ during an autopsy
   c. classifying a type of bacterial cell
   d. watching how the pupils in the eyes react to light

2. Acromegaly means which of the following?
   a. a large stomach
   b. enlarged extremities
   c. an inflamed stomach lining
   d. a large acrobat

3. The breakdown of sugar in the body for energy is called
   a. anabolism
   b. catabolism
   c. dogabolism
   d. hyperbolism

4. Which of the following is a measurement system based on the power of 10?
   a. English system
   b. British Imperial system
   c. metric system
   d. weights and measures system

5. The cause of a disease is referred to as the
   a. prognosis
   b. diagnosis
   c. pathology
   d. etiology

Fill in the Blank

6. Ted's knee injury occurred at last night's football game. Today his doctor wants to make a small incision and use a device to "look around the joint" to assess the damage. What is the term for this device? ____________

7. ______________ is the study of the structures of the body, and ______________ is the study of the functions of these structures.

8. For years, Ali never learned to swim because of her unnatural fear of the water, which is called ____________

9. Pulse and temperature represent two ______________ signs of the body.

10. Raheem had blood work done that showed a normal number of white blood cells (WBCs) and red blood cells (RBCs). What are the respective medical terms for these cell types?

    __________________________ __________________________

Short Answer

11. Explain the difference between diagnosis and prognosis.

12. Knowing that difficulty swallowing is called dysphagia, what do you think the function of a phagocyte is?

13. Contrast negative and positive feedback loops.

14. Describe one example of homeostasis in your body.

Suggested Activities

1. Using a medical dictionary, find five new medical terms and give their definition and pronunciation.

   ______________________ ____
   ______________________ ____
   ______________________ ____
   ______________________ ____
   ______________________ ____

2. Make up 3 × 5 inch note cards with five word roots discussed in this chapter and see how many medical words you can make using either prefixes or suffixes in the tables. For example, the word root arthr/o can be used to make the following: arthritis, arthralgia, arthroscope, and arthroplasty. Confirm that you made a real word by looking it up in a medical dictionary.

> **1-3** Now that you have completed your journey through this chapter, please go to the CD-ROM for interactive games and puzzles concerning the medical terms and concepts contained in this chapter. By playing the games you will reinforce your learning of medical terminology in a fun way.

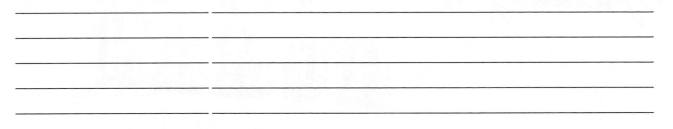

Greetings from

THE HUMAN BODY

Reading the Map

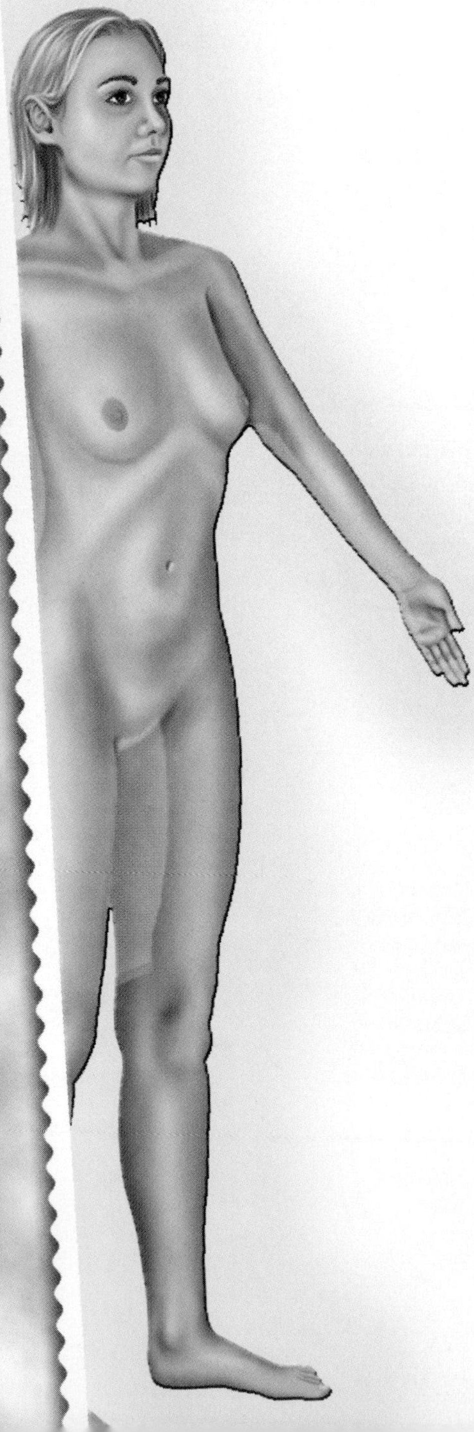

Now that we have a basic understanding of the native language and some basic anatomy and physiology concepts, how will we successfully navigate through an unfamiliar city or country? We must, of course, study maps so we can plan our visit and know where we are going. The same effort is required to learn the "terrain" of the human body. This chapter provides the major external map of the human body that serves as a guide for future chapters, which map in detail the internal regions. The medical directional terms and body locations are a foundation upon which to build as we journey together through this wondrous creation called the human organism. Isn't it ironic that if there is one thing we should know better than anything else, it should be our own bodies? To borrow from an old saying, by the end of our journey through this textbook, you will know your entire body like the back of your hand.

Chapter 2

LEARNING OBJECTIVES

At the end of your journey through this chapter, you will be able to:

- List and describe the various body positions
- Define the body planes and associated directional terms
- Locate and describe the body cavities and their respective organs
- List and describe the anatomical divisions of the abdominal region
- Identify and locate the various body regions

MULTIMEDIA APPLICATIONS

CD-ROM Interactive Exercises

- Additional video information on body positions, 2-1
- Videos on ultrasound, MRIs, and other diagnostic imaging, 2-2
- Interactive drag-and-drop exercise to reinforce body cavities, 2-3
- Interactive drag-and-drop exercise to reinforce anterior and posterior body regions, 2-4
- Interactive games and puzzles, 2-5

www.prenhall.com/colbert

- Professional Profiles
    - Radiologic Technology
    - Surgical Technology
- Related Internet Links
- Additional Review Questions

Pronunciation Guide

Correct pronunciation is important in any journey so that you and others are completely understood. Here is a "see and say" Pronunciation Guide for the more difficult terms to pronounce in this chapter.

abdominopelvic cavity (ab dom ih noh PELL vik KAV ih tee)
antecubital (An tee CUE bi tal)
buccal (BUCK al)
caudal (KAWD al)
cephalic (seh FAL ik)
coronal plane (kor ROHN al)
cranial (KRAY nee al)
crural (CRUR al)
distal (DISS tal)
dorsal (DOR sal)
gluteal (GLOO tee al)
mediastinum (me dee ah STY num)
midsagittal plane (mid SAJ ih tal)
pleural cavities (PLOO ral)
superficial (super FISH al)
thoracic cavity (tho RASS ik KAV ih tee)
transverse (tranz VERS)

THE MAP OF THE HUMAN BODY

When reading a map, you need certain universal directional terms, such as north, east, south and west, to help you understand and use the map. A map is often made to represent a specific region so that more details can be included about that particular region, making it easier to explore. Likewise, scientists have created standardized body directional terms and split the body into distinct regions, sections, and cavities so that we can more clearly and rapidly locate and discuss anatomical features. Having certain anatomical landmarks on the body also provides needed points of reference. For example, the spinal cord is a major anatomical landmark for many structures in the center of our bodies.

If a patient states, "I have pain in my stomach," does that really tell you a lot of information? Location of pain can help in determining what is wrong with a patient. It is helpful to know the type of pain (dull, sharp, or stabbing) and *exactly* where in that region the pain is located to help determine its cause. For example, pain in the general stomach area can indicate a variety of problems, including an ulcer, heart attack, appendicitis, indigestion, or liver problems. Knowing the exact region can help a clinician better determine the exact problem.

2-1 There are even more positions in health care, including the lateral, Trendelenburg, Sims, dorsal recumbent, and lithotomy positions. For more information on this subject and to view videos, please go to your CD-ROM for this chapter.

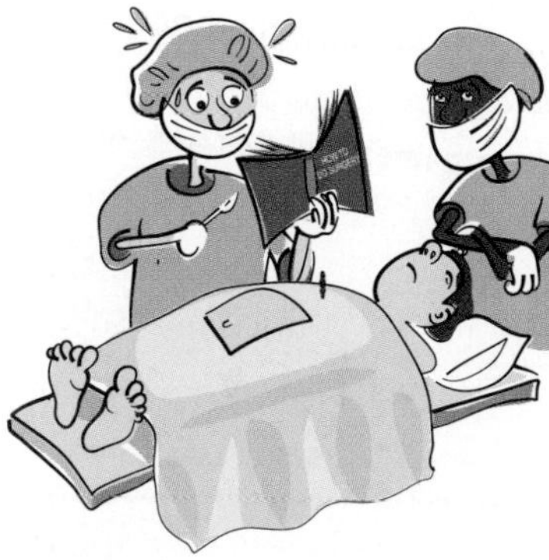

"Make a lateral incision in the medial aspect of the RUQ of the abdomen . . . boy, I wish I had paid attention to directional terms in medical school!"

"Here, let me show you. I learned directional terms and medical terminology from *Anatomy and Physiology for Health Professionals: An Interactive Journey*."

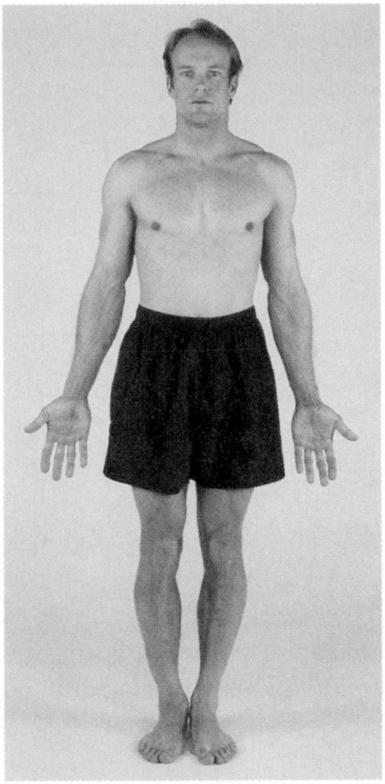

FIGURE ■ 2–1

The anatomical position.

Body Positions

The body can assume many positions and therefore have different orientations. To standardize the orientation for the study of anatomy, scientists developed the **anatomical position.** The anatomical position, as shown in Figure 2–1 ■, is a human standing erect, face forward, with feet parallel and arms hanging at the side, and with palms facing forward.

anatomical position *(an ah TOM ih kal)*

Other body positions that are important to discuss because of clinical assessments and treatments in health care are the **prone, supine,** and **Fowler's** positions. The supine position is laying face *upward,* or on your back. The prone position is laying face *downward,* or on your stomach. The Fowler's position is sitting in bed with the head of the bed elevated 45 to 60 degrees. This position is often used in the hospital to facilitate breathing and for comfort of the bedridden patient while eating or talking. See Figure 2–2 ■ for these body positions.

supine position *(sue PINE)*

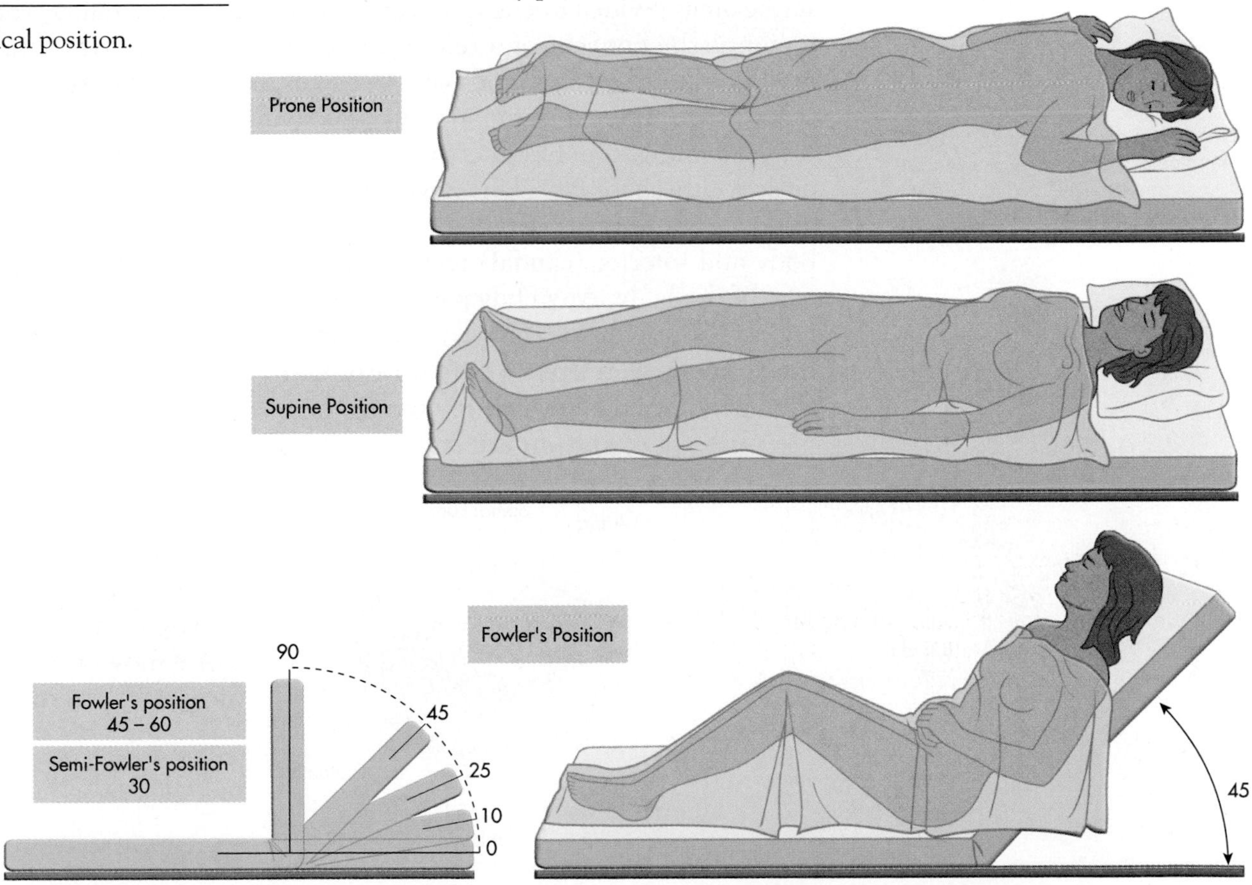

FIGURE ■ 2–2

Common patient positions.

TEST YOUR KNOWLEDGE 2-1

Answer the following questions:

1. Try standing in the actual anatomical position.
2. Give the best body position (prone, supine, or Fowler) for the following circumstances:

getting a back massage ____________________

watching television in bed ____________________

eating in a hospital bed ____________________

watching the stars at night ____________________

Body Planes and Directional Terms

Sometimes it is necessary to divide the body or even an organ or tissue sample into specific sections to further examine it. A plane is an imaginary line drawn through the body or organ to separate it into specific sections. For example, in Figure 2–3 ■, we see the **transverse plane** or **horizontal plane,** dividing the body into top (**superior**) and bottom (**inferior**) sections. This can also be called **cross-sectioning** the body. Cross-sectioning is often done with tissue and organ samples to further examine internal structures.

Transverse *(tranz VERS)*

cranial *(KRAY nee al)*
cranio = *skull*

cephalic *(seh FAL ik)*
cephalo = *toward the head*

caudal *(KAWD al)*
cauda = *tail*

-ic and *-al* are adjective endings that mean "pertaining to"

midsagittal *(mid SAJ ih tal)*

Notice in Figure 2–3 that certain directional terms can be used to describe areas divided by the transverse plane. One more analogy that relates to a map is the concept of a reference point. If you were traveling from Colorado to Florida, you would have to travel in a southeasterly direction. Colorado is your starting point and serves as your reference point. However, if you were traveling from Florida to Colorado, you would travel in a northwesterly direction because Florida is now your point of reference. In Figure 2–3, you can see that superior (**cranial** or **cephalic**) means toward the head or upper body and inferior (**caudal**) means away from the head or toward the lower part of the body. Any body part can be either superior or inferior depending upon your reference point. For example, the knee is superior to the ankle if the ankle is the reference point. Turning this around, the ankle is inferior to the knee if the knee is the reference point. Two other terms from this illustration are *cranial*, which refers to the skull, and **caudal,** which refers to body parts near the tail (tailbone).

The **median plane,** or **midsagittal plane,** divides the body into right and left halves. Figure 2–4 ■ shows this plane and the directional terms associated

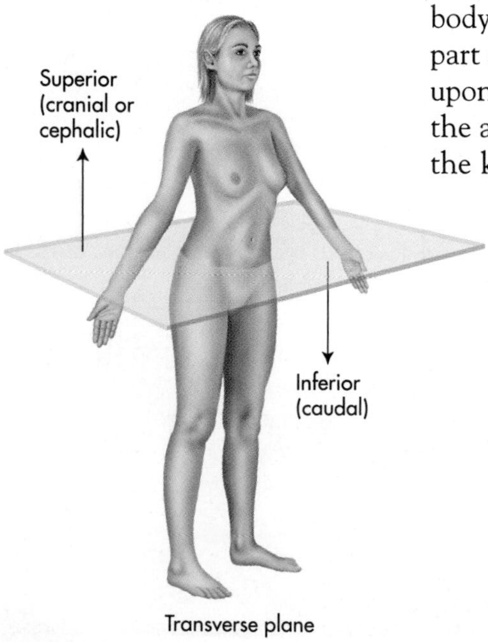

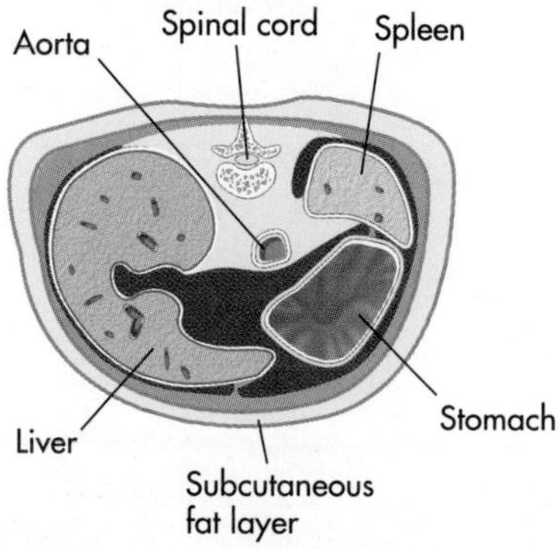

FIGURE ■ 2–3

Transverse plane and a cross-sectional view of the upper abdominal region.

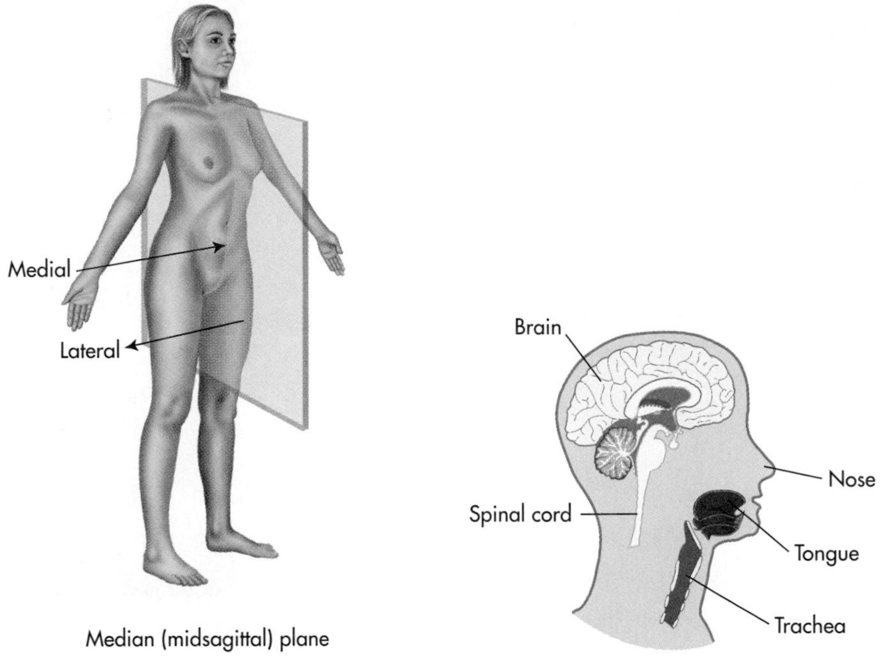

FIGURE ■ 2–4

Midsagittal or median plane along with a sagittal view of the head.

with it. **Medial** refers to body parts located near the middle or midline of the body. **Lateral** refers to body parts located away from midline (or on the side). If a technician were to section and examine an organ, he or she might make a midsaggital cut (cut the organ into equal right and left halves) in order to examine the internal parts of the organ or might simply make several saggital (vertical or lengthwise) cuts to slice the organ into smaller sections for closer examination.

medial *(MEE dee al)*
lateral *(LAT er al)*

coronal *(kor ROHN al)*
proximal *(PROK sim al)*

The **frontal plane,** or **coronal plane,** divides the body into front and back sections. **Anterior** and **ventral** refer to body parts toward or on the front of the body, and **posterior** and **dorsal** refer to body parts toward or on the back of the body. Figure 2–5 ■ demonstrates the coronal plane and associated directional terms. Remember, if during your trip you stop at the beach, you will know it is not safe to swim if you see a shark's *dorsal* fin sticking out of the water.

Clinical Application

DO YOU KNOW YOUR LEFT FROM YOUR RIGHT?

By now, it should be clear that a precise, standardized language with directional terms is needed to study anatomy and physiology and apply it in a health care setting. Something as simple as left and right can become critical. For example, suppose you are a surgical technologist and are ordered to put a tag around a patient's right leg to designate it as the leg to be amputated in an upcoming surgery. If you approach the patient from the bottom of the bed and place the tag on the leg on YOUR right side, you have erroneously placed it on the patient's left leg, and this could have disastrous results. The take-home message is that left and right *always* refer to the patient's left and right, *not yours.*

2-2 Go to the CD-ROM to view videos about and images of ultrasound, MRI, and other diagnostic imaging techniques used to visualize the interior of the body.

Additional Directional Terms

There are some additional directional terms that are important in health care. **Proximal** refers to body parts close to a point of reference of the body. This is con-

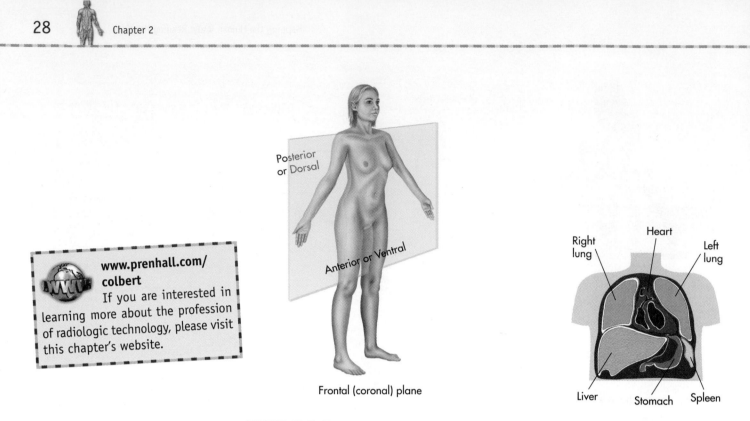

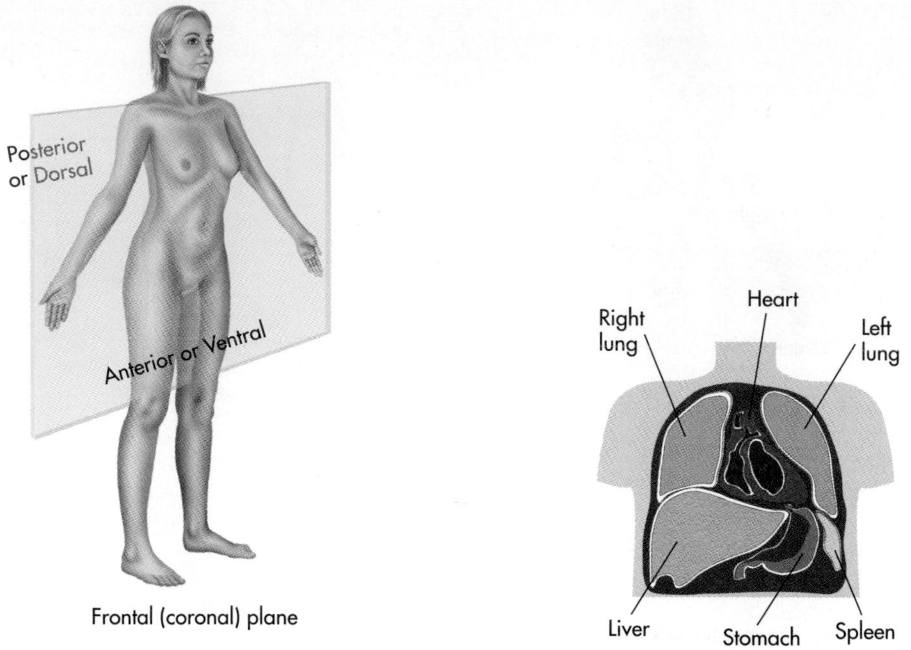

FIGURE ■ 2–5

Frontal or coronal plane along with a coronal view of the chest and stomach.

www.prenhall.com/colbert
If you are interested in learning more about the profession of radiologic technology, please visit this chapter's website.

distal *(DISS tal)*

trasted by **distal,** which refers to body parts away from a point of reference. For example, using your shoulder as a reference point, your elbow is proximal to your shoulder, while your fingers are distal to your shoulder. **External** means on the outside, and **internal** refers to structures on the inside. Did you know that your external skin is actually the body's largest organ? Most other organs are located internally within body cavities.

Superficial means toward or at the body surface. When a clinician draws blood from you, he or she looks for superficial veins that are easy to see and easy to access with the needle. **Deep** means away from the body surface. The large veins in your legs are deep veins and are more protected than superficial veins because injury to them can be more critical to survival than can injury to a smaller, superficial blood vessel. **Central** refers to locations around the center of the body (torso and head), and **peripheral** refers to the extremities (arms and legs) or surrounding or outer regions (see Table 2–1).

Applied Science

X-RAYS, CT SCANS, AND MRIs

Positions are also important in the radiologic sciences. X-rays are high-energy radiation that penetrates the body and gives a two-dimensional view of the bones, air, and tissues in the body. The standard X-ray (much like a photograph) can be enhanced with the use of computers to give much greater detail and contrast and to allow for a more realistic three-dimensional view. For example, if a golf ball–sized tumor in the lung was shown on a standard chest X-ray, you would have no idea of its actual depth because it would look flat, like a quarter. Computed tomography (CT) scanning uses a narrowly focused X-ray beam that circles rapidly around the body. The computer constructs thin-slice images and combines them to give much greater detail and allow for a more three-dimensional view, much like a loaf of sliced bread gives a better idea of the total shape of the loaf than does a single slice. The CT scan reveals the true depth of the quarter-shaped tumor shown on the regular X-ray. A magnetic resonance imager (MRI) produces even greater detail of tissue structures, even down to individual nerve bundles. Another possible advantage of the MRI is a decrease in radiation exposure.

cyanosis *(sigh ah NOH siss)*
cyano = *blue*
osis = *condition of*

www.prenhall.com/colbert Surgical technologists must have a command of medical directional terms used during surgical procedures. If you are interested in learning more about this profession, please visit the website for this chapter.

Clinical Application

CENTRAL VERSUS PERIPHERAL CYANOSIS

Cyanosis is a condition of bluish colored skin that is usually the result of low levels of oxygen in the blood. Peripheral cyanosis presents as bluish fingers and toes and may indicate the need for oxygen therapy depending on the condition of the patient. Peripheral cyanosis is sometimes difficult to detect in people with dark skin. Central cyanosis is much more serious and presents as bluish discoloration of the torso and inside the mouth. See Figure 2–6 ■, which illustrates central and peripheral cyanosis.

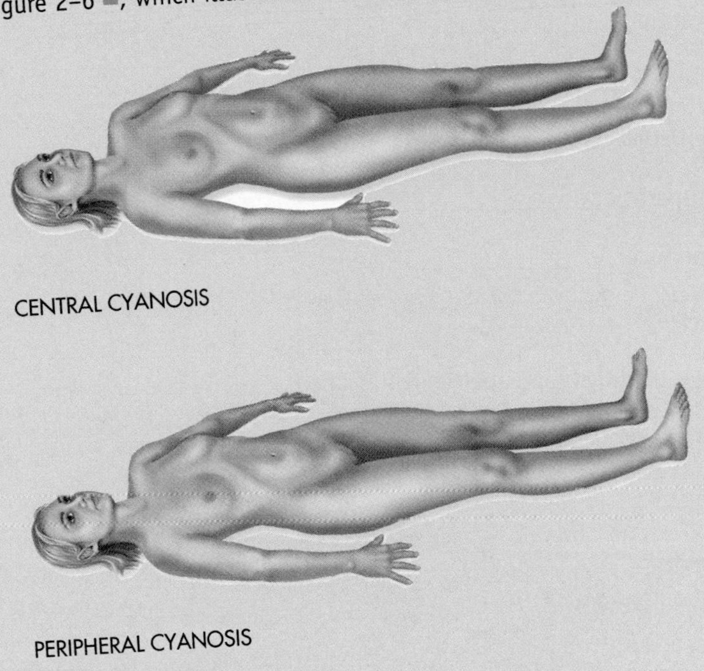

FIGURE ■ 2–6
Contrast of central versus peripheral cyanosis.

TABLE 2–1 Directional Terms

DIRECTIONAL TERM	MEANING	USE IN A SENTENCE
proximal	near point of reference	The wrist is *proximal* to the fingers.
distal	away from point of reference	The shoulder is *distal* to the fingers.
external	on the outside	The *external* defibrillator is used on the outside of the chest.
internal	on the inside	He received *internal* injuries from the accident.
superficial	at the body surface	The cut was only *superficial.*
deep	under the body surface	The patient had *deep* wounds from the chainsaw.
central	locations around center of body	The patient had *central* chest pain.
peripheral	surrounding or outer regions	The patient had *peripheral* swelling of the feet.

TEST YOUR KNOWLEDGE 2-2

Answer the following questions:

1. Give the opposite directional term:

superior ______________

posterior ______________

caudal ______________

ventral ______________

distal ______________

external ______________

superficial ______________

peripheral ______________

medial ______________

2. A spinal tap is performed on the (______________) portion of the body.

3. The plane that divides the body into upper and lower regions is called the ______________ plane.

4. Cutting an organ into two equal halves (right and left) requires a ______________ incision.

5. A scratch on the surface of the skin is called a ______________ wound.

6. The wrist is ______________ to the hand and ______________ to the elbow.

7. The nose is ______________ to the mouth.

8. A pain in your side can also be referred to as ______________ pain.

9. If your hands and feet are swollen with fluid (edema), you are said to have ______________ edema.

2-3 To reinforce the concept of body cavities and their locations, please go to your CD-ROM for an interactive drag-and-drop labeling exercise.

Body Cavities

thoracic cavity
(thoh RASS ik KAV ih tee)

abdominopelvic cavity
(ab dom ih noh PELL vik KAV ih tee)

cranial cavity
(KRAY nee al KAV ih tee)

spinal cavity *(SPY nal KAV ih tee)*

The body has two large spaces or cavities that house and protect organs. Located in the back of the body is the dorsal cavity and in the front, the ventral cavity. Figure 2–7 ■ illustrates these cavities. The larger anterior cavity is subdivided into two main cavities called the **thoracic cavity** and **abdominopelvic cavity.** These cavities are physically separated by the large, dome-shaped muscle called the diaphragm that is used for breathing. The thoracic cavity contains the heart, lungs, and large blood vessels. The heart has its own small cavity called the pericardial cavity. The abdominopelvic cavity contains the digestive organs, such as the stomach, intestines, liver, gallbladder, pancreas, and spleen in the upper or abdominal portion. The lower portion, called the pelvic cavity, contains the urinary and reproductive organs and the last part of the large intestine. A posterior or dorsal cavity is located in the back of the body and consists of the **cranial cavity,** which houses the brain, and the **spinal cavity,** which contains the spinal cord.

There are also smaller body cavities that designate specific areas, and these are further explored in upcoming chapters. For example, the nasal cavity is the space behind the nose, the oral or buccal cavity is the space within the mouth, and the orbital cavity houses the eyes.

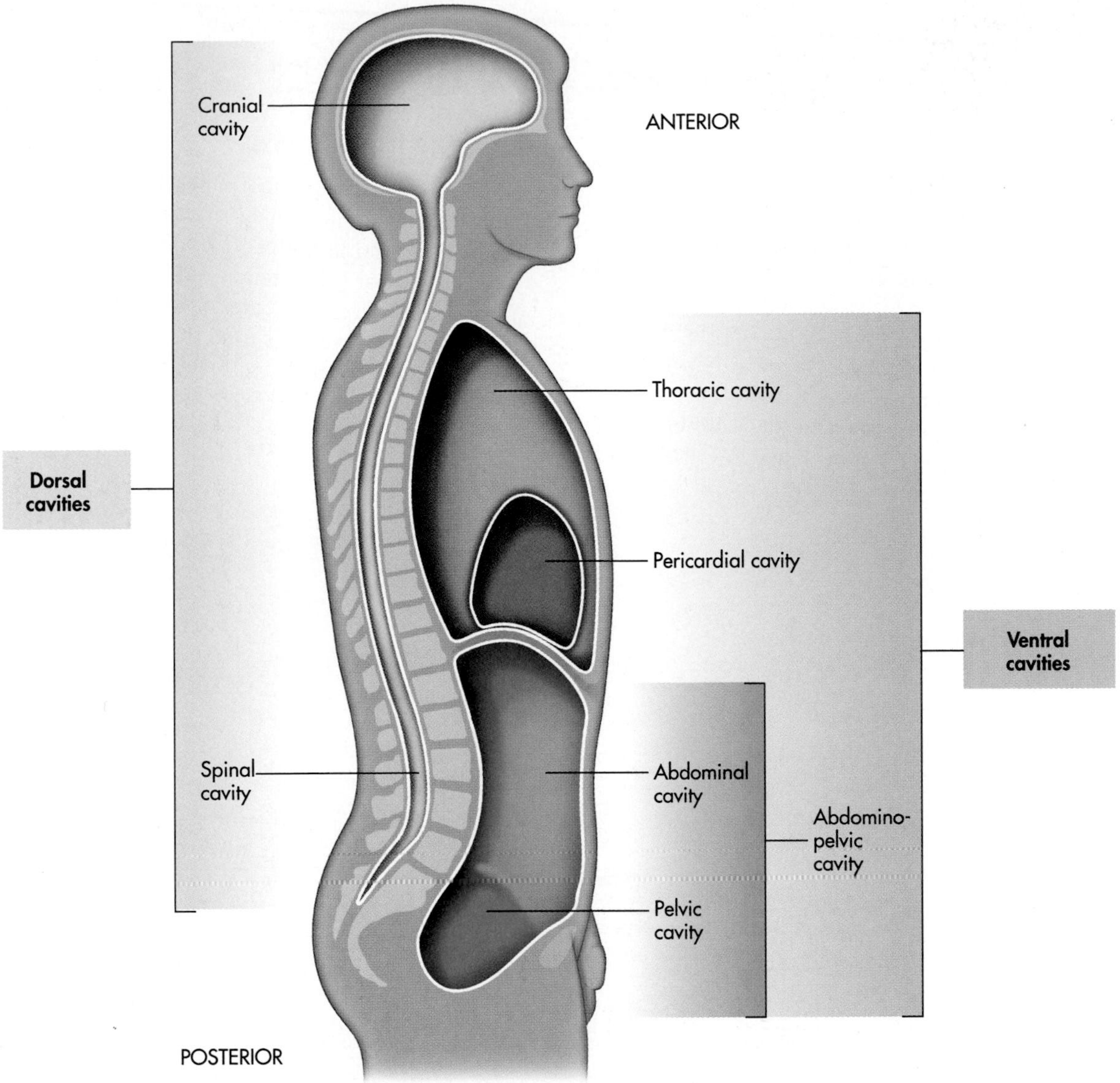

FIGURE ■ 2–7

Main body cavities.

TEST YOUR KNOWLEDGE 2-3

Identify the major body cavity where the following organs are located.

heart ________________

spinal cord ________________

stomach ________________

lungs ________________

reproductive organs ________________

brain ________________

Clinical Application

THE CENTRAL LANDMARK: THE SPINAL COLUMN

The spinal or vertebral column is a major, centrally located anatomical landmark and has five sets of vertebrae (spinal bones) labeled for the region of body location (see Figure 2–8 ■). The seven cervical (C) vertebrae are located in the neck; the 12 thoracic (T) vertebrae are located in the chest; the five lumbar (L) vertebrae are located in the lower back; and the five fused sacral (S) vertebrae (sacrum) are located near the final coccyx vertebra (tailbone). For example, the T5 vertebra is used to help locate on a chest X-ray the area where the right and left lung begin to branch. You'll learn even more about the spinal column and cord in Chapter 5, "The Skeletal System," and Chapters 8 and 9, "The Nervous System" (Parts I and II).

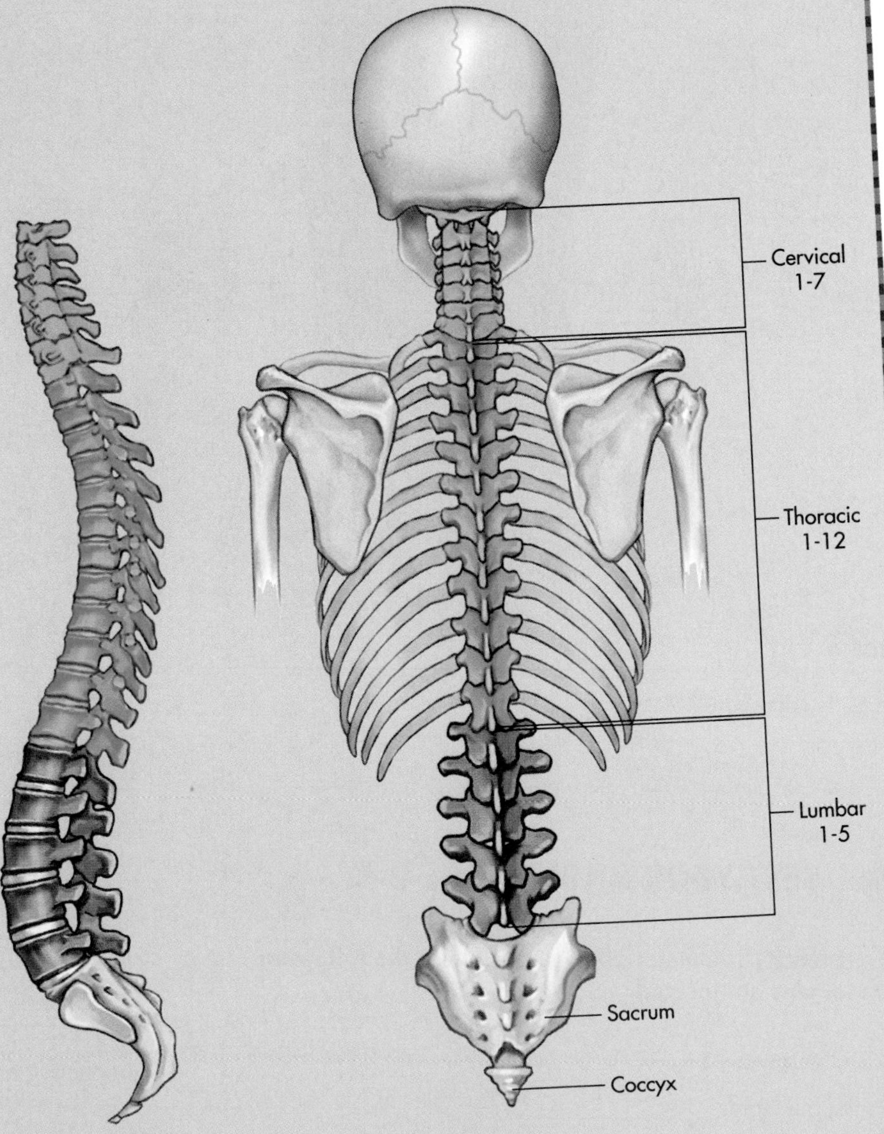

FIGURE ■ 2–8

The spinal column.

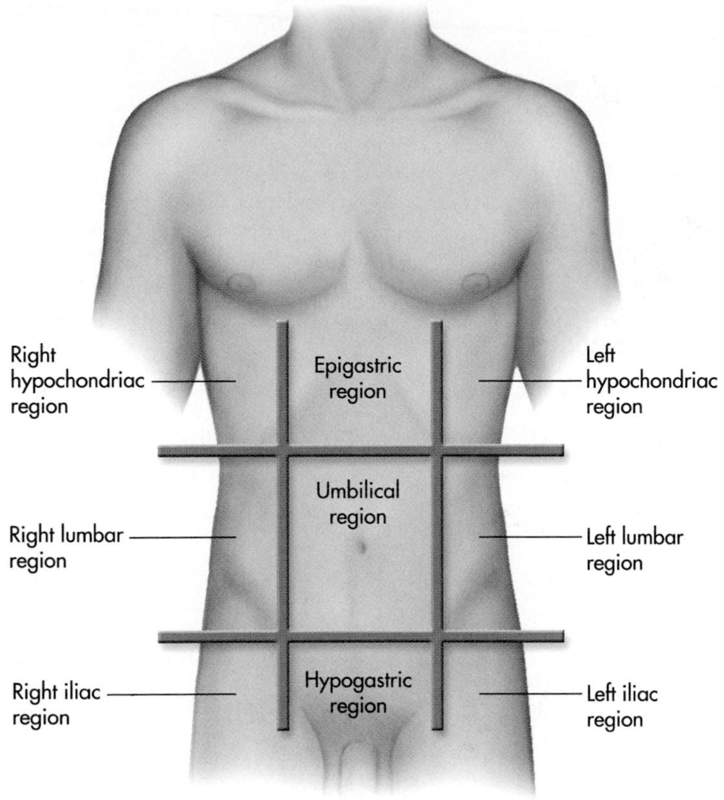

FIGURE ■ 2–9

The nine divisions of the abdominal region.

Body Regions

The abdominal region houses a number of organs. Anatomists have divided this region according to Figure 2–9 ■. Notice that understanding directional terms assists in locating the regions. For example, the **epigastric** region (epi, above; gastric, stomach) is located superior to the umbilical region. The right and left **hypochondriac** regions are located on either side of the epigastric region and contain the lower ribs. The centrally located **umbilical** region houses the naval or belly button. You may not remember your umbilical cord being cut as a newborn, but your belly button is a reminder that it occurred. Lateral to this region are the right and left lumbar regions at the level of the **lumbar** vertebrae. The hypogastric region lies inferior to the umbilical region and is flanked by the right and left iliac or inguinal regions. The **inguinal** region is where the thigh meets the body trunk and is also called the groin region.

epi = *above*
gastric = *stomach*
hypo = *below*
chondriac = *refers to ribs*
umbilical = *bellybutton*

lumbar = *lower back*

inguinal = *referring to groin*

2-4 Go to the CD-ROM for more interactive practice with drag-and-drop exercises focused on the various anterior and posterior body regions.

Clinical Application

HERNIAS

You may have heard of an umbilical (belly button) bulge, or inguinal hernia, and now you know exactly where such hernias are located. Just what is a hernia? A hernia is a tear in the muscle wall that allows a structure (usually an organ) to protrude through it. Sometimes this can be a minor nuisance, but a hernia can also be very dangerous if the blood flow is restricted to the portion of the organ that is protruding. Restricted blood flow can lead to death of the tissue and to serious consequences. Death of a tissue is called **necrosis.** Figure 2–10 ■ shows an inguinal and umbilical hernia with a protrusion of the intestines.

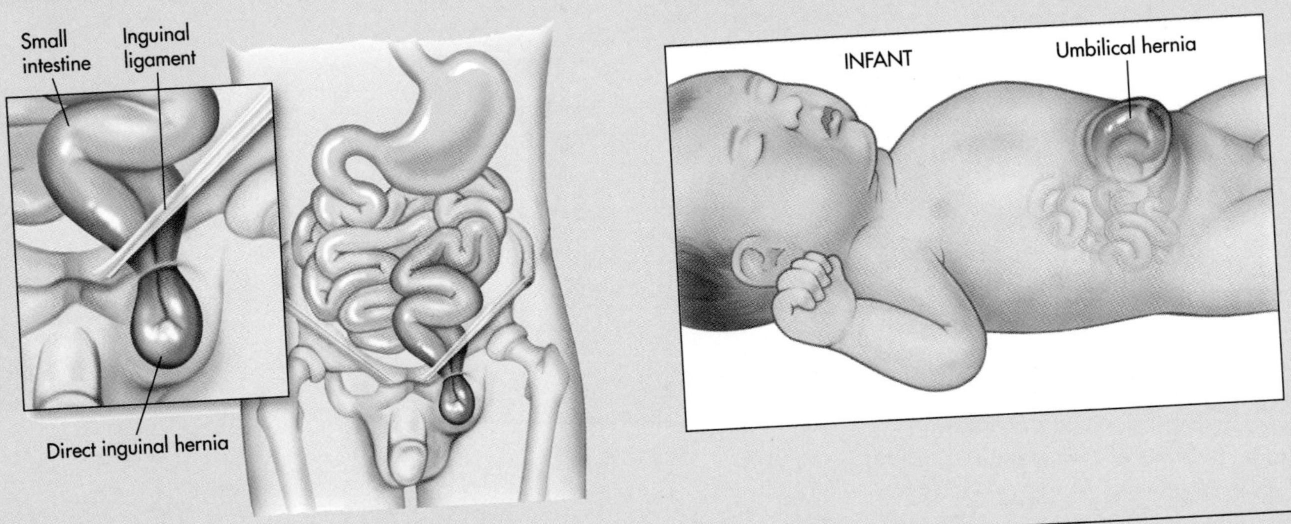

FIGURE ■ 2–10

Illustrations of inguinal and umbilical hernias.

A more practical way for health professionals to compartmentalize the abdominal region is to separate it into anatomical quadrants. Figure 2–11 ■ illustrates these quadrants, which are helpful in describing the location of abdominal pain. Knowing the organs located in the quadrant where the pain occurs can provide a clue to what type of problem the patient has. For example, tenderness in the right lower quadrant (RLQ) can be a symptom of appendicitis, because that is where the appendix is located. RUQ (right upper quadrant) pain may mean a liver or gallbladder problem.

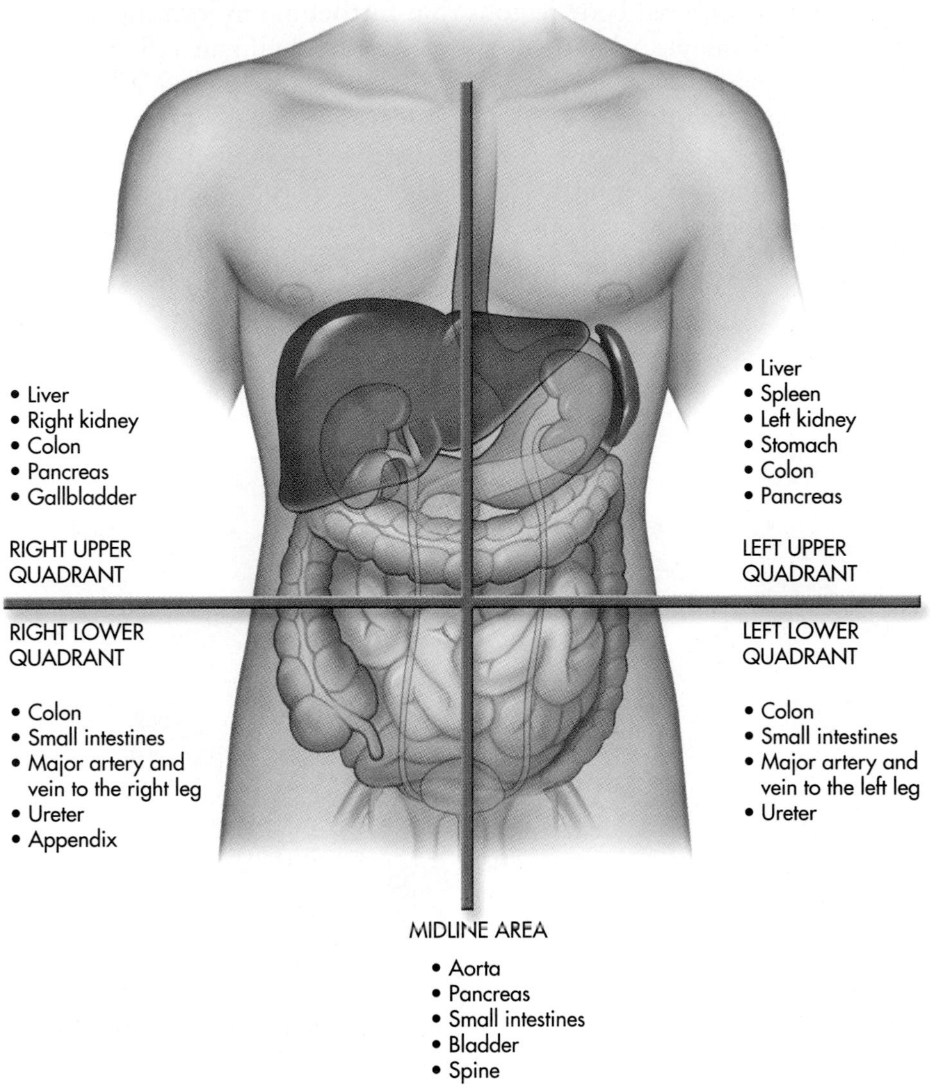

FIGURE ■ 2–11

The clinical division of the abdominal region into quadrants with related organs and structures

Amazing Body Facts

PSOAS TEST

This test—with its strange name—is one way to help determine if a patient has appendicitis. The patient is placed in a supine position and instructed to raise his or her right leg while the practitioner places a hand on the patient's right thigh and gives a slight opposing downward force. If it is appendicitis, the patient will usually experience pain in the right lower quadrant.

There are additional body regions that further aid in locating areas and structures. For example, what if you were asked to obtain an axillary temperature on an infant? Just where is the brachial or femoral pulse? What part of the body does carpal tunnel syndrome affect? See Figure 2–12 ■ for other common body regions and parts that are discussed in later chapters. In addition, review Table 2–2 for further practical examples of the medical importance of the various body regions.

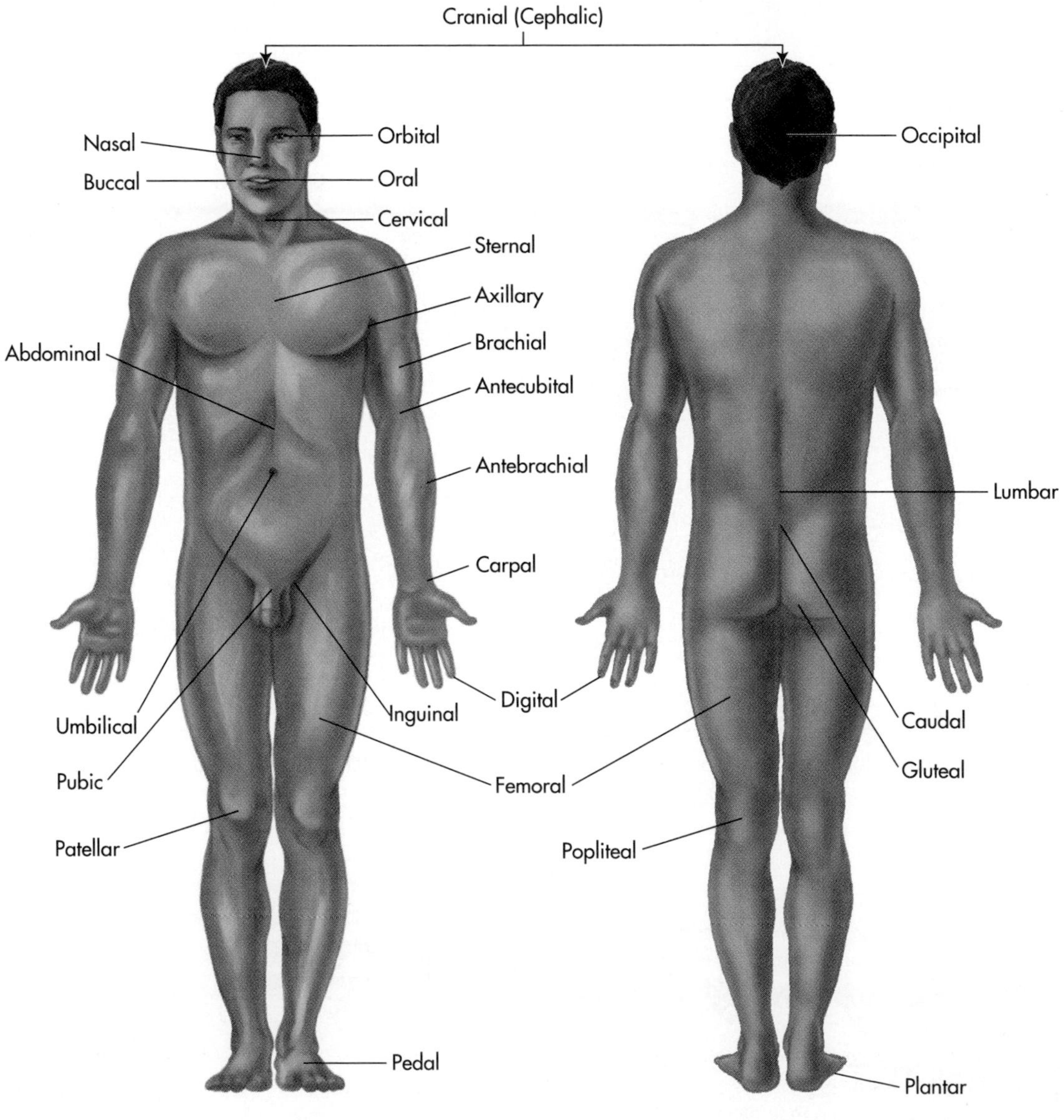

FIGURE ■ 2–12

Anterior and posterior body regions.

TABLE 2–2 Examples of Body Regions and Their Location

BODY REGION	LOCATION	MEDICAL EXAMPLE
antebrachial	forearm	between the wrist and elbow
antecubital	depressed area in front of elbow	area used to draw blood or start an IV
axillary	armpit	can be used to take temperature
brachial	upper arm	take blood pressure
buccal	cheek	check buccal region for central cyanosis
carpal	wrist	carpal tunnel syndrome
cervical	neck	cervical collar needed for neck injuries
digital	fingers	place digital oxygen sensors
femoral	upper inner thigh	check femoral pulse for effective CPR
gluteal	buttocks	the buttock is an injection site
lumbar	lower back	lumbar pain often occurs on long car trips
nasal	nose	medications can be given by nasal spray
oral	mouth	oral route is most common route for medications
orbital	eye area	orbital injury can cause damage to sight
patellar	knee	patellar injuries are very common in sports
pedal	foot	people with heart problems may have pedal edema (swelling)
plantar	sole of foot	plantar warts can be painful
pubic	genital region	the pubic region is often checked for body lice
sternal	breastbone area	the sternal area is used for CPR
thoracic	chest	the thoracic area is used to listen to heart and lung sounds

TEST YOUR KNOWLEDGE 2-4

Fill in the blank with the appropriate medical term for the body region. These can have more than one answer.

1. People who chew smokeless tobacco or snuff are more susceptible to _______________ cancer.
2. Antiperspirant sprays are usually used in the _______________ region.
3. Belly button rings are usually found in the _______________ region.
4. If you sit too long at your desk, you can develop _______________ pain.
5. During physicals, your reflexes are checked with a little rubber hammer that taps your _______________ region.

SUMMARY

Snapshots from the Journey

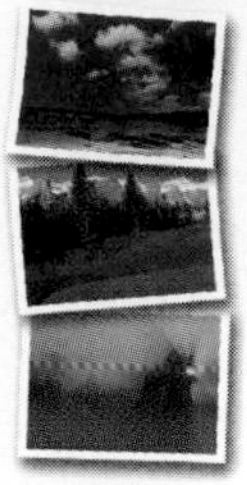

- The body can assume many different positions, and to standardize the study of anatomy, scientists often reference the anatomical position. In the anatomical position, the person stands with face and toes forward, hands at sides, and palms facing forward. Other positions, such as the prone, supine, and Fowler positions, are used in health care for assessment and treatments.
- The body can be divided by the use of planes into different sections. For example, the transverse, or horizontal plane divides the body into superior and inferior sections. The median, or midsagittal, plane divides the body into equal right and left halves, and the frontal, or coronal, plane divides the body into anterior and posterior sections.
- Directional terms, such as internal and external, proximal and distal, superficial and deep, central and peripheral, help us to navigate the body.
- It is important to always remember that directions such as right and left are referenced from the *patient's* perspective and NOT yours.
- The body has several cavities that house anatomical structures (mainly organs). For example, the cranial cavity houses the brain, the thoracic cavity houses the heart and lungs, the abdominopelvic cavity houses the digestive and reproductive organs, and the spinal cavity houses (guess what) the spinal cord.
- The body has many specific regions. For example, the umbilical region is found around your naval, or belly button, and the femoral region is located in the upper inner thigh area.
- The directional terms, anatomical landmarks, body regions, and body cavities are all important to know so that health care professionals can communicate in specific terms that leave no room for confusion.

Case Study

A 50-year-old female patient presents with sternal pain radiating to the left brachial area. Peripheral cyanosis is noted in the digital areas, and she exhibits pedal edema. No epigastric pain is noted. She reports that she became dizzy and fell, bruising the right orbital region, and she received superficial cuts to the right patellar region. The physician orders an IV to be started in the left antecubital space. Please answer the following questions in common lay terms.

a. Where would you suggest placing a bandage?
b. Where did her pain begin?
c. Where does the pain move to?
d. Does she have stomach pain?
e. Where will the IV be started?
f. What part of her body is swollen?

REVIEW QUESTIONS

Multiple Choice

1. A massage therapist would ask you to assume which position for a back massage?
   a. prone
   b. supine
   c. Fowler
   d. lotus

2. Which of the following is *not* in the abdominopelvic cavity?
   a. stomach
   b. liver
   c. reproductive organs
   d. heart

3. Carpal tunnel syndrome occurs in what region of the body?
   a. head
   b. cheek
   c. armpit
   d. wrist

4. The midsaggital plane divides the body into
   a. top and bottom
   b. front and back
   c. upper and lower
   d. left and right

5. An organ contained in the RLQ would be:
   a. appendix
   b. heart
   c. lungs
   d. brain

Fill in the Blank

1. A standard position in which a human stands erect, face forward, with feet parallel, arms at sides, and palms forward, is called the ______________ position.

2. The ______________ position is laying face upward and on your back.

3. The mouth is located ______________ to the nose, whereas the nose is located ______________ to the mouth.

4. The organ found in the cranial cavity is the ______________.

5. ______________ indicates blueness of the extremities and therefore affects the peripheral areas of the body.

Short Answers

1. List the organs found in the abdominal cavity.

2. Contrast the differences between the prone, supine, and Fowler positions.

3. List and describe two specific body regions that are found on the legs.

4. List and describe the location of the nine abdominal regions using directional terms.

Suggested Activities

1. Using a white t-shirt, draw and label the abdominal quadrants and the related organs.

2. Play pin the tail on the donkey by guiding the blindfolded person using only medical directional terms.

2-5

Now that you have completed your journey through this chapter, please go to the CD-ROM for interactive games and puzzles concerning the medical terms and concepts contained in this chapter. By playing the games you will reinforce your learning of medical terminology in a fun way.

Greetings from THE CELLS

The Raw Materials and Building Blocks

As we continue our journey, chances are that we will visit a city. A city is a complex combination of structures and systems. A brick or cement block is a basic structure upon which these buildings are constructed. The human body is also a complex combination of structures and systems, and a cell is the basic building block upon which the body is built. Just as there are different types, shapes, and sizes of building blocks, there are different types, shapes, and sizes of cells. Blood cells, skin cells, nerve cells, and so on, are all different from each other. We will learn more about each kind of cell in later chapters.

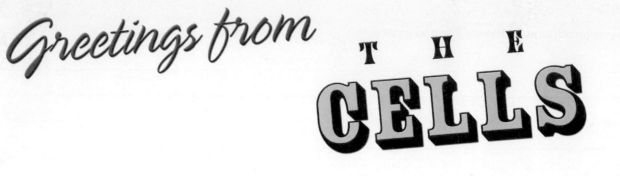

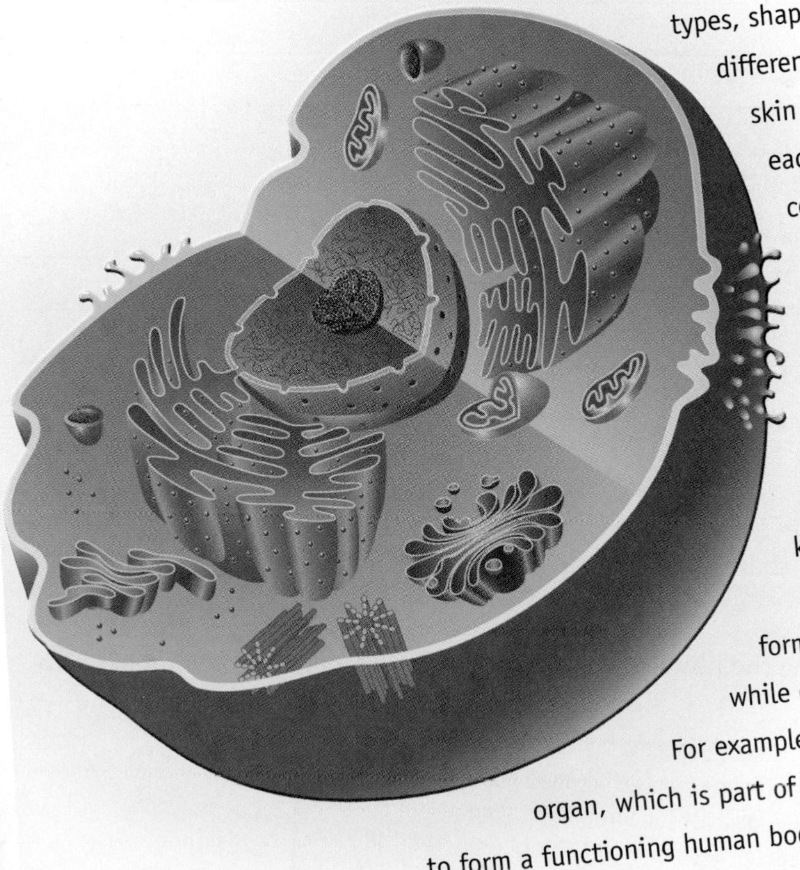

Although a cement block is a basic building block, it could not exist without sand, lime, and water, the components necessary to make cement. As this chapter explains, cells also consist of component parts, tiny cell structures called organelles that are needed to perform specific functions to keep the cell alive.

On a more involved level, cells of a similar type form tissue that functions to work together in an organ, while organs perform specific functions to create a system. For example, cardiac cells form heart tissues, which form the heart organ, which is part of the circulatory system. Finally, systems work together to form a functioning human body! When you think about it, we are very much like a city. Cities need transportation systems, control systems, systems to import food and water and export waste, and heating and cooling systems.

Chapter 3

LEARNING OBJECTIVES

At the end of your journey through this chapter, you will be able to:

- List and describe the various parts of a cell
- Explain the function of each organelle found within the cell
- Explain the process of cellular mitosis
- Describe the types of active and passive transport within cells
- Describe the structures required for cell motility
- Differentiate between bacteria, viruses, fungi, and protozoa

MULTIMEDIA APPLICATIONS

CD-ROM Interactive Exercises

- Animation of cellular parts and structure, 3-1
- Microbiology and proper hand washing and gloving techniques, 3-2
- Interactive games and puzzles, 3-3

www.prenhall.com/colbert

- Professional Profiles
  - Cytology
  - Lab Technician
- Related Internet Links
- Additional Review Questions

Pronunciation Guide

Correct pronunciation is important in any journey so that you and others are completely understood. Here is a "see and say" Pronunciation Guide for the more difficult terms to pronounce in this chapter.

benign (bee NINE)
capsid (CAP sid)
centrioles (SEN tree oles)
centrosomes (SEN tre soams)
chromatin (CROW ma tin)
cilia (SILL ee ah)
cytoplasm (SIGH toe plazm)
deoxyribonucleic acid (dee OK see RYE bow new clee ick AHsid)
endocytosis (en Doe Sigh TOE sis)
endoplasmic reticulum (EN doh PLAZ mic ri TIH cue lum)
exocytosis (EX oh sigh TOE sis)
flagella (flah GELL ah)
fungi (FUN jie)
Golgi apparatus (GOAL jee app ah RA tuss)
lysosomes (LIE seh soams)
malignant (mah LIG nant)
metastasis (meh TASS tah siss)
mitochondria (my teh CAHN dree ah)
mycelia (my SEE lee ah)
organelles (ore ga NELLS)
osmosis (ahz MOE sis)
phagocytosis (FAG oh sigh TOH sis)
pinocytosis (pin oh se TOH sis)
protozoa (pro toe ZOE ah)
ribonucleic acid (rie bow new KLEE ic)
ribosomes (RIE beh Soams)
vesicle (VESS ih kle)

OVERVIEW OF CELLS

Cells are units formed from chemicals and structures and are found in all living things. Some organisms are composed of only a single cell. Practically all of the cells in our body are microscopic in size, ranging from about one third to one thirteenth the size of the dot on this exclamation point! What is amazing is that certain nerve cells can be two feet in length or longer! When we refer to cells as the "building blocks" of our bodies, we immediately think of brick-shaped objects. However, cells can be flat, round, threadlike, or irregularly shaped. While the approximately *7.5 trillion* cells found in the human body vary in size, shape, and purpose, they normally work together to allow for proper functioning of processes necessary for life, such as digestion, respiration, reproduction, movement, and production of heat and energy. Figure 3–1 ■ represents a typical cell with its major components. We now discuss the individual components.

Applied Science

ATOMS AND MOLECULES

Although cells are composed of small structures called organelles, it is important to note that these organelles are composed of even smaller substances. Atoms, which are the tiny building blocks of all matter, combine to form molecules such as water, sugar, and proteins, which are then used to build cellular structures and facilitate cellular functions.

CELL STRUCTURE

Even though cells in our bodies can vary greatly in size, shape, and function, they share certain common traits. As previously stated, we consider cells the basic building blocks of the human body. However, to better understand them, let's look at cells as miniature cities with a variety of systems, structures, and or-

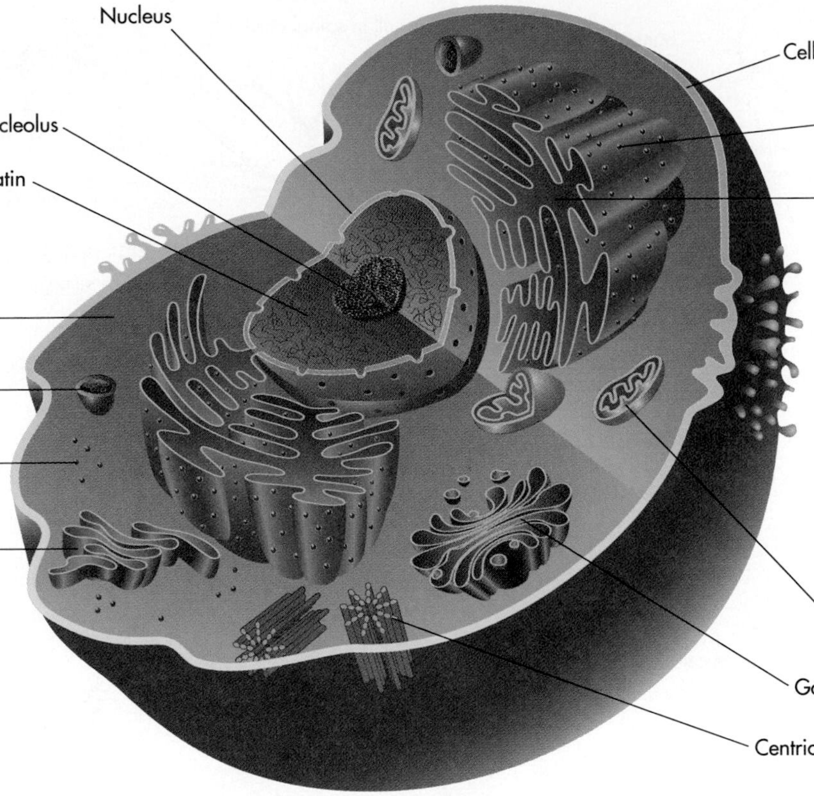

FIGURE ■ 3–1

Cellular components.

ganizations that are necessary for proper function. Almost all human cells possess a nucleus (except mature red blood cells), organelles, cytoplasm, and a cell membrane. Each component of a cell has a special purpose.

Cell Membrane

We can think of the **cell membrane** as the city limits. This is a defined boundary that possesses a definite shape and actually holds the cell contents together. The cell membrane acts as a protective covering. For a city to thrive, people and materials must be able to travel in and out of the city. A cell membrane is responsible for allowing materials in and out of the cell. What is interesting is that the membrane allows only certain things into or out of the cell. Because it chooses what may pass through, we call it a *selectively permeable* (or *semipermeable*) membrane.

In addition, the cell membrane has identification markers on it to show that it comes from a certain person, much like *PA* is an "identification marker" that tells us Pittsburgh is in Pennsylvania. If a foreign cell shows up in an individual (such as in a transplanted organ), the body signals an attack on that cell or group of cells. For all that it is responsible for, the cell membrane is only 3/10,000,000 of an inch thick. Each cell, regardless of its shape or function, must have a cell membrane in order to maintain its integrity and survive. See Figure 3–2 ■, which shows examples of various cell types found within the human body.

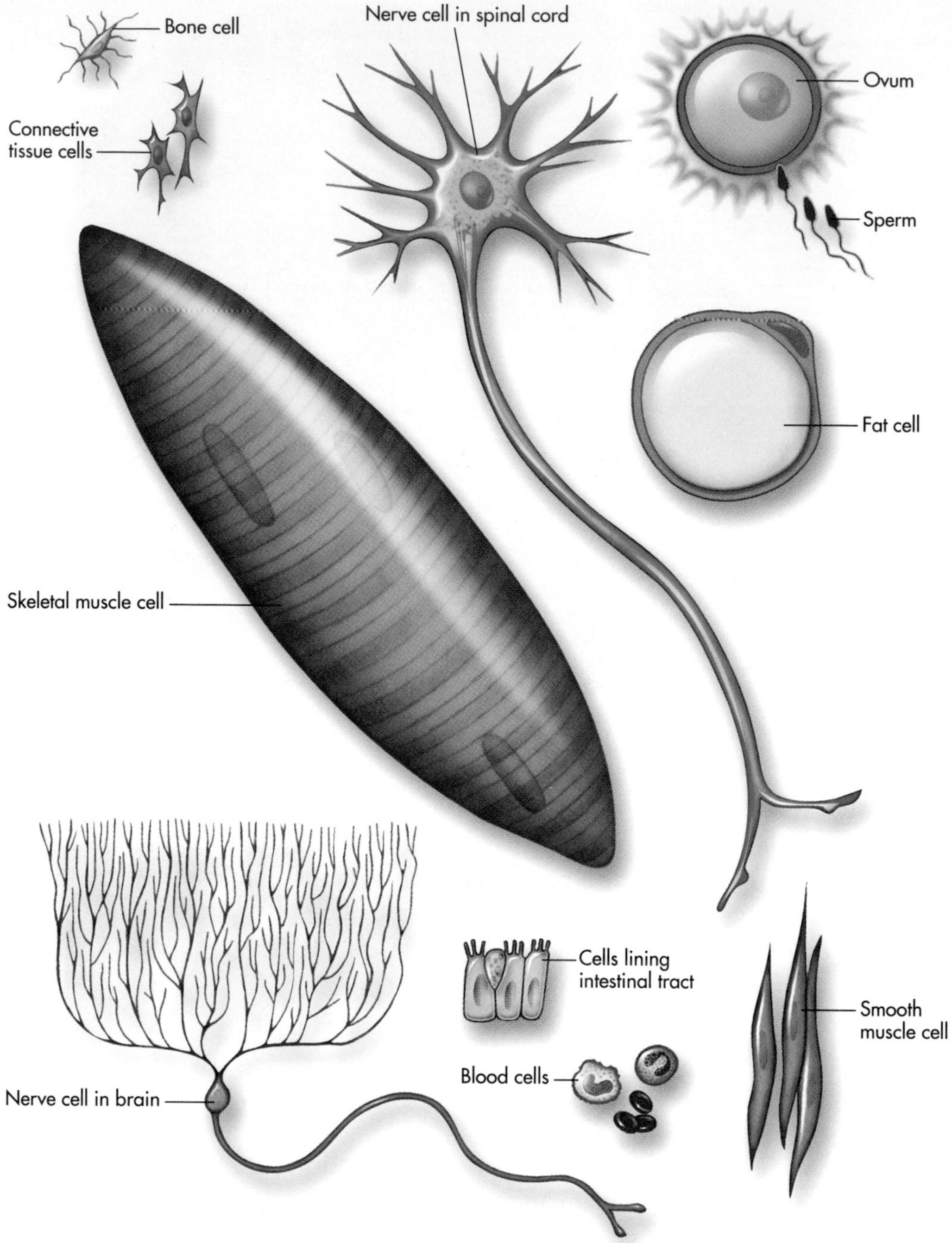

FIGURE ■ 3–2

Various types of cells within the human body.

Transport Methods

If we think of the cell membrane as the city limits or a boundary, we need to discuss how things get across this boundary. It can be done in two broad ways. **Passive transport** and **active transport** describe the movement of materials across the cell membrane. *Passive transport*, as the words suggest, requires no extra form of energy to complete. It is similar to having a yo-yo in your hand and simply letting go. The yo-yo simply falls as it unwinds from the string. No input of energy is needed. *Active transport* requires some addition of energy to make it happen. Throwing your yo-yo requires an addition of energy from your arm to make it happen.

PASSIVE TRANSPORT

Passive transport can be further divided into four types:

- diffusion
- facilitated diffusion
- osmosis
- filtration

> **Learning Hint**
>
> **CONCENTRATION GRADIENT**
>
> If a substance moves from higher concentration to lower concentration, it is said to be moving *with* the concentration gradient (difference). For example, if you are in a long grocery store line "concentrated" with people and three new lanes opens up, the people will quickly move from the highly concentrated line to the lower concentrated areas (the new open lanes). Soon, you will notice, all lines will equalize, demonstrating that even people move with a concentration gradient and reach equilibrium.

Diffusion Diffusion is our most common means of passive transport by which a substance of higher concentration travels to an area of lesser concentration. The difference between these two concentrations is called the concentration gradient. This is like dumping a packet of powdered drink mix into a pitcher of water. The water gradually assumes the color and flavor of the powder until the entire contents of the container are the same color and taste (nature likes a nice, equal balance!). Another example may be one of your classmates overusing perfume or cologne. Once in the classroom, the smell diffuses from high concentration on the individual to low concentration throughout the classroom. He or she may need to be reminded of the old saying that perfume should never announce your presence before your arrival.

Diffusion is necessary in the transportation of oxygen from the lungs and into the blood. It is also needed to transport the waste (carbon dioxide) from the blood to the lungs and eventually out into the air. This vital process is further discussed in Chapter 13, (The Respiratory System). See Figure 3–3 ■ for examples of diffusion.

Facilitated Diffusion Facilitated diffusion is a variation of diffusion in which a substance is helped in moving across the membrane, similarly to an usher helping you to your seat at a ball game. Glucose is the substance that is often helped in the body. You may wonder, if it is helped, how can it be considered *passive* transport? It best can be thought of as a situation in which the glucose was already moving in an attempt to cross the membrane and conveniently encounters an already revolving door. Once it steps into the door, it is quickly "pushed" along until it comes out on the other side of the membrane. See Figure 3–4 ■, which illustrates facilitated diffusion.

Osmosis Osmosis is another form of passive transport in which water travels through a selectively permeable membrane to equalize concentrations of a substance. The substance that is dissolved in the water is called the *solute*. Remember that nature likes things balanced and equal. Water

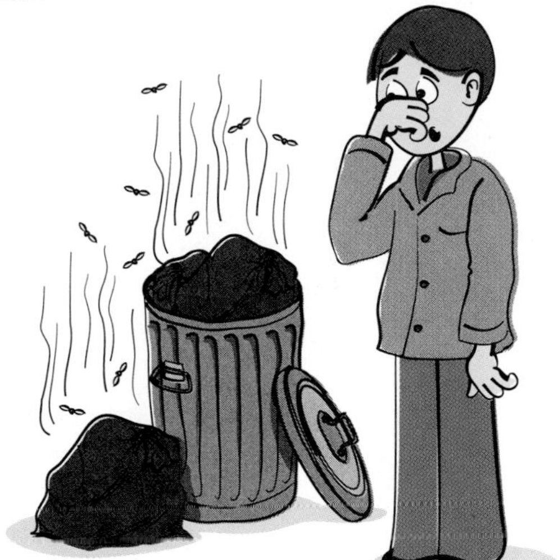

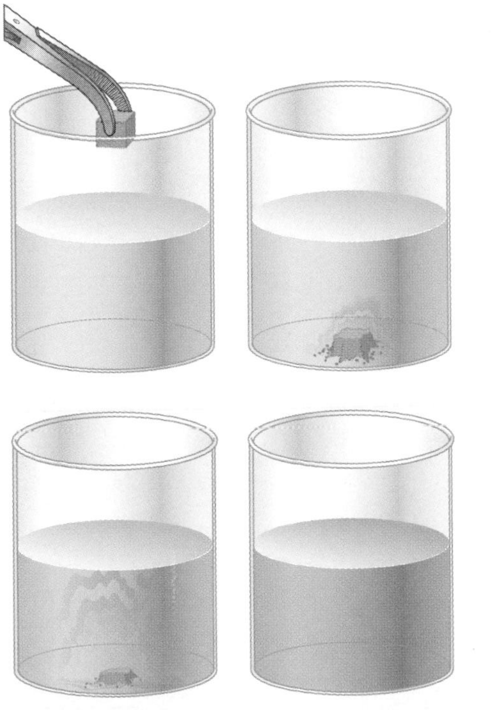

FIGURE ■ 3–3

Two examples of diffusion.

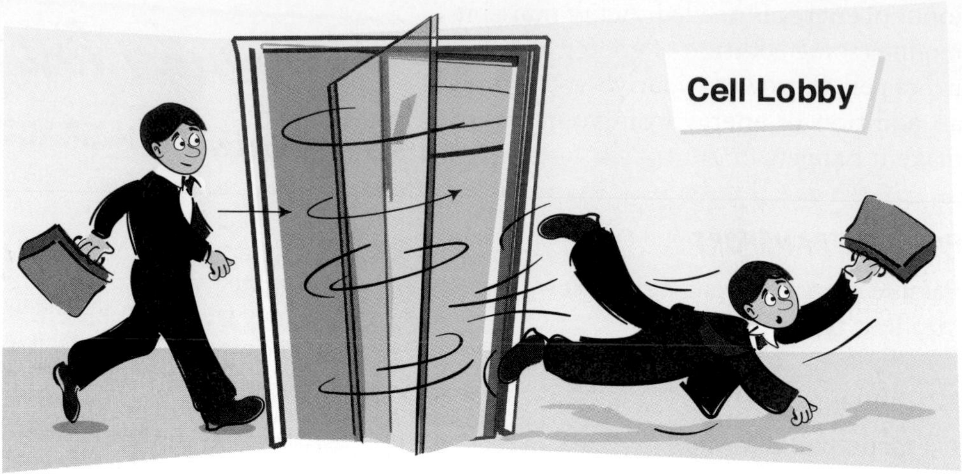

FIGURE ■ 3–4

Facilitated diffusion.

tends to travel across a membrane from areas that have a low concentration of a solute to areas that have a higher concentration of the solute until the concentration is the same on both sides of the membrane. Keep in mind that the water is moving with *its* concentration gradient. See Figure 3–5 ■ for a visual description. This ability of a substance to "pull" water toward an area of higher concentration of the solute is called **osmotic pressure.** The greater the concentration of the solute, the greater the osmotic pressure it exerts to bring in water.

Filtration Filtration is the final member of the passive transport group. This method differs from osmosis in that pressure is applied to force water and its dissolved materials across a membrane. Filtration caused by pressure is similar to a rush of people being pushed through the turnstiles during rush hour

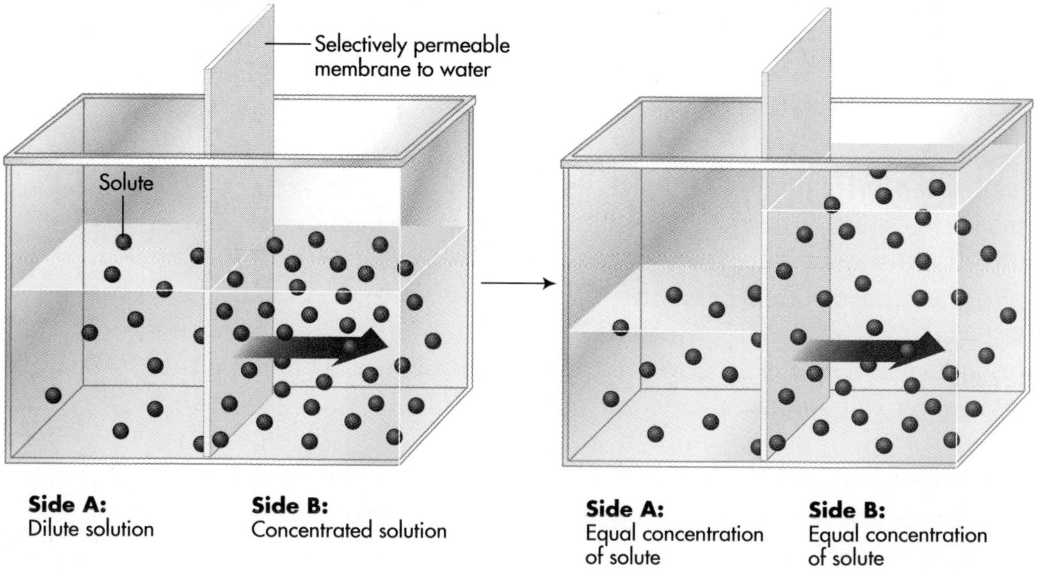

FIGURE ■ 3–5

Osmosis: Water moves from an area of low solute concentration to an area of higher solute concentration.

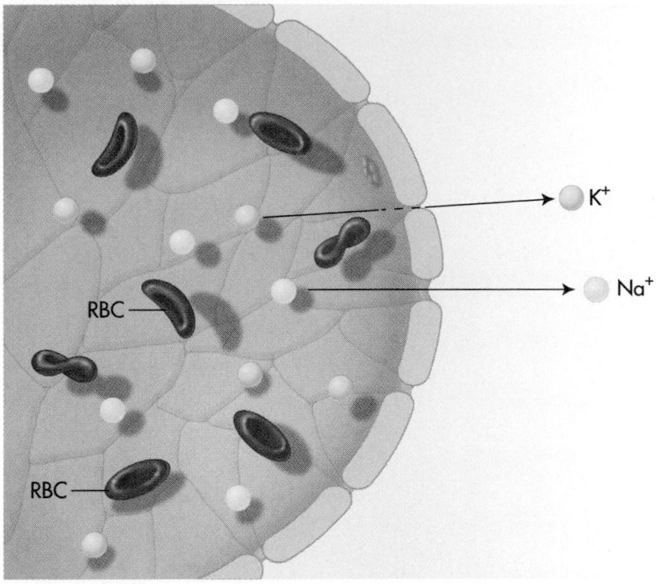

FIGURE ■ 3–6

The process of filtration in the kidneys, where smaller solutes such as the electrolytes sodium and potassium pass through the membrane, while the larger blood proteins and cells normally do not.

or the effect you get when you squeeze the trigger on a squirt gun. The major supplier of force in the body is the pumping of the heart, which forces blood flow into the kidneys where filtration takes place. This concept is expanded in Chapter 16, "The Urinary System." For now, see Figure 3–6 ■, which illustrates the process of filtration.

TEST YOUR KNOWLEDGE 3-1

Fill in the blanks:

1. This form of passive transportation is like combining drink mix and a pitcher of water: ______________.
2. When considering osmosis, water travels across a semipermeable membrane from an area of ______________ concentration of solute to an area of ______________ concentration of solute.
3. ______________ allows only certain sizes of particles to pass through.
4. The act of removing carbon dioxide from the blood to the lungs is achieved through ______________.
5. Glucose is often transported by ______________.

ACTIVE TRANSPORT

Active transport can be broken down into three types:

- active transport pumps
- endocytosis
- exocytosis

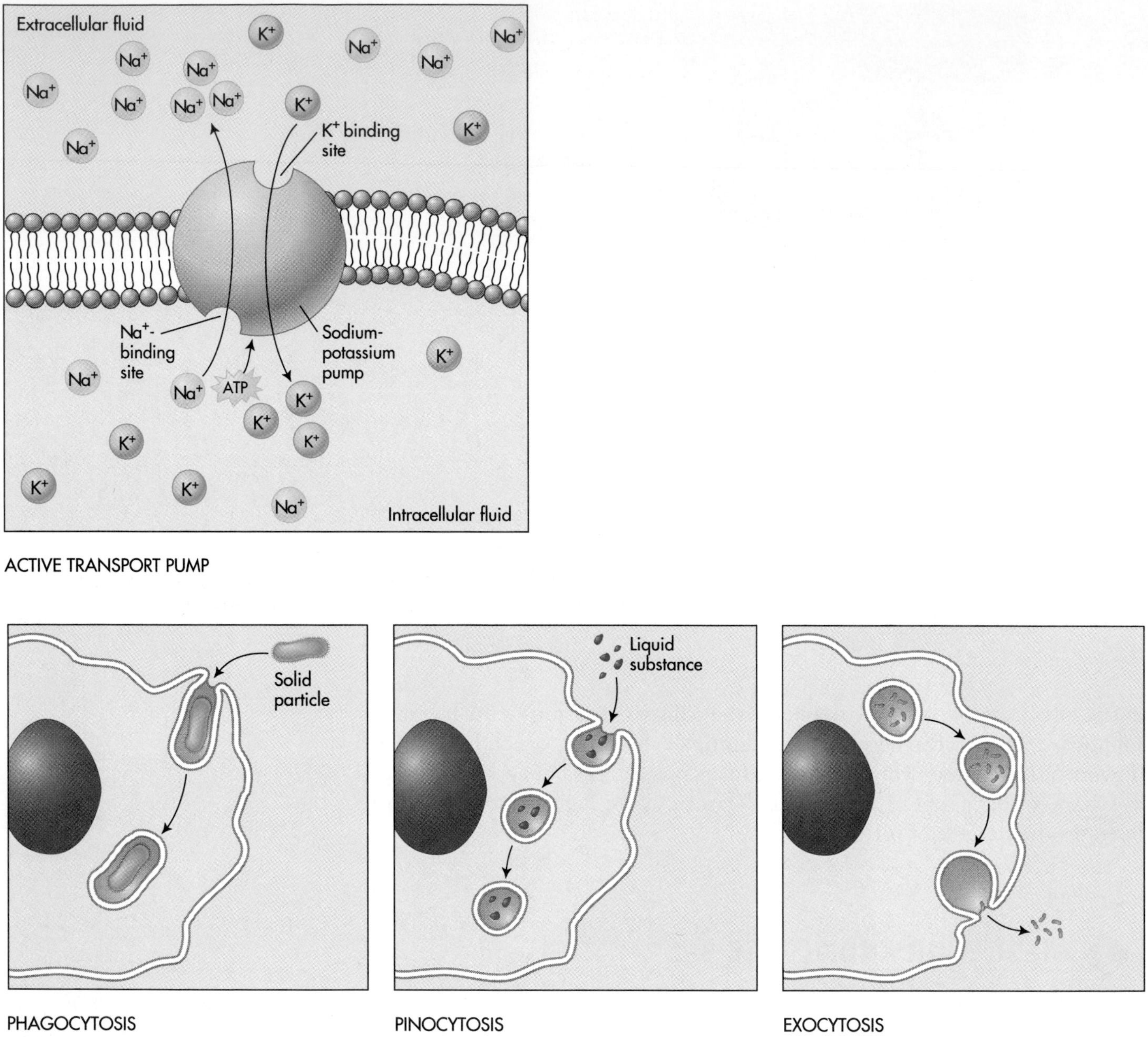

FIGURE ■ 3–7

Types of active transport in and out of cells.

Active Transport Pumps Active transport pumps require the addition of energy in the form of an energy molecule called adenosine triphosphate, or ATP (which we soon discuss) to move a substance. Energy is needed because the cell is trying to move a substance into an area that already has a high concentration of that substance. It's kind of like trying to put six pounds of sugar into a five pound bag! It can be done, but you have to apply a lot of pressure (energy). A common example in our cells is the need to transport potassium (K+). Cells contain a good amount of potassium. The only way to get more into a cell is to apply energy to "push" it in.

Endocytosis **Endocytosis** is utilized by the cells for the *intake* of liquid and food when the substance is too large to diffuse across the cell membrane. The cell membrane actually surrounds the substance with a small portion of its membrane, forming a chamber, or **vesicle,** which then separates from the membrane and moves into the cell. If it is a solid particle being transported, we call it **phagocytosis.** That is also the term that describes what white blood cells do to bacteria to prevent infections in our bodies. If the intake involves water, it is called **pinocytosis.**

endocytosis *(en DOE sigh TOE sis)*
endo = *within*
cyt = *cell*
osis = *condition*

phago = *eating*

pino = *to drink*

Exocytosis In some situations, the cell needs to transport substances *out* of itself. This is called **exocytosis.** Some cells may produce a substance needed outside the cell. Once this substance is made, it is surrounded by a membrane forming a vesicle (bladder or sac) and moves to the cell membrane. This vesicle becomes a part of the cell membrane and expels its load out of the cell. For further explanation of active transport, see Figure 3–7 ■.

Please see Table 3–1, which puts all of the methods of transport together for your viewing pleasure.

exocytosis *(Ex oh sigh TOE sis)*
exo = *outside*

TEST YOUR KNOWLEDGE 3-2

Complete the following:

1. Differentiate between phagocytosis and pinocytosis.
2. Tell whether the following processes are active or passive:
   a. endocytosis ______________
   b. facilitated diffusion ______________
   c. osmosis ______________
   d. phagocytosis ______________
   e. filtration ______________

Cytoplasm

Living organisms require balanced environments in which to thrive. Humans require the right mixture of oxygen and nitrogen; sea creatures require the right balance of salt and water; a chick embryo requires albumen, or "egg white," in which to develop. Likewise, the internal parts of a cell require a special environment, called **cytoplasm,** in order to survive.

Nucleus and Nucleolus

The nucleus has been described as the "brain of the cell." In our case, we will consider it to be City Hall: a control center. City Hall dictates the activity of the city departments much as the nucleus dictates the activities of the organelles

TABLE 3–1 Methods of Cellular Transportation

CELLULAR TRANSPORTATION METHODS	DESCRIPTION
Passive Transportation (no energy required)	
diffusion	moving a substance from an area of high concentration to an area of low concentration
facilitated diffusion	substance is assisted via "revolving door" in a direction it was already traveling from an area of high concentration to an area of low concentration
osmosis	water travels across a membrane from areas that have a low concentration of a solute to areas that have a higher concentration of solute until the concentration is the same on both sides of the membrane
filtration	pressure is applied to force water and dissolved materials across a membrane
Active Transport (energy required)	
active transport pumps	require additional energy in form of ATP to move substances against the concentration gradient (from low concentration to high concentration)
endocytosis	ingesting substances that are too large to diffuse across the cell membrane
phagocytosis	form of endocytosis in which *solid* particles are being brought into the cell via vesicles
pinocytosis	form of endocytosis in which *liquid* is being brought into the cell via vesicles
exocytosis	transportation of material outside of the cell

in the cell. Since City Hall is crucial to the city's function, security is important to protect it from attack or damage. That is why metal detectors are installed at the doors. The nucleus of a cell is similar. It is surrounded by a double-walled nuclear membrane. Even though this membrane is composed of two layers, it has large pores that allow certain materials to pass in and out of the nucleus.

Somewhere in City Hall are blue prints of the city showing the buildings, streets, water and gas lines, and so forth. The nucleus also contains "blueprints"—and "building codes" too. **Chromatin** is the material found in the nucleus that contains DNA (**deoxyribonucleic acid**). DNA contains the specifications (blueprints), for the creation of new cells. Chromatin eventually forms chromosomes, which contain **genes.** Genes determine our inherited characteristics (remember Aunt Pearl saying how much you look like your Uncle Elmer?).

A spherical body made up of dense fibers called the **nucleolus,** is found within the cell nucleus. Its major function is to

www.prenhall.com/colbert
Cytology is a general term used for the study of cells. However, in health care there are a variety of areas of specialization when studying cells. Go to the book's website to learn more about areas of specialization in cytology and to view a video about laboratory technicians, which profiles the various professional areas.

synthesize the **ribonucleic acid (RNA)** that forms ribosomes. Now we have the blueprints, but what about the materials that we need? Who's in charge of getting these materials together? That's where **ribosomes** and **centrosomes** come into play. Figure 3–8 ■ shows the cell membrane, cytoplasm, nucleus, and nucleolus. We will continue to rebuild the cell's infrastructure as we discuss their specific functions.

Ribosomes

Ribosomes are organelles that are found on the endoplasmic reticulum or floating around in the cytoplasm. Ribosomes are made of RNA and assist in the production of enzymes and other proteins that are needed for cell repair and reproduction. Following our analogy, ribosomes can be considered building material suppliers for remodeling and repair.

Centrosomes

In a city, completely new structures often are needed to replace old ones. Therefore, the cell needs a building contractor to build new structures. The **centrosomes** fill this need. Centrosomes contains **centrioles** that are involved in the division of the cell. Cellular division, or reproduction, will be discussed once we

centrosomes *(SEN tre soams)*
centrioles *(SEN tree oles)*

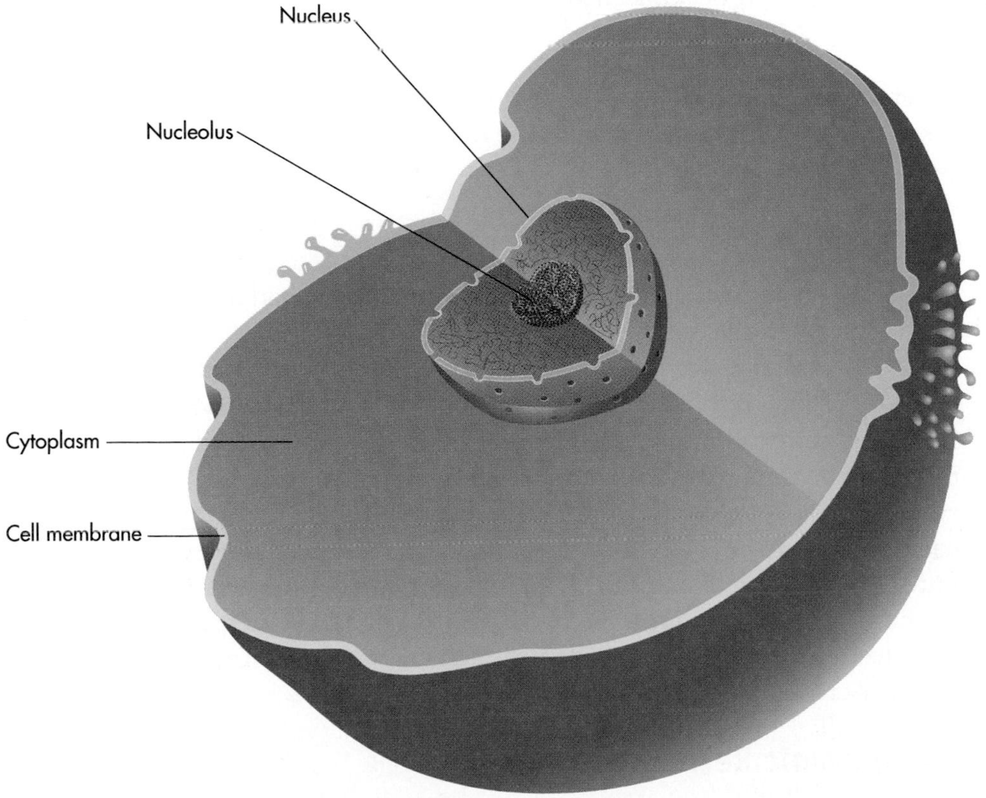

FIGURE ■ 3–8

The cell membrane, cytoplasm, nucleus, and nucleolus.

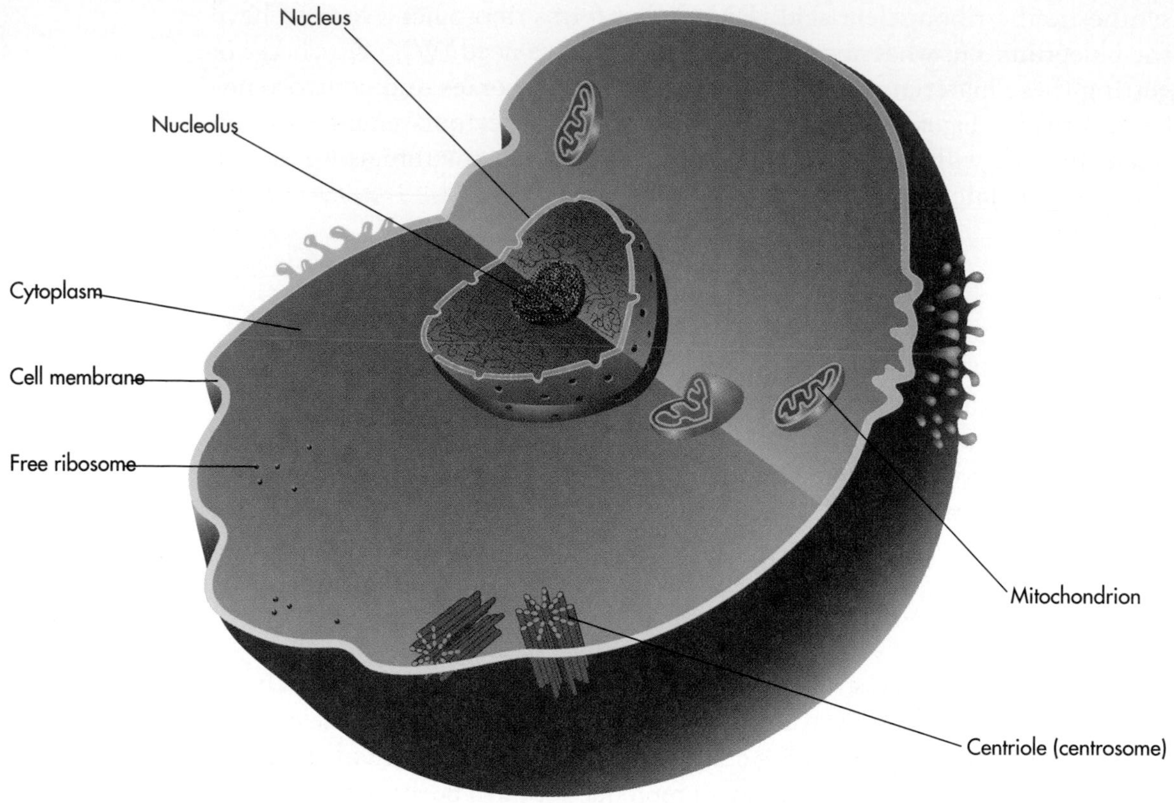

FIGURE ■ 3–9

The cell membrane, cytoplasm, nucleus, nucleolus, ribosomes, centrosomes, and mitochondria.

cover all the cell parts. Centrioles are tubular shaped and usually found in pairs. See Figure 3–9 ■, which now adds the nucleus, nucleolus, ribosomes, and centrosomes to the cell.

Mitochondria

mitochondria *(my teh CAHN dree ah)*

Could you possibly imagine what it would be like if we had no electricity in our city? Things would come to a standstill. The **mitochondria,** tiny bean-shaped organelles, act as power plants to provide up to 95 percent of the body's energy needs for cellular repair, movement, and reproduction. As a city's need for power increases, more power plants are built. Similarly, if a given cell type is very active and needs more power, there are a larger number of mitochondria in that cell. Liver cells, which are quite active, can have up to 2,000 mitochondria in each cell. Sperm cells "swim" with a tail (flagellum), so they need only a single mitochondria coiled around the tail for energy. Special enzymes in the mitochondria help to take in oxygen and use it to produce energy. While our city uses electricity for most of its power, the cell uses adenosine triphosphate (ATP), which is created by the mitochondria (see Figure 3–9).

Endoplasmic Reticulum

endoplasmic reticulum *(EN doh PLAZ mic ri TIH cue lum)*

Although there are paths, walkways, and sidewalks in our city, the main structure for travel is a road system. The **endoplasmic reticulum** is a series of channels set up in the cytoplasm that are formed from folded membranes. The endoplasmic reticulum has two distinct forms. One has a sandpaper-like surface, the result of ribosomes on its surface, which we call the *rough* endoplasmic reticulum, and it is responsible for the synthesis of protein. Once the protein is synthesized, it is sent to the Golgi apparatus for processing. The second form has no ribosomes on its surface, making it appear smooth, so we call it the *smooth* endoplasmic reticulum (complex stuff, huh?). The smooth endoplasmic reticulum synthesizes lipids (fats) and steroids. Think of this as a series of dirt and paved roads with butcher shops and food processing plants along the way (see Figure 3–10 ■).

Golgi Apparatus

Golgi apparatus *(GOAL jee app ah RA tuss)*

Cities have factories with their own fleet of trucks. The **Golgi apparatus** is very similar to these factories. This organelle looks like a bunch of flattened, membranous sacs. Once the Golgi apparatus receives protein from the endoplasmic reticulum, it further processes and stores it as a shippable product, much like a packaging plant does. Not only does it prepare the protein for shipping, a part of the Golgi apparatus surrounds the protein that then separates itself from the main body of this organelle. That portion, with its load, then travels to the cell membrane where it releases (secretes) the protein! This is an actual example of exocytosis. Cells that constitute organs with a high level of secretion or storage (like the digestive system) contain higher numbers of the Golgi apparatus. Salivary glands and pancreatic glands, for example, are made of cells containing many Golgi apparati.

Lysosomes

lysis = *to break down*

All cities create waste that must be removed. Cells are no different. **Lysosomes** are vesicles containing powerful enzymes that take care of cleaning up intracellular debris and other waste. Lysosomes are multitalented. They also aid in maintaining health by destroying unwanted bacteria through the process of phagocytosis. Please see Figure 3–10, which contains all the organelles.

3-1 For an animation of the parts and structure of a cell, please go to your CD-ROM for this chapter.

Other Interesting Parts

cytoskeleton *(SIGH toe SKELL eh ton)*

Similar in some ways to the skeleton, the **cytoskeleton** is a network of microtubules and interconnected filaments that provide shape to the cell and allow the cell and its contents to be mobile.

vesicle *(VESS ih kle)*

Vesicles, often created by the golgi apparatus, can be thought of as little trucks. They can be loaded up with substances, travel to another site in the cell or cell membrane, and then drop off their loads.

flagella *(flah GELL ah)*

Suppose we could build cities that float on large bodies of water. How would we propel them to new locations? Certain cells can solve this problem through the use of **flagella.** Flagella are whip-shaped tails that move some cells in a fashion similar to that of a tadpole.

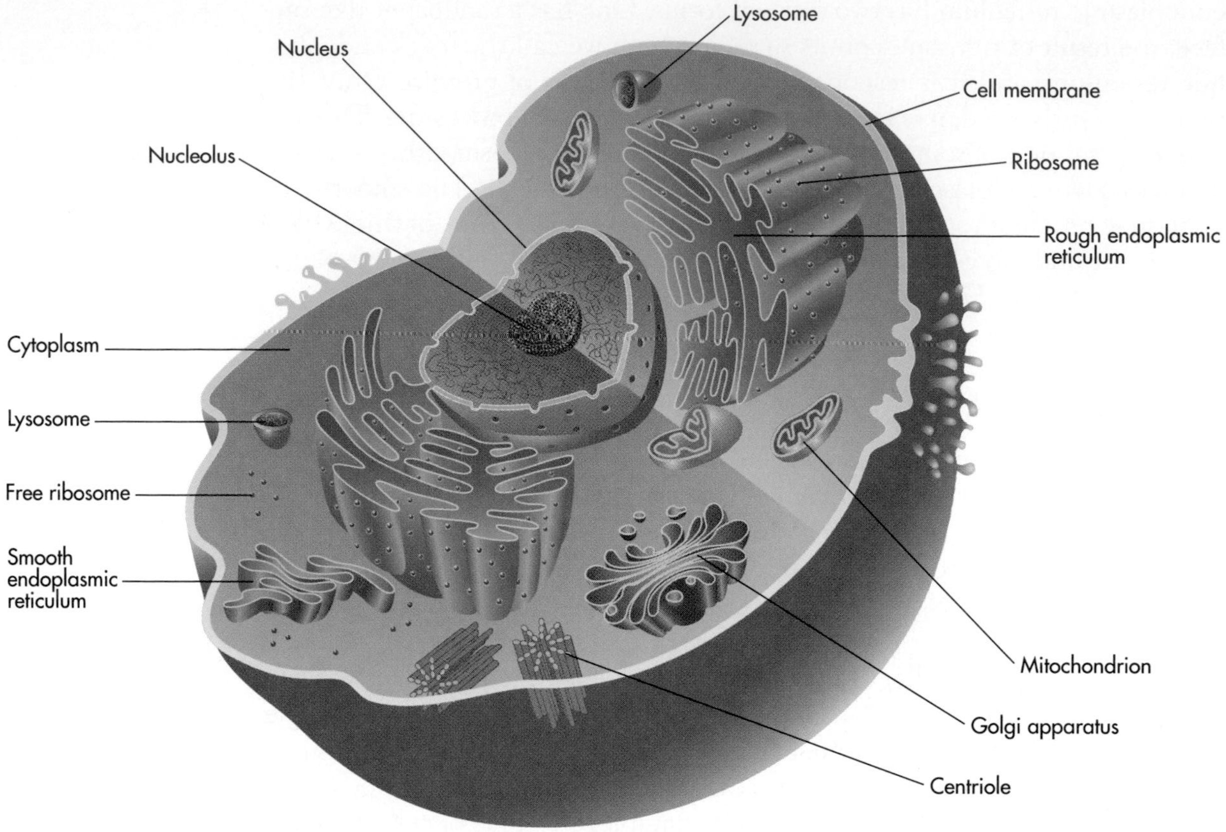

FIGURE ■ 3–10

The cell membrane, cytoplasm, nucleus, nucleolus, ribosomes, centrosomes, mitochondria, endoplasmic reticulum, Golgi apparatus, and lysosomes.

cilia = *(SILL ee ah)*

Applied Science

CELL ENERGY AND ATP: THE ENERGY MOLECULE

We all know that we need to eat to obtain energy, but how does energy get from food to cells? In simple terms, the body takes in food and breaks it down (digestion). During this process, energy is released from the food. Now, the problem is that cells can't use this energy directly. Only food converted to glucose (simple sugar) can be used to make energy. Glucose can be used by your cells during a series of chemical reactions called *cellular respiration*. During cellular respiration, glucose is combined with oxygen and is transformed in your mitochondria into the high energy molecule called Adenosine Triphosphate (ATP). ATP is made up of a base, a sugar, and three (hence, *tri*phosphate) phosphate groups. The phosphate groups are held together by high-energy bonds. When a bond is broken, a high level of energy is released. Energy in this form can be used by the cells. When a bond is used, ATP becomes **ADP** (**adenosine diphosphate**), which has only two phosphate groups. ADP now is able to go and pick up another phosphate and form a high-energy bond so energy is stored and the process can begin again! Life is good.

The future may offer new ways of transporting people and materials. For example, perhaps cities will install moving sidewalks, similar to those in some airports. Certain cells have solved such transport problems already through the use of **cilia.** Cilia are short, microscopic, hairlike projections located on the outer surface of some cells. They begin a wavelike motion that carries particles in a given direction. The action is comparable to when a band member jumps into a crowd and is moved by the wave action of the audience's arms. This is something NOT recommended by the authors. This is one way our lungs stay clean from the dust particles and germs that we inhale every day.

TEST YOUR KNOWLEDGE 3-3

Choose the best answer:

1. What organelle most closely follows the given analogy?

_____ city hall

_____ road system

_____ power plant

_____ packing and shipping plant

_____ the "cell propeller"

Mitosis

Cellular reproduction is the process of making a new cell. Cellular reproduction is also known as **cell division,** because one cell divides into two cells when it reproduces. Cells can only come from other cells. When cells make *identical* copies of themselves *without the involvement* of another cell that is called **asexual reproduction.** Most cells are able to reproduce themselves asexually whether they are animal cells, plant cells, or bacteria.

a = *without*

The cells that make up the human body are a type of cell known as a **eukaryotic cell.** Eukaryotic cells have a nucleus, cellular organelles and usually, several chromosomes in the nucleus. (Reminder: the genetic material of the cell, DNA, is bundled into "packages" of chromatin known as chromosomes.) Since chromosomes carry all the instructions for the cells, all cells must have a complete set after reproduction. These instructions include how the cell is to function within the body and blueprints for reproduction. No matter whether a cell has one chromosome, like bacteria, or 46 chromosomes, like humans, all the chromosomes must be copied before the cell can divide.

eukaryotic cell *(you care ee AH tic SELL)*

Let's start off with the simple cellular division of a bacterium. Bacterial cells, which do not have a nucleus or organelles, reproduce very easily, through a process known as *binary fission*. Bacterial cells simply copy their DNA, divide up the cytoplasm and split in half!

> *Amazing Body Facts*
>
> **BACTERIAL REPRODUCTION**
>
> Bacteria can reproduce so rapidly that they can double their population every hour! No wonder a bacterial infection can get out of hand so fast.

Now let's go to the more complex cellular reproduction. Eukaryotic cells, like yours, must go through a more complicated set of maneuvers in order to reproduce. Not only do your cells have to duplicate all 46 of their chromosomes, they have to make sure that each cell gets all of the chromosomes and all of the right organelles. The process of sorting the chromosomes, so that each new cell gets the right number of copies of all of the genetic material, is called **mitosis.** Mitosis is the only way that eukaryotic cells can reproduce asexually.

mitosis *(my TOE sis)*

The Cell Cycle

The total life of a eukaryotic cell can be divided into two major phases known as the **cell cycle.** Most of the cell cycle is devoted to a phase known as **interphase.** During interphase, a cell is not dividing, but is performing its normal function along with stockpiling needed materials and preparing for division by also copying DNA and making new organelles. Only a brief portion of the cell cycle, the **mitotic phase,** is devoted to actual cell division. The mitotic phase is divided into two major portions. Mitosis is the division and sorting of the *genetic material*, while **cytokinesis** is the division of the *cytoplasm*.

cytokinesis *(SIGH toe kih NEE Suss)*

Mitosis, the division of the genetic material, is the most complicated part of cell division for a eukaryotic cell. What further complicates mitosis is that the process is further divided into four specific phases. As you'll soon see, the four phases are based on the position of the chromosomes relative to the new cells. They are: **prophase, metaphase, anaphase,** and **telophase.** To put all these processes and phases in perspective, please refer to the flowchart in Figure 3-11 ■.

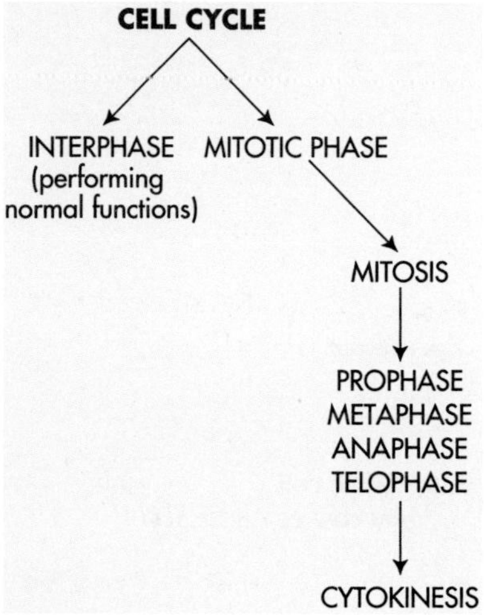

FIGURE ■ 3–11

Flow Chart of the cell cycle.

THE PHASES OF MITOSIS

Let's proceed step by step through the four phases of mitosis using Figure 3-12 ■ as a reference.

1. Prophase (pro = before) - the nucleus disappears, the chromosomes become visible, a set of chromosomal anchor lines or guide wires, the spindle, forms.
2. Metaphase (meta = between), the chromosomes line up in the center of the cells.
3. Anaphase (an = without), the chromosomes split and the spindles pull them apart.
4. Telophase (telo = the end), the chromosomes go to the far end of the cell, the spindle disappears and the nuclei reappear.

During or directly after telophase, cytokinesis happens and the cell divides in half. The original cell was the mother cell that has now formed into two new identical daughter cells. Thus mitosis, asexual reproduction in eukaryotic cells, results in two new daughter cells identical to the original mother cell.

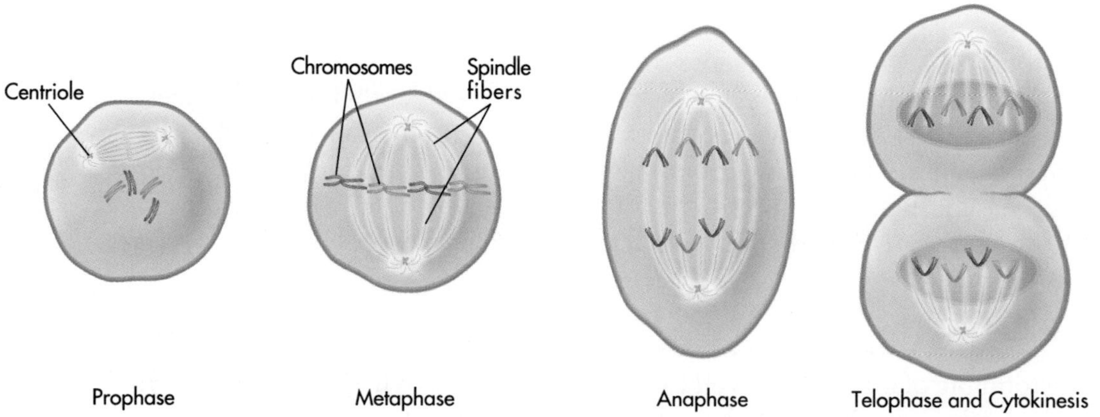

FIGURE ■ 3–12

Phases of mitosis.

MITOSIS IN YOUR BODY

Mitosis, asexual cellular reproduction, serves many purposes in your body. Any time your cells need to be replaced, mitosis is the method used to replace them. Many of your tissues are replaced on a regular basis. Bone, epithelium, skin, and blood cells all replace themselves on a regular basis. Repair and regeneration of damaged tissue is accomplished by mitosis as well. If you cut your hand, the skin is replaced, first by collagen, but eventually, by the original tissue. Mitosis increases in cells near the injury so that the damaged or destroyed cells can be replaced. A broken bone is replaced in much the same way.

Growth is also accomplished by mitosis. Lengthening of bones as you grow, increases in muscle mass due to exercise, indeed, most ways that tissue gets bigger, are due to mitosis of cells in the tissues or organs. Without mitosis, your body would not be able to grow or replace old or damaged cells.

Sexual reproduction is different from mitosis. **Meiosis** is the term for the division of cells in order for reproduction to occur. This process will be discussed in Chapter 17, "The Reproductive System."

> *Learning Hint*
>
> **MITOSIS VERSUS MEIOSIS**
>
> These words sound and look alike and are therefore often confused. Remember, meiosis produces gametes or sexual cells which contain half of the chromosomes because the sexual union of male and female will contribute the other half. Mitosis (I reproduce myself) is asexual and produces exact copies of the cell and the full complement of chromosomes since no union is needed.

TEST YOUR KNOWLEDGE 3-4

Choose the best answer:

1. Cells are reproducing themselves during this portion of the cell cycle
   a. metaphase
   b. mitotic phase
   c. meiotic phase
   d. manic phase

2. During this phase of mitosis the nucleus disappears and the spindle appears
   a. prophase
   b. metaphase
   c. anaphase
   d. telophase

3. During this phase of mitosis the chromosomes begin to pull apart
   a. prophase
   b. metaphase
   c. anaphase
   d. telophase

4. Which of the following is not a function of asexual reproduction?
   a. tissue repair
   b. replacement of cells
   c. tissue growth
   d. cloning humans

Clinical Application

MITOSIS RUN AMOK

When the body is healthy, cells grow in an orderly fashion: they grow at the appropriate rate in the appropriate number, shape, and alignment. Sometimes conditions are altered in the body (either internally or externally) that trigger changes in the way the cells grow. Cell growth can become wild and uncontrolled, leading to too many cells being produced and resulting in a lump, or tumor. Generally, tumors are classified as either benign or malignant. **Benign** tumors typically grow slowly and push healthy cells out of the way. Usually, benign tumors are not life-threatening. **Malignant,** or cancerous, tumors grow rapidly and invade rather than push aside healthy cell tissue. Cancer actually means "crab" (remember your Zodiac signs?) and is a good description of cancer cells in that they spread out into healthy tissue like the legs and pincers of a crab. Cancerous tumors also differ from benign tumors in that parts of a cancerous tumor can break off and travel through the blood system or the lymphatic network and start new tumors in other parts of the body. This breaking off and spreading of malignant cells is called **metastasis.** One reason that lung cancer is so deadly (more women die from it than from breast cancer) is that it can metastasize for a fairly long time before it is even diagnosed in lungs. By the time it is discovered, tumors may be growing in the liver and brain and in other parts of the body, making survival very difficult.

benign *(bee NINE)*
malignant *(mah LIG nant)*

MICROORGANISMS

As in any city, you have a large and diverse population. While the vast majority of the population are good citizens who provide positive contributions to the city, there are some who can cause problems. The same can be said for the world of microorganisms. The following "microcitizens" of our city will now be discussed:

- bacteria
- viruses
- fungi
- protozoa

Bacteria

bacteria *(back TEER ee ah)*
pathogen *(PATH oh jenn)*
path/o = *disease*
gen = *producing*

When you hear the word **bacteria,** you probably first think of an organism that produces disease, or what is called a **pathogen.** You are somewhat correct in assuming so because bacteria make up the largest group of pathogens. Some bacterial pathogens even release toxic substances in your body. Bacteria grow rapidly and reproduce by splitting in half, sometimes doubling as rapidly as every 30 minutes!

You will learn throughout this book that bacteria are often harmless and, in fact, essential for life. These bacteria live within or on us, and are part of what we call our **normal flora.** For example, certain bacteria in your intestine help to digest food, and some help to synthesize vitamin K, which helps clot blood so we don't bleed to death when we get a cut or scrape. See Figure 3–13 ■, which shows examples of various types of bacteria.

normal flora *(FLOOR ah)*

Viruses

An even more basic pathogen is a **virus** (see Figure 3–14 ■). Viruses (from a Latin term meaning "poison") are infectious particles that have a core containing genetic material (codes to replicate) surrounded by a protective protein coat called a **capsid.** Some viruses have an additional layer, or membrane, surrounding the capsid. Viruses are interesting because they cannot grow, "eat," or reproduce by themselves. They must enter another cell (host cell) and hijack that cell's parts, energy supply, and materials to do all of the aforementioned activities! In addition, each virus must target specific cells in the body to claim as hosts. For example,

> *Amazing Body Facts*
>
> **MAGNETOTAXIS: SOME BACTERIA RESPOND TO MAGNETIC FIELDS**
>
> Believe it or not, some bacteria can sense and respond to a magnetic field. These types of bacteria are sensitive to Earth's magnetic field and orient themselves to this force! This ability to move in response to magnetic forces is called *magnetotaxis*. This discovery was made by Richard Blakemore as he observed bacteria living in sulfide-rich mud from a lake. As he changed the position of the mud, the bacteria would reorient themselves to Earths's magnetic field. Upon further examination, Blakemore determined that these bacteria possessed particles of iron oxide, a magnetic metal compound that is stored in a cell structure called *magnetosome*.

Capsid *(CAP sid)*

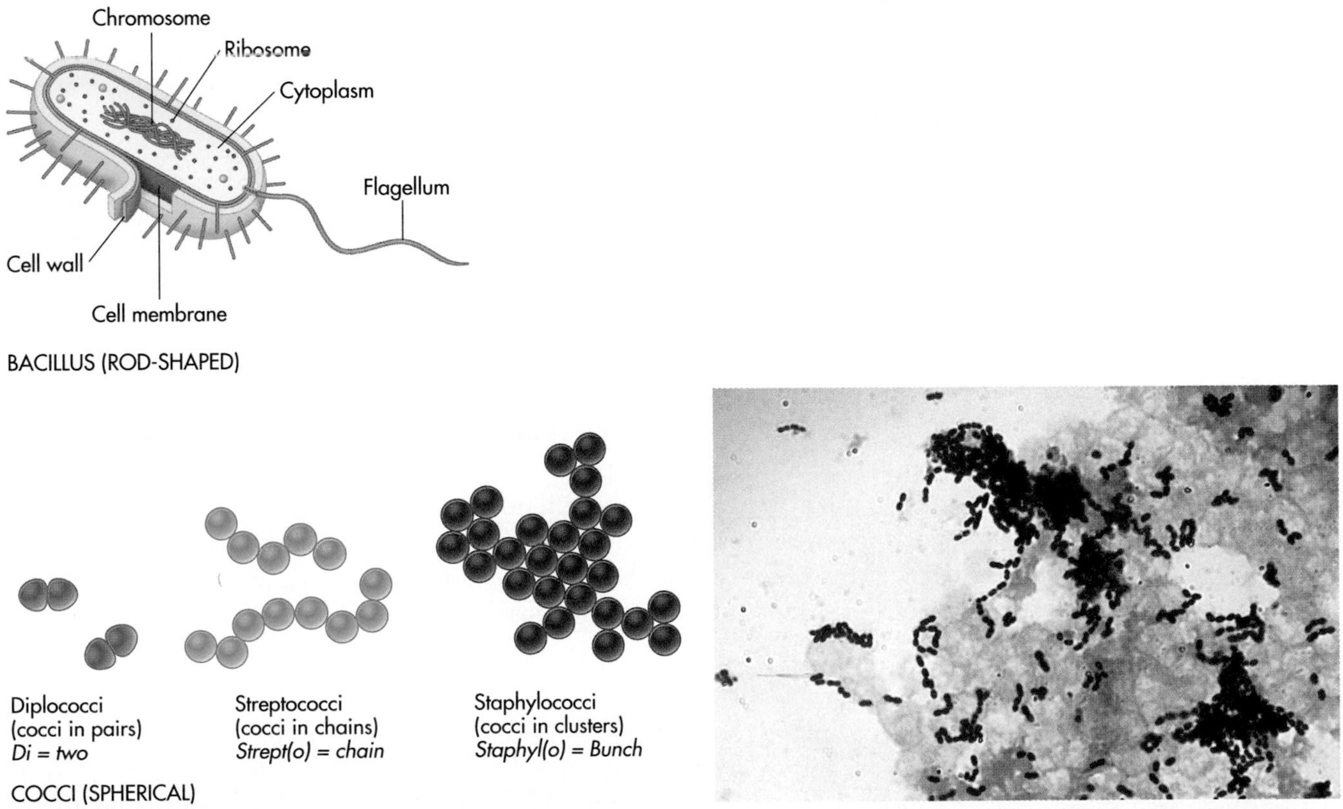

FIGURE ■ 3–13

Types of bacteria.

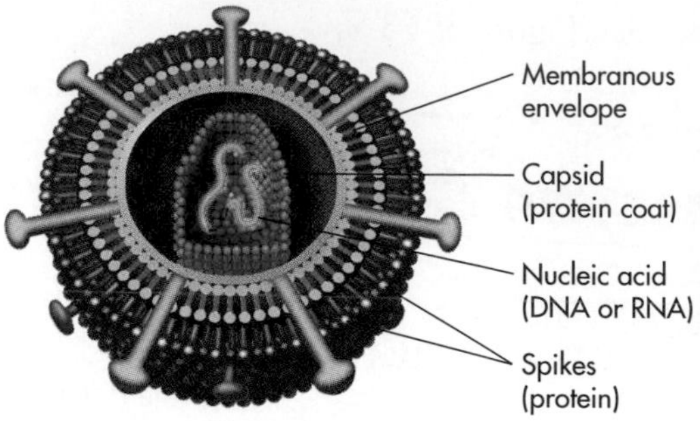

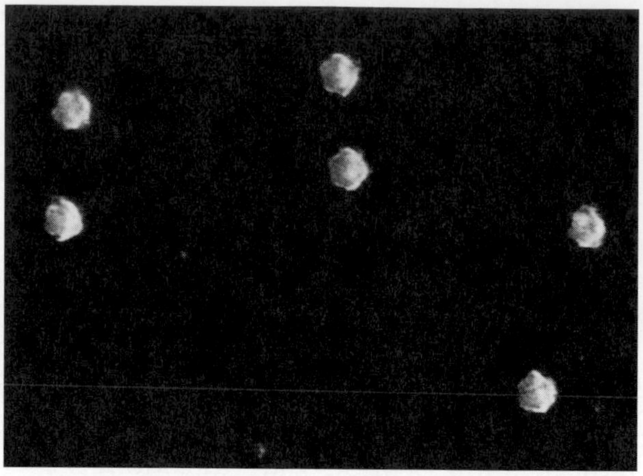

FIGURE ■ 3–14

A virus.

the viruses that cause a cold target the cells found in the respiratory system, and the viruses that cause herpes target cells that are found in the tissues of our nervous system. Most of the upper respiratory infections that people get are caused by viruses and, like all viral infections, they do not respond to antibiotics.

It is interesting to note (or disturbing for those of you who worry about everything) that viruses can stay dormant in the body and become active once again later in life. This is true for all of us who have had chicken pox. Those viruses stay in the body and may later become active and cause a potentially painful skin condition called *shingles*, caused by the herpes zoster virus. It is also interesting to note that the actual virus is relatively easy to kill by itself, but once it becomes part of a cell, it is hard to kill without harming the individual cell.

Fungi

fungi *(FUN jie)*
mycelia *(my SEE lee ah)*

anti = *against*
bios = *life*

Note

While antibiotic technically mean "against all life," it usually refers to antibacterial agents and is therefore used to treat bacterial infections. There are specific antiviral agents for viral infections.

Fungi, the plural form of fungus, can be either a one-celled or multicelled organism. These plantlike organisms have tiny filaments, called **mycelia,** that travel out from the cell to find and absorb nutrients. Like bacteria, fungi, such as edible mushrooms, can be good, but in certain situations they can also cause problems (see Figure 3–15 ■). Fungi also can spread through the release of **spores.** Normally, we are not affected by fungi, but if the body has a problem with its immune system, then fungi have a chance to cause an infection. If tissue becomes damaged, fungi can more easily create an infection. Wind may pick up and carry spores that can be inhaled, potentially causing lung infections. Interestingly, you can inhale fungi spores and still not develop an infection. It is estimated that up to 80 percent of the population in certain regions of the United States have tested positive for the inhalation of certain fungi! Examples of fungal infections are athlete's foot and a mouth fungus called thrush or candidiasis.

Protozoa

Protozoa *(pro toe ZOE ah)*

Protozoa are one-celled animal-like organisms that can be found in water, such as ponds, and in soil. Disease caused by these microorganisms can result from swallowing them (such as by drinking contaminated water) or from being bitten by insects that carry them in their bodies (such as malaria-carrying mosquitoes). See Figure 3–16 ■.

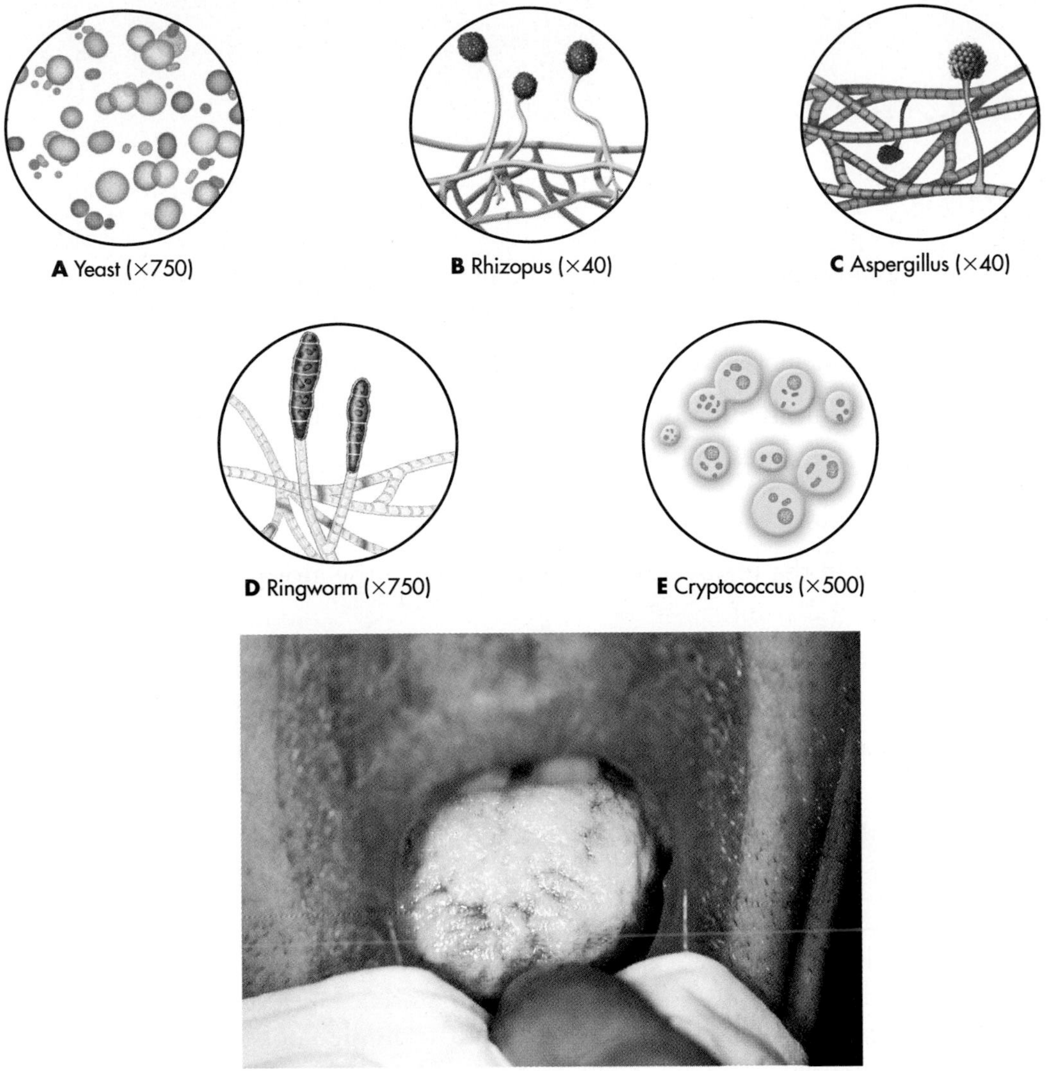

FIGURE ■ 3–15

Types of fungi and a fungal infection of the tongue. (Photo Source: Courtesy of Jason L. Smith, MD.)

> **3-2** If you would like more information on microbiology, pathogenic organisms, and ways to prevent the spread of disease, please go to your CD-ROM. In addition, a video demonstrates the proper hand-washing and gloving techniques to minimize the spread of infection. Don't forget the interactive games created just for this chapter!

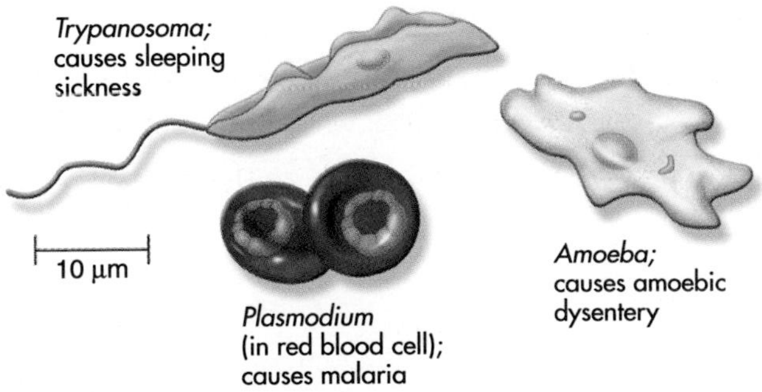

FIGURE ■ 3–16

Protozoa.

SUMMARY

Snapshots from the Journey

- All living organisms are made of one or more cells. Cells are the fundamental units of living organisms.
- Even though cells are the fundamental units, they are composed of a variety of parts that are necessary for proper cellular function. These small parts are called organelles.
- Substances can cross the cell membrane via passive or active transport.
- Passive transport can occur through diffusion, facilitated diffusion, osmosis, or filtration.
- Active transport can occur through active transport pumps, endocytosis, or exocytosis.
- One form of cellular movement is through the use of flagella.
- Cilia found in the lungs aid in the removal of foreign particles in the airways through rhythmic movement.
- Cells and tissues grow, are replaced and are repaired by asexual reproduction. Cells make identical copies of themselves. This takes place all over your body whenever tissues grow or are repaired.
- Some tissues, like epidermis, blood and bone replace themselves continually, always by asexual reproduction.
- The life of the cell can be depicted as a cell cycle. Only about 10% of the cell cycle is devoted to mitosis. The rest of the time the cell is in interphase, preparing to divide and carrying on day to day cellular activities.
- Asexual reproduction in eukaryotic cells is accomplished by a relatively complex process called mitosis and cytokinesis. Mitosis, the division of the genetic material, takes place in four phases, prophase, metaphase, anaphase and telophase. Cytokinesis is the division of the cytoplasm and organelles. Mitosis produces two daughter cells, identical to each other.
- Meiosis is the sexual reproduction of cells. If an organism is going to reproduce sexually it must use specialized cells called gametes with only half the typical number of chromosomes for that organism. The chief difference between mitosis and meiosis is mitosis is asexual and produces the exact number of chromosomes where meiosis is sexual and combines two cells with half of the needed chromosomes.
- Not all bacteria are bad. In fact, the body needs bacteria to survive.
- Although a virus is not a one-celled organism, it needs another cell to replicate.
- Fungi can be single-celled or a multicelled organism and can cause infections in the body. Spores can be immune to a harsh environment, thus allowing fungi to spread.
- Protozoa are one-celled and can cause disease through ingestion or through insect bites.

Case Study

Given the following mini-scenarios, identify what type of microorganism may be the causative agent.

a. Two young boys complain of a stomach ache and severe diarrhea after drinking pond water.

b. Julia is a 13-year-old with a compromised immune system due to an inherited disease. Two days after returning home from a school field trip to a mushroom factory, Julia complains of shortness of breath and is diagnosed with a respiratory infection.

c. Bob has had a stubborn cold for three days and is given an antibacterial agent. However, he doesn't respond to the treatment and the cold persists.

REVIEW QUESTIONS

Multiple Choice

1. The cell membrane can best be described as
   a. permeable to all materials
   b. nonpermeable
   c. rigid
   d. semipermeable

2. All of the following are passive forms of transport *except*
   a. facilitated diffusion
   b. exocytosis
   c. osmosis
   d. filtration

3. With a greater concentration of a solute, what will happen to osmotic pressure?
   a. it will become less
   b. it will become greater
   c. it will remain the same
   d. there is no relation between osmotic pressure and the concentration of solute.

4. Where are the specifications for the creation of new cells found?
   a. DNA
   b. RNA
   c. ATP
   d. ADP

5. Which microorganism can cause disease?
   a. bacteria
   b. fungi
   c. virus
   d. all of the above

Matching

1. Match the following organelles with their function:

_____ nucleus	a. the "powerhouse" of the cell
_____ cell membrane	b. processing, packaging, and shipping of materials
_____ golgi apparatus	c. the gatekeeper of the cell
_____ mitochondria	d. the "brain" of the cell
_____ cytoplasm	e. the internal environment
_____ lysosome	f. sanitation engineers

Short Answer

1. List and describe the four methods of passive transport.

____

____

____

____

2. Why do viruses need cells?

____

____

____

____

3. How does passive transport differ from active transport?

____

____

____

____

4. Discuss how cells can provide motility for themselves.

____

____

____

____

5. Contrast the process of mitosis and meiosis.

____

____

____

____

Suggested Activities

1. Research the various cell types within the body and see how many you can list.

2. Research five sexually transmitted diseases (STDs) and list the causative microorganism for each.

> **3-3** Now that you have completed your journey through this chapter, please go to the CD-ROM for interactive games and puzzles concerning the medical terms and concepts contained in this chapter. By playing the games you will reinforce your learning of medical terminology in a fun way.

Greetings from

TISSUES AND SYSTEMS

The Inside Story

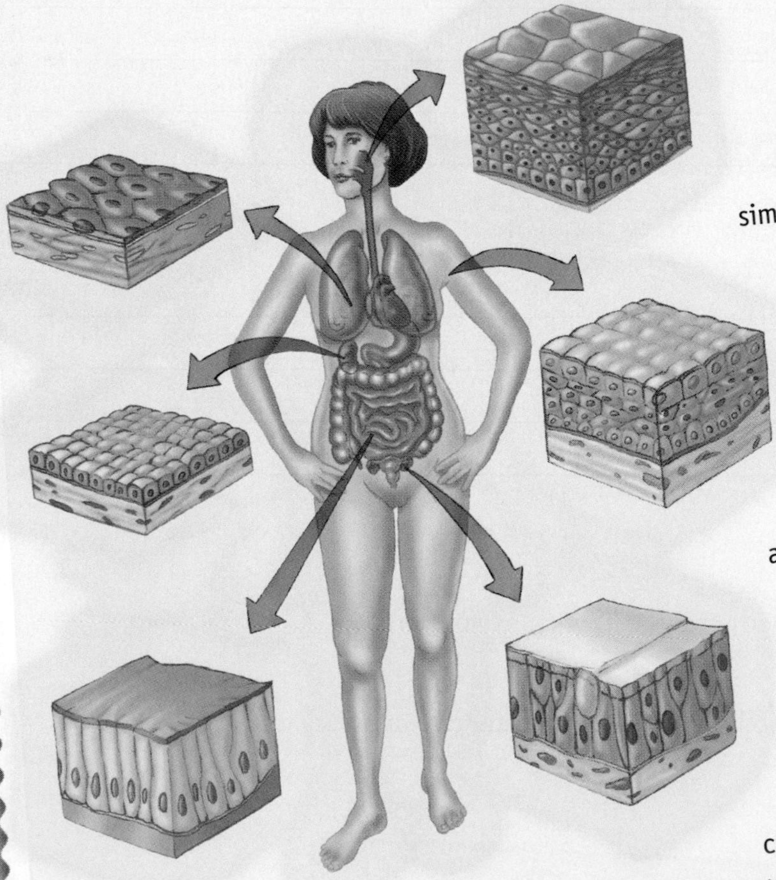

Previously, we discussed cells as the basic building blocks of the body. In this chapter, we explore **tissues**, which are collections of similar cells. We can consider cells to be individual employees. At the next level, we can think of tissue as a group of employees who have the same or similar educational background, such as radiologic technicians, at a hospital. A combination of tissues designed to perform a specific function or several functions is called an **organ**. This could be compared to an X-ray department in the hospital, where specific functions such as X-rays, CT scans, MRIs, and barium swallows (a procedure, not a bird!) are performed. Organs that work together to perform specific activities, often with the help of accessory structures, form what we call **systems**. We can compare a system to a hospital that provides a service (health care) to the citizens of our city through the combination of all of the departments: laboratory, nursing, respiratory care, physical therapy, dietetics, housekeeping, and so on. This chapter provides an overview of tissues, organs, and systems, which will be expanded upon in later chapters.

Chapter 4

LEARNING OBJECTIVES

At the end of your journey through this chapter, you will be able to:

- Explain the relationship between cells, tissues, organs, and systems
- List and describe the four main types of tissues
- Identify and describe the various body membranes
- Differentiate the three main types of muscle tissues
- Describe the main components of nerve tissue
- List and describe the main functions of the body systems

MULTIMEDIA APPLICATIONS

CD-ROM Interactive Exercises

- Videos on melanoma and skin cancer, 4-1
- Interactive exercises: Body systems identification and labeling of main components, 4-2
- Interactive games and puzzles, 4-3

www.prenhall.com/colbert

- Professional Profile: Histotechnology
- Related Internet Links
- Additional Review Questions

Pronunciation Guide

Correct pronunciation is important in any journey so that you and others are completely understood. Here is a "see and say" Pronunciation Guide for the more difficult terms to pronounce in this chapter.

cuboidal (cue BOYD al)
cutaneous membranes (cue TAY nee us)
epithelial tissue (ep ih THEE lee al)
genitourinary (gen i toe YOUR in air EE)
glia (GLEE ah)
meninges (men IN jeez)
neuroglia (noo ROH glee ah)
neurons (NOO ron)
parietal (pah RYE eh tal)
serous membrane (SEER us)
skeletal muscle (SKELL eh tal)
squamous (SKWAY muss)
stratified (STRAT ih fied)
striated muscle (STRY ate ed)
synovial membrane (sin OH vee al)
transitional (tran ZISH ion al)
visceral (VISS er al)

OVERVIEW OF TISSUES

Just as there are many different types of cells with various functions and responsibilities, tissues come in different shapes and sizes, again with the structure dependent upon the function. Let's begin to explore the different tissue types.

Tissue Types

histo = *tissue*

Tissue is a collection of similar cells that act together to perform a function. Imagine individual cells as bricks. Placing these bricks (cells) in a specific pattern creates the functional wall (tissue) of a building. There are many different types of tissues depending upon the required function. The four main types of tissues are

- epithelial
- connective
- muscle
- nervous

We will now discuss these major types of tissue and their subdivisions.

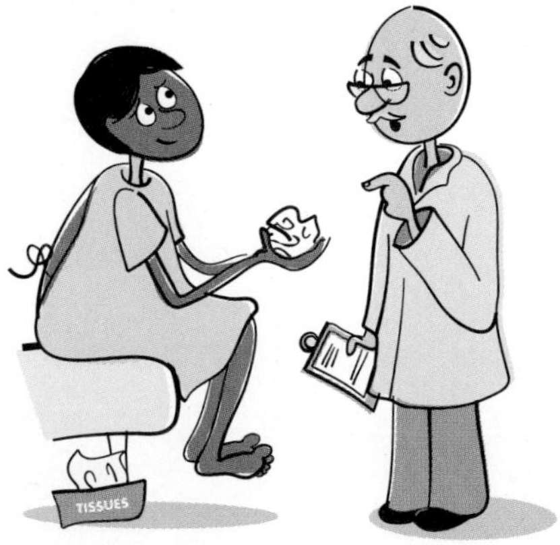

"No Mr. Smith, that is not the kind of tissue sample we need."

EPITHELIAL TISSUE

Similar in purpose to the plastic wrap we use to keep food fresh or to cover bowls in the refrigerator, epithelial tissue not only covers and lines much of the body but also covers many of the parts found in the body. The cells in this form of tissue are packed tightly together, forming a sheet that usually has no blood vessels in it. The epithelium in the bowel is an exception, where capillaries do exist.

squamous *(SKWAY muss)*

cuboidal *(cue BOYD al)*

We can further classify epithelial cells by their shape and arrangement. These cells can be flat or scalelike (**squamous**), cube-shaped (**cuboidal**), columnlike (*columnar*), or stretchy and variably shaped (**transitional**). If these cells are arranged in a single layer and are all the same type of cell, we classify them as *simple*. If they are arranged in several layers, we say they are **stratified,** and they are named by the type of cell that is on the outer layer (such as stratified columnar). The function required of the cell dictates which type of cell formation is utilized. For example, simple squamous cells are utilized in the lungs because of their flat, thin design, which makes for easy transfer of oxygen from the lungs to the blood. Figure 4–1 ■ shows the types and locations of epithelial tissues. These are further discussed in later chapters.

transitional *(tran ZISH ion al)*

stratified *(STRAT ih fied)*

Amazing Body Facts

SKIN AND VITAMIN PRODUCTION

You know that you get vitamins and minerals from the foods you eat and the supplements you take, but did you know that your skin produces vitamin D when you are exposed to sunlight?

Membranes Generally, *membranes* are sheetlike structures found throughout the body that perform special functions. Although membranes can be classified as or-

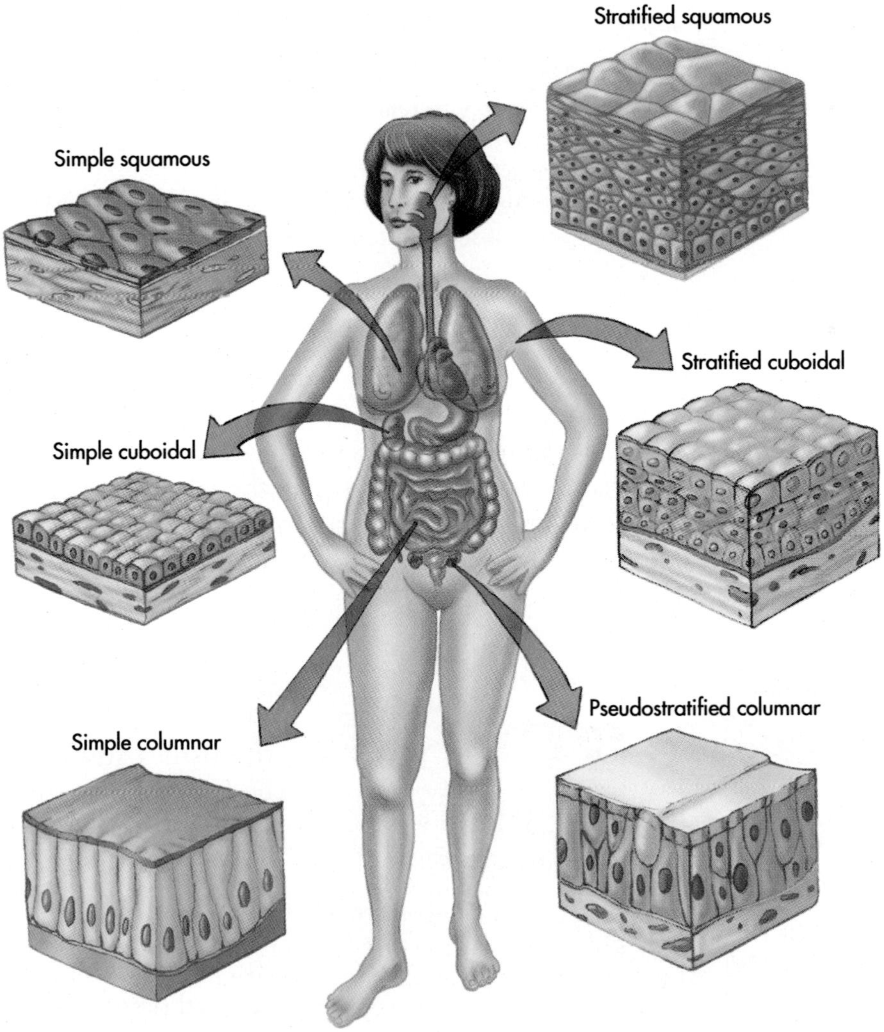

FIGURE ■ 4–1

Types and locations of epithelial tissues.

serous membranes *(SEER us)*

parietal = *(pah RYE eh tal) "wall; therefore, the parietal membrane lines the wall of the cavity.*

visceral *(VISS er al)*

viscero = *organs; therefore, visceral membranes enclose organs.*

muc/o; myx/o = *combining forms indicating relative to mucus*

TABLE 4–1 Types of Epithelial Membranes

1. cutaneous	• Functions like a tarp placed over a boat • the main organ of the integumentary system, commonly known as your skin • makes up approximately 16 percent of the total body weight • skin is largest, visible organ
2. serous	• A two layered membrane with a potential space in between • Comprised of the parietal and visceral layers
parietal	• lines the wall of the cavities in which organs reside • produces serous fluid, which reduces friction between different tissues and organs (Without this friction-reducing fluid, each beat of your heart and every breath you take would be uncomfortable. The effect is similar to running water over a sheet of plastic placed on the grass. You can run, jump onto the plastic, and slide. Imagine how that would feel without the water running over the plastic!)
visceral	• wraps around the individual organs • Also produces serous fluid, which reduces friction between different tissues and organs
3. mucous	• Lines openings to the outside world, such as your digestive tract, respiratory system, and urinary and reproductive tracts • Called mucous membranes because they contain specialized cells that produce mucus (Mucus can act as a lubricant like the oil in a car. Mucus also serves several other important purposes besides grossing you out, as you will see in future chapters.)

gans, we discuss them along with tissues for ease of explanation. Membranes classified as *epithelial* membranes possess a layer of epithelial tissue and a bottom layer of a specialized connective tissue. Epithelial membranes are classified into three general categories, as you can see in Table 4–1.

Figure 4–2 ■ shows the location of the serous and mucous membranes of the body.

Amazing Body Facts

BLOOD AND LYMPH AS CONNECTIVE TISSUES

Even though blood and lymph are fluid, they are considered to be connective tissue because they are a liquid mixture comprised of a group of cells that have specialized functions. These fluid connective tissues contain specialized cells and dissolved proteins suspended in a watery substance. We expand upon these two very important tissues in later chapters.

CONNECTIVE TISSUE

Connective tissue is the most common of the tissues and is found throughout the body more than any other form. That is because it is found in organs, bones, nerves, muscles, membranes, and skin. Connective tissue's job is to hold things together and provide structure and support. Fine, delicate webs of loosely connected tissue (areolar tissue) hold organs together and help to hold other connective tissues together. Fat is also a connective tissue known as adipose tissue. Although we always seem to want to lose fat, we truly need some fat in our bodies

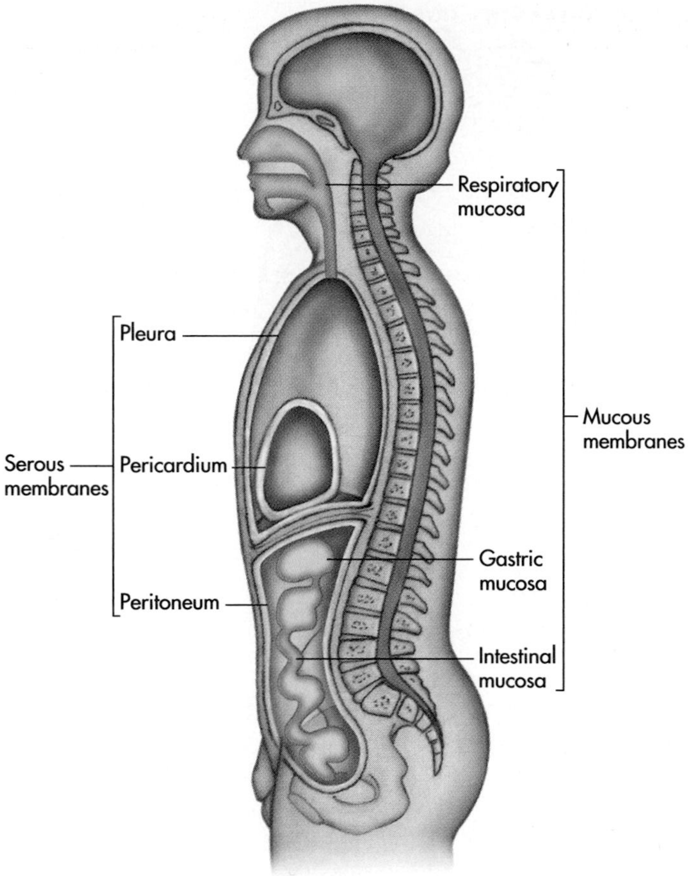

FIGURE ■ 4–2

Location of serous and mucous membranes.

Learning Hint

MUCOUS ISN'T ALWAYS MUCUS

"A rose by any other name is still a rose" might work well in Shakespeare's plays, but mucous isn't always mucus. Although they sound the same, mucous and mucus are two different things. Mucous is an adjective that describes the type of membrane that produces *mucus*, the actual substance.

for proper functioning. Connective tissue can also be more densely packed and form strong cordlike structures similar to wire cables on suspension bridges. Tendons and ligaments are composed of dense connective tissue. The skin also needs to be densely packed to form a protective barrier, and it therefore uses dense connective tissue. Because connective tissue is so versatile and found throughout the body, we will discuss it in more depth in the relevant chapters. Please see Figure 4–3 ■, which illustrates the various types of connective tissues and shows some of the places where they are found.

The membrane type associated with connective tissue is the **synovial** membrane. This important membrane type is found in the spaces between bone joints and produces a slippery substance called synovial fluid, which greatly reduces friction when joints move. Imagine runners without synovial membranes: their knees would burst into flames during track meets. Figure 4–4 ■ shows a synovial joint and membrane.

synovial *(sin OH vee al)*

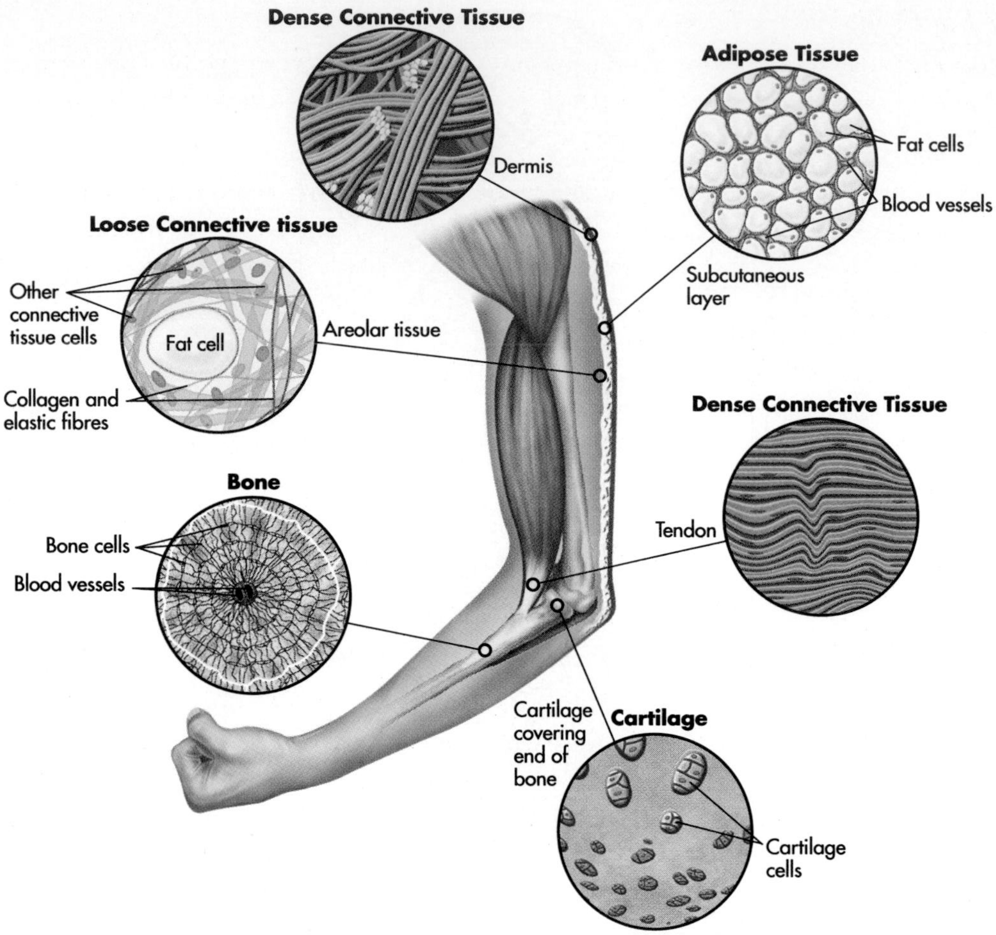

FIGURE ■ 4–3

Types and locations of connective tissues.

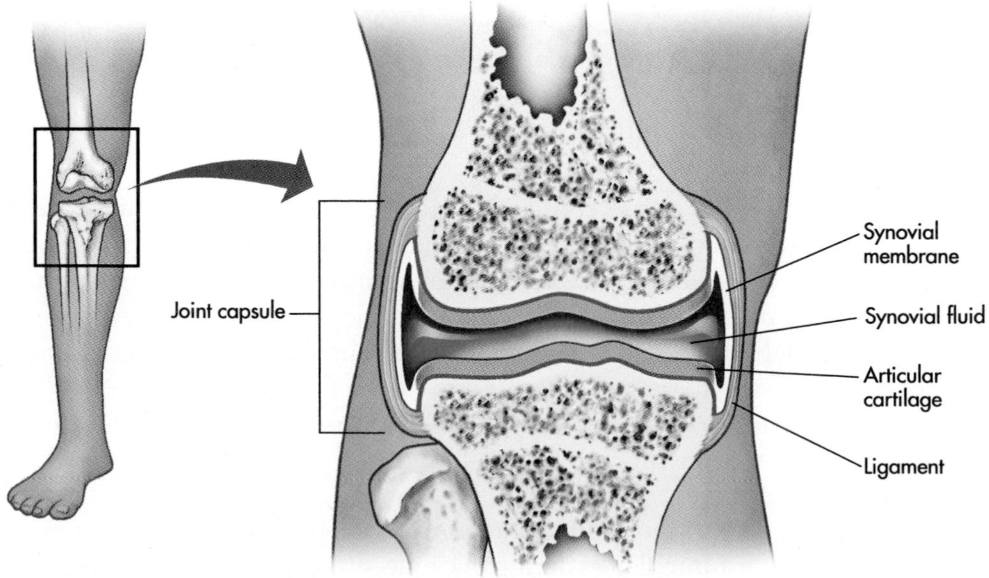

FIGURE ■ 4–4

The synovial joint.

MUSCLE TISSUE

Muscle tissue provides the means for movement by and in the body. This form of tissue has the ability to shorten itself (contractility). There are three types of muscle tissue: **skeletal, cardiac,** and **smooth.**

Skeletal Muscle Skeletal muscle (often described as **striated** because of its striped appearance) is attached to bones and causes movement by contracting and relaxing. It also surrounds certain openings of the body, such as the mouth, and controls the size of the opening. Unless you are a ventriloquist, it is very hard to speak clearly without moving your lips. The cells that make up this tissue type are long and fiberlike with many nuclei in each cell. Our brain thinks about moving or speaking and causes the correct muscle to contract or relax as necessary. Since this is a conscious effort, we call these muscles *voluntary* muscles.

striated *(STRY ate ed)*

Cardiac Muscle Cardiac muscle is found in the walls of the heart. Our hearts beat without our conscious thought. Since cardiac muscle contracts and relaxes without conscious thought, this muscle type is considered *involuntary* muscle tissue. The cells in this tissue type interlock with each other, promoting more efficient contraction, as you will learn in Chapter 12, The Cardiovascular System.

Smooth Muscle Smooth muscle tissue forms the walls of hollow organs, such as in our digestive system (which is why it is often called *visceral* tissue) and blood vessels. Since we don't have to consciously think about digesting food, we consider this muscle type to also be involuntary muscle tissue. Cells forming this tissue are not as long and fibrous as skeletal muscle, and each cell has only one nucleus. Figure 4–5 ■ shows the various types of muscle tissue.

Note

smooth muscle is named such due to no striations.

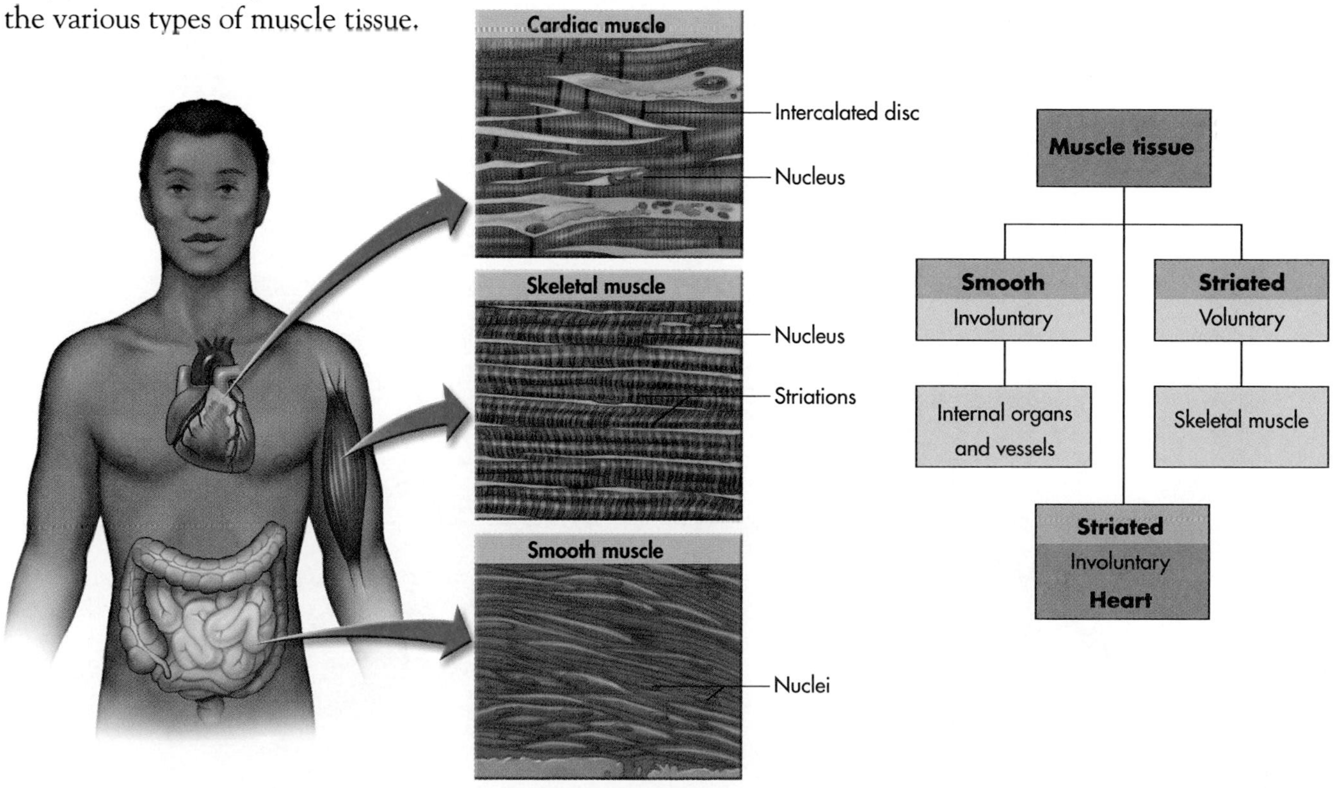

FIGURE ■ 4–5

Labeled diagram and flowchart of the three muscle tissue types.

NERVOUS TISSUE

neuro = *nerves*

neurons *(NOO ron)*

glia = *(GLEE ah) glue, hence the name for cells that holds the nerve cells together*

dendr/o = *tree, hence the name of the branching dendrite structure*

meninges *(men IN jeez)*

Nerve tissue acts as a rapid messenger service for the body, and its messages can cause actions to occur. There are two types of nerve cells. **Neurons** are the conductors of information, and **glia** (sometimes called **neuroglia**) cells function as support by helping to hold the neurons in place. The branchlike formations that make up part of the neuron, called **dendrites**, receive sensory information. The trunk-shaped structure, called the axon, transports information *away* from the cell body. The membranes associated with covering the brain and spinal cord are called **meninges.** Many nerves have an insulating layer called the myelin sheath, which is further discussed in Chapter 8, The Nervous System, Part One. Figure 4–6 ■ shows the two types of nerve cells.

www.prenhall.com/colbert
The allied health profession that specializes in the study of tissues is histotechnology. To learn more about this professional career, please visit the book's companion website for this chapter.

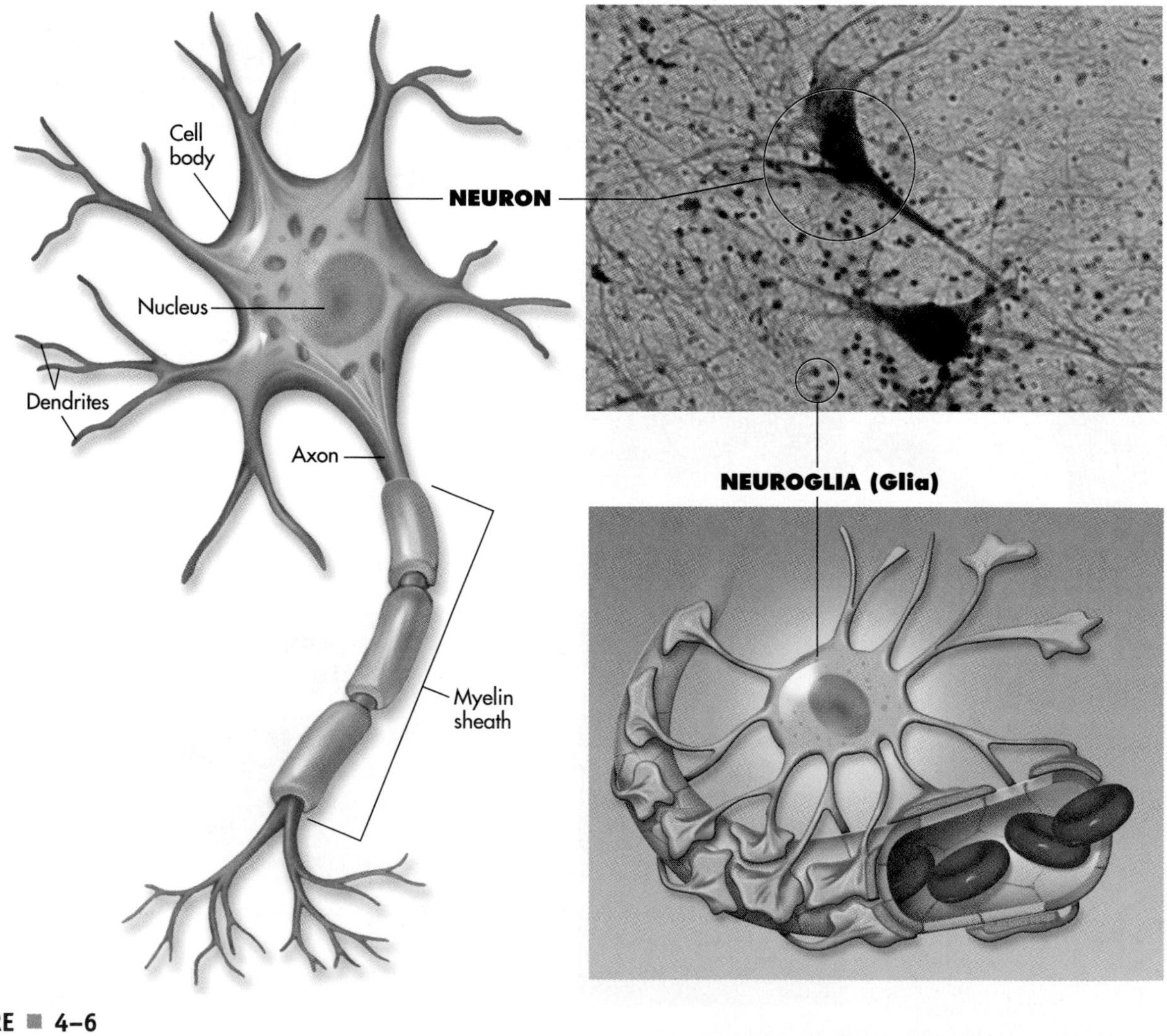

FIGURE ■ 4–6

The two main types of nerve cells.

TEST YOUR KNOWLEDGE 4-1

Complete the following:

1. List and describe the four types of epithelial cells.

   ____

2. Lubrication for joints is produced by which type of membrane?

   ____

3. Why is connective tissue so prominent in the body?

   ____

   ____

   ____

4. Explain the difference between the terms mucous and mucus.

   ____

   ____

   ____

Clinical Application

MELANOMA

Melanoma, a skin cancer, has had a rapid increase in the rate of incidence in the past several decades. Melanoma is significant for two main reasons. First, it has a very high mortality rate and, in fact, is the cancer with the most rapidly increasing mortality rate. It accounts for approximately 75 percent of all skin cancer deaths. It is the most common form of cancer in people aged 25 to 29. In 1935, one of every 1,500 individuals was diagnosed with melanoma. Now it is about one person in every 75. Second, it is one of our more preventable cancers. The culprit? Excessive sun exposure and tanning! Although the classic patient has fair skin, blue eyes, and blonde or red hair, more darkly pigmented individuals are also at risk, but at a somewhat lower rate. The effects of blistering sunburns have an additive effect. This means that each childhood sunburn you had increases your chance of developing melanoma in adulthood. Protection from excessive sun and early detection are keys to survival.

melano = *black*
oma = *tumor*

4-1 To view videos on melanoma and skin cancer, see your CD-ROM.

ORGANS

As mentioned earlier, a hospital department is made up of employees who work together to perform specific functions, much like an organ. An organ is the result of two or more types of tissues organizing in such a way as to accomplish a task that the tissues cannot do on their own. Some organs occur singly, such as the heart, and some occur in pairs, such as the lungs. It is interesting to note that we can survive quite well with only one healthy organ from a paired group (such as a lung or kidney). Your heart, lungs, stomach, liver, and kidneys are all examples of organs found in your body. It is important to understand that there are regular organs and *vital* organs. Vital organs are the ones that you can't live without. Your heart, brain, and lungs are vital organs. Organs that you can live without include your appendix, spleen, and gallbladder. Some vital organs come in pairs, so if one is damaged or removed, you can still survive. Lungs and kid-

TABLE 4–2 Systems and Organs of the Human Body

BODY SYSTEM	ORGANS IN THE SYSTEM	COMBINING FORM	MEDICAL SPECIALTY
Integumentary	Skin	dermat/o, cutane/o	**dermatology** (der mah **TALL** oh jee)
	Hair	trich/o	
	Nails	ung/o	
	Sweat glands	sud/o, hidr/o	
	Sebaceous glands	seb/o	
Musculoskeletal	Muscles	my/o, muscul/o	**orthopedics** (or thoh **PEE** diks)
	Bones	oste/o	
	Joints	arthr/o	
Endocrine	Thyroid gland	thyr/o	**endocrinology** (en doh krin **ALL** oh jee)
	Pituitary gland	pituit/o	**internal medicine**
	Testes	test/o, orchi/o	
	Ovaries	ovari/o, oophor/o	**gynecology** (guy neh **KOL** oh jee)
	Adrenal glands	adren/o	
	Pancreas	pancreat/o	
	Parathyroid glands	parathyroid/o	
	Pineal gland	pineal/o	
	Thymus gland	thym/o	
Cardiovascular	Heart	cardi/o	**cardiology** (car dee **ALL** oh jee)
	Blood	hemat/o, hem/o	**hematology** (hee mah **TALL** oh jee)
	Arteries	arteri/o	**internal medicine**
	Veins	phleb/o, ven/o, veni/o	
Lymphatic and Immune	Spleen	splen/o	**immunology** (im yoo **NALL** oh jee)
	Lymph	lymph/o	
	Thymus gland	thym/o	
Respiratory	Nose	nas/o, rhin/o	**otorhinolaryngology** (oh toh rye noh lair ing **GALL** oh jee)
	Pharynx	pharyng/o	**thoracic** (tho **RASS** ik) **surgery**
	Larynx	laryng/o	
	Trachea	trache/o	
	Lungs	pneum/o	**pulmonology** (pull mon **ALL** oh jee)
	Bronchial tubes	bronch/o	**internal medicine**

neys are a good example. Table 4–2 is a nice, quick reference to the various organs of the body.

SYSTEMS

A body system is formed by organs that work together to accomplish something more complex than what a single organ can do on its own. Take the heart, for example. Even if your heart is functioning perfectly, you would die without all of the other parts that make up the cardiovascular system. Much like a road system in the city, you need the arteries, veins, and blood to get vital oxygen and nutrients to the cells and to remove the waste products produced by those cells.

Although we discuss the body systems separately, it is extremely important that you understand that all of the body systems are interrelated, often depending on each other for proper functioning.

TABLE 4–2 Systems and Organs of the Human Body (*continued*)

BODY SYSTEM	ORGANS IN THE SYSTEM	COMBINING FORM	MEDICAL SPECIALTY
Gastrointestinal	Mouth	or/o	**gastroenterology** (gas troh en ter **ALL** oh jee)
	Pharynx	pharyng/o	**internal medicine**
	Esophagus	esophag/o	
	Stomach	gastr/o	
	Small intestine	enter/o	
	Colon	col/o colon/o	**proctology** (prok **TOL** oh jee) procto = anus
	Liver	hepat/o	
	Gallbladder	cholecyst/o	
	Pancreas	pancreat/o	
Urinary	Kidneys	nephr/o, ren/o	**nephrology** (neh **FROL** oh jee)
	Ureters	ureter/o	**urology** (yoo **RALL** oh jee) uro = urine
	Bladder	cyst/o, vesic/o	
	Urethra	urethr/o	
Reproductive	Ovaries	oophor/o	**gynecology** gynec/o = woman
	Uterus	uter/o, hyster/o	**obstetrics** (ob **STET** riks)
	Fallopian tubes	salping/o	
	Vagina	vagin/o	
	Mammary glands	mamm/o	
	Testes	orchid/o	
	Prostate	prostat/o	
	Urethra	urethr/o	
Nervous	Brain	encephal/o	**neurology** (noo **RAL** oh jee)
	Spinal cord	myel/o, spin/o	**neurosurgery** (noo roh **SIR** jer ee)
	Nerves	neur/o	
Special senses	Eye	ocul/o, ophthalm/o	**ophthalmology** (off thal **MALL** oh jee)
	Ear	ot/o	**otolaryngology** (oh toh lair ing **GALL** oh jee)

Skeletal System

Throughout your journey, you will see many different kinds of buildings. The one thing all of the buildings have in common is some sort of skeletal structure for support. Most people think that the skeleton's only job is to provide support and structure to the body, much like the framework of a house, but it does much more. The bones of the skeleton protect organs such as the brain; in combination with muscles, it provides movement; it acts as a storage vault for a variety of minerals, such as calcium and phosphorus; AND it also produces blood cells! That's pretty impressive stuff! The main components of this system are bones, joints, ligaments, and cartilage. Please see Figure 4–7 ■ that shows the main components of the skeletal system.

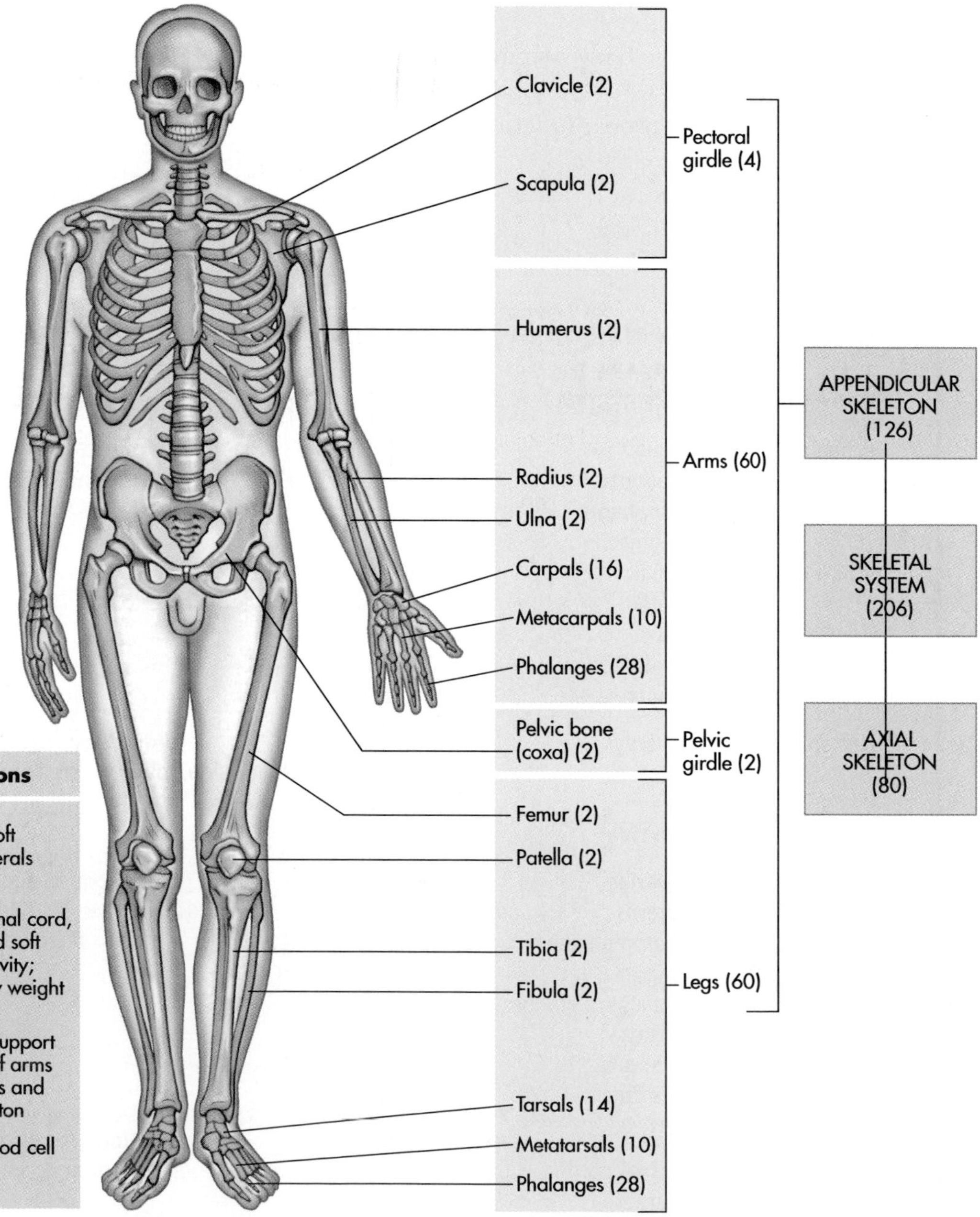

Organ	Primary Functions
Bones (206), Cartilages, and Ligaments	Support, protect soft tissues; store minerals
Axial Skeleton (skull, vertebrae, sacrum, ribs, sternum)	Protects brain, spinal cord, sense organs, and soft tissues of chest cavity; supports the body weight over the legs
Appendicular Skeleton (limbs and supporting bones)	Provides internal support and positioning of arms and legs; supports and moves axial skeleton
Bone Marrow	Primary site of blood cell production

FIGURE ■ 4–7

The skeletal system.

Muscular System

"All of this dry reading makes me thirsty. I think I'll go get something to drink." The muscular system is responsible for getting you up and over to that refrigerator (see Figure 4–8 ■). This voluntary action is made possible by skeletal muscles that are attached to your bones. Two general classifications of muscle are *voluntary* (of which we just had an example) and *involuntary*. Involuntary muscles perform without consciously being told to do so. The smooth muscle found in the walls of organs, often called *visceral muscle*, and the muscle found in the heart, called cardiac muscle, are examples of involuntary muscles. Smooth muscle is also found in blood vessels and airways, where it helps control the diameter of passageways. So, the main parts of the muscle system are skeletal, smooth, and cardiac muscles. We were just kidding about the "dry" reading and know you're anxious to "move" onto the next system.

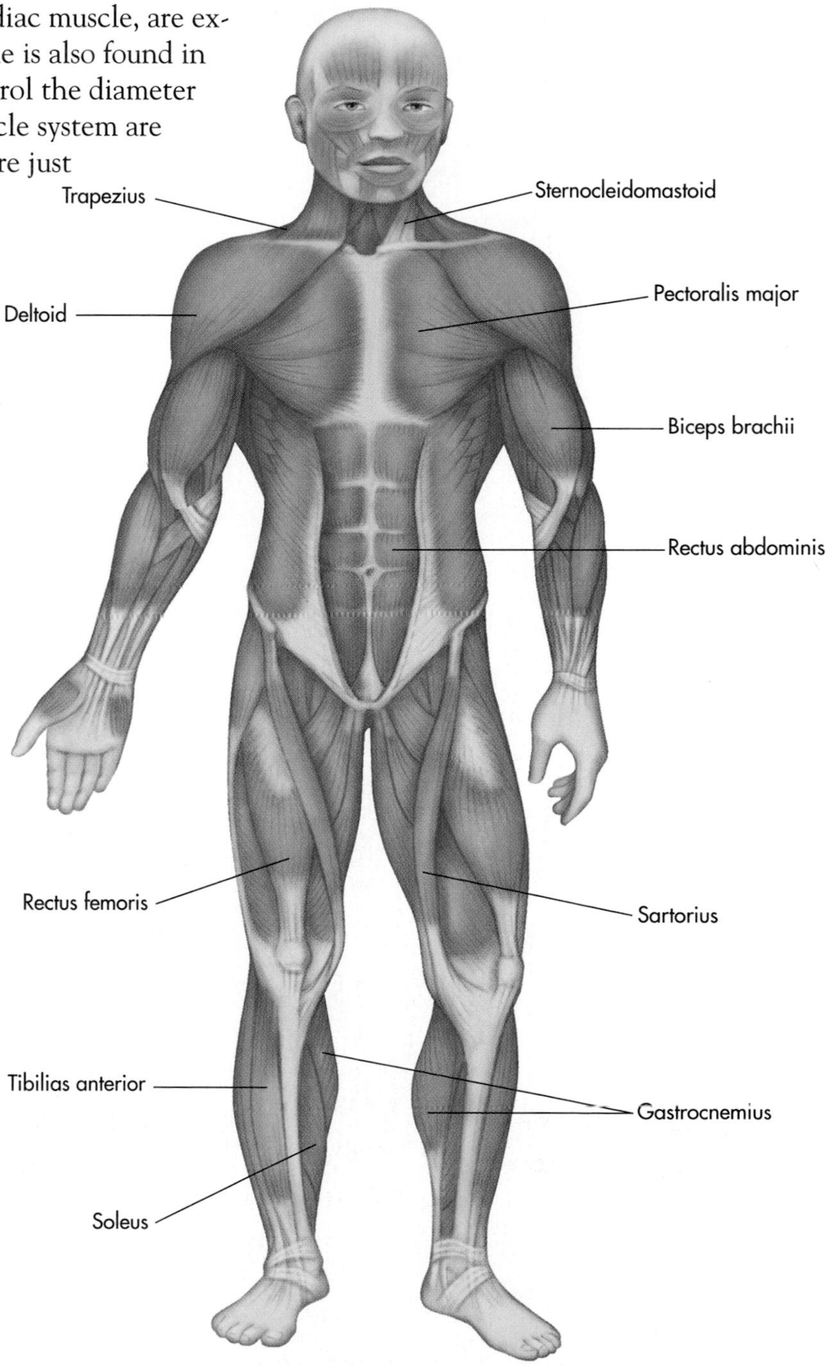

Organ	Primary Functions
Skeletal muscles (700)	Provide skeletal movement, control openings of digestive tract, produce heat, support skeletal position, protect soft tissues

FIGURE ■ 4–8

The muscular system.

Integumentary System

All cities must have first responders, such as paramedics, police, firefighters, and safety inspectors, who cover and protect the city and its inhabitants. The body's first line of protection is your skin. Skin is the main part of the integumentary system. Beside protecting your body from invasion, the integumentary system also helps to regulate body temperature through sweating, shivering, and changes in the diameter of blood vessels in the skin. Much of the sensory information received from the outside world (heat, cold, pain, pressure, etc.) comes from sensors in the skin. Glands in the skin help to lubricate and waterproof the skin and also inhibit the growth of unwanted bacteria. The main components of this system include skin, hair, sweat glands, sebaceous glands, and nails (see Figure 4–9 ■).

Nervous System

Much like the activities of City Hall, the nervous system is the rapid messenger system of the body that both receives and sends messages for activities to occur. The messages conducted by the nervous system are stimulated by the body's internal and external environments. This is important not only so we may experience the world around us but to also protect us from harm. The nervous system also monitors what is going on inside the body. How do we know when we were hungry or when we have had enough to eat? This information is obtained through **sensations**, which are conscious feelings or an awareness of conditions that occur inside and outside of the body. These sensations are

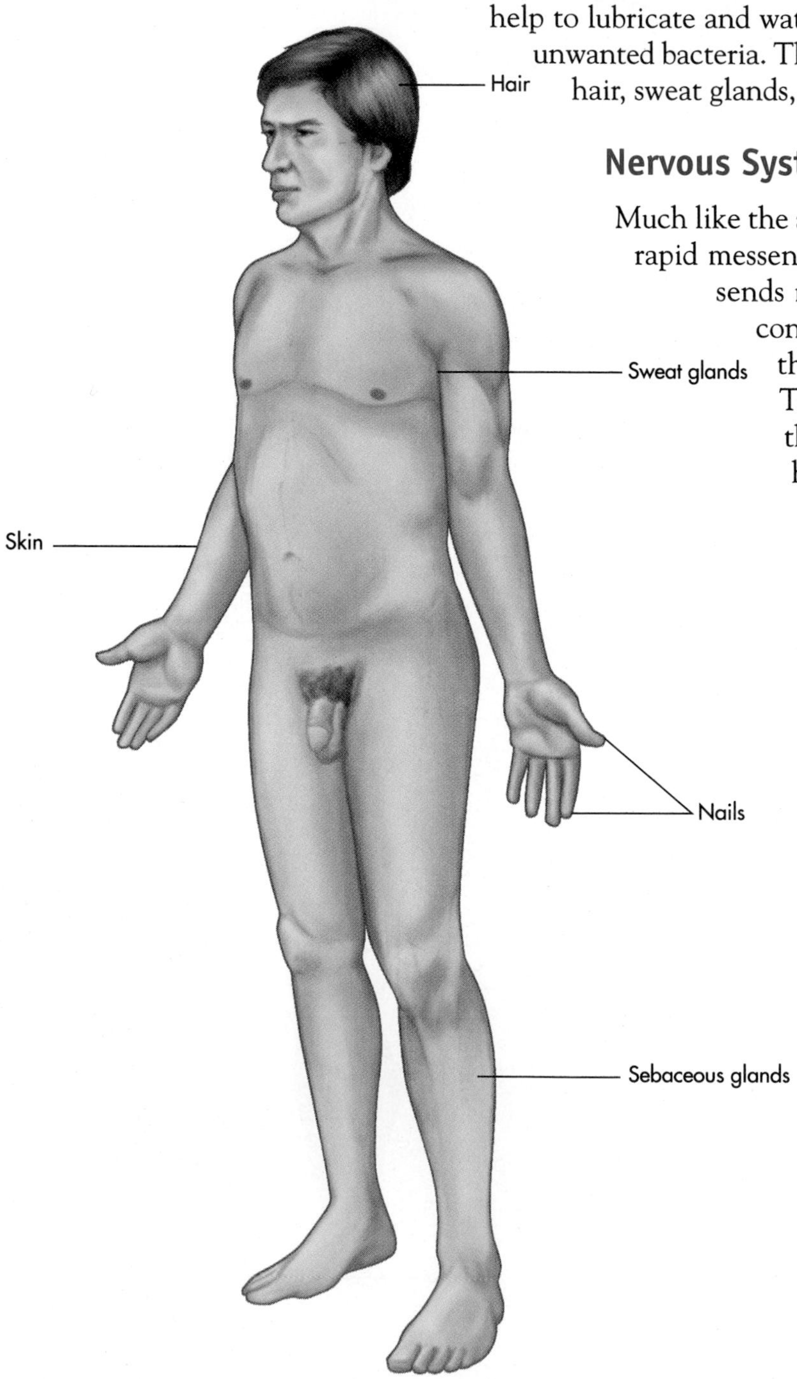

Organ	Primary Functions
Skin	
Epidermis	Covers surface, protects underlying tissues
Dermis	Nourishes epidermis, provides strength, contains glands
Hair Follicles	Produce hair
Hair	Provide sensation, provide some protection for head
Sebaceous glands	Secrete oil that lubricates hair
Sweat Glands	Produce perspiration for evaporative cooling
Nails	Protect and stiffen tips of fingers and toes
Sensory Receptors	Provide sensations of touch, pressure, temperature, pain

FIGURE ■ 4–9

The integumentary system.

caused by stimulation of our sensory receptors. So, then, the three main functions of the nervous system are sensory (receiving messages), processing and interpreting messages, and motor (acting on those messages). The main parts of the nervous system are the nerve cells (glial cells and neurons), the spinal cord with its spinal fluid, peripheral nerves, and, of course, the brain. Since we are dealing with sensations, our special sensory organs include the eyes (sight), nose (smell), tongue (taste), and ears (for hearing *and* balance). We will place the special senses in their own chapter later in this book. See Figure 4–10 ■, which depicts the nervous system.

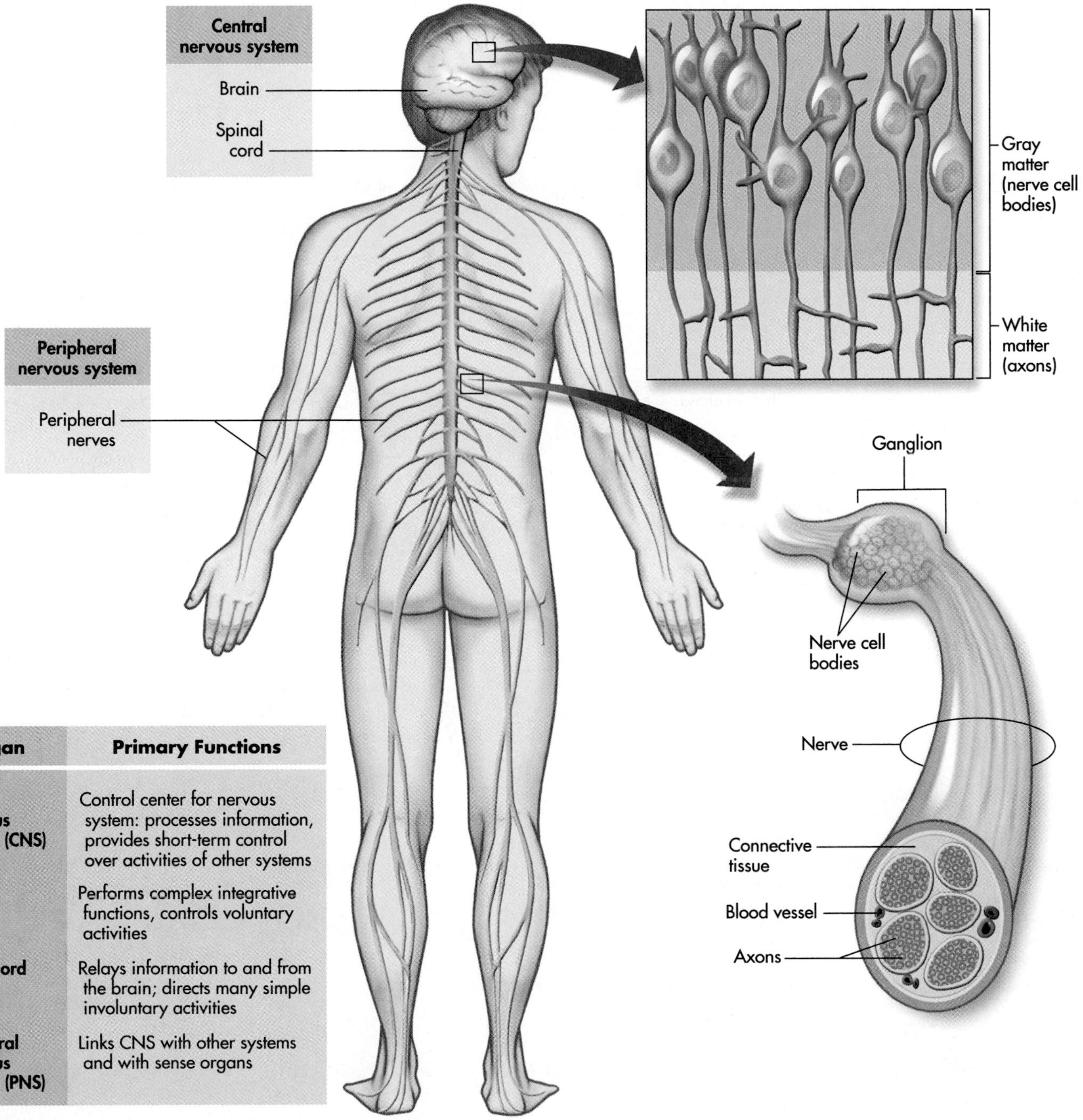

Organ	Primary Functions
Central Nervous System (CNS)	Control center for nervous system: processes information, provides short-term control over activities of other systems
Brain	Performs complex integrative functions, controls voluntary activities
Spinal cord	Relays information to and from the brain; directs many simple involuntary activities
Peripheral Nervous System (PNS)	Links CNS with other systems and with sense organs

FIGURE ■ 4–10

The nervous system.

Endocrine System

While not as quick acting as the nervous system, the endocrine system also acts as a control center for virtually all of the body's organs (see Figure 4–11 ■). This control is accomplished through endocrine glands that release chemical substances called hormones that are circulated through the cardiovascular system. The endocrine system helps to regulate the body's metabolic processes that utilize carbohydrates, fats, and proteins, and it plays an important role in the rate of growth and reproduction. In addition, the endocrine system helps to regulate the fluid

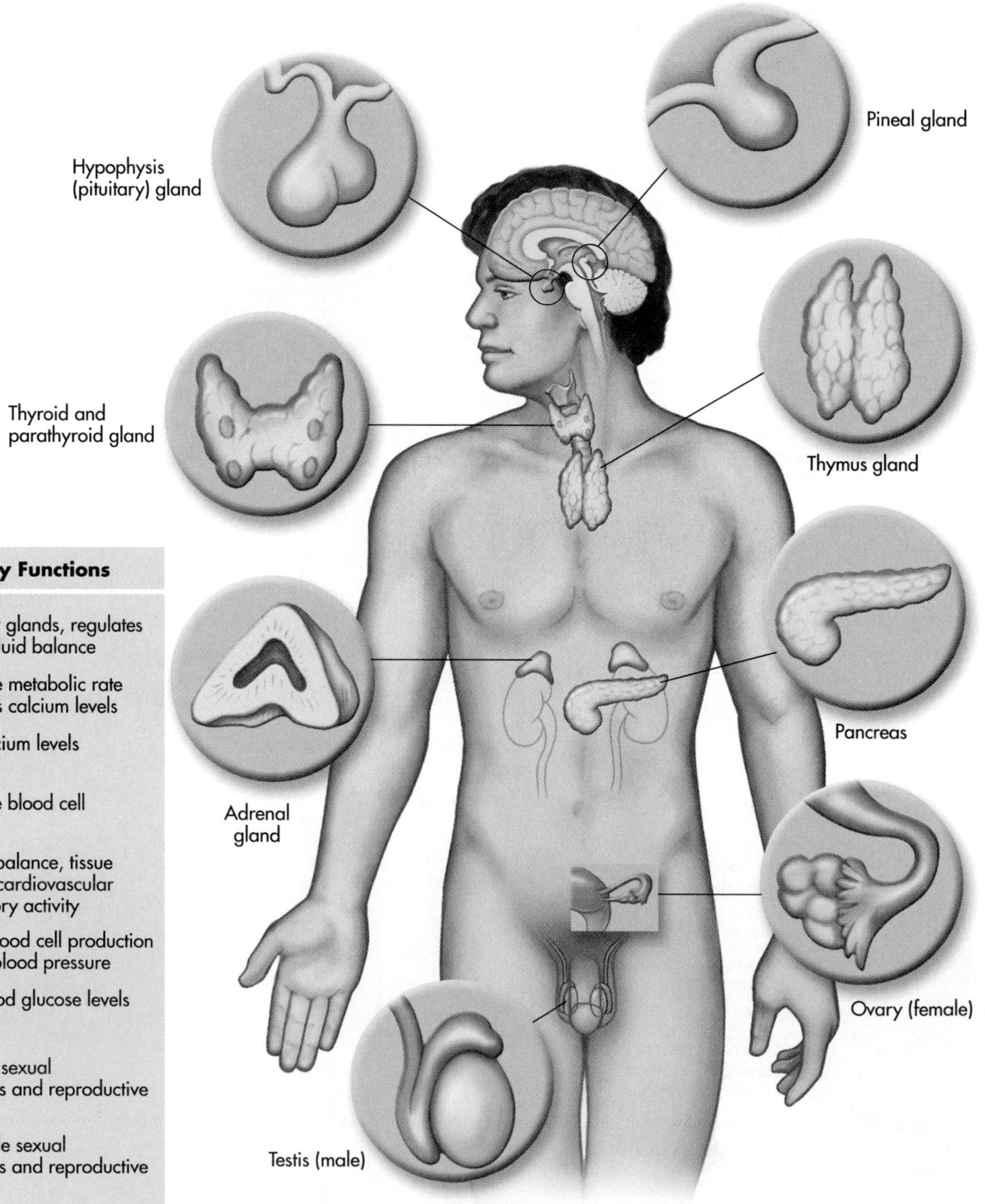

Organ	Primary Functions
Pituitary Gland	Controls other glands, regulates growth and fluid balance
Thyroid Gland	Controls tissue metabolic rate and regulates calcium levels
Parathyroid Gland	Regulates calcium levels (with thyroid)
Thymus	Controls white blood cell maturation
Adrenal Glands	Adjust water balance, tissue metabolism, cardiovascular and respiratory activity
Kidneys	Control red blood cell production and elevate blood pressure
Pancreas	Regulates blood glucose levels
Gonads	
Testes	Support male sexual characteristics and reproductive functions
Ovaries	Support female sexual characteristics and reproductive functions

FIGURE ■ 4–11

The endocrine system.

and electrolyte balances of the body. If that weren't enough, the hormones produced by the endocrine system help you to deal with general stress and the stresses produced by infection and trauma! The main parts of the endocrine system include the hypothalamus, pineal, pituitary, thyroid, parathyroid, thymus, adrenal glands, the pancreas and the gonads (testes in males and ovaries in females), plus a variety of hormones.

Cardiovascular System

cardio = *heart*

vasculo = *blood vessels*

Often referred to as the circulatory system, the cardiovascular system is the main transportation system to each cell of our body, much like the roads, sidewalks, and subways of our city. Please see Figure 4–12 ■. Through this system, water, oxygen, and a variety of nutrients and other substances necessary for life are transported to the cells, and waste products are transported away from the cells. Also like our city, these routes can become clogged or blocked, causing major problems. Imagine what happens to a busy four-lane highway if two of the lanes are shut down because of construction or an accident. The traffic slows and pressure builds up due to the congestion, much like the blood flow does when the arteries become partially obstructed. The buildup of pressure (hypertension) can be very dangerous. The main components of this system are the heart, arteries, veins, capillaries, and, of course, the blood.

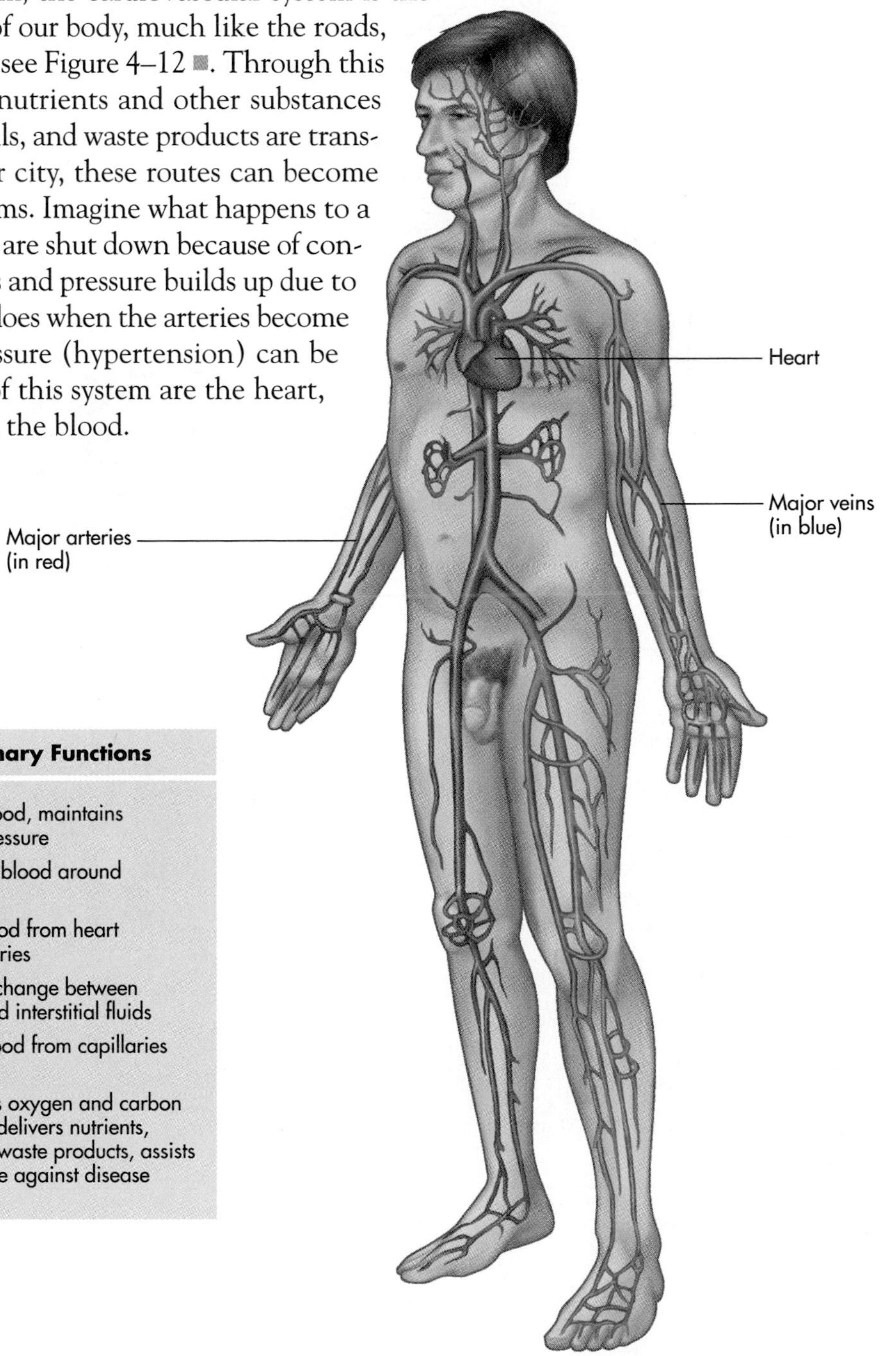

Organ	Primary Functions
Heart	Pumps blood, maintains blood pressure
Blood Vessels	Distribute blood around the body
Arteries	Carry blood from heart to capillaries
Capillaries	Site of exchange between blood and interstitial fluids
Veins	Return blood from capillaries to heart
Blood	Transports oxygen and carbon dioxide, delivers nutrients, removes waste products, assists in defense against disease

FIGURE ■ 4–12

The cardiovascular system.

Respiratory System

Think about a time you went swimming and stayed a little too long underwater, and you will remember how important our respiratory system is! We all know the old concept of being able to live weeks without food and days without water, but think about how long you would last without oxygen. Without conscious effort, your lungs move approximately 12,000 quarts of air a day! Our respiratory system, much like the ventilation system in an office building, not only supplies us with fresh oxygen but performs several other important functions as well. Our lungs eliminate the carbon dioxide created as a result of cellular metabolism. The respiratory system filters, warms, and moistens air as it is inhaled. The mucous lining of the airway helps trap foreign particles and germs. This system also helps to maintain the proper acid-base balance of the blood and aids in the elimination of ingested alcohol. The main parts of the respiratory system are the pharynx, larynx, trachea, bronchial tubes, and lungs (see Figure 4–13 ■).

Organ	Primary Functions
Nasal Cavities	Filter, warm, humidify air; detect smells
Pharynx	Chamber shared with digestive tract; conducts air to larynx
Larynx	Protects opening to trachea and contains vocal cords
Trachea	Filters air, traps particles in mucus; cartilages keep airway open
Bronchi	Same as trachea
Lungs	Include airways and alveoli; volume changes responsible for air movement
Alveoli	Sites of gas exchange between air and blood

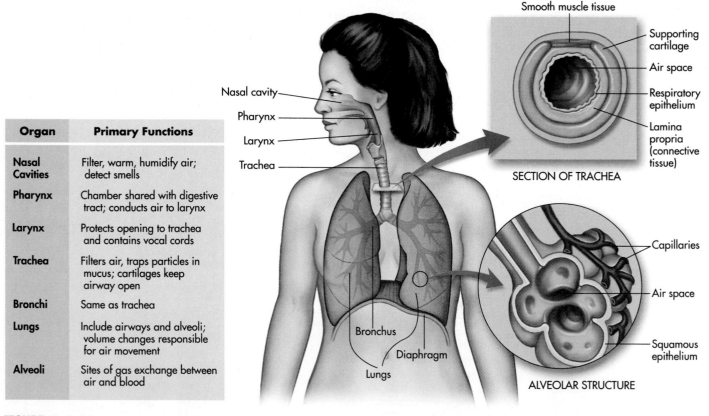

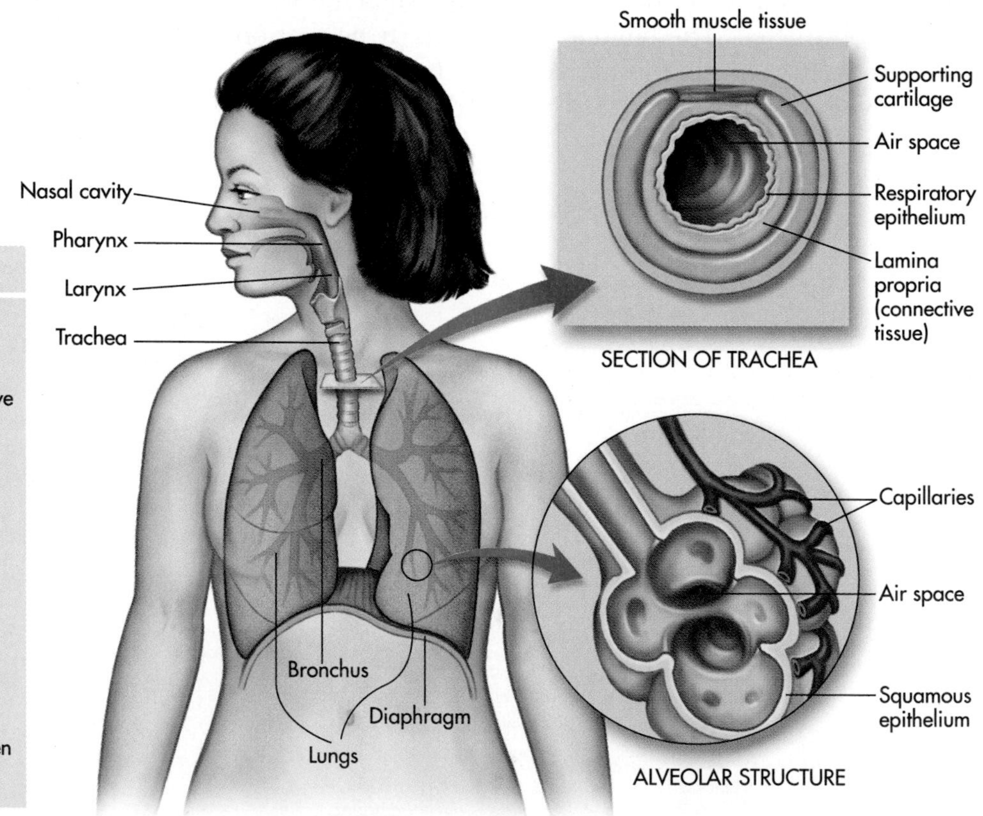

FIGURE ■ 4–13

The respiratory system.

Lymphatic and Immune System

Much like the storm drain system of our city, this very important, but often forgotten, system is responsible for helping to maintain proper fluid balance in our body and to protect it from infection. Excess fluid that may collect in places it shouldn't in the body is brought back into the lymphatic system, cleaned and processed, and then recirculated. Special structures called lymph nodes act as filters to capture unwanted infective agents. Lymph vessels and ducts, lymph nodes, the thymus gland, tonsils, and the spleen are the major parts of the immune system. In addition, the immune portion of the lymphatic system produces specialized infection-fighting white blood cells called lymphocytes. The immune system is the police force of the human body, patrolling for harmful invaders (see Figure 4–14 ■).

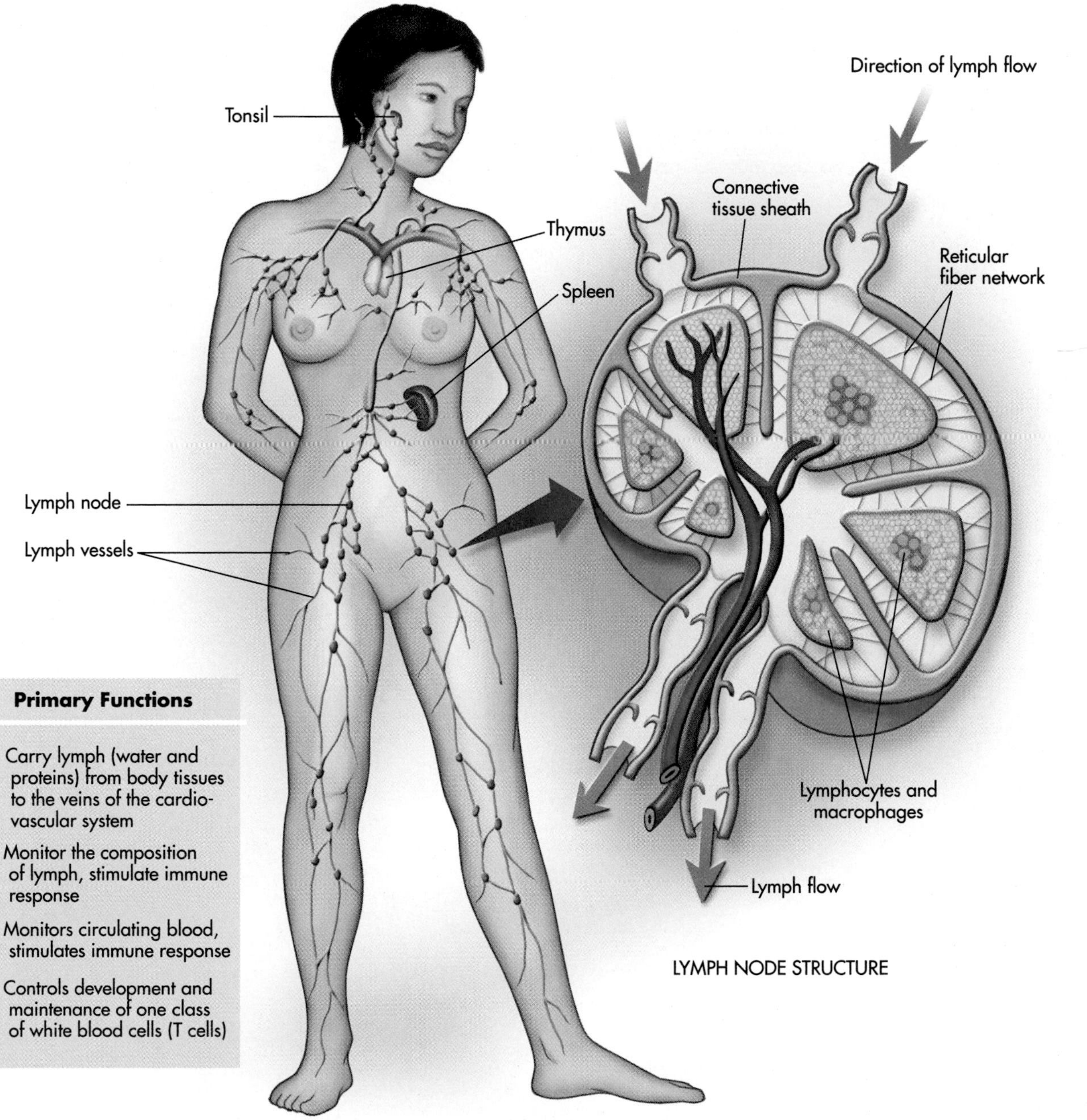

Organ	Primary Functions
Lymphatic Vessels	Carry lymph (water and proteins) from body tissues to the veins of the cardiovascular system
Lymph Nodes	Monitor the composition of lymph, stimulate immune response
Spleen	Monitors circulating blood, stimulates immune response
Thymus	Controls development and maintenance of one class of white blood cells (T cells)

FIGURE ■ 4–14

The lymphatic system.

Gastrointestinal, or Digestive, System

The digestive system (often called the GI system by savvy health care professionals) breaks down raw materials (food), both mechanically and chemically, into usable substances. Please see Figure 4–15 ■. Once these usable substances are created, this system absorbs them for transportation to the cells of the body. Materials that aren't used, as well as cellular waste, are transported out of the body by this system, much like the waste disposal and sewage system of our city.

Organ	Primary Functions
Salivary Glands	Provide lubrication, produce buffers and the enzymes that begin digestion
Pharynx	Passageway connected to esophagus
Esophagus	Delivers food to stomach
Stomach	Secretes acids and enzymes
Small Intestine	Secretes digestive enzymes, absorbs nutrients
Liver	Secretes bile, regulates blood chemistry
Gallbladder	Stores bile for release into small intestine
Pancreas	Secretes digestive enzymes and buffers; contains endocrine cells
Large Intestine	Removes water from fecal material, stores waste

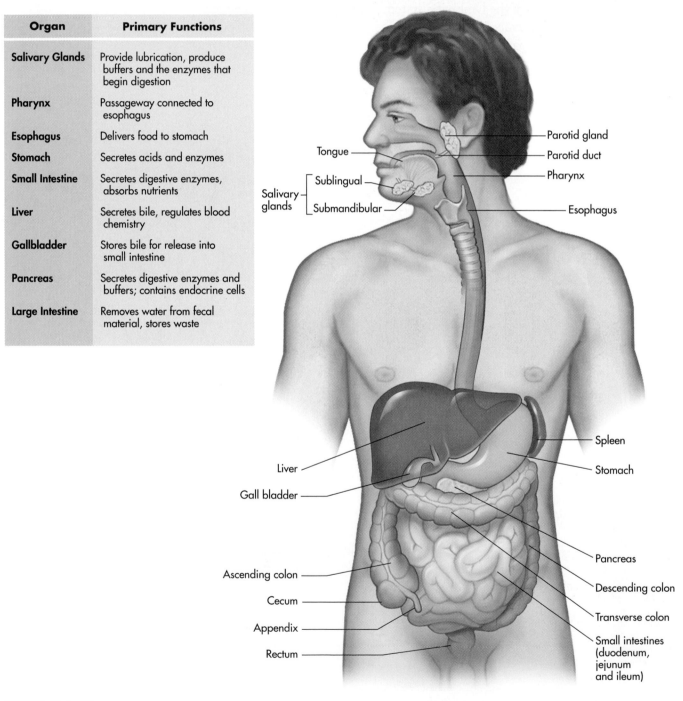

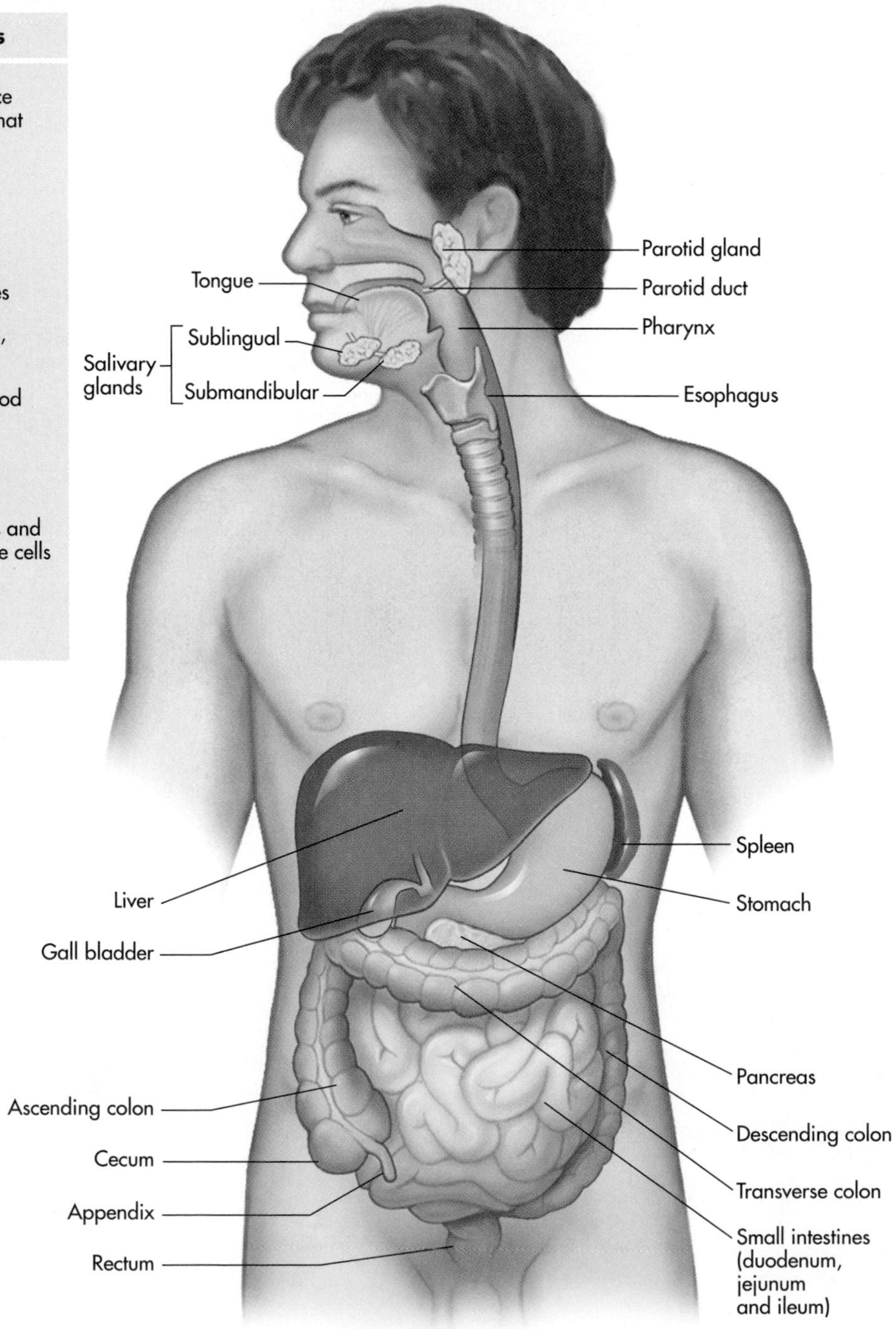

FIGURE ■ 4–15

The digestive system.

The main parts of the digestive system are the mouth, pharynx, esophagus, stomach, intestines, accessory organs, and anal canal.

Urinary System

While the digestive system plays a large role in the elimination of certain digested waste, the urinary system plays an important role in the elimination of waste products such as forms of nitrogen. In addition, electrolytes, drugs and other toxins, and excessive water are removed. This system is crucial for maintaining the proper balance of water you have in your body and regulating your blood pressure. The urinary system helps regulate the number of red blood cells and the acid-base and electrolyte balance of blood. The main parts of the urinary system are the kidneys, ureters, urinary bladder, and urethra (see Figure 4–16 ■).

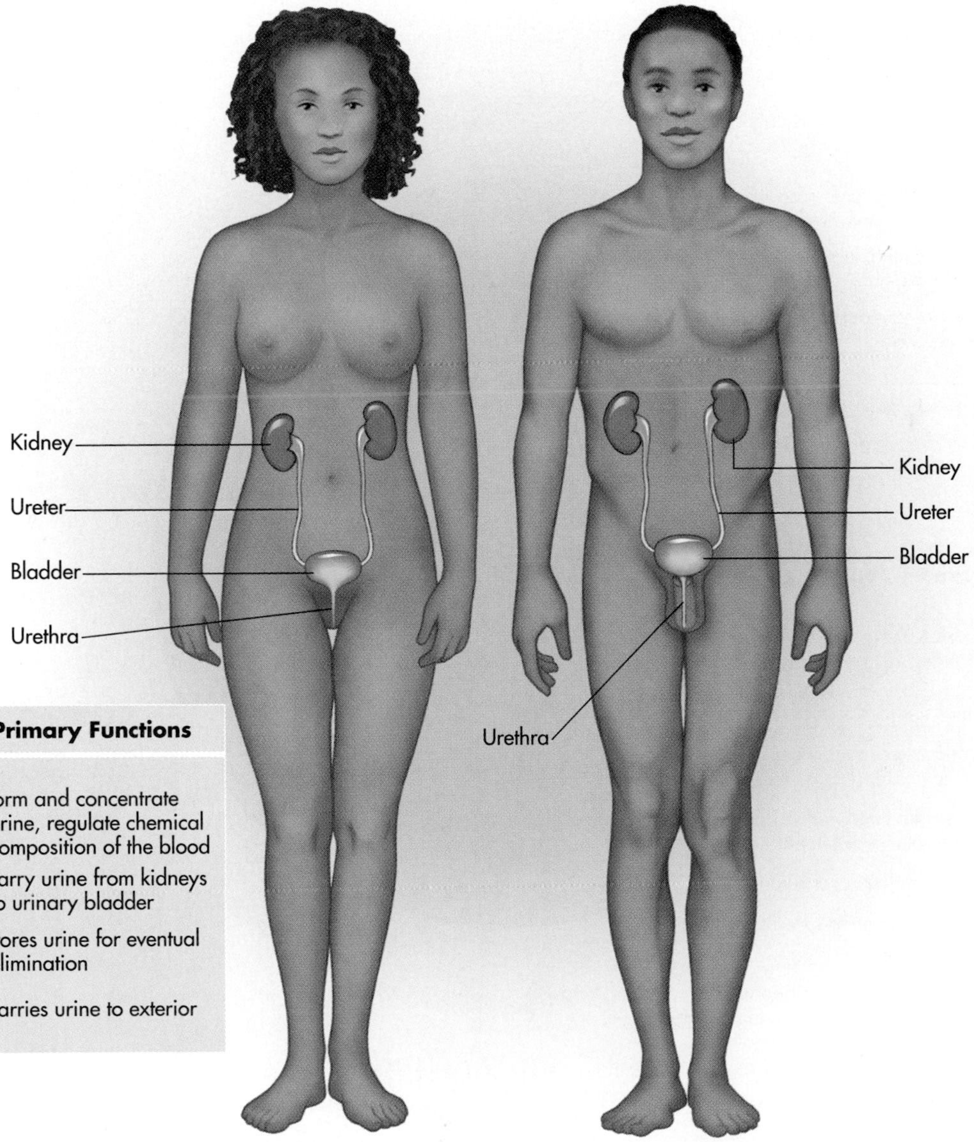

Organ	Primary Functions
Kidneys	Form and concentrate urine, regulate chemical composition of the blood
Ureters	Carry urine from kidneys to urinary bladder
Urinary bladder	Stores urine for eventual elimination
Urethra	Carries urine to exterior

FIGURE ■ 4–16

The male and female urinary systems.

Reproductive System

genitourinary
(gen i toe YOUR in air EE)

We build new cities or new buildings to accommodate growing needs or to replace worn out structures. The reproductive system does the same thing. Quite simply, without this system, we would not exist. The reproductive system is often combined with the urinary system to create the **genitourinary,** or **GU** system. Humans require a male and female to produce offspring. The male is needed to provide sperm that contains certain genetic traits of that individual, while the female provides an egg with her traits and a place for

Organ	Primary Functions (female)
Ovaries	Produce ova (eggs) and hormones
Uterine Tubes	Deliver ova or embryo to uterus; normal site of fertilization
Uterus	Site of development of offspring
Vagina	Site of sperm deposition; birth canal at delivery; provides passage of fluids during menstruation
External Genitalia	
Clitoris	Erectile organ, produces pleasurable sensations during sexual act
Labia	Contain glands that lubricate entrance to vagina
Mammary Glands	Produce milk that nourishes newborn infant

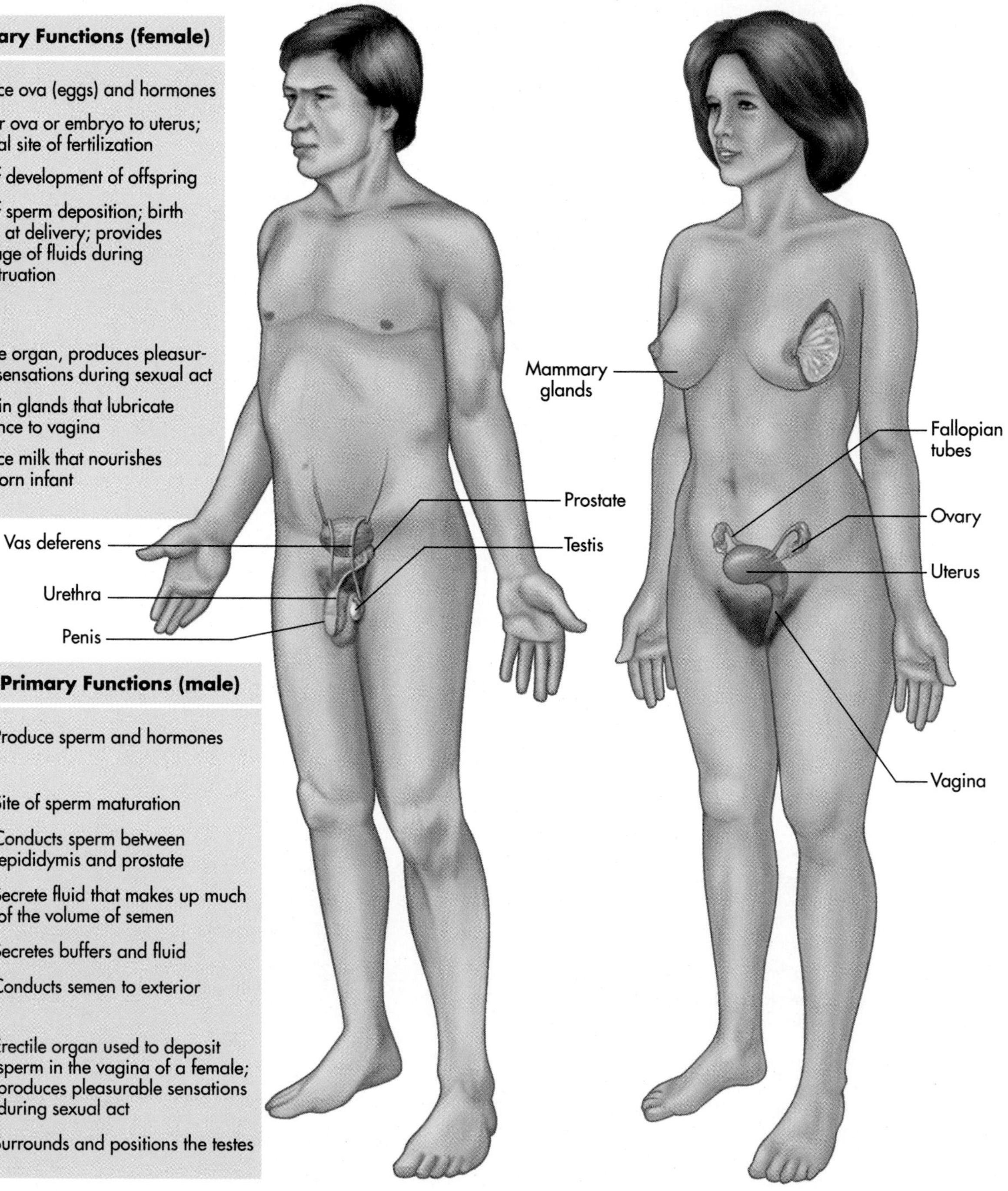

Organ	Primary Functions (male)
Testes	Produce sperm and hormones
Accessory Organs	
Epididymis	Site of sperm maturation
Ductus deferens (sperm duct)	Conducts sperm between epididymis and prostate
Seminal vesicles	Secrete fluid that makes up much of the volume of semen
Prostate	Secretes buffers and fluid
Urethra	Conducts semen to exterior
External Genitalia	
Penis	Erectile organ used to deposit sperm in the vagina of a female; produces pleasurable sensations during sexual act
Scrotum	Surrounds and positions the testes

FIGURE ■ 4–17

The male and female reproductive systems.

the fertilized egg to grow to maturity. The main female parts of this system are the ovaries, eggs, fallopian tubes, uterus, and vagina. For men, the main parts are the testes, sperm, and penis (see Figure 4–17 ■).

4-2 Now that we have briefly discussed the body systems, go to your CD-ROM for an interactive activity identifying the various systems along with their major components.

TEST YOUR KNOWLEDGE 4-2

List the correct system for the following activities

1. exchanges carbon dioxide for oxygen

   ____

2. eliminates nitrogen, drugs, and excessive water from the body

   ____

3. main storage for calcium

   ____

4. maintains body temperature and provides much of the sensory information from the external world

   ____

5. protects the body from invading pathogens

   ____

6. moves blood through the body

   ____

7. converts food to energy

   ____

8. with the help of the sun, produces vitamin D

   ____

SUMMARY

Snapshots from the Journey

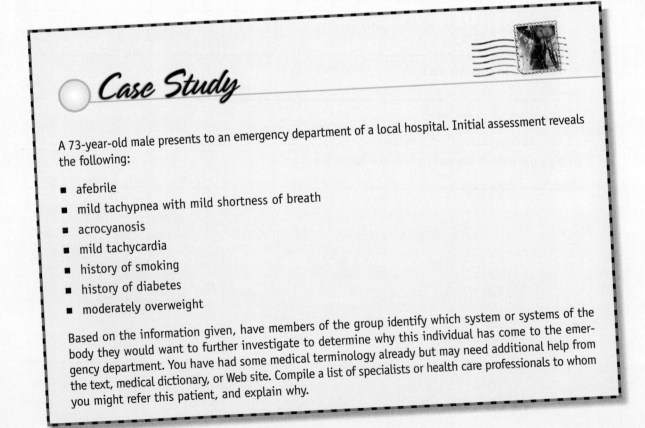

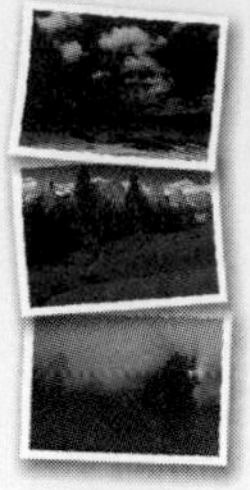

- Cells are the basic building blocks of the body.
- Tissue is a collection of similar cells that act together to perform a function. The four main types of tissues are epithelial, connective, muscle, and nervous.
- Membranes are sheetlike structures found throughout the body; they perform specific functions.
- The four major membrane types are cutaneous, serous, mucous, and synovial.
- Tissues that combine to perform a specific function or functions are called an organ.
- Organs that work together, often with the help of accessory structures, to perform specific activities create a system.
- There are 11 major body systems: skeletal, muscular, integumentary, nervous, endocrine, cardiovascular, respiratory, lymphatic/immune, gastrointestinal, urinary, and reproductive. Even though these are distinct systems, they are interrelated, and their relationships are highlighted in upcoming chapters.

Case Study

A 73-year-old male presents to an emergency department of a local hospital. Initial assessment reveals the following:

- afebrile
- mild tachypnea with mild shortness of breath
- acrocyanosis
- mild tachycardia
- history of smoking
- history of diabetes
- moderately overweight

Based on the information given, have members of the group identify which system or systems of the body they would want to further investigate to determine why this individual has come to the emergency department. You have had some medical terminology already but may need additional help from the text, medical dictionary, or Web site. Compile a list of specialists or health care professionals to whom you might refer this patient, and explain why.

REVIEW QUESTIONS

Multiple Choice

1. Blood can be classified as which type of tissue?
   a. connective
   b. cardiac
   c. nerve
   d. muscle

2. This membrane lines body cavities and covers the organs found in those cavities.
   a. cutaneous
   b. serous
   c. mucous
   d. mucus

3. This muscle type has interlocking cells for more efficient contraction.
   a. skeletal
   b. neuroglial
   c. cardiac
   d. smooth

4. The acid-base balance found in your body is mainly controlled by the following system:
   a. skeletal
   b. urinary
   c. endocrine
   d. none of the above

5. Which of the following organs belong to the digestive system?
   I. urethra
   II. gallbladder
   III. spleen
   IV. small intestine

   a. I, II
   b. I, III, IV
   c. III, IV
   d. II, IV

Fill in the Blank

1. The system that coordinates all the body's functions is the ______________ system.

2. The ______________ system is the "motion" system.

3. Cartilage is a specific type of ______________ tissue.

4. The layer of serous membrane that covers specific organs is called the ______________ layer.

5. The skin is composed of ______________ ______________ tissues.

Short Answer

1. List in order from simplest to most complex the following: organs, cells, systems, tissues.

2. What is the purpose of dendrites?

3. What is the purpose of synovial fluid?

4. Contrast the three types of muscle tissues and identify where they are found.

Suggested Activities

1. Choose one system to research. Identify all the tissue types and membranes found within that system and describe the individual tissue and membrane functions.

2. Create five to ten multiple-choice quiz questions related to this chapter and have a quiz show contest.

4-3 Now that you have completed your journey through this chapter, please go to the CD-ROM for interactive games and puzzles concerning the medical terms and concepts contained in this chapter. By playing the games you will reinforce your learning of medical terminology in a fun way.

Greetings from THE SKELETAL System

The Framework

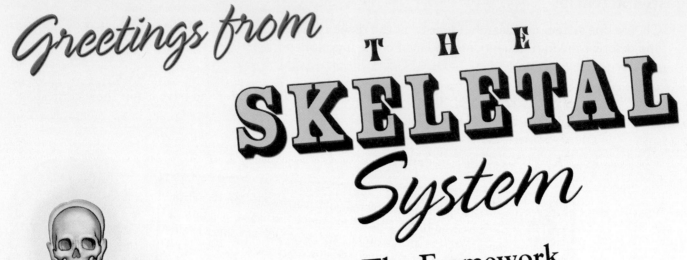

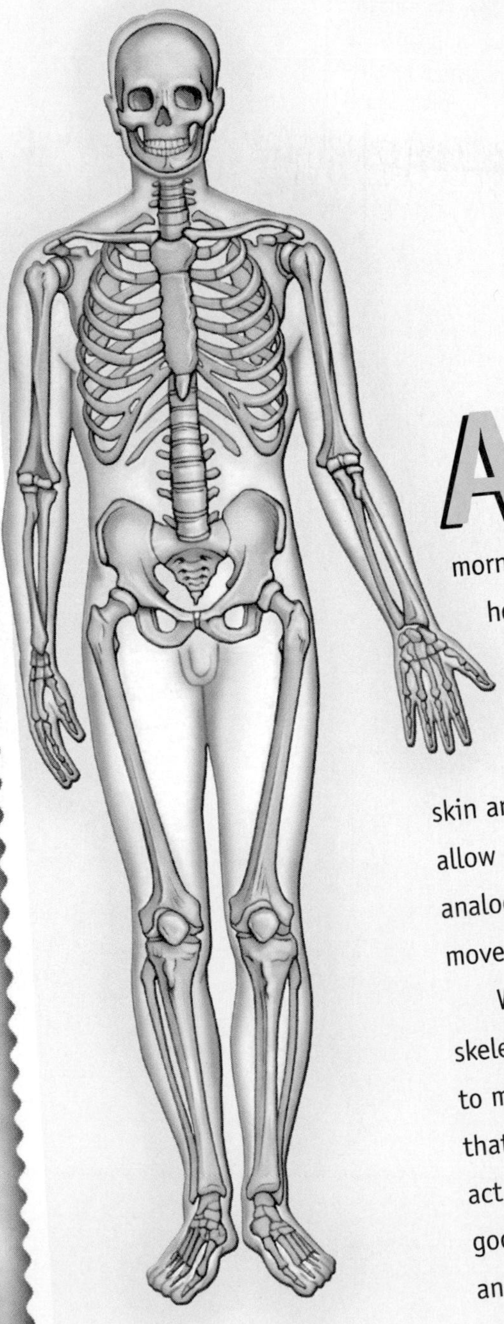

As we continue our journey, we may stop to visit friends or relatives and perhaps stay overnight. Their house will protect us from the elements and provide a safe place to sleep. Our hosts will offer us a good breakfast in the morning from the stored goods within. Although we cannot see the framework that holds up the house, without it everything would fall apart. We can think of the human body as a house. The wood framework is the skeleton, composed of bones that provide shape and strength. That is why we are beginning the system chapters with the body's own framework, upon which the muscles and skin are layered much like stone or siding. Mounted on the framework are hinges that allow doors to swing open and shut and windows that glide to open or close. These are analogous to the joints and muscles attached to the skeleton that allow for body movement.

What's the first thing you think of when someone asks about the function of the skeleton? From our analogy, you would probably say, "to provide support and allow us to move." But the skeleton does so much more. As explained in this chapter, the bones that make up your skeleton also protect the soft body parts, produce blood cells, and act as a storage unit for minerals and fat—much like our hosts' home, which stored goods within for that scrumptious breakfast! In this chapter, we discuss the makeup and importance of the 206 bones in the adult skeleton as well as cartilage, ligaments, and joints. And now it's time to "bone up" on the skeletal system.

Chapter 5

LEARNING OBJECTIVES

At the end of your journey through this chapter, you will be able to:

- Describe the functions of the skeletal system
- Identify and describe the anatomy and physiology of bone
- Locate and describe the various bones within the body
- Differentiate between bone, cartilage, ligaments, and tendons
- Locate and describe the various joints and types of movement of the body
- Explain common diseases and disorders of the skeletal system

MULTIMEDIA APPLICATIONS

CD-ROM Interactive Exercises

- Interactive drag-and-drop exercise: Labeling the parts of a bone, 5-1
- Animation on joint classification and movement, 5-2
- Animations of various types of skeletal body movements, 5-3
- Interactive drag-and-drop labeling of the major bones of the skeletal system, 5-4
- Interactive drag-and-drop of labeling of bones of the skull, 5-5
- Animation on how bone fractures heal, 5-6
- Videos on arthritis and osteoporosis, 5-7
- Interactive games and puzzles, 5-8

www.prenhall.com/colbert

- Professional Profile: Radiologic Technologists
- Related Internet Links
- Additional Review Questions

Pronunciation Guide

Correct pronunciation is important in any journey so that you and others are completely understood. Here is a "see and say" Pronunciation Guide for the more difficult terms to pronounce in this chapter.

appendicular skeleton (app en DIK yoo lahr SKELL eh ton)
arthritis (ahr THRYE tiss)
articulation (AHR tick you lay shun)
axial skeleton (AK see al SKELL eh ton)
cancellous bone (CAN cell us)
diaphysis (dye AFF ih siss)
epiphyseal plate (eh piff ih SEE al)
epiphysis (eh PIFF ih siss)
medullary cavity (MED uh lair ee)
osseous tissue (OSS see us)
ossification (OSS siff ih cay shun)
osteoarthritis (OSS tee oh ahr THRYE tiss)
osteocytes (OSS tee oh site)
osteons (OSS tee ons)
periosteum (pair ee OSS tee um)
synovial fluid (sin OH vee al)
trabeculae (tra BECK you lay)
vertebrae (VER teh bray)

SYSTEM OVERVIEW: MORE THAN THE "BARE BONES" ABOUT BONES

The skeleton has many more uses than to just scare people on Halloween. It is a wondrous structure that serves more functions than simply providing a framework for the human body. It also produces blood cells, provides protection for organs, helps us to breathe, acts as a warehouse for mineral storage, and, along with the muscular system, allows for movement.

General Bone Classification

The primary components of the skeleton are bones. Although they may seem lifeless and are composed of nonliving minerals such as calcium and phosphorus, they are very much alive, constantly building and repairing themselves. This is kind of ironic because the word *skeleton* is derived from the Greek word meaning "dried-up body."

We can classify bone types according to their shape:

- long bones
- short bones
- flat bones
- irregular bones

Long bones are longer than they are wide and are found in your arms and legs. *Short bones* are fairly equal sized in width and length, similar to a cube, and are mostly found in your wrists and ankles. *Flat bones* are thinner bones that can be either flat or curved and are platelike in nature. Examples of flat bones are the

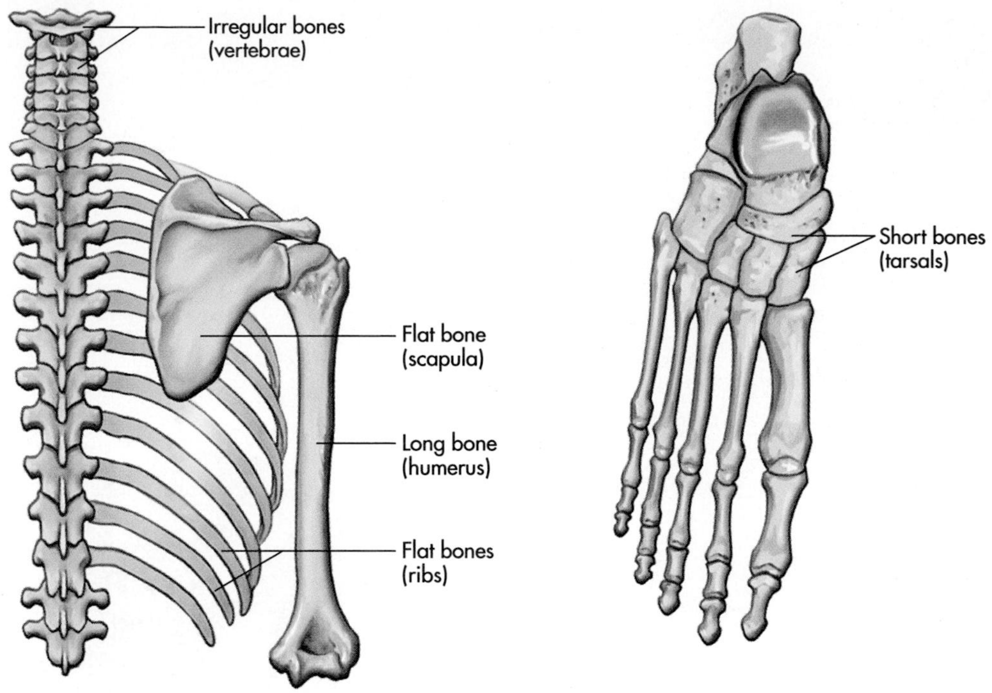

FIGURE ■ 5–1

Various bone shapes.

skull, ribs, and breastbone (**sternum**). *Irregular bones* are like the parts of a jigsaw puzzle. These are the odd-shaped bones needed to connect to other bones. Some examples of irregular bones are the hip bones and the **vertebrae** that make up your spine. See Figure 5–1 ■ for a view of the various bone shapes.

sternum *(STER num)*

vertebrae *(VER teh bray)*

Basic Bone Anatomy

Let's look at the overall construction of a bone by examining a long bone in Figure 5–2 ■. Bone is covered with **periosteum,** which is a tough and fibrous connective tissue. This cover contains blood vessels, which transport blood and nutrients into the bone to nurture the bone cells. It also contains lymph vessels and nerves. In addition, the periosteum acts as anchor points for ligaments and tendons, which we discuss later. Note in Figure 5–2 that both ends of the long bone increase in size. Each bone end is called an **epiphysis.** The region between or "running through" the two ends is called the **diaphysis.**

You can see that the diaphysis is hollow. This hollow region is called the **medullary cavity** and acts as a storage area for bone marrow, much like a kitchen cabinet that contains food is hollow but well stocked. There are two kinds of bone marrow, yellow and red. Yellow marrow has a high fat content. In emergencies—for instance, in the event of massive blood loss—when you need more red blood cells, some of the yellow marrow can convert to red bone marrow to help in red blood cell production.

periosteum *(pair ee OSS tee um)*
peri = *around*
osteum = *bone*

epiphysis *(eh PIFF ih siss)*
epi = *over or upon*
diaphysis *(dye AFF ih siss)*
dia = *through*
medullary cavity *(MED uh lair ee)*

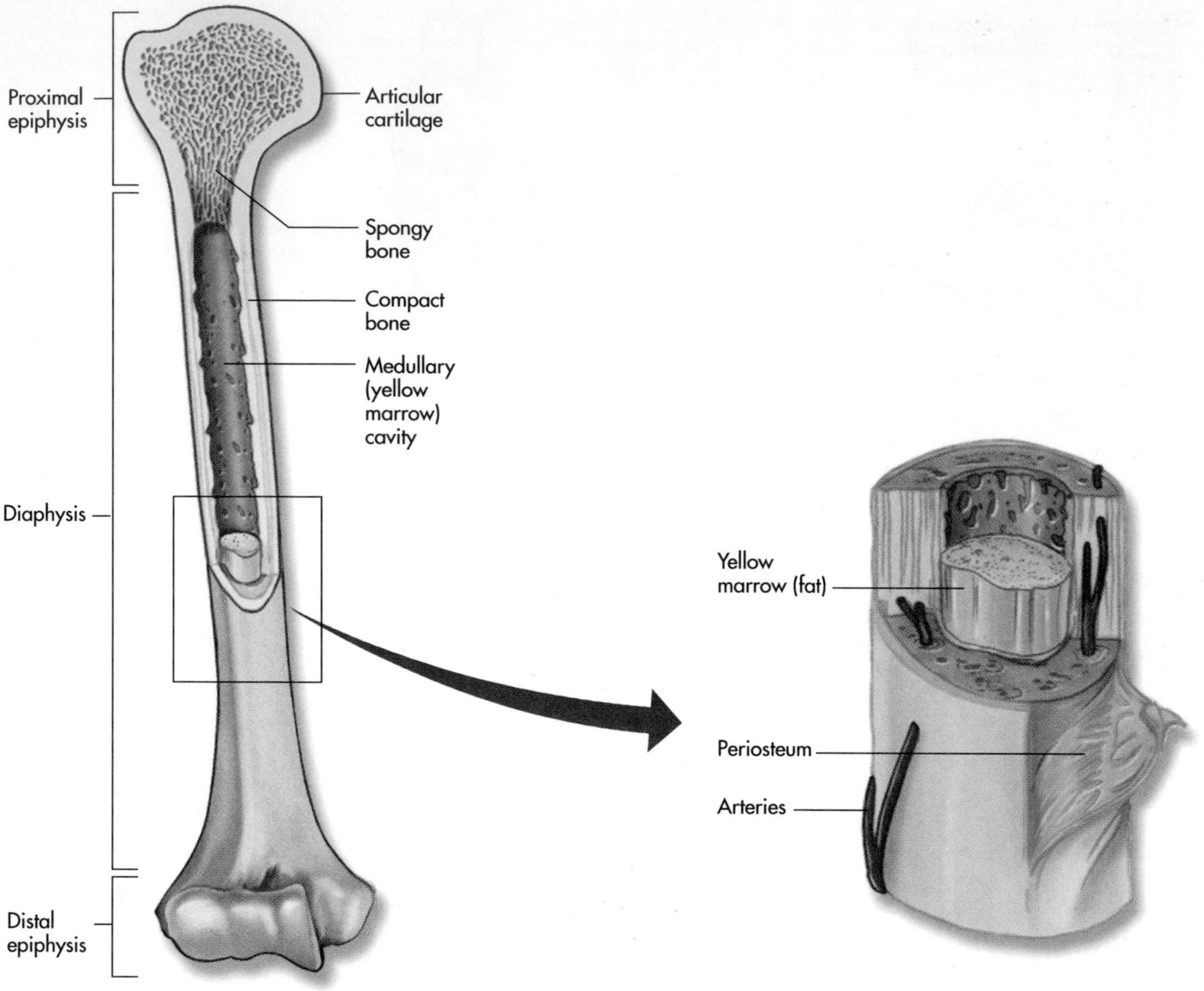

FIGURE ■ 5–2

Basic bone anatomy.

Bone Tissue

osteons *(OSS tee ons)*
osteocytes *(OSS tee oh site)*

There are two types of bone tissue: compact and spongy. **Compact bone** is a dense, hard tissue that normally composes the shafts of long bones and the outer layer of other bones. Microscopic examination reveals that the material of compact bone is tightly packed. This makes for a dense and strong structure. This material forms microscopic cylindrical-shaped units called **osteons,** or *haversian systems*. Each unit has mature bone cells (**osteocytes**) forming concentric circles around blood vessels. The area around the osteocytes is filled with protein fibers, calcium, and other minerals. The osteons run parallel to each other with blood vessels laterally connecting with them to ensure sufficient oxygen and nutrients for the bone cells.

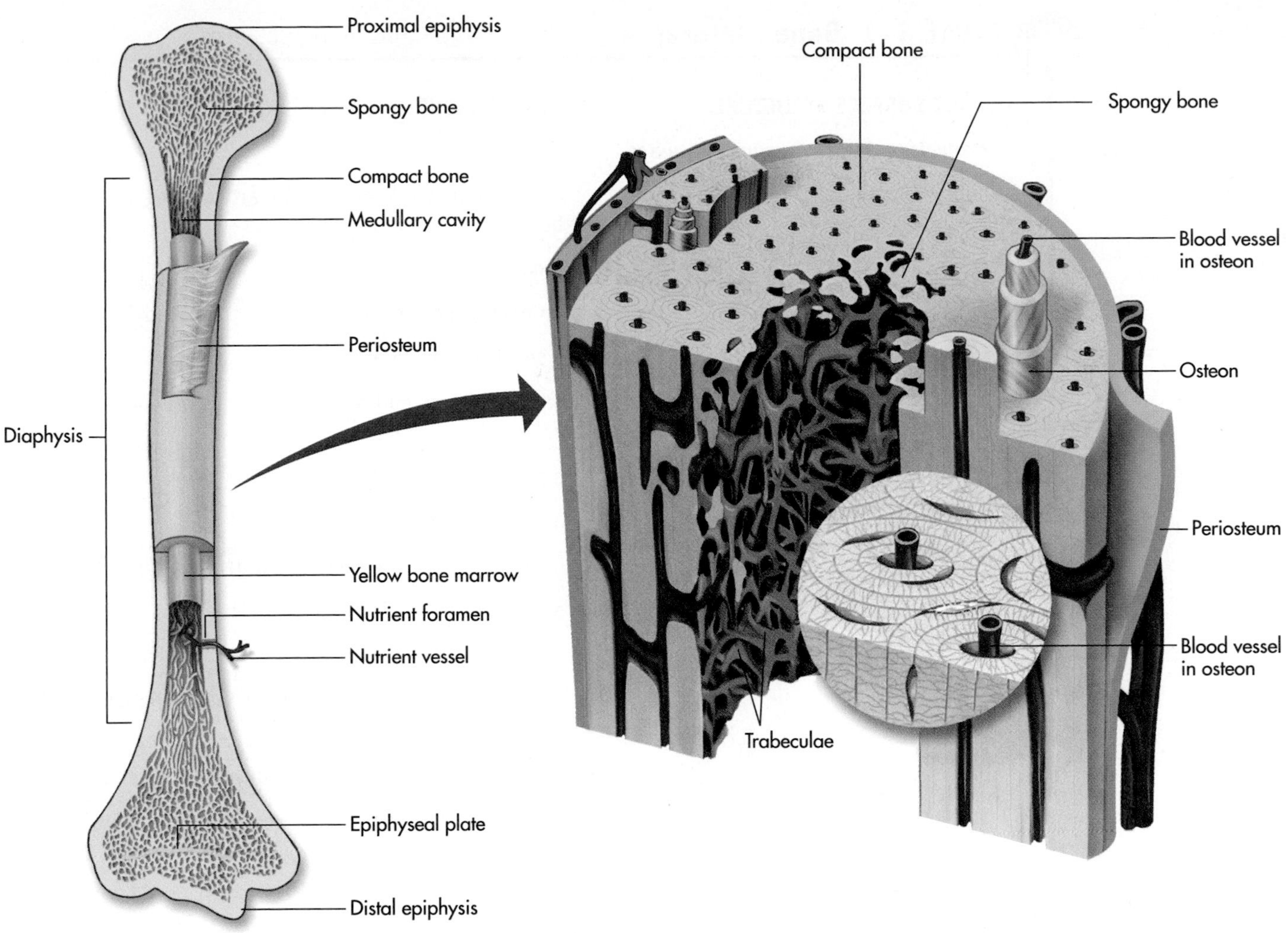

FIGURE ■ 5–3

Comparison of compact and spongy bone.

Spongy (or **cancellous**) bone is different than compact bone. Instead of haversian systems, spongy bone tissue is arranged in bars and plates called **trabeculae.** Irregular holes between the trabeculae give the bone a spongy appearance. Spongy bone is lined with **endosteum**, a tissue similar to periosteum. This serves two purposes: it helps make the bones lighter in weight and it provides a space for red bone marrow, which produces red blood cells (see Figure 5–3 ■).

cancellous bone *(CAN cell us)*

trabeculae *(tra BECK you lay)*

Surface Structures of Bones

Bone is not perfectly smooth. If you examine one closely, you will find a variety of projections, bumps, and depressions. Generally, projecting structures act as points of attachment for muscles, ligaments, or tendons, while grooves and depressions act as pathways for nerves and blood vessels. Both projecting

TABLE 5–1 Bone Features

BONE SURFACE STRUCTURES	DESCRIPTIONS
Projecting Structures and Processes	
condyle	a large, rounded knob, usually articulating with another bone
crest	a narrow ridge
epicondyle	an enlargement near or superior to a condyle
facet	a small, flattened area
head	an articulating end of a bone that is rounded and enlarged
process	a prominent projection
spine	a sharp projection
trochanter	located only on the femur; a larger version of a tubercle
tubercle	a knoblike projection
Depressions and Openings	
foramen	a passageway through a bone for blood vessels, nerves, and ligaments; a hole
fossa	either a groove or shallow depression
meatus	a tube or tunnellike passageway through bone
sinus	a hollow area

structures and depressions can work together as joining or articulation points to form joints such as the ball and socket joint in the hip. Table 5–1 lists many of these bone features.

hemopoiesis *(HEME ah poy ee sus)*
heme = *blood*
poiesis = *to make*

Amazing Body Facts

RED BONE MARROW AND RED BLOOD CELLS

The areas of bone with red bone marrow, which produces red blood cells, are found in the skull, clavicles (collar bones), vertebrae of the spinal column, sternum (breast bone), ribs, and pelvis and in the spongy bone that makes up the epiphysis of the long bones. The production of red blood cells, known as *hemopoiesis*, is truly an incredible process! Since red blood cells last only about 120 days, red blood cell production is a constant job in order to maintain the 25,000,000,000,000 (give or take a few) red blood cells contained in the human body. As a result, it has been calculated that approximately 3 million new red blood cells are created every second! What's more, your body can step up production to 10 times that rate in cases of severe blood loss. If the red marrow can't maintain the needed production, some of the yellow marrow can be converted to red marrow to assist.

TEST YOUR KNOWLEDGE 5-1

Complete the following:

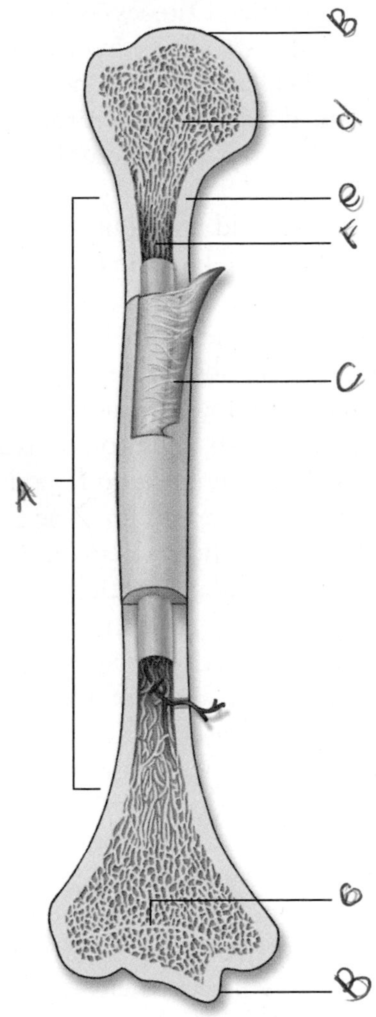

1. Label the following diagram:
   a. diaphysis
   b. proximal and distal epiphysis
   c. periosteum
   d. spongy bone
   e. compact bone
   f. medullary cavity
   g. epiphyseal plate

2. Where are the locations and what is the purpose of red bone marrow?

3. Discuss three functions of bone in your body.

4. Mature bone cells in compact bone are called
   a. marrowcytes
   b. osteocytes
   c. riflecytes
   d. monocytes

5. The end of a long bone is called the
   a. epiphysis
   b. periosteum
   c. diaphysis
   d. knob

Bone Growth and Repair

Ossification, or osteogenesis is the formation of bone in the body. Bones grow *longitudinally* in order to develop height, and they grow *horizontally* (wider and thicker) so they can more efficiently support body weight and any other weight we support when we work or play. There are four types of cells involved in the formation and growth of bone:

ossification *(OSS siff ih cay shun)*

- osteoprogenitor cells
- osteoblasts
- osteocytes
- osteoclasts

Osteoprogenitor cells are nonspecialized cells found in the periosteum, endosteum, and central canal of compact bones. Nonspecialized cells can turn into other types of cells as needed. **Osteoblasts** are the cells that actually form

osteo = *bone*
progeny = *offspring*
blast = *immature stage of cell development*

5-1 For a drag-and-drop exercise in labeling parts of the bone, go to your CD-ROM for this chapter.

bones. They arise from the nonspecialized osteoprogenitor cells and are the bone cells that secrete a matrix of calcium with other minerals that give bone its typical characteristics. **Osteocytes** are considered mature bone cells that were originally osteoblasts. In other words, osteoblasts surround themselves with a matrix of calcium to then become the mature osteocytes. So bone is built up or formed by osteoprogenitor cells becoming osteoblasts, which surround themselves with a mineral matrix to become full-blown ostecytes or bone cells.

clast = *causing breakage into parts*

Not only does the body constantly build bone but it must also constantly be able to tear down old bone. This is the job of the **osteoclast.** It is believed that osteoclasts originate from a type of white blood cell called a monocyte that is found in red bone marrow. Amazingly, the osteoclasts' job is to tear down bone material and help move calcium and phosphate into the blood! You can think of osteoblasts and osteoclasts as employees of a house remodeling company: the osteo**b**lasts are masons laying down brickwork to make new exterior walls, and the osteo**c**lasts are tearing out the inside to remodel! As explained shortly, the job the osteoclasts do is very important for bone growth and repair.

intra = *within*

Bone development and growth begins when you are growing in the womb through intramembranous and endochondral ossification. *Intramembranous* ossification occurs when bone develops between two sheets composed of fibrous connective tissue, such as in the development of your skull. Cells from connective tissue turn into osteoblasts and form a matrix that is similar to the trabeculae of spongy bone while other osteoblasts create compact bone over the surface of the spongy bone. As discussed previously, once the matrix surrounds the osteoblasts, they become osteocytes, and this is how bones of the skull develop.

endo = *within*
chrondal = *referring to cartilage*

The majority of your skeletal bones are created through **endochondral** ossification in which shaped cartilage is replaced by bone. Refer to Figure 5–4 ■. In this situation, which begins several months before birth, periosteum surrounds the diaphysis of the "cartilage" bone as the cartilage itself begins to break down. Osteoblasts come into this region and create spongy bone in an area that is then called the *primary ossification center*. Meanwhile, other osteoblasts begin to form compact bone under the periosteum. Here is where the osteoclasts come into play. Their job is to break down the spongy bone of the diaphysis to create the medullary cavity. After you are born, the epiphyses on your long bones continue to grow. However, shortly after birth, secondary ossification of this area begins with spongy bone forming and not

Amazing Body Facts

AGING AND BONE BUILDING

Even in adults, bone continues to be broken down and rebuilt. In fact, about 10 percent of the body's bone is torn down and rebuilt each year! Your bones continue to increase in mass well into your 20s. The osteoclasts break down and remove worn-out bone cells and deposit calcium into the blood. They last for approximately three weeks. Osteoblasts then pull the calcium out of the blood, form and surround themselves with that mineralized matrix we talked about, and mature into osteocytes. Because of this continual breakdown of old and creation of new bone, adults actually need more calcium in their diets than do children! The process of breaking down and rebuilding bone continues well into a person's 40s so there normally is no net gain or loss of bone mass.

This continuing process allows your body to sculpt bone into shapes that accommodate the body's activity. For example, exercise, such as running or weight lifting, causes calcium to stay in the bone, making it thicker, denser, and stronger than those of a sedentary person (couch potato) or an individual who is in outer space. Continuous or repeated actions or postures tend to cause bone to be resculpted. For example, due to constant squatting, a certain pattern of bumps forms on the bones of the hips, shins, and knees. As a result of this pattern, it was determined that Neanderthal man squatted rather than sat.

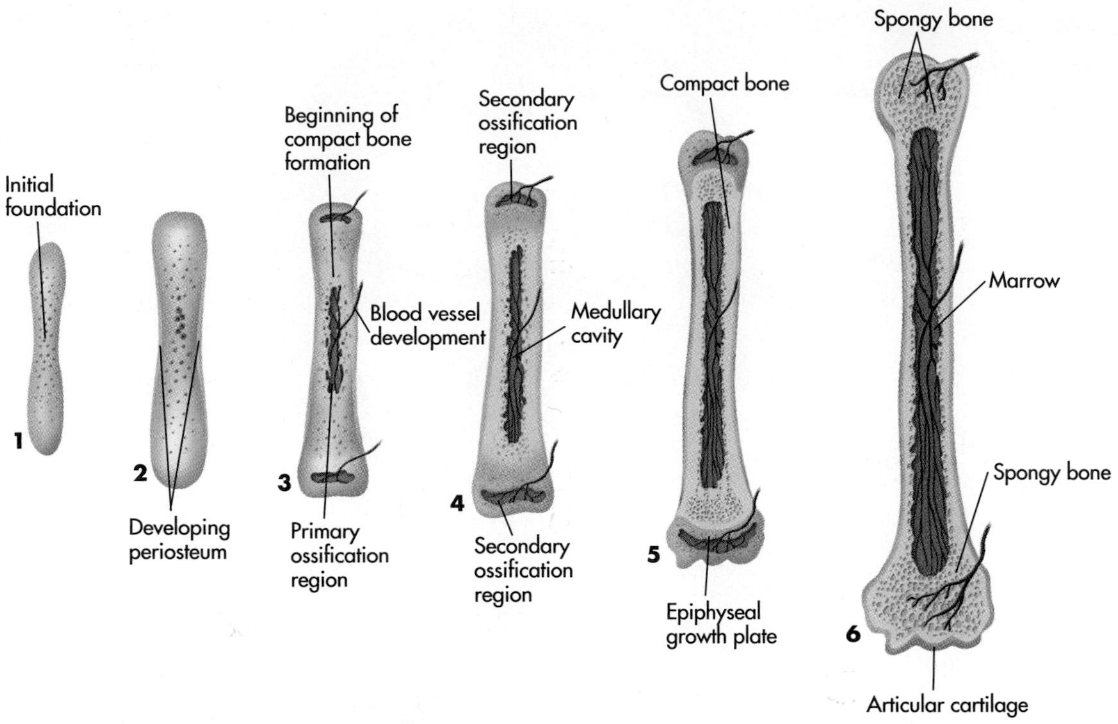

FIGURE ■ 5–4

Endochondral ossification of long bone.

breaking down. A thin band of cartilage forms an **epiphyseal plate** (often called the *growth plate*) between the primary and secondary ossification centers. This plate is important because, as long as it exists, the length and width of the bone will increase. As explained in Chapter 10, "The Endocrine System," hormones control the growth of bones, which means that eventually the plates become ossified, thereby stopping bone growth.

epiphyseal plate *(eh piff ih SEE al)*

Cartilage

Cartilage is a special form of dense connective tissue that can withstand a fair amount of flexing, tension, and pressure. We find cartilage playing many roles throughout the body. The flexible parts of your nose and ears are cartilage (imagine how many people would have broken off ears and noses if it weren't for cartilage!).

cartilage *(KAR tih lij)*

Cartilage also makes a flexible connection between bones. For example, the cartilage between the breast bone and ribs allows your chest to flex and give so you don't break your ribs when you run into things or collide with another player during a football game. Something as simple as taking a deep breath could become be a major struggle if it weren't for this flexibility.

This amazing tissue also acts as a cushion between the bones. As you can see in Figure 5–5 ■, *articular cartilage* is located on the ends of bones and acts as a shock absorber, preventing the bone ends from grinding together as they move. In addition at this location, a small sac, called the **bursa,** contains a lubricant called **synovial fluid.** Even with cartilage and synovial fluid protect-

bursa *(BER sah)*
synovial fluid *(sin OH vee al)*

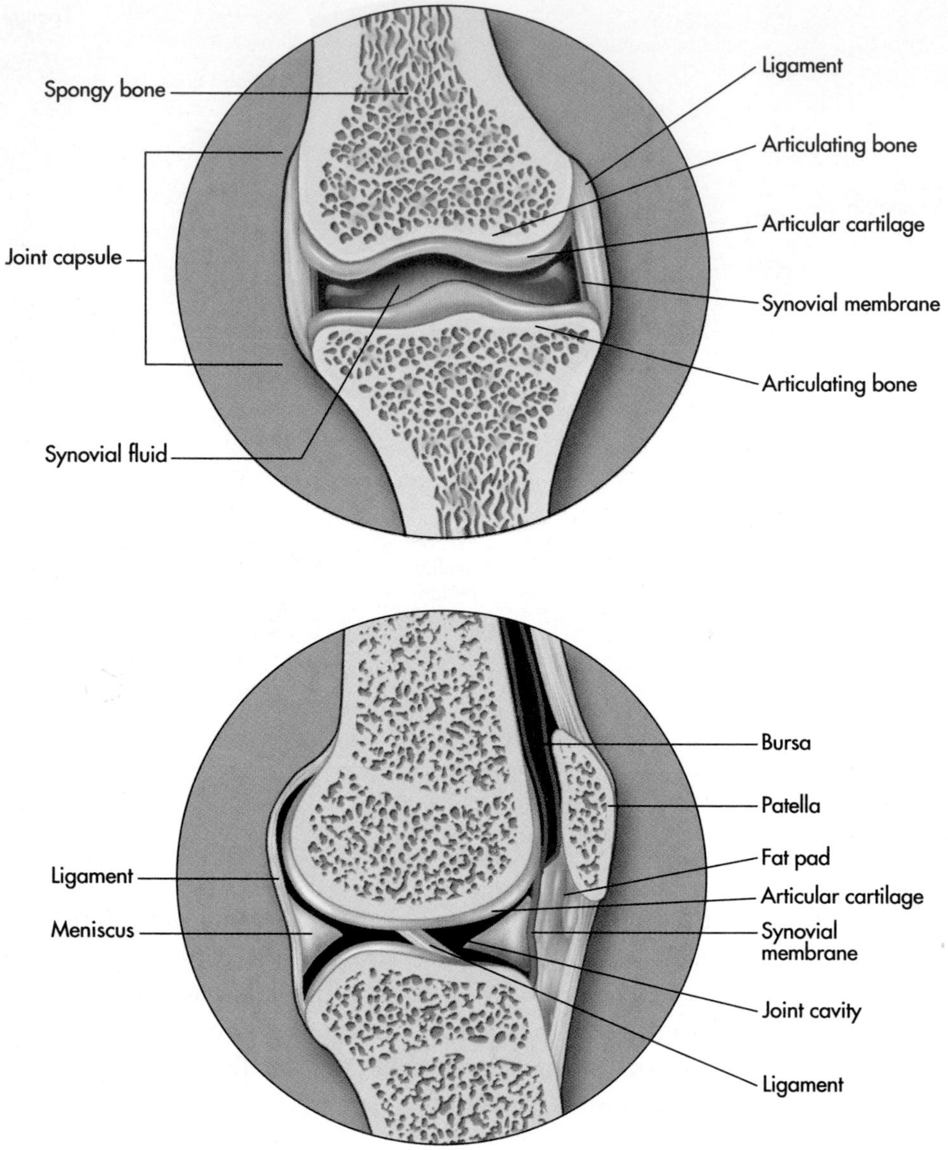

FIGURE ■ 5–5

Articular cartilage and synovial joint.

ing the area between bones, joints can wear out and become inflamed, resulting in a condition called **arthritis,** or **osteoarthritis.**

arthritis *(ahr THRYE tiss)*
arth = *joint*
itis = *inflammation of*
osteoarthritis *(OSS tee oh ahr THRYE tiss)*
oste = *bone*
Articulation *(AHR tick you lay shun)*

Joints and Ligaments

Without **joints,** the body could not move. When two or more bones *join* together, a joint, or an **articulation,** is formed. Freely moving joints have to be held together and yet still be moveable. This is accomplished through the use of another specialized connective tissue called a **ligament.** (Again, see Figure 5–5.) Ligaments are very tough, whitish bands that connect from bone to bone and can withstand pretty heavy stress. Do not confuse ligaments with **tendons.** While ligaments hold bone to bone, tendons are cordlike structures that attach muscle to bone. There are several types of joints, and each works in a specific way.

TEST YOUR KNOWLEDGE 5-2

Choose the best answer:

1. A term that can be used to describe the formation of bone is:
   a. ossification
   b. periosteum
   c. bonafide
   d. osteclasts
2. These cells actually form bones:
   a. osteoclasts
   b. pericytes
   c. generator cells
   d. osteoblasts
3. Another name for the "growth plate" is:
   a. tectonic plate
   b. epiphyseal plate
   c. upper palate
   d. periostium plate
4. This special connective tissue composes your ears and nose:
   a. tendons
   b. ligaments
   c. cartilage
   d. cartridge
5. This lubricant helps to prevent wear between the joints:
   a. pleural fluid
   b. synovial fluid
   c. mucous
   d. petroleum jelly
6. These structures attach bone to bone;
   a. ligaments
   b. tendons
   c. cords
   d. articulations

Joints are classified either by function or structure. In terms of function, joints can be immobile, can move a little, or can move freely. For example, skull sutures are immobile, the pubic symphysis between your pelvic bones moves a little, and your elbow moves freely. If we characterize joints by structure, we divide them based on the type of connective tissue that links the bones together. **Fibrous joints** are held together by short connective tissue strands. They are either immobile or slightly movable. The sutures in your skull are fibrous joints. **Cartilaginous joints** are held together by cartilage disks. The pubic symphysis and the joints between your ribs and sternum are cartilaginous joints. Cartilaginous joints are either immobile or slightly movable. Finally, **synovial joints** are joined by a joint cavity lined with a synovial membrane and filled with synovial fluid. All synovial joints are freely moving. Synovial joints are constructed in various ways that determine how they can move.

- *Pivot joints* (which act like a turnstyle) are the type of joint found in your neck and forearm. Pivot joints can only rotate.
- *Ball and socket joints* are located in your hips and shoulders and can perform all types of movement, including rotation.
- *Hinge joints* are found in your knees and elbows. They can either open or close.
- *Gliding joints* are the flat, or slightly curved, platelike bones found in your wrists and ankles. Gliding joints slide back and forth.

5-2 For some excellent animations on joint classification and how they move, go to your CD-ROM for this chapter!

- *Saddle joints* have a bone shaped just like a saddle and another bone similar to a horse's back. This joint type is found in the base of your thumb. Saddle joints rock up and down and side to side.
- *Condyloid joints* occur as a result of an oval-shaped bone end fitting into an elliptical cavity in the other end so there is movement from one plane to another but no rotation. The knuckles of your finger are condyloid joints.
- *Ellipsoidal joints* provide two axes of movement through the same bone, like the joint formed at the wrist with both the radius and ulna.

To better visualize these various joints, look at Figure 5–6 ■.

Movement Classification

Since joints allow for various types of movement, these individualized movements can also be classified, as you can see in the examples in Figure 5–7 ■. *Flexion* occurs when a joint is bent, decreasing the angle between the involved

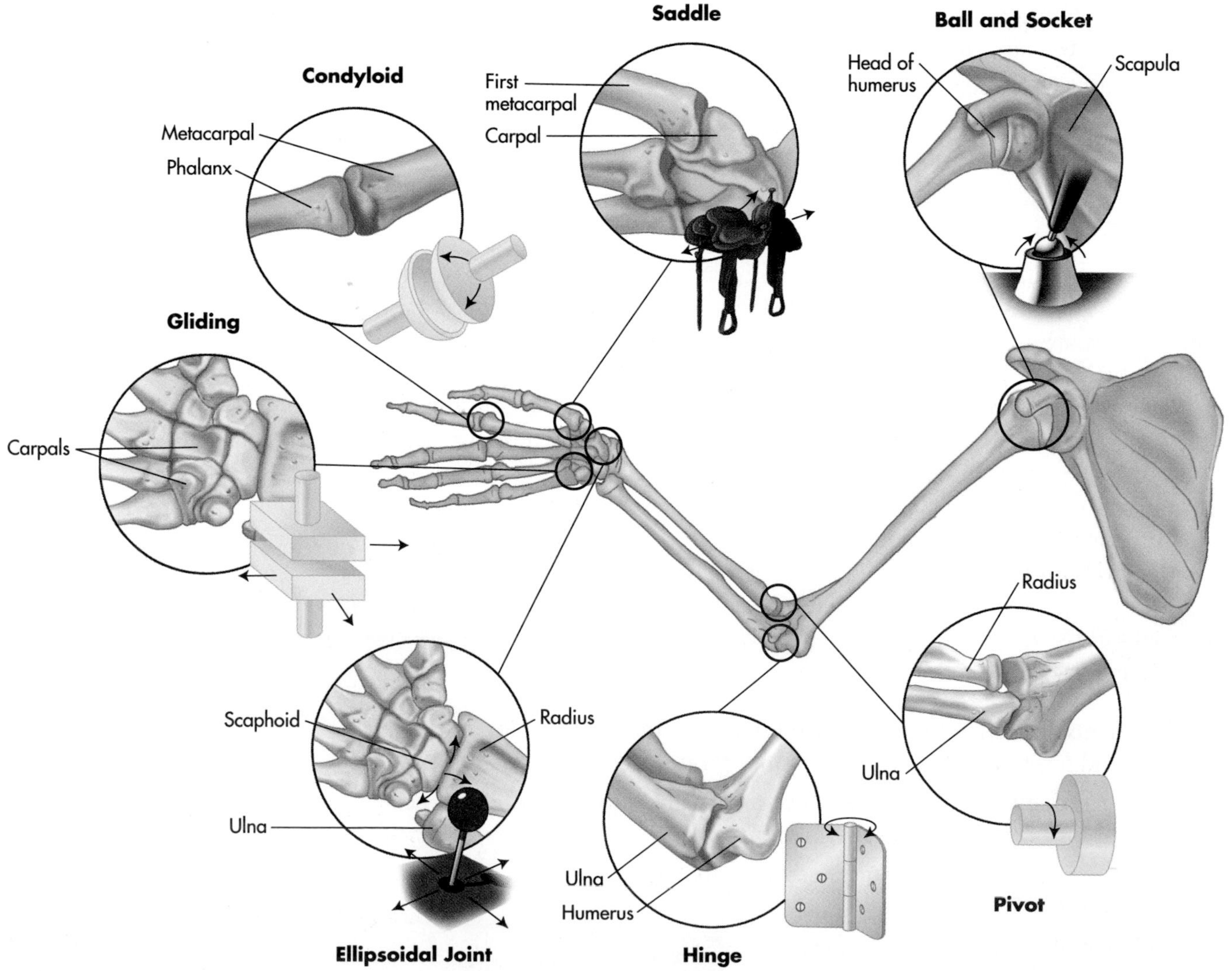

FIGURE ■ 5–6

Types of joints.

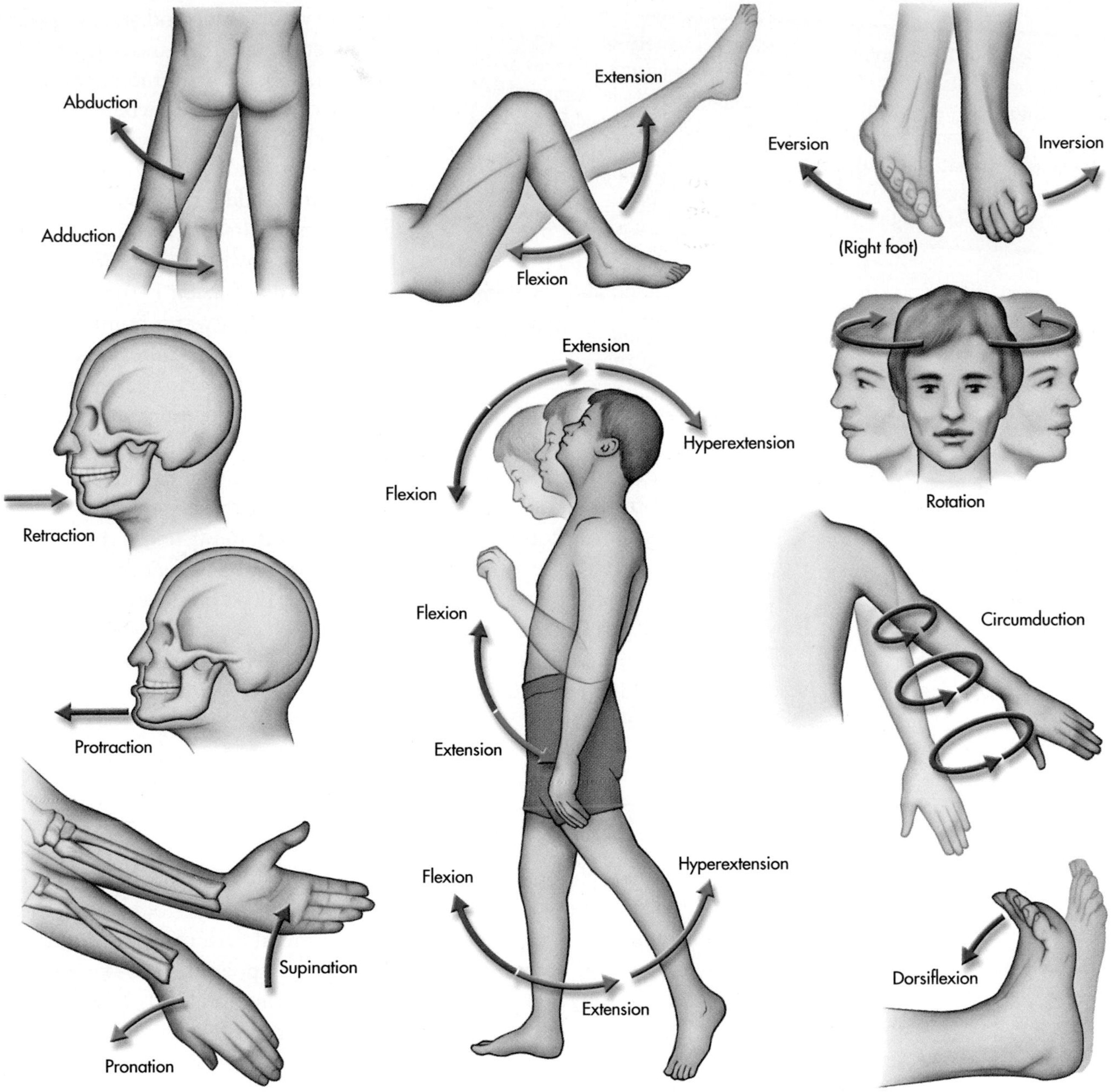

FIGURE ■ 5–7

Classification of joint movements.

bones, as when the leg is bent at the knee. *Extension* is a result of straightening a joint so the angle between the involved bones increases, as occurs with a kicking motion. Ballerinas utilize *plantar flexion* when they dance on their toes. *Dorsiflexion* occurs when the foot is bent up toward the leg. If the joint is forced to straighten beyond its normal limits, *hyperextension* occurs.

> **5-3** To see a video on the types of movement made by the human body, go to your CD-ROM for this chapter.

Abduction and *adduction* can be confusing. **Ab**duction means to move *away* from the body's midline (think, "**B**e gone!"

Radiologic Technologist is a title for a variety of health care professionals who utilize radiation to make images of bones and other body parts. Radiographers prepare patients for X-rays, take the "picture," and develop the X-ray film so physicians can read (analyze) them. For more information about these areas of health care, visit the companion Web site for links to the American College of Radiology and the American Society of Radiologic Technologists.

5-4 For more detailed views of the skeletal system (appendicular and axial) and drag-and-drop labeling exercises, go to your CD-ROM for this chapter.

as you move your arm up and away to swat a bee). A**dd**uction means to move *toward* the midline of the body. To remember adduction, think of your a**dd**ress, where packages and mail come *to* you. Then when you move your arm back toward yourself after swatting at a bee, you are a**dd**ucting your arm.

Inversion results when the sole of one foot is turned inward so it points to the other foot, while *eversion* is the opposite: the foot is turned outward, pointing away from the opposite foot. *Supination* occurs when the hand is turned to the point where the palm faces upward; *pronation* turns the palm downward. Although you may not have heard of *circumduction*, you have seen this combination of movements in the circular arm movement that a softball pitcher utilizes.

Protraction is the motion of drawing a part forward. *Retraction* is the motion of drawing backward. Figure 5–7 shows the protraction and retraction of the jaw. The movements are analogous to a turtle sticking his head out (protracting) and drawing it back in (retracting) to the shell.

Finally, *rotation* is when a bone "spins" on its axis. An example is when your head rotates (looking left and right) before you cross the street.

THE SKELETON

axial skeleton
(AK see al SKELL eh ton)

appendicular skeleton
(app en DIK yoo lahr SKELL eh ton)

Anatomically, the skeleton can be divided into two main sections. The **axial skeleton** includes bones of the bony thorax, spinal column, hyoid bone, bones of the middle ear, and skull. This part of the skeletal system protects the organs of the body and is composed of 80 bones. The **appendicular skeleton** is, as its name implies, the region of your appendages (arms and legs), as well as the connecting bone structures of the hip and shoulder girdles, and contains 126 bones (see Figure 5–8 ■). Interestingly, nearly half of the total number of your bones can be found in your hands and feet!

Special Regions of the Skeletal System

The skeleton consists of many different special regions. These distinctions make it easier to locate and discuss the hundreds of bones and associated components in this system. In this section, we make a quick tour of each region, beginning at the top.

THE HUMAN SKULL

The skull protects and houses the brain and has openings needed for our sensory organs, such as the eyes, nose, and ears. It also forms the mouth, which is a common passageway for both the digestive and respiratory systems. The skull contains fibrous connective tissue joints called *suture* lines that hold the bony

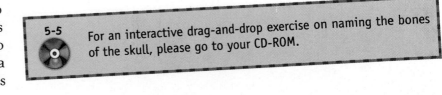

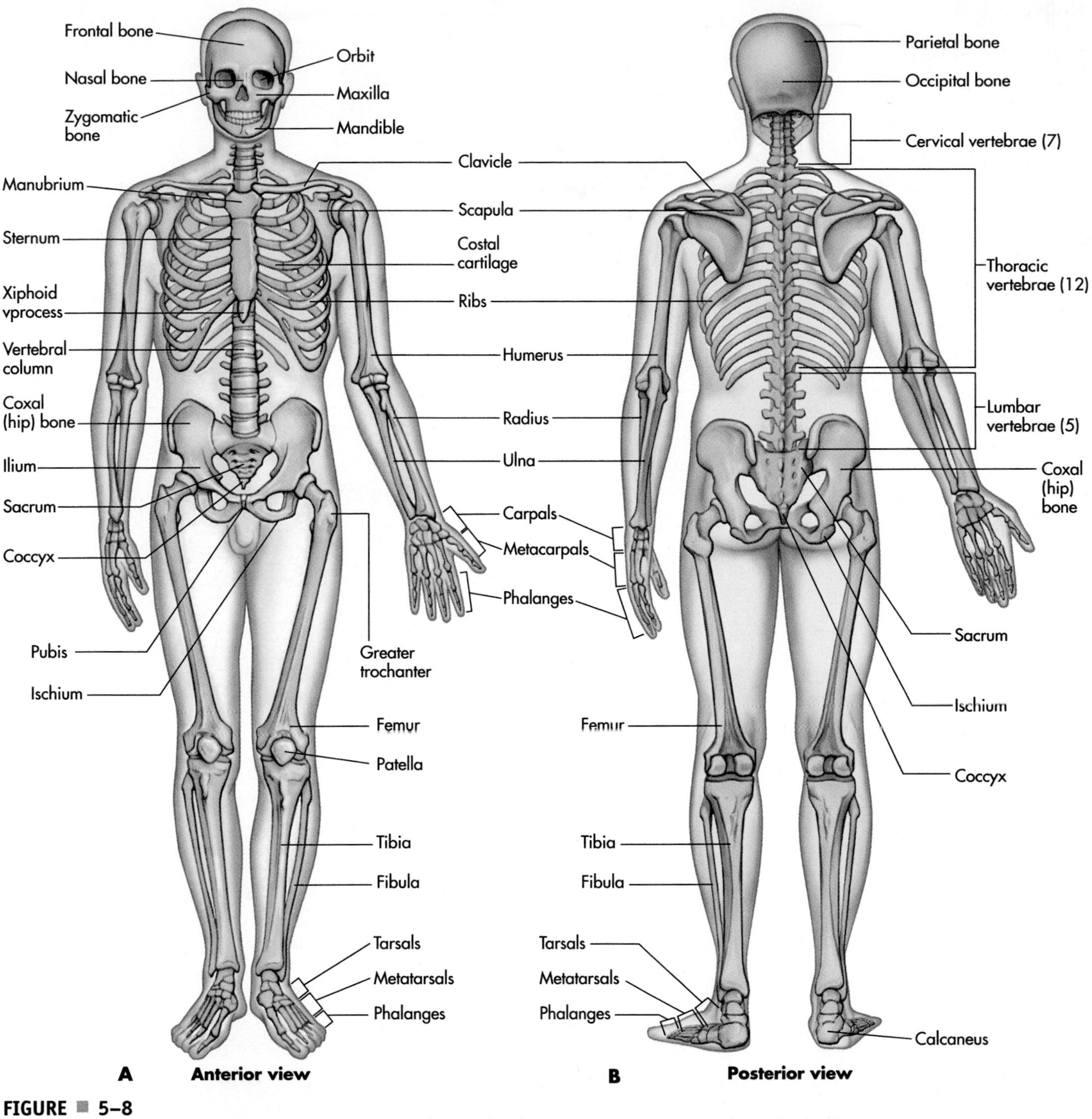

FIGURE ■ 5–8

The anterior and posterior human skeleton.

plates of the skull together. While these joints are not actually moveable, they do provide some degree of flexibility, which is important to absorb shock from a blow to the head, thus decreasing the chance of a skull fracture. Figure 5–9 ■ shows the bones of the skull in greater detail.

> 5-5
> For an interactive drag-and-drop exercise on naming the bones of the skull, please go to your CD-ROM.

FIGURE ■ 5–9

Bones of the skull.

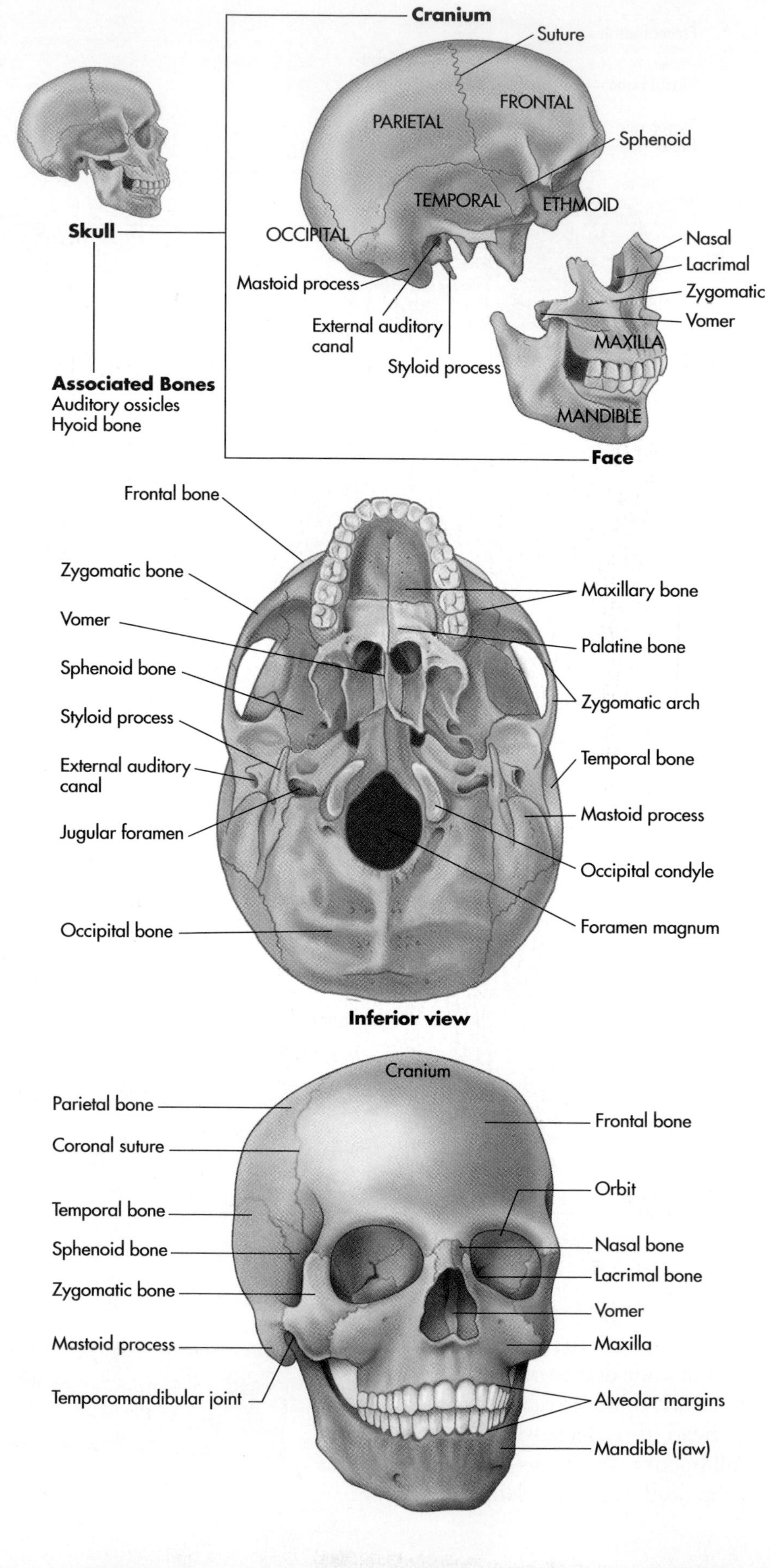
Cranium
Suture
FRONTAL
PARIETAL
Sphenoid
TEMPORAL
ETHMOID
OCCIPITAL
Skull
Nasal
Lacrimal
Zygomatic
Vomer
Mastoid process
External auditory canal
MAXILLA
Styloid process
Associated Bones
Auditory ossicles
Hyoid bone
MANDIBLE
Face
Frontal bone
Zygomatic bone
Maxillary bone
Vomer
Palatine bone
Sphenoid bone
Zygomatic arch
Styloid process
Temporal bone
External auditory canal
Mastoid process
Jugular foramen
Occipital condyle
Occipital bone
Foramen magnum
Inferior view
Cranium
Parietal bone
Frontal bone
Coronal suture
Orbit
Temporal bone
Nasal bone
Sphenoid bone
Lacrimal bone
Zygomatic bone
Vomer
Mastoid process
Maxilla
Temporomandibular joint
Alveolar margins
Mandible (jaw)

THE BONY THORAX

The bones of the chest form a thoracic "cage" that provides support and protection for the heart, lungs, and great blood vessels (see Figure 5–10 ■). This cage is flexible because of cartilagenous connections that allow for movement during the process of breathing. The sternum, or breastbone, is the anatomical location for conducting compressions of the heart during cardiopulmonary resuscitation (CPR). The sternum is composed of three distinct areas. The *manubrium* is the superior portion, and the *body* is the largest, central portion. The *xiphoid* is the final and inferior portion that ossifies (hardens) by age 25 and can be broken off if CPR is improperly performed. During cardiac compressions, the heart is compressed anteriorly by the body of the sternum and posteriorly by the bones of the vertebral column.

The thoracic cage consists of 12 pairs of elastic arches of bone called ribs. The ribs are attached by cartilage to allow for their movement when we breathe. The true ribs are pairs 1 to 7 and are called *vertebrosternal* because they connect anteriorly to the sternum and posteriorly to the thoracic vertebrae of the spinal column. Pairs 8 to 10 are called the false ribs, or *vertebrocostal,* because they connect to the costal cartilage of the superior rib and again posteriorly to the thoracic vertebrae. Rib pairs 11 and 12 are called the floating ribs because they have no anterior attachment.

THE SPINAL COLUMN

The spinal, or vertebral, column protects the spinal cord which is the superhighway for information coming to and from the central nervous system. The individual bones, or vertebrae, are numbered and classified according to the body region where they are located (see Figure 5–11 ■). For example, there are seven vertebrae found in the cervical or neck region, and they are numbered C-1 though C-7 respectively.

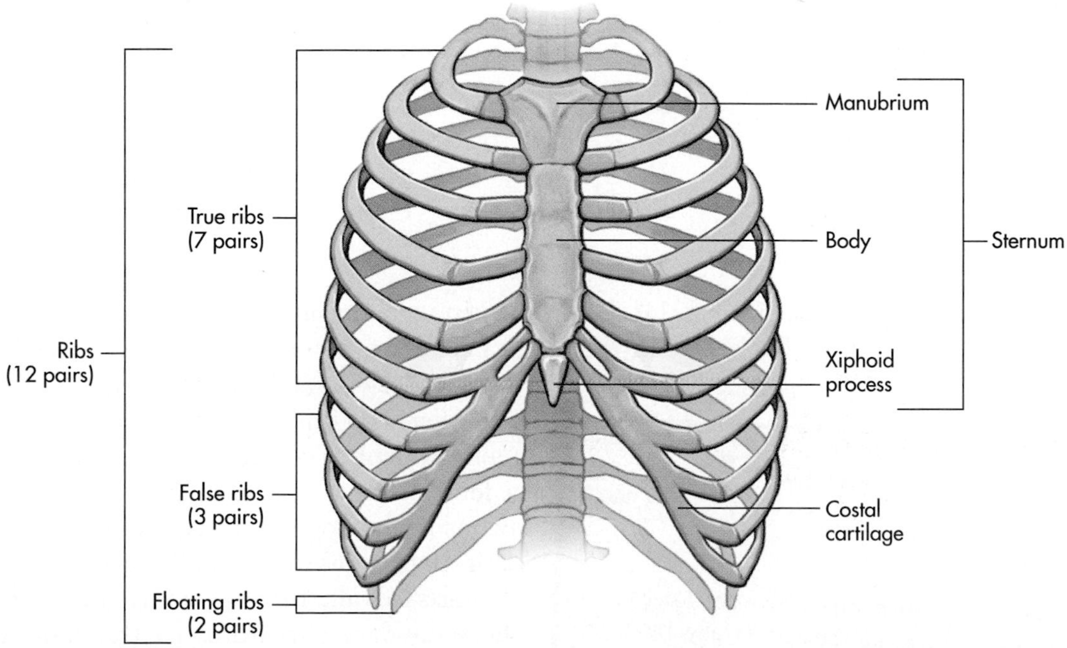

FIGURE ■ 5–10

The bony thorax.

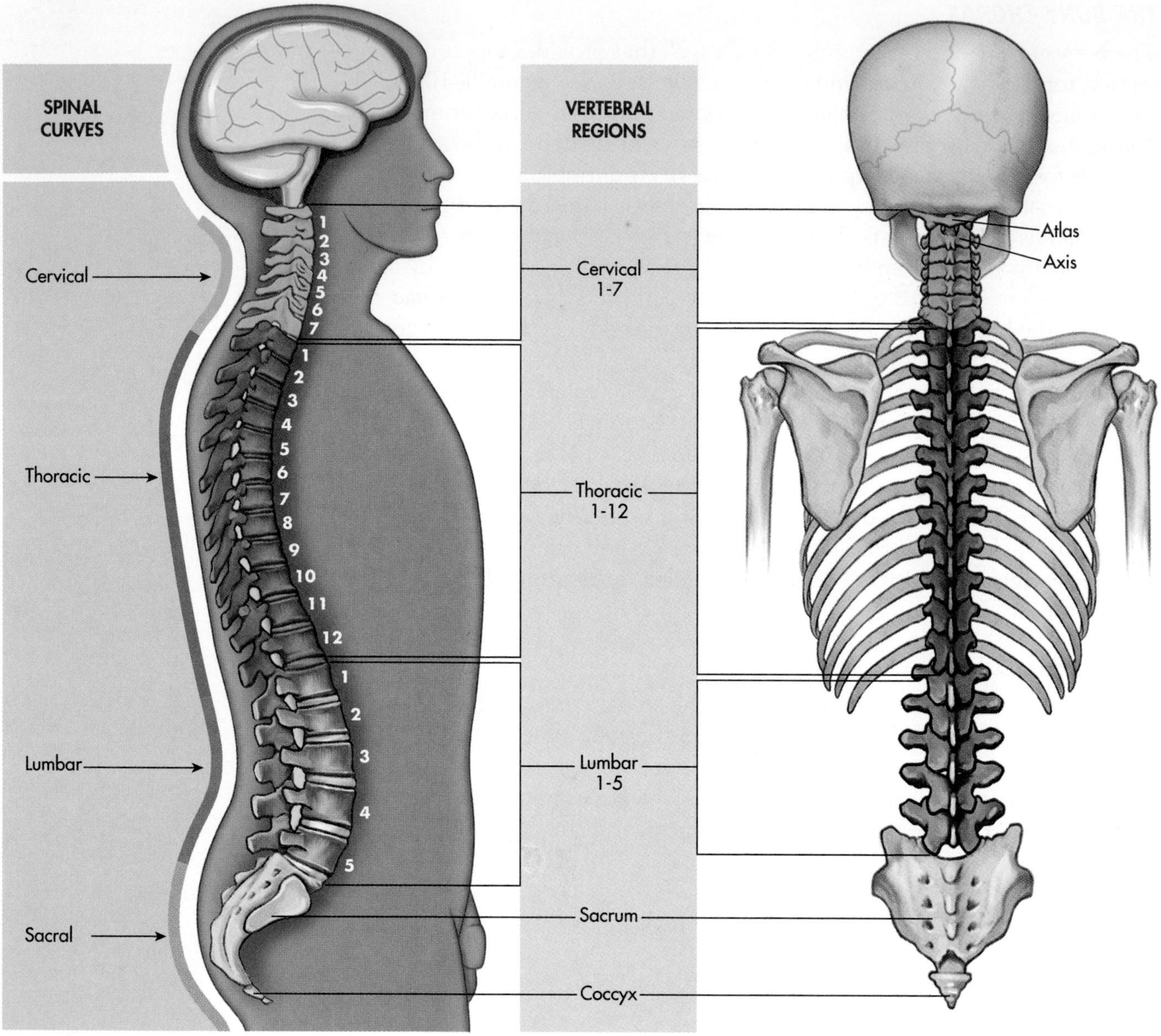

FIGURE ■ 5–11

The spinal column.

As seen in Figure 5–11, there are seven vertebrae in the neck region, twelve in the upper back, five in the lower back, five fused vertebrae in the mid-buttock region, and three to five small bones at the very end (tailbone). At birth, the vertebral column is concave to the front, like a fetal position (primary curvature) but bends in the opposite direction as the infant starts to raise and holds its head as well as starts to walk. In other words, there will be secondary curvatures by the time a child is 2. From 2 years onward, the vertebral column develops a secondary cur-

> *Learning Hint*
>
> **NUMBER OF VERTEBRAE**
>
> To remember the number of vertebrae in each region, think of 7 days in a week for cervical and 12 months in a year for thoracic. Finally, the lumbar region has the same number of vertebrae as digits on your hand (5).

vature in the neck, a primary curvature in the upper back, a secondary curvature in the lower back, and a primary curvature in the mid-buttocks and tailbone regions. If the body is not in balance, whether due to congenital deformity, trauma, poor posture, or disease, these curvatures may be exaggerated, leading to kyphosis (humpback, usually in the thorax) or lordosis (swayback, usually in the lumbar region). Scoliosis is when there is a sideways bend and sway in the spinal column. Figure 5–12 ■ illustrates these conditions.

> **5-6** For an animation on how bones heal, visit your CD-ROM for this chapter

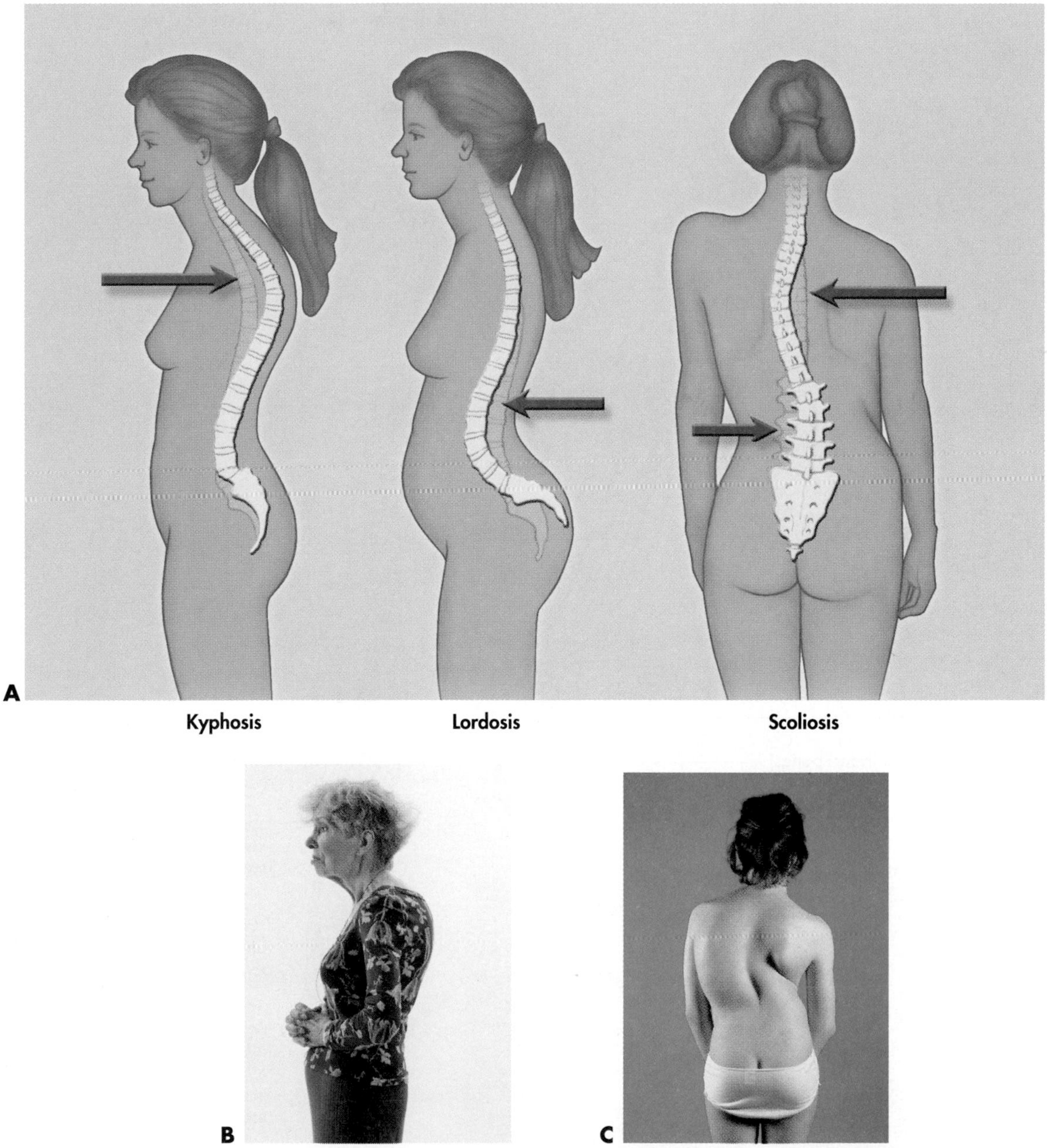

FIGURE ■ 5–12

Spinal disfigurements. (A) Spinal disfigurements compared to healthy spinal curves. (B) Kyphosis. (Source: Phototake NYC.) (C) Scoliosis. (Source: Photo Researchers, Inc.)

UPPER AND LOWER EXTREMITIES

The appendicular region consists of the arms and legs. Since these areas perform most of the body movement, the greatest number of sport-related injuries occur here. Please see Figure 5–13 ■, which shows the bones of the upper and lower extremities. These figures show the bony landmarks of the limbs and girdles, which will be beneficial in learning and understanding where the muscles discussed in Chapter 6 will attach.

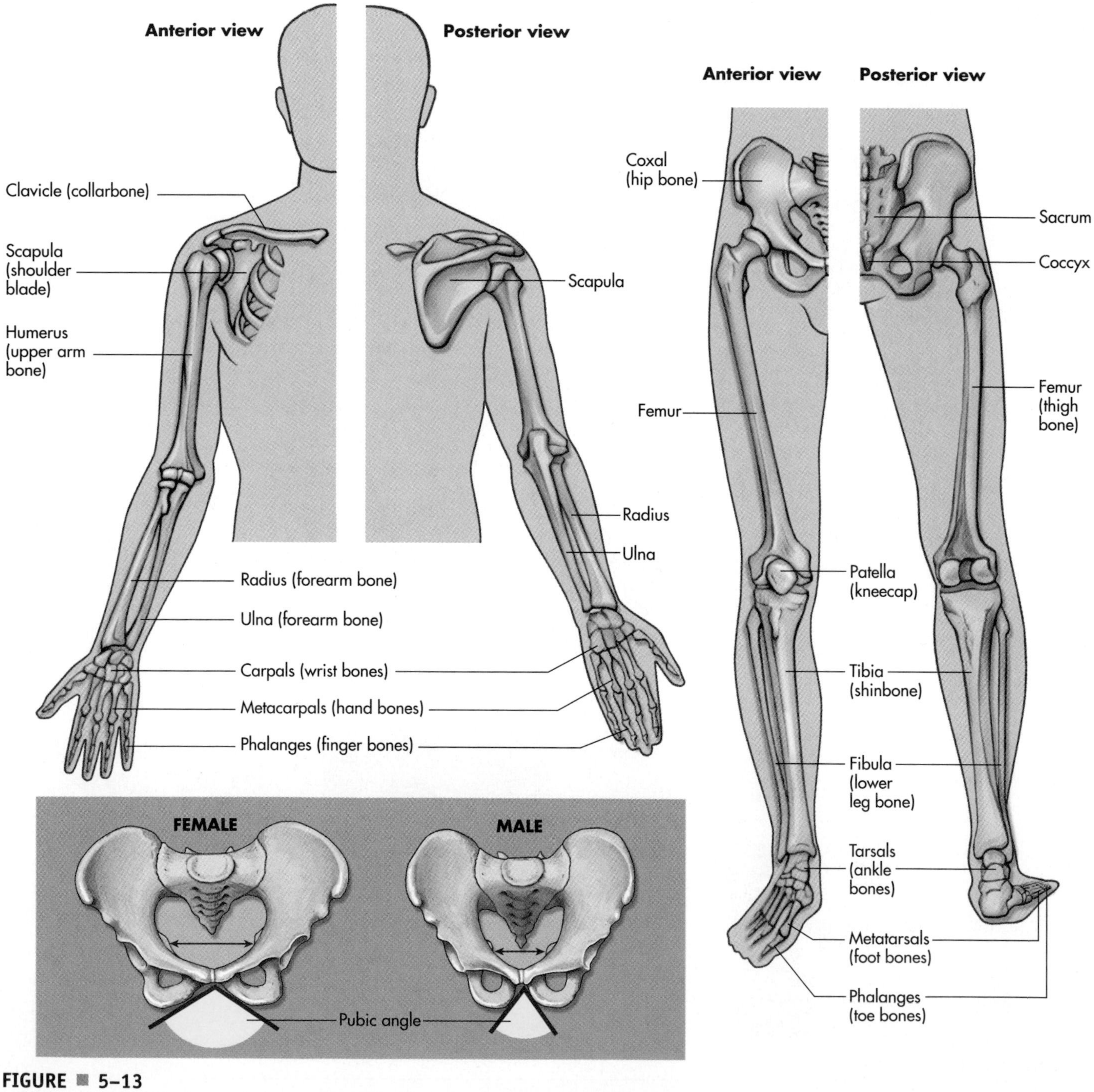

FIGURE ■ 5–13

Bones of the upper and lower extremities.

Notice that the pelvic girdle in women is different than in men. Women have a greater pubic angle that facilitates childbirth and also a relatively broad girdle to support the extra weight of the child. This difference can be used to identify the sex of a skeleton, such as in a murder case or an archeologic find.

TEST YOUR KNOWLEDGE 5-3

Answer the following:

1. What is the difference between the axial skeleton and the appendicular skeleton?
2. Which of the following bones is considered to be part of the axial skeleton?
   a. humerus
   b. patella
   c. femur
   d. sternum
3. The number of vertebra in the thoracic region is
   a. 5
   b. 7
   c. 12
   d. 120
4. Describe the difference between flexion and extension.

Flexion - move toward body
extension - move away

COMMON DISORDERS OF THE SKELETAL SYSTEM

All good things must come to an end, and the same can be said about the health of your skeletal system. In general, as the body ages, the cartilage and bones deteriorate. Although this is a natural process that we will all encounter, in some cases, we can slow the process down.

As the body ages, the chemical composition of cartilage changes. The bluish tint and flexibility of young skeletal cartilage changes to a more brittle, opaque-yellow colored form. Calcification or hardening of cartilage leads to brittleness. Articular cartilage, once it becomes brittle, doesn't function as well as young, healthy cartilage and can become arthritic. **Arthritis** is an inflammatory process of the joint or joints. The related tendons and ligaments also become less flexible, causing a decrease in the range of motion in joints.

Bone mass also changes with age. In our 50's, the skeleton begins to change: the breakdown of bone becomes greater than the formation of new bone. At the cellular level, the osteoclasts are tearing down more bone than the osteoblasts are forming. As a result, we see total bone mass beginning to gradually decrease. A micro-

5-7 For more information about bone diseases, go to your CD-ROM, which features videos concerning arthritis and osteoporosis.

Clinical Application

BONE FRACTURES

Chances are that you have broken a bone or know someone who has broken a bone in the past, but did you know that not all breaks are the same? Although there are a variety of fractures, the following are the more common ones. Please refer to the illustrations for further clarification.

A *hairline* fracture, which looks like a piece of hair on the X-ray, is a fine fracture that does not completely break or displace the bone. A *simple* or *closed* fracture is a break without a puncture to the skin. An individual in an accident who has a bone that is severely twisted may receive a *spiral* fracture. *Greenstick* fractures are incomplete breaks, which more often occur in children because they have softer, more pliable bones (like sapling branches) than adults (like seasoned twigs). If a bone is crushed to the point that it becomes fragmented or splintered, that is classified as a *comminuted* fracture. A fracture in which the bone is pushed through the skin is referred to a *compound* or *open* fracture. These fractures are particularly nasty because deep tissue has the potential to be exposed to bacteria once the bone is set into place, and, hence, the chance for infection in addition to the break is increased. See Figure 5-14 ■ for examples of common fractures.

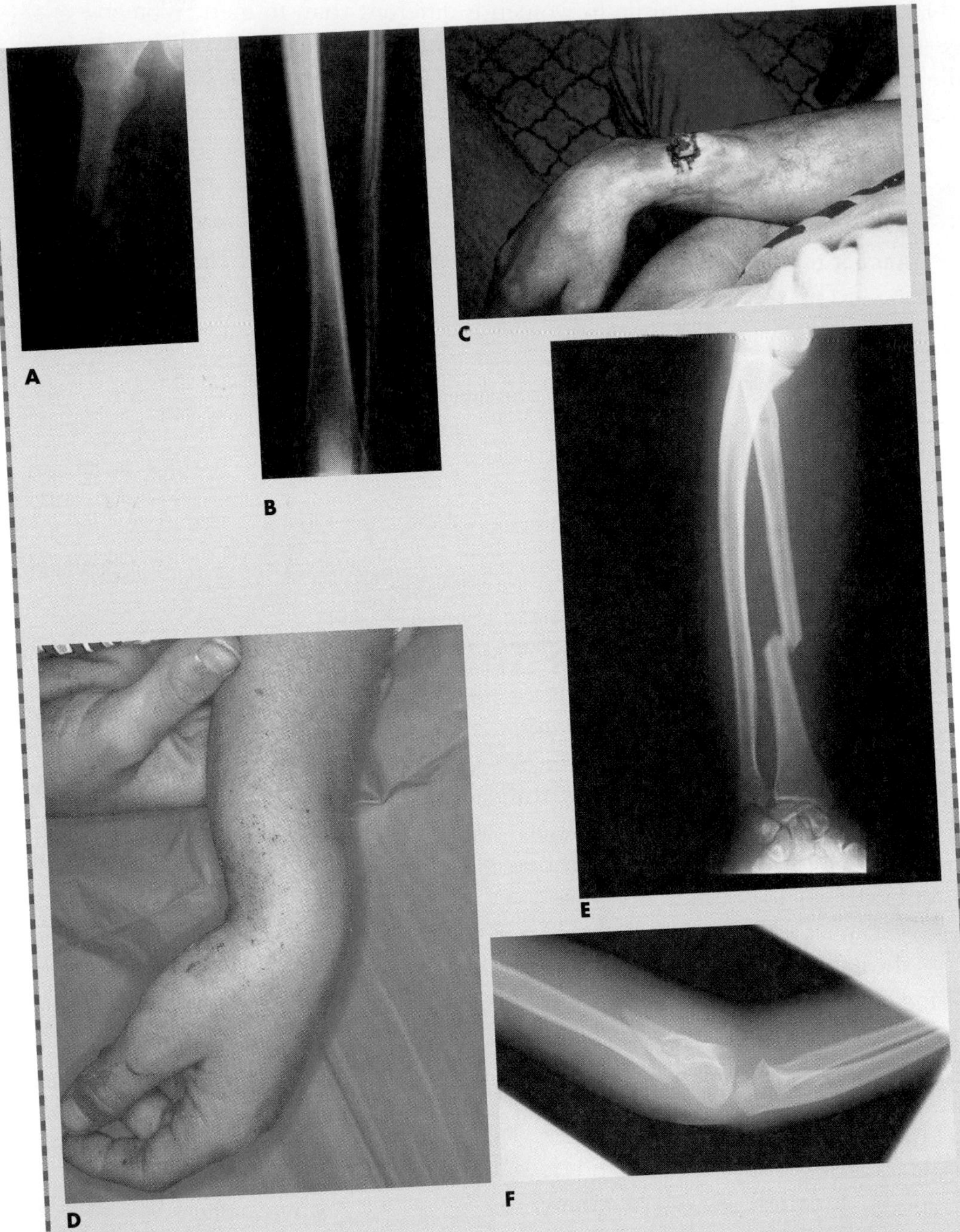

FIGURE 5–14

(A) Femur, AP view, comminuted fracture. (B) Tibia, simple, transverse fracture. (C) Open fracture of the wrist. (D) Displaced fracture of the distal radius. (Source: Charles Stewart & Associates.) (E) X-ray of complete fracture of the radius. (Source: James Stevenson/Science Photo Library/Photo Researchers, Inc.) (F) Fractured humerus. (Source: Charles Stewart & Associates.)

scopic examination of bones going through this process reveals increasing holes in the bone. This bone is lighter in weight and weaker than healthy bone, thereby making it more prone to breakage. Men appear to lose less than 25 percent of their bone mass, whereas women experience a 35 percent loss on average. This condition of decreasing bone density, known as **osteoporosis,** is a

TABLE 5–2 Bone Disorders

CLASSIFICATION	EXAMPLE(S)
Congenital disorders	abnormal curvature of the spine (kyphosis, lordosis, scoliosis), cleft palate, clubfoot
Degenerative disorders	osteoporosis
Infection	osteomyelitis
Nutritional disorders	osteomalacia (vitamin D deficiency), rickets (vitamin D deficiency), scurvy (vitamin C deficiency)
Secondary disorders	endocrine system dysfunction: gigantism, pituitary dwarfism
Trauma	bruises, fractures
Tumors	chondrosarcomas, myelomas, osteosarcomas

congenitus = *born together (the child and the condition)*

osteoporosis *(OSS tee oh poor OH siss)*
osteo = *bone*
porosis = *condition of porous nature*

osteomalacia *(OSS tee oh mah LAY she ah)*
malacia = *softening*

chondrosarcoma *(KON droe sar KOE ma)*
chondr = *cartilage*
oma = *tumor*
sarcoma = *tumor of connective tissue*

serious problem. As recently as 2003, about 3.6 *million* Americans suffered with this disease, and 6.3 *million* related doctor visits were made.

Even though bone mass loss is a natural process of aging, it can be slowed by a healthy lifestyle. It is important to consume the proper amount of dietary calcium to build strong bones in the first place. Proper calcium intake during the formative years, including the teenage years, and continued calcium consumption as the body ages, is crucial. Vitamin D is important because it allows your body to absorb ingested calcium from the digestive tract. As previously discussed, exercise (especially weight-bearing forms) also plays a vital role in developing and maintaining bones, so stay active. And, surprisingly, the excessive use of caffeine and cigarette smoking can reduce bone density. Individuals who, for a lifetime, consume two cups of black caffeinated coffee per day tend to show an increased loss of bone density, while cigarette smokers have shown a loss of 5 percent to 8 percent bone mineral density.

While osteoporosis and arthritis are big concerns, there are many more potential disorders of bones and joints. As you can see in Tables 5–2 and 5–3, these disorders can generally be classified by the following causative agents: congenital, degenerative, nutritional, secondary disorders, infection, inflammation, trauma, and tumors.

TABLE 5–3 Joint Disorders

CLASSIFICATION	EXAMPLE(S)
Degenerative disorders	osteoarthritis
Infection	gonococcal arthritis, rheumatic fever, septic arthritis, viral arthritis
Inflammation	bursitis, arthritis
Secondary disorders	immune system dysfunction: rheumatoid arthritis; metabolic dysfunction: gout
Trauma	ankle and foot injuries, dislocations, hip fractures, knee injuries

SUMMARY

Snapshots from the Journey

- In addition to providing support and protection for the body, the skeleton also produces blood cells and acts as a storage unit for minerals and fat.
- The 206 bones of the skeleton can be classified according to their shapes: long bones, short bones, flat bones, and irregular bones.
- Bone is covered with periosteum, which is a tough, fibrous connective tissue. In long bones, each bone end is called an *epiphysis*, and the shaft is called the *diaphysis*. The hollow region within the diaphysis is called the *medullary cavity* and stores yellow marrow.
- Compact bone is a dense, hard tissue that normally composes the shafts of long bones or is found as the outer layer of the other bone types. Spongy bone is different in that it contains irregular holes that make it lighter in weight and provides a space for red bone marrow, which produces red blood cells.
- Ossification is the formation of bone in the body. *Osteoprogenitor* cells are nonspecialized cells that can turn into *osteoblasts*, which are the cells that actually form bones. *Osteocytes* are considered mature bone cells that were originally osteoblasts. Osteoclasts originate from a type of white blood cell called a *monocyte*, found in red bone marrow. Osteoclasts break down bone material and help move calcium and phosphate into the blood.
- A thin band of cartilage forms an epiphyseal plate (often referred to as the *growth plate*), and as long as it exists, the length and width of the bone will increase.
- Cartilage is a special form of dense connective tissue that can withstand a fair amount of flexing, tension, and pressure and makes a flexible connection between bones, as between the breastbone and ribs. It also acts as a cushion between bones.
- Various types of joints join two or more bones and provide various types of movement. The point at which they join is called an articulation. Ligaments are very tough, whitish bands that connect from bone to bone to hold the joint together and can withstand heavy stress.
- The skeleton can be divided into two main sections. The axial skeleton includes bones of the bony thorax, spinal column, hyoid bone, bones of the middle ear, and skull. The appendicular skeleton is the region of your appendages (arms and legs) as well as the connecting bone structures of the hip and shoulder girdles.
- As we age, the chemical composition of cartilage changes, causing it to become more brittle. Articular cartilage that ages or becomes injured can lead to arthritis, which is an inflammatory process of the joint or joints. Bone mass also gradually decreases with age, beginning in a person's 50s. Even though this is a natural process of aging, it can be slowed by a healthy lifestyle.

Case Study

A somewhat frail 76-year-old female visits her physician's office for an annual check-up. Her social history shows she smokes a pack of cigarettes a day and she is a heavy coffee drinker. She has had several fractured bones in the last five years that required medical attention. During initial examination, measurements show that the patient has lost approximately an inch of height over the past year. She has also lost several pounds but states she still wears the same size clothes.

a. What possible bone disease do you think she is exhibiting?

b. Describe the bone changes in this condition on a macro and cellular level.

c. What treatments and/or lifestyle changes would you suggest?

REVIEW QUESTIONS

Multiple Choice

1. Your elbow is an example of which type of joint?
   a. hinge joint
   b. ball-and-socket joint
   c. gliding joint
   d. fibrous joint

2. The sternum is the correct medical term for which bone?
   a. shin bone
   b. breastbone
   c. shoulder blade
   d. collar bone

3. The end of a long bone is the
   a. diplodicus
   b. epiphysis
   c. condylcorn
   d. perla

4. As long as this exists, your bones will increase in length and width:
   a. Torger center
   b. ossifier
   c. Mantoux membrane
   d. epiphyseal plate

5. The aging process, excessive caffeine, and cigarette smoking can each contribute to this bone disease:
   a. ligamental stenosis
   b. osteoporosis
   c. cartilentious dementia
   d. ossification

Fill in the Blanks

1. Name three large appendicular bones: ______________, ______________, and ______________.
2. List three places where cartilage is found in the body: ______________, ______________, and ______________.
3. ______________ is a liquid found in joints that keeps them lubricated.
4. The specialized cells that constantly rebuild bone are called ______________.
5. These specialized cells are needed to tear down bone: ______________.

Short Answer

1. Describe the difference in function between tendons and ligaments.

____

____

____

____

2. List three functions of the skeletal system.

____

____

____

____

3. What happens to our skeletal system as we age?

____

____

____

____

4. What are the functions of cartilage?

____

____

____

____

Suggested Activities

1. Using art paper, cut out, label, and assemble bones to create a full-sized skeleton.

2. Act out various range-of-motion exercises and perform and identify different joint movements.

3. Visit the library and research how the human skeleton has evolved, also noting the differences between male and female skeletons, posture changes, and changing shapes of various bones.

5-8 Now that you have completed your journey through this chapter, please go to the CD-ROM for interactive games and puzzles concerning the medical terms and concepts contained in this chapter. By playing the games you will reinforce your learning of medical terminology in a fun way.

Greetings from THE MUSCULAR System

Movement for the Journey

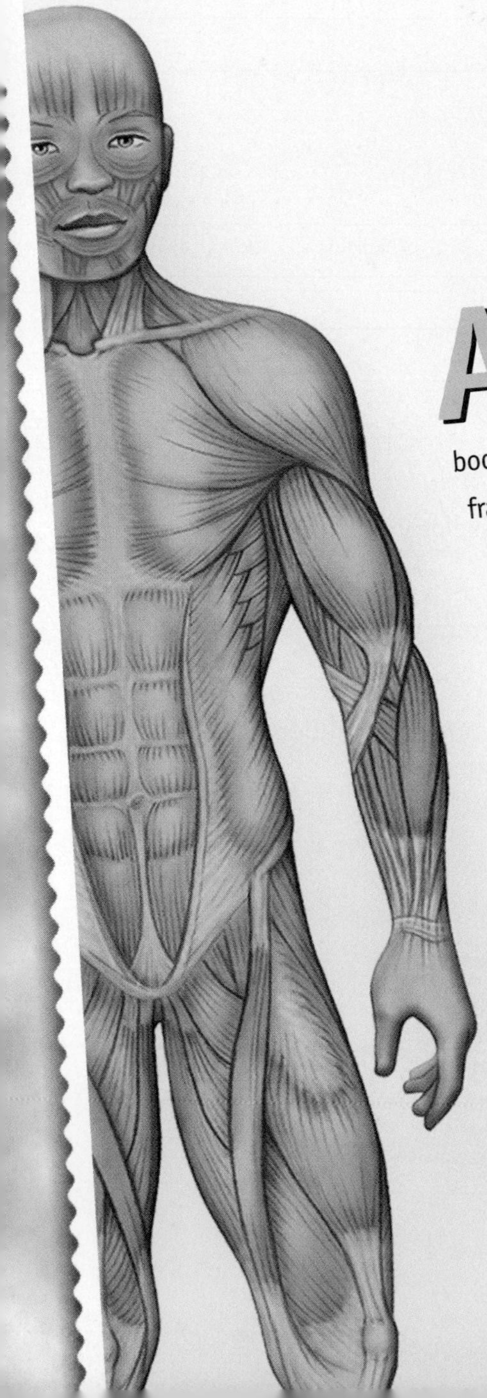

As we continue our journey of exploration, we obviously need a transportation method to reach our destination. We can go by a plane, train, or automobile. However, no matter what transportation system we use, we must utilize the body's muscular system to get to the vehicle. While the skeletal system provides the framework for the human body, the body also needs a system that allows movement, or locomotion, which is the job of the muscular system. The movement we are most familiar with is the use of our external muscles to walk, run, or lift objects. This external movement allows us to explore all the wonderful sites throughout our journey and, yes, even to turn the pages as we journey through this book. However, movement is also required within the body. This internal movement occurs when food, air, waste products, and body fluids such as blood must all be transported within our bodies. For example, if you drink some bad water on our journey, the smooth muscles in your digestive tract will rapidly pass it through your system to be expelled in the form of urgent diarrhea. Different types of specialized muscles within the muscular system allow for both external and internal movement. This chapter defines and contrasts the different muscle types needed for external and internal body movement.

Chapter 6

LEARNING OBJECTIVES

At the completion of your journey through this chapter, you will be able to:

- Differentiate the three major muscle types
- Discuss the function of tendons and ligaments
- Explain the difference between voluntary and involuntary muscles
- Describe the various types of skeletal muscle movement
- Identify and explain the components of a muscle cell
- Describe the chemical activities required for muscle movement
- Contrast the activity of cardiac, smooth, and skeletal muscle
- Discuss common disorders of the muscular system

MULTIMEDIA APPLICATIONS

CD-ROM Interactive Exercises

- Interactive 3-D animation of labeled muscle groups of specified regions: head and neck; upper limb, forearm, and hand; shoulder and arm; trunk and abdomen; pelvis, hip and thigh; lower limb and foot, 6-1
- Interactive drag-and-drop exercise of myofibril structures, 6-2
- Animation of cellular muscle contraction, 6-3
- Videos of various massage therapy techniques, 6-4
- Videos of muscle atrophy and muscular dystrophy, 6-5
- Interactive games and puzzles, 6-6

www.prenhall.com/colbert

- Professional Profiles:
  - Kinesiology
  - Physical Therapy
  - Occupational Therapy
  - Massage Therapy
- Related Internet Links

Pronunciation Guide

Correct pronunciation is important in any journey so that you and others are completely understood. Here is a "see and say" Pronunciation Guide for the more difficult terms to pronounce in this chapter.

acetylcholine (ah SEET ul KOE leen)
actin (ak TIN)
adenosine triphosphate (ah DEN oh sin)
ataxia (ah TAK see ah)
atrophy (AT roh fee)
diaphragm (DYE ah fram)
electromyography (ee lek troh my OG rah fee)
fibromyalgia (fie bro my AL jeuh)
flaccid (FLAS sid)
flexion (FLEK shun)
glycogen (GLIE co jin)
Guillian-Barré syndrome (Gey ya bar RAY)
hypertrophy (high PER troh fee)
intercalated discs (in ter KUH late ed)
muscular dystrophy (MUSS kyoo lahr DISS troh fee)
myalgia (my AL jee ah)
myasthenia gravis (my as THEE nee ah)
myofibril (my oh FIE bril)
myosin (MY oh sin)
rigor mortis (RIG er MORE tiss)
sarcomeres (SAR koh meres)
sphincters (SFING ters)
tetanus (TET an nuss)
tonus (TONE us)

OVERVIEW OF THE MUSCULAR SYSTEM

Because of the numerous functions they must perform, muscles come in many shapes and sizes. The structure of the muscle matches its function, as you will shortly see.

Types of Muscles

Muscle is a general term for all contractile tissue. The term muscle comes from the Latin word *mus*, which means "mouse," because the movement of muscles looks like mice running around under our skin. The contractile property of muscle tissue allows it to become short and thick in response to a nerve impulse and then to relax once that impulse is removed. This alternate contraction and relaxation is what causes movement. Muscle cells are elongated and resemble fibers such as in clothing. Muscular tissue is constructed of bundles of these muscle fibers. These fibers are approximately the diameter of human hair. Under the direction of the nervous system, all of the muscles provide for motion of some type for your body.

The body has three major types of muscles: **skeletal, smooth,** and **cardiac.** We begin with a general description and comparison of these three muscle types and then get more specific about each type.

Skeletal muscles are voluntary muscles, which means they are under conscious control and derive their name because they are attached to the bones of the skeletal system. The fibers in skeletal muscles appear to be striped and are therefore called *striated* (striped) muscle. These muscles allow us to perform external movements—running, lifting, or scratching, for example. These are the muscles we try to develop through exercise and sports and also so we look good at the beach.

Unlike skeletal muscle, smooth muscle is involuntary and not under our conscious control. It is also called smooth muscle because it does not have the striped appearance of skeletal muscles. This involuntary muscle is found within certain organs, blood vessels, and airways. Because it is the muscle of organs, it is sometimes called *visceral muscle*. Smooth muscle allows for the internal movement of food (*peristalsis*) in the case of the stomach and other digestive organs. Smooth muscle also facilitates the movement of blood by changing the diameter of the blood vessels (vasoconstriction and vasodilation), and also the movement of air by changing the diameter of the airways found in our lungs.

The third type of muscle is the specialized cardiac muscle, which has a striated appearance. This muscle type is found solely in the heart. It makes up the walls of the heart and causes the heart to contract. These contractions cause the internal movement (circulation) of blood within the body. Fortunately, cardiac muscle, like smooth muscle, is an involuntary muscle. Imagine if we had to think each time in order for our heart to beat. Figure 6–1 ■ contrasts the three types of muscles found within the body. We will now explore each of these types of muscles in further depth.

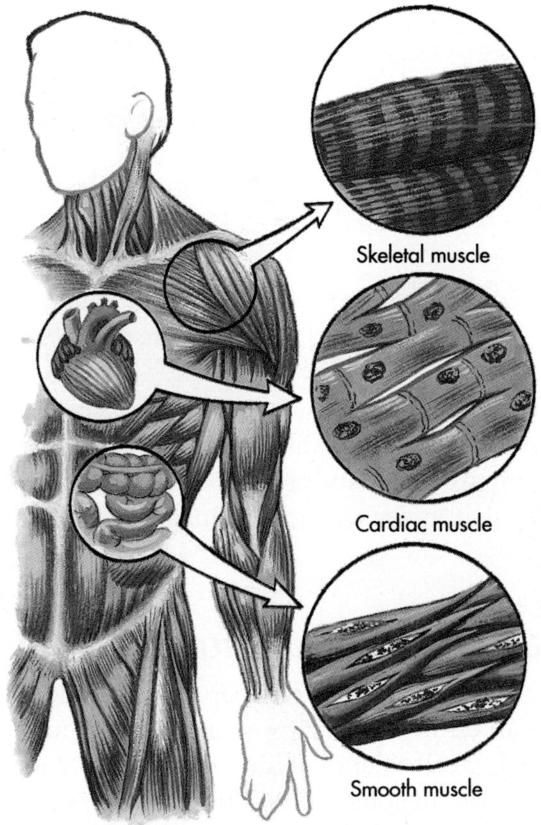

FIGURE ■ 6–1

The three types of muscle: Skeletal, Cardiac, and Smooth.

TEST YOUR KNOWLEDGE 6-1

Choose the best answer:

1. The biceps muscle is an example of a
   a. smooth muscle
   b. cardiac muscle
   c. skeletal muscle
   d. dinosaur muscle

2. Smooth muscle is found in all the following *except*
   a. airways
   b. digestive system
   c. blood vessels
   d. heart

3. Which types of muscles are striated?
   a. smooth and cardiac
   b. cardiac and skeletal
   c. skeletal and smooth
   d. smooth only

Amazing Body Facts

MUSCLES

- Muscles make up almost half the weight of the entire body.
- The size of your muscles depends on how much you use them and how big you are. This is why ice skaters have large leg muscles.
- Individual elongated muscle cells can be up to 12 inches, or 30 centimeters, in length.
- At about the age of 40, the number and diameter of muscle fibers begin to decrease, and by age 80, 50 percent of the muscle mass may be lost

Skeletal Muscles

Skeletal muscles are attached to bones and provide movement for your body. Remember from Chapter 5, The Skeletal System **tendons** are fibrous tissues that usually attach skeletal muscle to bones and that **ligaments** attach bone to bone. Note that some muscles can attach to a bone or soft tissue without a tendon. Such muscles use broad sheets of connective tissue called *aponeurosis*. This type of connection is found, for example, in some facial muscles and the tongue.

Skeletal muscle is also known as voluntary muscle because its movement can be controlled by conscious thought. The numerous skeletal muscles found throughout the body are responsible for movement, maintaining our body posture, and heat generation. See Figure 6–2 ■, which shows some of the major muscles found in the human body.

SKELETAL MUSCLES OF SPECIFIC BODY REGIONS

Many times on a journey, we need a roadmap for reference. These roadmaps are often big maps of an entire state. However, there are also inserts of specific cities that give much greater detail. Think of Figure 6–2 as our "state map" of the anterior and posterior major muscles. The following series of "city maps" will provide you with greater detail.

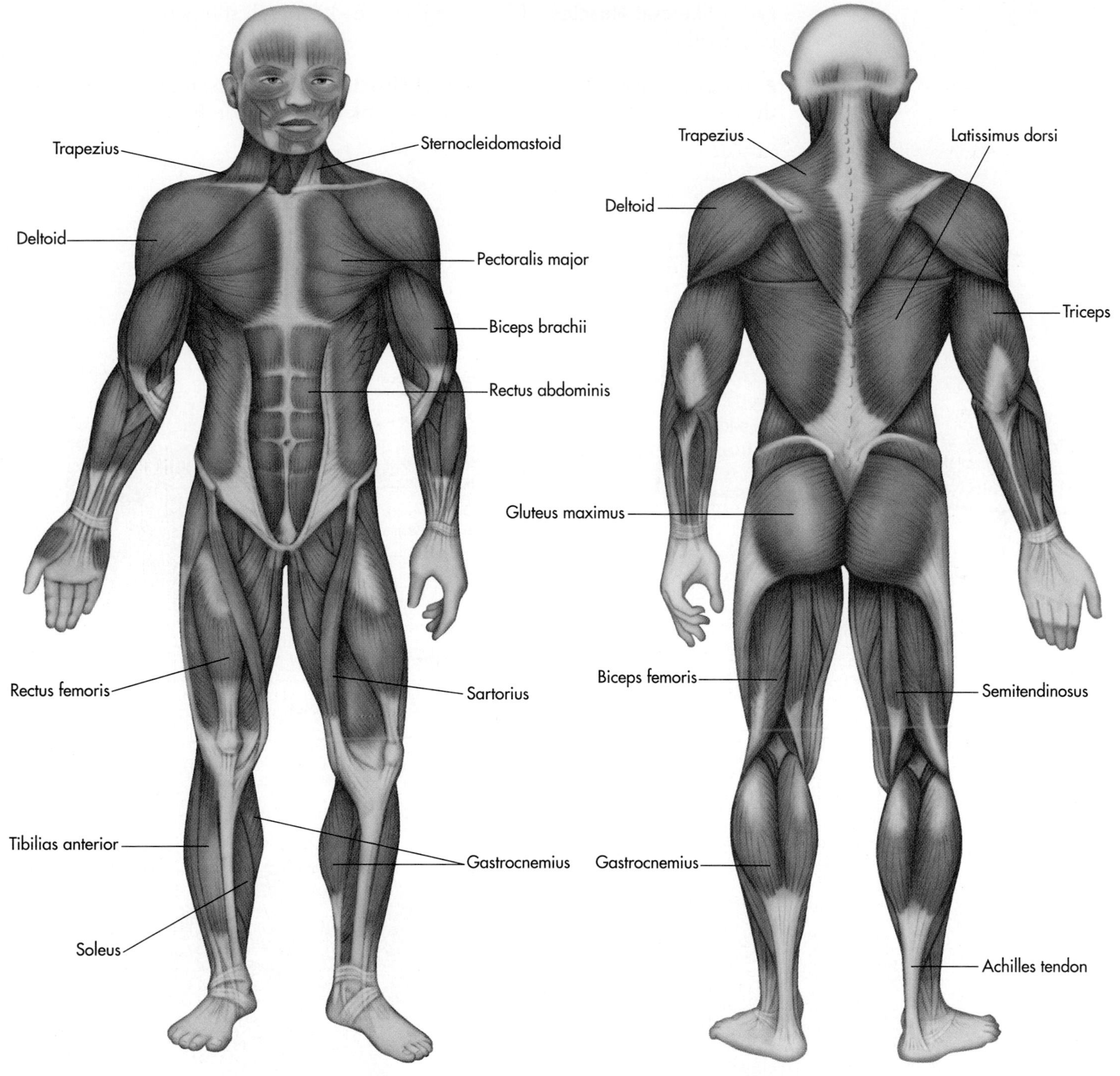

FIGURE ■ 6–2

Anterior and posterior view of major muscles.

Facial Skeletal Muscles Please see Figure 6–3 ■ which shows the facial skeletal muscles.

Anterior and Posterior Trunk Skeletal Muscles Now, take an in-depth look at the muscles of the anterior and posterior trunk of the body in Figure 6–4 ■.

> **6-1** To view 3-D labeled animations of more specific muscles of body regions in greater detail, please go to your CD-ROM for this chapter. The distinct regions covered are the head and neck; upper limb, forearm, and hand; shoulder and arm; trunk and abdomen; pelvis, hip, and thigh; and lower limb and foot. In addition, you can play an interactive drag-and-drop exercise to label various muscles.

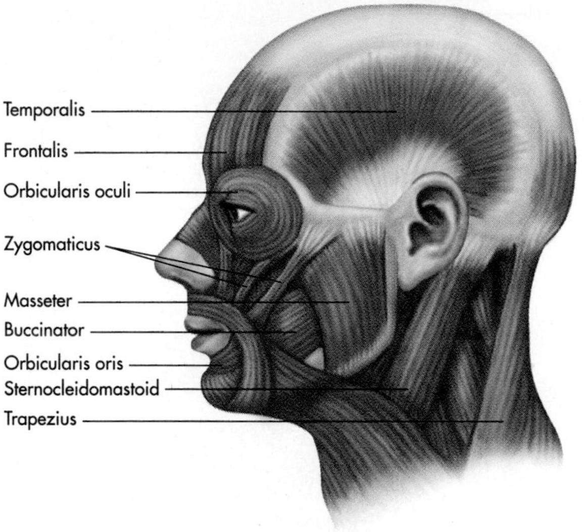

FIGURE ■ 6–3

Skeletal facial muscles.

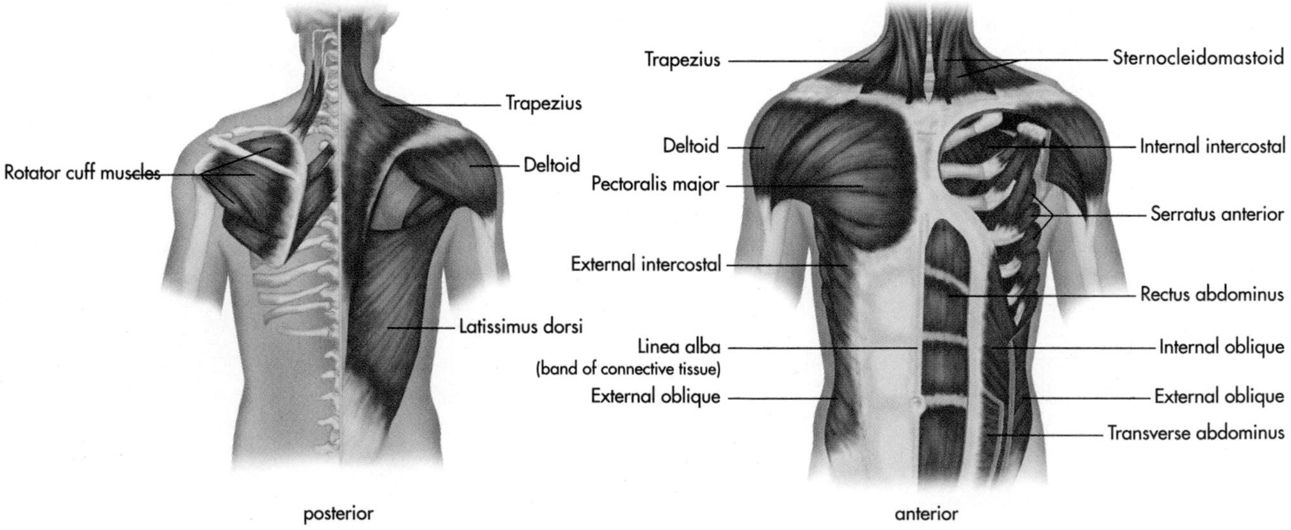

FIGURE ■ 6–4

Skeletal muscles of the posterior and anterior trunk.

Skeletal Muscles of the Arm and Shoulder Moving out to the peripheral area of the body, we now zoom in on the skeletal muscles of the hand, arm, and shoulder in Figure 6–5 ■.

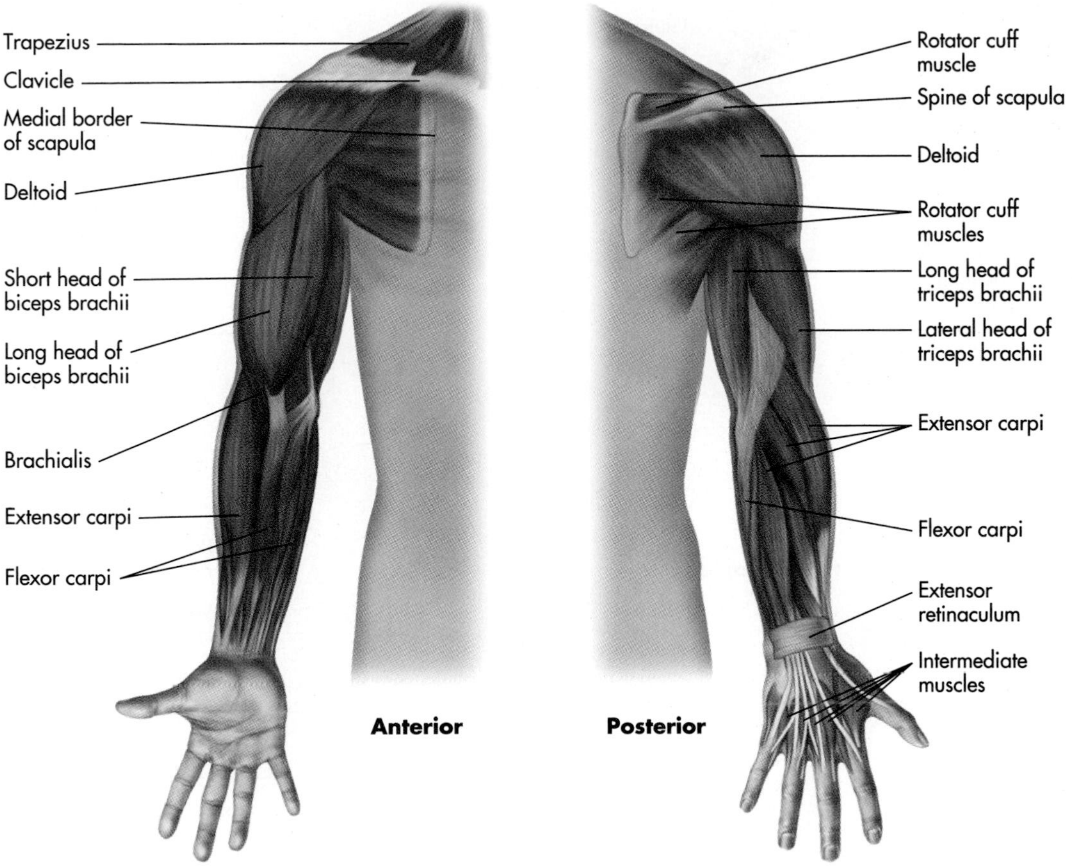

FIGURE ■ 6–5

Skeletal Muscles of the shoulder, arm, and hand.

Skeletal Muscles of the Legs We finish our tour with the skeletal muscles of the hip and leg in Figure 6–6 ■.

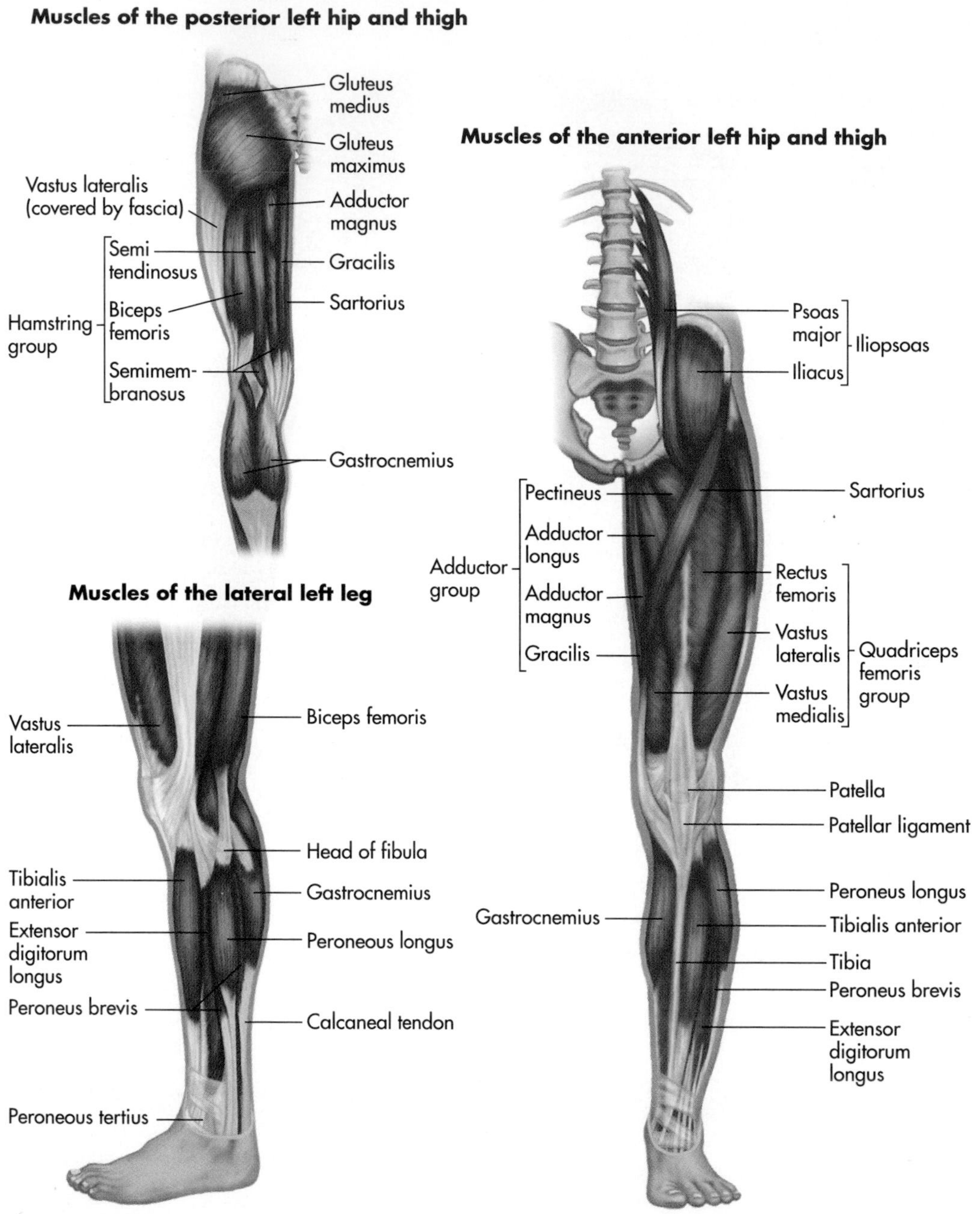

FIGURE ■ 6–6

Skeletal muscles of the hip and leg.

SKELETAL MUSCLE MOVEMENT

The body requires several different types of movement for various tasks. This movement is accomplished through the coordination of the contraction and relaxation of various muscles.

Contraction and Relaxation

Movement of the body is a result of the contraction (shortening of the muscle fibers) of certain muscles and the relaxation of others. Consider the act of bending your arm so your fingers touch your shoulder. To really learn the concept, actually bend your arm and touch your fingers to your shoulder while resting your other hand on your biceps muscle. In order to do this, your forearm is drawn to your shoulder as a result of the contraction of your biceps. Did you feel the shortening and bulging of the biceps? Muscles, either by themselves or in muscle groups that cause movement, are known as **agonists** or **primary movers.**

agonist *(AG on ist)*

The chief muscle causing the movement is the primary mover, and in this example it is the biceps muscle. Typically, as your muscle contracts, one of the bones will move (lower forearm) while the other (humerus) will remain stationary. The end of the muscle that is attached to the stationary bone is the **point of origin,** and in this example, it is at the shoulder area. The muscle end that is attached to the moving bone is the **point of insertion;** in this example, it is near the elbow (see Figure 6–7 ■).

Other muscles can assist this movement, such as some of the muscles in the hands and wrist. These are called **synergistic** muscles because they assist the primary mover. To straighten out that same arm requires you to relax your biceps

synergistic *(sin er GIS tic)*

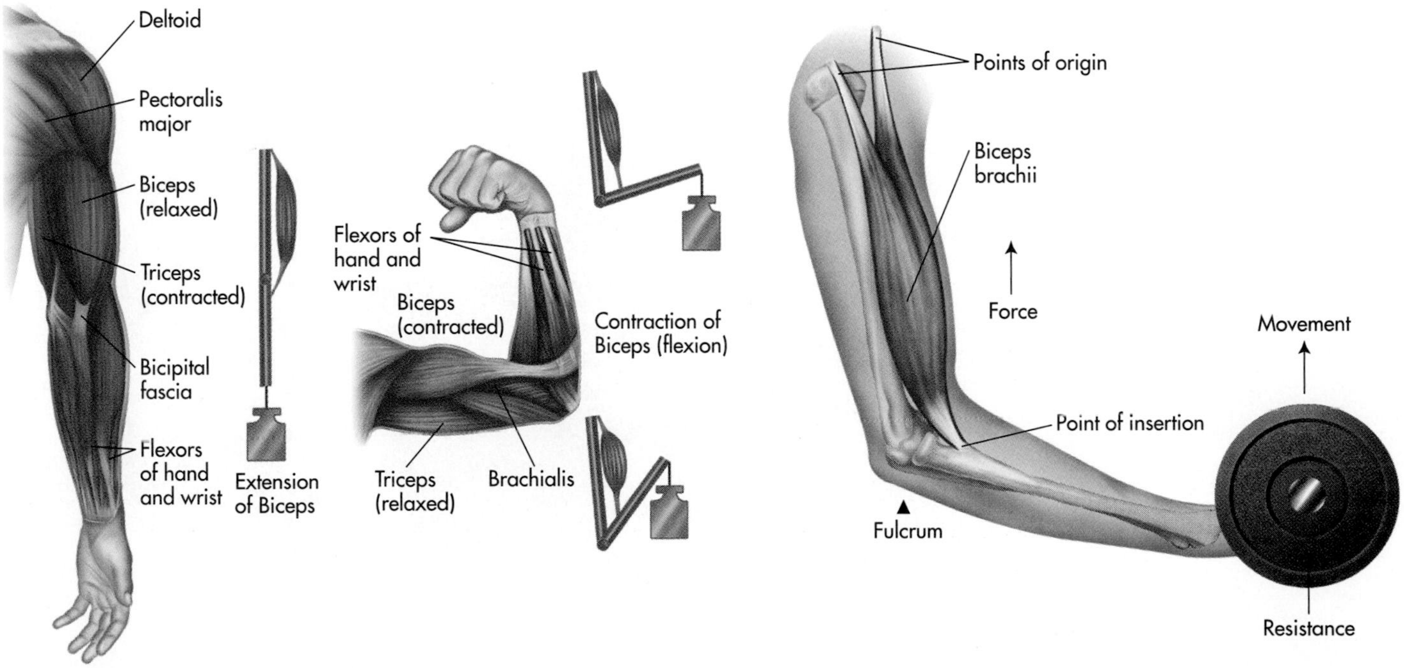

FIGURE ■ 6–7

Coordination of antagonist muscles to perform movement.

muscle and to contract the triceps muscles. Since these muscles cause movement in the opposite direction when they contract, they are called **antagonists.** This brings us to an important concept. All movement is a result of contraction of primary movers and relaxation of *opposing* muscles. In our example, you cannot forcefully contract the biceps muscles and straighten out your arm. Try it. Again, see Figure 6–7 for the illustration of the antagonistic muscles of the biceps and triceps.

One very important skeletal muscle that controls our breathing is the **diaphragm.** This dome-shaped muscle separates the abdominal and thoracic cavities and is responsible for performing the major work of bringing atmospheric air into our lungs. Exactly how this process occurs is discussed in detail in Chapter 13, The Respiratory System. The diaphragm is unique in that it is under both voluntary and involuntary control. You don't have to think each time you breathe, but you can voluntarily change the way you breathe. Figure 6–8 ■ shows the major muscle of breathing.

Movement Terminology

abduction *(ab DUK shun)*
  ab = *away, as in abduct or abnormal*

adduction *(add DUK shun)*
  ad = *toward*

Certain terms are utilized to describe the direction of body movement. In Chapter 5, we discussed movement as it relates to joints in the skeletal system. In this chapter, we briefly discuss movement as it relates to muscles. **Rotation** describes circular movement that occurs around an axis. Rotation occurs, for example, when you turn your head from left to right or right to left. **Abduction** means to move *away* from the midline of the body. When you raise your arm to point when giving directions, you are performing abduction. **Adduction** occurs when you produce a movement that moves *toward* the midline of the body.

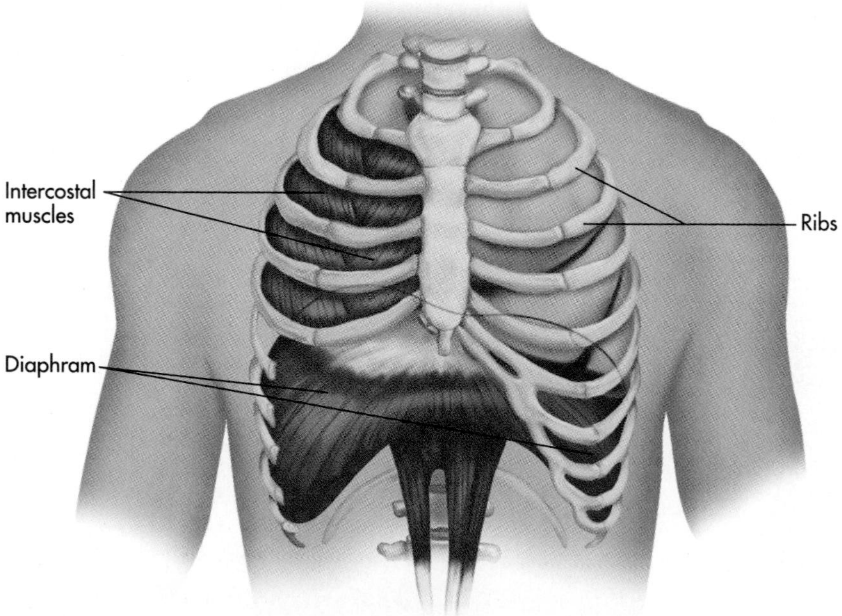

FIGURE ■ 6–8

The diaphragm: The major muscle of breathing.

When you bring your arm back down to your side from pointing, you are performing adduction.

extension *(eks TEN shun)*

flexion *(FLEK shun)*

Extension is a term used for *increasing* the angle between two bones connected at a joint. Extension is needed when you kick a football. In this situation, extension occurs when your leg straightens out during the kick. The muscle that straightens the joint is called the **extensor muscle. Flexion** is the opposite of extension. In this situation, you *decrease* the angle between two bones. Flexion occurs when you bend your legs to sit down. Flexion and rotation occur when you get your arm into position to arm wrestle. The muscle that bends the joint is called the **flexor muscle.** In this case a picture is worth a thousand words or at least the 124 words used to explain these concepts. Figure 6–9 ■ illustrates these movements.

Applied Science

KINESIOLOGY

Kinesiology is the study of muscles and movement. A kinesiologist is one who studies movement and can employ therapeutic treatment (kinesitherapy) by specific movements or exercises. Go to the companion Web site to learn more about the profession of kinesiology.

TEST YOUR KNOWLEDGE 6-2

Give the correct body movement term for the following activities:

1. looking right and left at a stop sign ______________
2. doing a split ______________
3. Patting yourself on the back for labeling all these activities correctly ______________
4. the first movement in curling a weight ______________
5. returning the weight from the curled position to your side ______________

MUSCULAR MOVEMENT AT THE CELLULAR LEVEL

Exactly how is muscular contraction and relaxation accomplished? How does the muscle tissue cause a coordinated and smooth contraction? Let's look in more detail at how muscles work.

The Functional Unit of the Muscle

We have talked about muscles on a macro, or very large, scale. For example, how does that large biceps you've developed from working out contract when you touch your shoulder? Now, let's explore the makeup of the individual muscle fiber to learn exactly how this contraction takes place. As stated previously, muscle consists of elongated cells called muscle fibers, which can be up to 12 inches, or 30 centimeters, in length. Each muscle fiber contains functional units

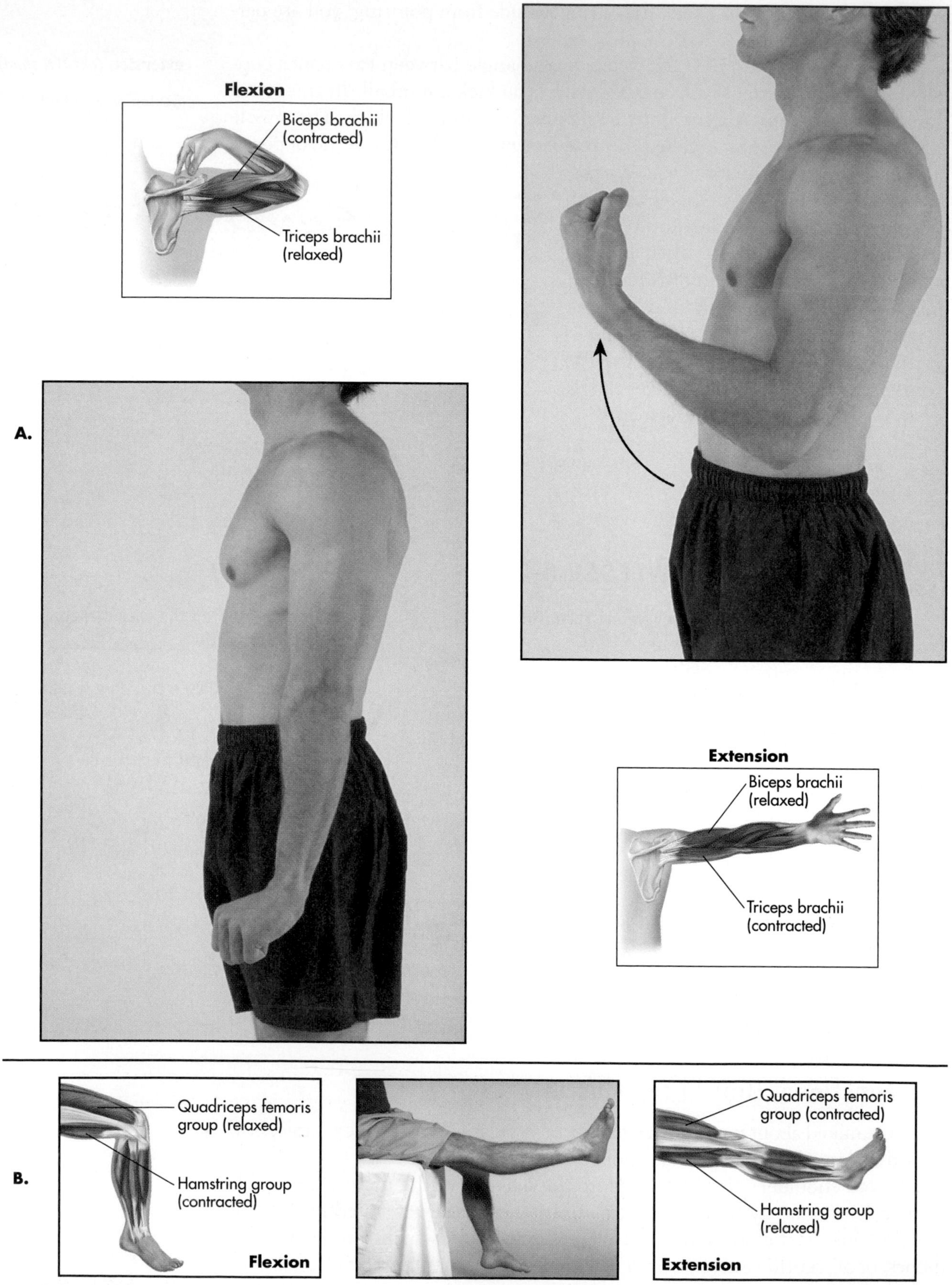

FIGURE ■ 6–9

The types of skeletal movement. (A) Flexion and extension of left forearm. (B) Flexion and extension of the leg.

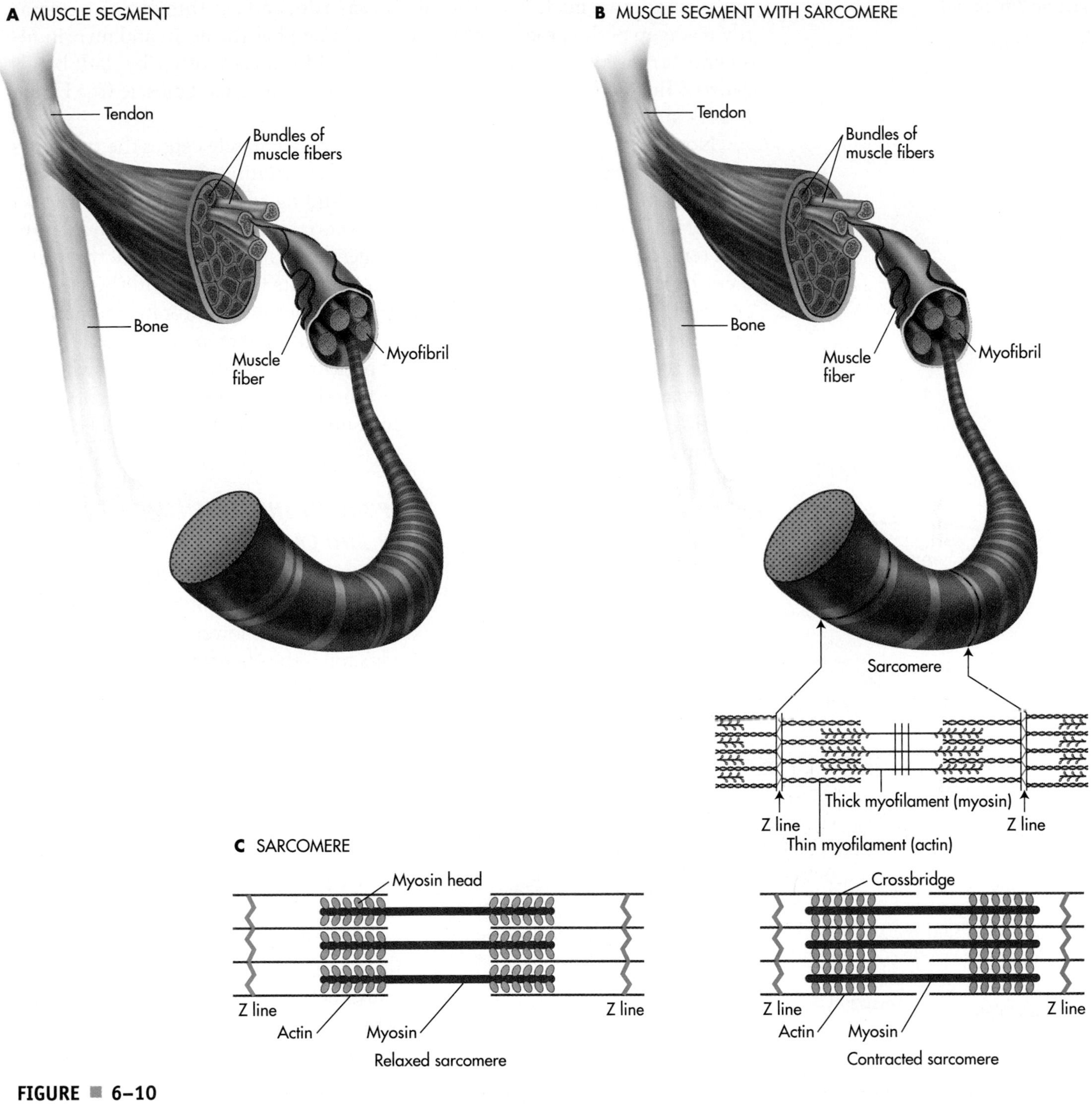

FIGURE ■ 6–10

(A) The muscle segment. (B) The muscle segment with sarcomere. (C) Relaxed and contracted sarcomeres.

called **myofibrils,** and several of these myofibrils can be bundled together to form a muscle cell. The muscle myofibril can be considered a strand of metal, and these strands of metal can be put together to form a cable, which would be a muscle segment (see Figure 6–10A ■).

myofibril *(my ah FIE bril)*
myo = *muscle*

In order for contraction to take place, each fiber must possess many functional contractile units called **sarcomeres.** Each fiber has the ability to contract because of the makeup of the sarcomere. Each sarcomere unit has two types of threadlike structures called thick and thin myofilaments. The thick

sarcomeres *(SAR ca meres)*

myosin *(MY oh sin)*

actin *(AK tin)*

myofilaments are made up of the protein **myosin,** and the thin ones are primarily made up of the protein **actin.** The sarcomere has the actin and myosin filaments arranged in repeating units separated from each other by dark bands called **Z lines,** which give the striated appearance to skeletal muscle (see Figure 6–10A and B).

Note in Figure 6–10C that the contraction of a muscle causes the two types of myofilaments to slide toward each other, shortening each sarcomere and, therefore, the entire muscle. Picture a tube sliding within a tube, such as on a trombone. This sliding filament action and corresponding contraction requires that temporary connections, or crossbridges, be formed between the thick filament heads (myosin heads) and the thin filaments (actin) to pull the sarcomere together. Once the crossbridges form, the myosin heads rotate and pull the actin toward the center of the sarcomere. When the sarcomere relaxes, the filaments return to their resting or relaxed position. Visualize a raised drawbridge, where cars cannot pass. In order to be functional, the cross-connection—or lowering of the drawbridge—must occur, similar to the crossbridges needed to be formed for a muscle contraction.

6-2 To perform an interactive drag-and-drop exercise on labeling myofibril structures, please go to your CD-ROM.

IMPORTANT INGREDIENTS: ATP AND CALCIUM

In the previous analogy of the drawbridge, consider that a toll must be paid in order for the bridge to lower and connect. The body's toll is the energy molecule **adenosine triphosphate** (ATP) and **calcium** (Ca), which are needed for contraction and relaxation. ATP provides the energy to help the myosin heads form and break the crossbridges with actin. When the muscle is relaxed, calcium is stored away from the actin and myosin in the **sarcoplasmic reticulum** (SR), which is a specialized series of interconnecting tubules and sacs that surround each myofibril. When the muscle is stimulated, calcium is released from the SR and causes actin, myosin, and ATP to interact, which causes the contraction. When calcium leaves the muscle and returns to the SR, the crossbridges are broken and the muscle relaxes.

Applied Science

INTERRELATEDNESS OF NEUROMUSCULAR SYSTEM

Contraction of a skeletal muscle requires the coordination of both the muscular and nervous systems. The initiation of a skeletal muscular contraction requires an impulse from a motor neuron of the nervous system to trigger a release of a neurochemical transmitter called **acetylcholine** (ACh), which opens the sodium channels and sets the process of muscle contraction into motion. This all occurs at the neuromuscular junction. The nervous system's role in this action and the neuromuscular connection are fully explored in Chapters 8 and 9.

acetylcholine *(ass SET ul KOE leen)*

When the nervous system tells the muscle to contract, the signal causes the muscle fiber to open what are called *sodium ion channels*. Sodium ions flow through these channels into the muscle fibers. This causes the muscle fibers to become excited and calcium is released from the sarcoplasmic reticulum. The calcium, now free in the cytoplasm of the muscle fiber, helps myosin bind with actin in the presence of ATP. The calcium is then pumped back into the sarcoplasmic reticulum for storage and the muscle now relaxes.

6-3 Cellular muscular contraction may be hard to visualize. Please go to your CD-ROM to see an animation of cellular-level muscle contraction that visually pulls all of these concepts together.

Have you ever heard of a dead body rising from a table or showing signs of movement? This may sound like the opening for a movie about zombies or the "undead." Actually, it is a normal physiologic process called **rigor mortis** that can be explained by science and not by science fiction.

rigor mortis *(RIG er MORE tiss)*

When a body dies, all the stored calcium cannot be pumped back into the sarcoplasmic reticulum. Therefore, excess calcium remains in the muscles throughout the body and causes the muscle fibers to shorten (contract) and stiffen the whole body. In addition, ATP is not present in a dead body to break the cross bridges. This stiffening process of the entire body is termed rigor mortis.

www.prenhall.com/colbert
Not only do the skeletal muscles facilitate movement but, integrated with the nervous system, they provide support for posture while standing or sitting. Promoting balance and posture, along with proper muscle function, is one of the responsibilities of physical therapists. Physical therapists perform many therapies, such as range of motion (ROM) exercises, to ensure full muscle movement. Occupational therapists assist patients in utilizing and adapting their muscle function to perform activities of daily living and improving their quality of life. Massage therapists work directly on the muscles to aid in their relaxation and optimal functioning. To learn more about these professions, please go to the Web site for this chapter.

TEST YOUR KNOWLEDGE 6-3

Fill in the blank.

1. The region between two Z lines is called a ______________.
2. The thick myofilament needed for muscle contraction is called ______________
3. The thin myofilament needed for muscle contraction is called ______________
4. The two ingredients needed for cross bridges to form and break are ______________ and ______________

VISCERAL OR SMOOTH MUSCLE

We've introduced the concept of smooth muscle earlier in this chapter, now let's take a closer look. **Visceral muscle,** or **smooth muscle,** is found in the organs (except the heart) of your body, such as your stomach and other digestive organs, and in the blood vessels and bronchial airways. The ability for smooth muscle to expand and contract plays a vital role in many of the body's internal workings. For example, the vital sign blood pressure can be affected by whether the blood vessels get larger in diameter (**vasodilate**) or get smaller in diameter (**vasoconstrict**). Vasodilation can lead to decreases in blood pressure due to smooth muscle relaxation in the vessel that allows it to enlarge. The enlarged vessel has less resistance to flow, and the blood pressure therefore goes down. Conversely, vasoconstriction can cause increased blood pressure due to the smooth muscle contraction that restricts the blood vessel.

vasodilate *(vase oh DIE late)*

vasoconstrict *(vase oh CON strict)*

Learning Hint

SMOOTH MUSCLE REGULATION OF BLOOD PRESSURE

In considering blood pressure, visualize a large highway. If one lane is taken away (vasoconstriction), the same number of cars must now fit through one less lane, leading to traffic congestion (increase in pressure). If you open up another lane (vasodilate), you relieve some of this pressure.

As another example, during an asthma attack, smooth muscles in the airways of the lungs constrict, making it difficult to get air in and out of the lungs. This is what causes the wheezing sound heard during an attack.

sphincters *(SFING ters)*

A special type of smooth muscle, called **sphincters,** are found throughout your digestive system. These donut-shaped muscles act as doorways to let materials in and out by alternately contracting and relaxing. For example, the sphincters of the stomach act like doors that open up to allow food in from the esophagus and also to allow food out into the small intestine. Have you ever swallowed a large amount of bread or stuffing and had it get stuck on the way down to your stomach? This is a painful reminder that there is a sphincter that must relax and open to allow food to enter your stomach. The muscles of the digestive system are discussed in greater depth in Chapter 15, The Gastrointestinal System.

Smooth, or visceral muscles, are involuntary muscles and do not contract as rapidly as skeletal muscles. Skeletal muscles, once stimulated, can contract 50 times faster than smooth muscle. Because of their slower activity and lower metabolic rate, smooth muscles receive only moderate amounts of blood. Once injured, smooth muscle rarely repairs itself and, instead, forms a scar.

CARDIAC MUSCLE

Cardiac muscle forms the walls of the heart. The contraction of cardiac muscle squeezes blood out of the chambers of the heart, causing the blood to circulate through your body. Cardiac muscle is involuntary muscle. Remember, this means that we don't have to consciously think about making our heart contract every time we need a heartbeat. Cardiac muscle fibers are somewhat shorter than the other muscle types. Since the heart must work constantly until you die, the cardiac muscles must receive a generous blood supply to get enough oxygen and nutrition, as well as to get rid of waste. In fact, cardiac muscle has a richer supply of blood than any other muscle in the body. The cardiac muscle fibers are connected to each other by **intercalated disks.** Because of this connection, as one fiber contracts, the adjacent one contracts, and so on. This is similar to the domino effect or the human wave at a football stadium if done correctly. A wave of contraction occurs, allowing blood to be squeezed out of the heart and into the body. This directed wave is important for a full and effective emptying of the blood within the heart. Imagine if everyone squeezed the tube of toothpaste in the middle: think of all the wasted toothpaste that would be left in the tube and how happy the toothpaste manufacturers would be. See Figure 6–11 ■.

Clinical Application

MUSCLE TONE

Have you ever had a cast on for an extended period of time? When it is removed, the arm or leg is much smaller and weaker than the limb without the cast. Why does this occur? Normally, all muscles exhibit muscle tone (**tonus**). Tonus is the partial contraction of a muscle with a resistance to stretching. Athletes who exercise regularly have increased muscle tone, making their muscles more pronounced. The muscle fibers in an athlete increase in diameter (**hypertrophy**) and become stronger. Hypertrophy refers to increased growth or development. When muscles are not used, they begin to lose their tone and become flaccid (soft and flabby). For example, if a patient is required to remain in bed (bedfast) for an extended period of time, his or her muscles waste away (**atrophy**) from the lack of use. One of the reasons patients are gotten out of bed as soon as possible is to prevent atrophy from occurring. If skeletal muscle is damaged, it can regenerate itself. However, if the damage is extensive, then a scar forms.

intercalated disk *(in ter KUH late ed)*
hyper = *greater than normal*
trophy = *growth or development*
a = *without*

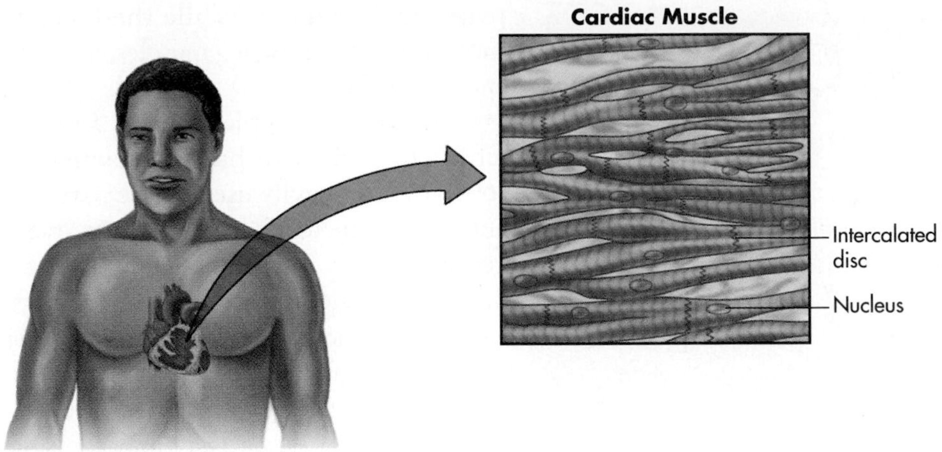

FIGURE ■ 6–11

Heart and intercalated disks.

Cardiac muscle does not regenerate after severe damage; this leads to tissue death such as occurs in a severe heart attack. If the blood supply going to the heart from the coronary arteries is blocked, cardiac muscle damage can occur, causing scarring of the heart. Scar tissue does not help the healthy muscles of the heart to contract. If the scarred area is extensive, the remaining cardiac muscle may not be sufficient to pump blood efficiently. An individual with scarred cardiac muscle may have a severely diminished cardiac output, which could lead to severe disability or even death.

MUSCULAR FUEL

Muscle, like all tissue, needs fuel in the form of nutrients and oxygen in order to survive and function. The body stores a carbohydrate called **glycogen** in the muscle. Glycogen is always on reserve waiting to be converted to a usable energy source. When needed, the muscle can convert glycogen to **glucose,** which releases energy for the muscle to function. Muscles with very high demands (such as leg muscles) also store fat and use it as energy. The release of energy also produces heat, and this is why strenuous or prolonged exercises can overheat our bodies.

glycogen *(GLIE co jin)*

glucose *(GLOO kohs)*

The higher-demand muscles not only use fat as an energy source, but have a much richer blood supply than do less demanding muscles. These muscles are needed for endurance, such as required by long-distance running. The richer blood supply carries extra oxygen to hardworking muscles, giving those muscles a darker color.

Some muscles, such as those in the hand, have fewer heavy demands placed on them and need only a small supply of blood. These muscles utilize the local blood supply for glucose and the glycogen stored within. They therefore have a lighter color. These muscles are faster but do not have the endurance capabilities that heavily used muscles have. Next time you take a long walk, keep

Applied Science

MAINTAINING A CORE BODY TEMPERATURE

Not only do muscles produce movement, but they help maintain posture, stabilize joints, and produce heat. Producing heat is important in maintaining the body core temperature. As the energy-rich ATP is used for muscle contraction, three fourths of its energy escapes as heat. This process helps to maintain body temperature by producing heat when muscles are utilized. This is why your temperature rises when exercising and also why you shiver when you are very cold. Shivering is your body's way of saying it is too cold and it needs to generate a lot of heat via many muscle contractions (shivering). In turn, this increases the body temperature.

pumping your hand. While the hand can move faster than the leg muscles, it will tire more quickly.

Another example can be found in chicken. Because its breast and wing muscles are not heavily used, those parts contain white meat. It's legs, however, endure constant use, and the meat is therefore dark. By contrast, a woodcock, a migratory bird that must fly long distances (endurance), has dark breast meat. Now you know why a chicken's breast meat is white. When is the last time you saw a chicken flying overhead?

COMMON DISORDERS OF THE MUSCULAR SYSTEM

myalgia *(my AL jee ah)*
fibromyalgia *(fie bro my AL je)*
algia = *pain*

Because there are so many muscles covering the entire body and they are constantly being used, many disorders occur within this system. Here are just a few examples. **Myalgia** means pain or tenderness in a muscle. **Fibromyalgia** may be one of the most common musculoskeletal disorders affecting woman under age 40, but it is still not fully understood. Symptoms include aches, pains, and muscle stiffness with specific tender points on anatomical regions of the body. The exact cause is unknown, and it is linked with other diseases such as chronic fatigue syndrome.

6-4 With physical activity and the daily stress of life, muscles often become sore and fatigued. Massaging techniques help to stimulate blood flow and relax tense muscles. To understand more about various massage techniques, please go to your CD-ROM to view videos showing several different methods of massage.

ataxia *(ah TAK see ah)*
a = *without*
tax/o = *coordination*

lysis = *destruction of*

Ataxia is a condition in which the muscles are irregular in their actions or there is a lack of coordination. **Paralysis** is the partial or total loss of the ability of voluntary muscles to move. Sometimes it might be temporary; other times it might be permanent. A muscle that involuntarily suddenly and violently contracts for a prolonged period of time is said to have a **spasm** or **cramp.** A spasm can occur in a single muscle or in a muscle group. **Sprains** are tears or breaks in ligaments, while **strains** are tears or injury in muscles and tendons. A common running exercise–related inflammatory condition of the extensor muscles and surrounding tissues of the lower leg is **shin splints.**

itis = *inflammation of*

electromyography *(elec troh my AH graf ee)*
electro = *electric*
myo = *muscle*
graphy = *graph*

A **hernia** occurs when there is a tear in the muscle wall and an organ of the body protrudes through that opening. **Tendinitis** is a condition in which tendons become inflamed. Muscular disorders can be diagnosed by **electromyography** (EMG), a test in which a muscle or group of muscles are stimulated with an electrical impulse. This impulse causes a muscle contraction. The strength of that muscle contraction is then recorded. Certain diseases can alter the strength of muscles.

Due to the close integration of the two systems, several diseases involve both the *nervous* system and the *muscular* system—hence, the term **neuromuscular** disease. **Myasthenia gravis** is a neuromuscular disease in which the patient exhibits gradually increasing profound muscle weakness. The first symptom of this disease is often the drooping of one or both of the upper eye lids. There is also progressive paralysis. Interestingly, tendon reflexes almost always remain. **Muscular dystrophy** is an inherited muscular disease in which muscle fibers degenerate and there is progressive muscular weakness. **Guillain-Barré syndrome** is a disorder of the *peripheral* nervous system that causes *flaccid* paralysis (limp muscles) and the loss of reflexes. Interestingly, the paralysis is usually *ascending*, meaning that it starts in the feet or lower extremities and progresses toward the head. Paralysis usually peaks within 10 to 14 days. Eventually, most patients return to normal, although it may take several weeks or months. **Tetanus,** on the other hand, creates rigid paralysis. With this disease, any type of minor stimulus can cause muscles to go into major spasm. The stimulus can be something as simple as a loud noise or turning on a light in a room. Tetanus is a result of toxins produced by a bacteria found in the ground and can be spread by any type of puncture, not just the "rusty nail" many were warned about when they were kids. Smooth and cardiac muscle conditions are discussed in upcoming chapters.

muscular dystrophy
(MUSS kyoo lahr DISS troh fee)
dys = *difficult*
trophy = *growth or nourishment*

Guillain-Barré syndrome
(Gey ya bar RAY)

Applied Science

A USEFUL APPLICATION OF A DEADLY TOXIN

Botulism is a potentially deadly disease caused by food poisoning with the *Clostridium botulinum* bacteria. Science has found a way to utilize the poison generated by this bacteria for medical and cosmetic treatment. Small amounts of botulinus toxin are injected into facial muscles to stop previously untreatable facial twitching. The toxin basically paralyzes the muscles. The same toxin is used to treat wrinkles without the use of surgery and is known as Botox injections.

tetanus *(TETT ah nuss)*

6-5 To view videos on muscle atrophy and muscular dystrophy, please go to your CD-ROM for this chapter.

SUMMARY

Snapshots from the Journey

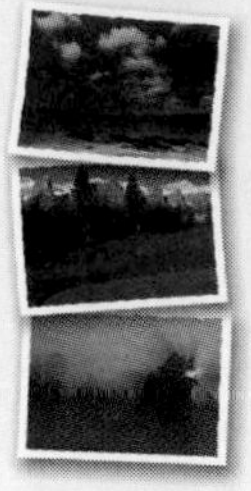

- The three main types of muscles are skeletal, smooth, and cardiac.
- Skeletal muscle is striated, or striped, voluntary muscle that allows movement, stabilizes joints, and helps maintain body temperature.
- Smooth muscle is a nonstriated involuntary muscle found in the organs of the body and linings of vessels; it facilitates internal movement within the body.
- Cardiac muscle is involuntary, striated muscle found only in the heart.
- All movement is a result of contraction of primary movers and relaxation of opposing muscles.
- Muscles usually attach to bones via tendons.
- Large muscles consist of many single muscle fibers comprised of myofibrils. The smallest functional contractile unit is called a sarcomere.
- Each sarcomere unit contains the two threadlike contractile proteins myosin and actin.
- Muscles contract as the actin and myosin protein filaments, in the presence of ATP and calcium, form crossbridges that cause the filaments to slide past each other, thereby causing the muscle to contract or shorten.
- There is an interrelation between the nervous and muscular systems in which the motor neuron of the nervous system initiates the activity of muscle contraction through the release of a neurotransmitter.
- There are many common diseases and conditions of the muscles, and because the nervous system is so closely related, there are also many common neuromuscular diseases.

Case Study

A 30-year-old patient complains of ascending flaccid paralysis that began with tingling in the toes and muscle weakness. This individual presented to the emergency department after the leg weakness became so profound that he could barely walk, and now he notices his arms weakening. Loss of reflexes were also noted.

a. What disease do you think this is? ______________________________
b. Knowing that this patient is losing the ability to use skeletal muscles, what life-threatening condition could occur? ______________________________
c. What vital signs must you monitor? ______________________________
d. Why is muscle atrophy a problem? ______________________________
e. What areas of patient care must be addressed? ______________________________
f. What is the likely prognosis? ______________________________

REVIEW QUESTIONS

Multiple Choice

1. Another name for voluntary muscle is
   a. skeletal
   b. smooth
   c. cardiac
   d. nonstriated

2. Which structure does *not* contain smooth muscle?
   a. blood vessels
   b. heart
   c. digestive tract
   d. bronchi

3. Most skeletal muscles attach to bones via
   a. ligaments
   b. joints
   c. flexors
   d. tendons

4. The state of partial skeletal muscle contraction is known as
   a. homeostasis
   b. muscle tone
   c. partialus contractus
   d. flexerus

5. Cardiac muscle
   I. is a voluntary muscle
   II. has intercalated disks to assist contraction
   III. regenerates after injury
   VI. lines the blood vessels

   a. I only
   b. I and II
   c. II only
   d. I, II, III, VI

Fill in the Blank

1. A sudden or violent muscle contraction is a ______________.

2. Partial or total loss of voluntary muscle use is ______________.

3. A tear in the muscle wall through which an organ can protrude is a ______________.

4. The body stores a carbohydrate called ______________ in the muscle; it can be converted to a usable energy source.

5. ______________ means pain or tenderness in the muscle.

Short Answers

1. List the three major muscle types and give an example of each.

____

____

____

____

2. Contrast the term hypertrophy and atrophy and give an example of how each situation could occur.

3. Explain how vasoconstriction and vasodilation affect blood pressure.

4. Explain the steps needed in a skeletal muscle contraction.

Suggested Activities

1. Pick a major muscle group and discuss how your life would be different if that group could not function properly due to a disease or accident.

2. Bodybuilding requires an extensive knowledge of muscles and muscle groups. Demonstrate five different exercises and the different muscles they would develop.

3. Pair off with a partner and perform various muscle movements showing rotation, abduction, adduction, extension, and flexion. See if your partner can accurately classify each motion.

6-6 Now that you have completed your journey through this chapter, please go to the CD-ROM for interactive games and puzzles concerning the medical terms and concepts contained in this chapter. By playing the games you will reinforce your learning of medical terminology in a fun way.

Greetings from THE INTEGUMENTARY System

The Protective Covering

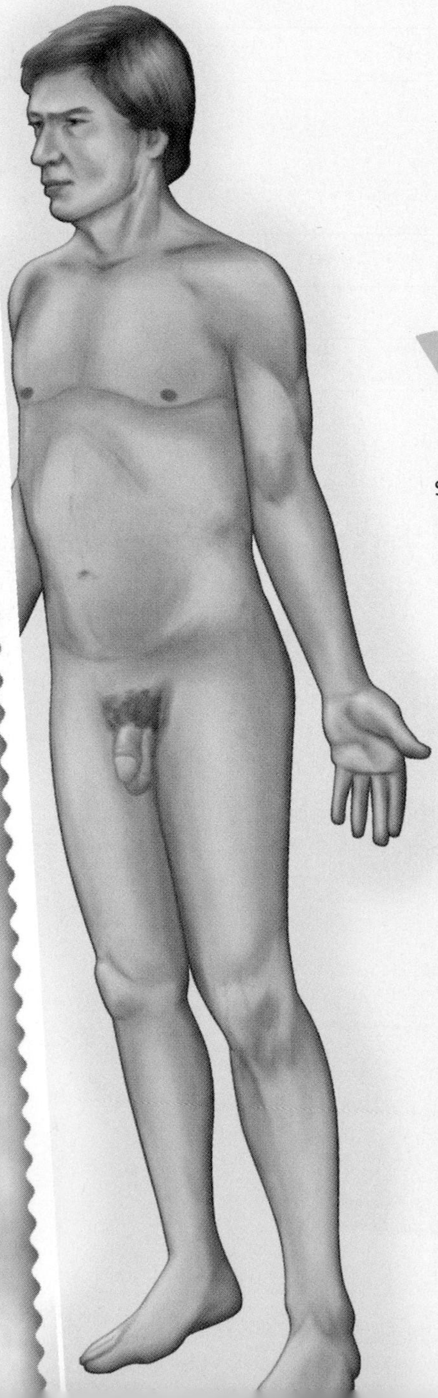

You learned in Chapter 5 that the skeletal system is like the framework of a building or house. But the framework is just one part of a building; the integrity of a house wouldn't last very long without shingles on its roof, siding of some sort, and windows, all of which help prevent the environment from doing damage to the main structures and inner workings. Like a house, the human body must be sheltered from the environment: that is the job of the integumentary system. Your skin forms a protective barrier to shield your body from the elements, guard against pathogens, and perform several other vital functions.

Think how important your skin is to your well-being and your ability to fully enjoy your journey. Without your skin, you would be unable to regulate your body temperature and would be uncomfortable in any environment. We paint our houses to protect them from the elements, likewise, we apply sun screen when we spend a day at the beach. While your skin is an important organ, there are several other accessory components such as nails, hair, and glands involved, hence, the name integumentary *system*.

Chapter 7

LEARNING OBJECTIVES

At the end of your journey through this chapter, you will be able to:

- Discuss the functions of the integumentary system
- List and describe the layers of the skin
- Explain the healing process of skin
- Describe the structure and growth of hair and nails
- Explain how the body regulates temperature through the integumentary system
- Discuss various common diseases of the integumentary system

MULTIMEDIA APPLICATIONS

CD-ROM Interactive Exercises

- Interactive drag-and-drop exercises: three layers of skin and the integumentary system, 7-1
- Animation on wound repair and the formation of scar tissue, 7-2
- Animation of pressure sores formation, prevention, and treatment, 7-3
- Interactive drag-and-drop exercise of the anatomical structures of a hair follicle, 7-4
- Videos and animations on diseases of the skin: decubitus ulcers, eczema, and skin cancer, 7-5
- Interactive games and puzzles, 7-6

www.prenhall.com/colbert

- Professional Profiles:
  - EMT-Paramedic
  - Nursing
- Related Internet Links
- Additional Review Questions

Pronunciation Guide

Correct pronunciation is important in any journey so that you and others are completely understood. Here is a "see and say" Pronunciation Guide for the more difficult terms to pronounce in this chapter.

- apocrine (APP oh crin)
- carotene (CARE eh teen)
- corium (CORE ee um)
- eccrine (EKK rin)
- epidermis (ep ih DER miss)
- epithelial cells (ep ih THEE lee al)
- keratin (KAIR ah tin)
- keratinization (KAIR ah tin eye ZAY shun)
- lesion (LEE zhun)
- lunula (LOO nyoo lah)
- melanin (MELL an in)
- melanocytes (mell AN oh sights)
- pustule (PUS tyool)
- sebaceous gland (see BAY shuss)
- sebum (SEE bum)
- squamous cells (SKWAY muss sells)
- stratum corneum (STRAY tum core NEE um)
- subcutaneous fascia (sub cue TAY nee us FAY she ah)

SYSTEM OVERVIEW

In this section, we will look at the functions and parts of the integumentary system. This system is the protective covering of the body and is the most exposed system. Get ready for this chapter to "get under your skin."

Integumentary System Functions

The integumentary system is comprised of the skin and its accessory components of hair, nails, and associated glands. Your integumentary system performs several vital functions besides protecting you from an invasion of disease-producing pathogens. This system helps keep the body from drying out, acts as storage for fatty tissue necessary for energy, and, with the aid of some sunshine, your skin produces vitamin D (needed to help your body utilize phosphorus and calcium for proper bone and teeth formation and growth). In addition, the skin provides sensory input (pleasant and unpleasant sensations involving pressure and temperature, for example) for your brain and helps regulate your body temperature.

The Skin

Your skin is quite a large organ, easily weighing twice as much as your brain, approaching 20 pounds in an average adult. In fact, the skin is the largest organ. It covers an area of about 20.83 square feet on an adult-sized body. A closer examination of a cross section of skin reveals three main layers of tissue:

- **epidermis**
- **dermis**
- **subcutaneous fascia** (also called the hypodermis layer because it lies *under* the dermis)

As we discuss these three layers, please refer to Figure 7–1 ■ for further clarification.

epidermis *(ep ih DER miss)*
epi = *upon*
dermis *(DER miss) true skin*

subcutaneous fascia *(sub cue TAY nee us FAY she ah)*
sub = *under*
cutane/o = *skin*
fascia = *band*

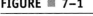

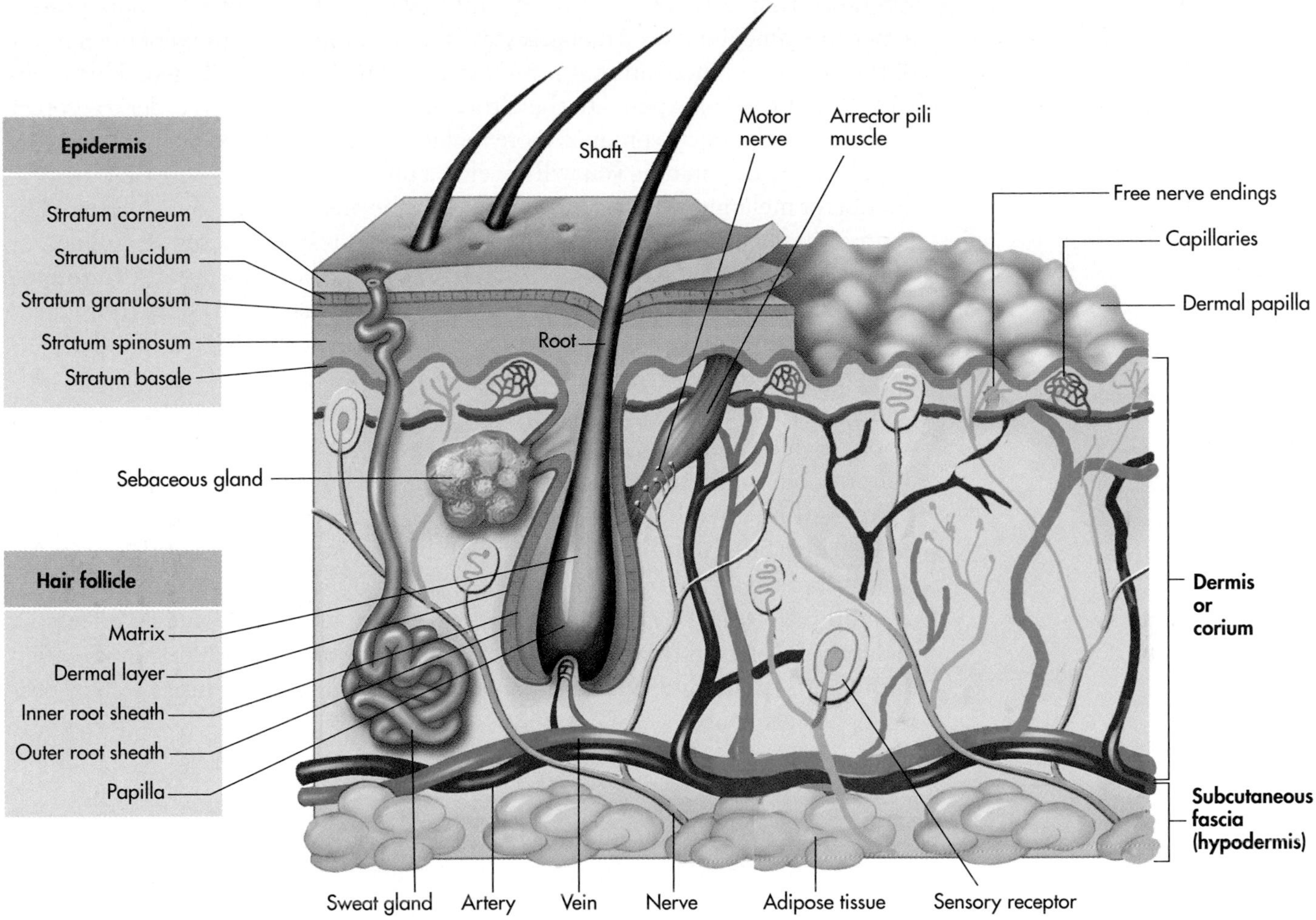

FIGURE ■ 7–1

The three layers of the skin.

EPIDERMIS

The epidermis is the layer of skin that we normally see. It is made up of five or six even smaller layers of stratified squamous epithelium. The epidermis is interesting for several reasons. First, it contains no blood vessels (avascular) or nerve cells. Second, the cells on the surface of this layer are constantly shedding, being replaced with new cells that arise from the deeper region called the **stratum basale** or basal layer of the epidermis in a process that takes 2 to 4 weeks. In fact, the outermost surface of skin is actually a layer of dead cells called **stratum corneum,** which are characteristically flat, scaly, keratinized (hardened) epithelial cells. Cells are born in the basal layer. As they are pushed toward the surface, they die and fill up with the protein, keratin. Through everyday activities such as bathing, drying off, and moving around, the body sloughs off *500 million* cells a day, equaling about *one and a half pounds* of dead skin a year! This continuous replacement of cells is very important because it allows your skin to quickly repair itself in cases of injuries.

Specialized cells called **melanocytes** are located deep in the epidermis and are responsible for skin color. Melanocytes produce **melanin,** which is the actual

a = *without*
vascular = *referring to vessels*

stratum corneum *(STRAY tum core NEE um)*
stratus = *to spread out*
kerat/o = *hard or horny*

melanocytes *(mell AN oh sights)*
melan/o = *black, extremely dark hue*
melanin *(MELL an in)*

substance that affects skin color. An interesting note is that all people possess about the same number of melanocytes. The variations of skin color are a result of the amount of melanin that is produced and how it is distributed. This is obvious when you are exposed to the ultraviolet rays of the sun. In order to protect your skin, melanocytes produce more melanin and, voila!, you've got a tan. You will also note that in time you will develop a tan line demonstrating that the production of melanin occurs only as needed, in the areas where needed. Regardless of an individual's skin tone or color, all skin types respond to sun exposure. For some of us, the melanin locates in patches on the skin, forming *freckles*. **Carotene,** which is another form of skin pigment, gives a yellowish hue to skin. Individuals with a pinkish hue derive that color from the hemoglobin in their blood.

carotene *(CARE eh teen)*

There are times when skin color can indicate an underlying disease. Although carotene gives a yellowish hue to skin, that is normal. In a situation where liver disease exists, the body can't excrete a substance call *bilirubin*. As bilirubin builds up in the body, *yellow jaundice* occurs, giving the skin a deeper yellow color. The changes in color are not as apparent on individuals with darker skin, but the yellowish color is easily seen in the whites of the eyes. Although bronze skin is associated with healthy outdoor living, individuals with a malfunctioning adrenal gland may have the same color due to excessive melanin deposits in the skin. Excessive bruising (black and blue marks called ecchymosis) could indicate skin, blood, or circulatory problems as well as possible physical abuse.

DERMIS

The layer right below, or inferior to, the epidermis layer is the thicker dermis layer, often called the **corium.** This layer of dense, irregular, connective tissue is considered the "true skin" and contains the following:

corium *(CORE ee um)*

- capillaries (tiny blood vessels)
- collagenous and elastic fibers
- involuntary muscles
- nerve endings
- lymph vessels (transport fluids from tissue to the blood system)
- hair follicles
- sudoriferous glands (sweat)
- sebaceous glands (oil)

Small "fingers" of tissue project from the surface of the dermis and anchor this layer to the epidermal layer. Fingerprints, toe prints, and other unique skin patterns also arise from this layer. Nerve fibers are located in the corium so the body can sense what is happening in the environment. Because this layer also possesses blood vessels, this is where your blush comes from when you get embarrassed!

Amazing Body Facts

(MORE A BOTHERSOME FACT OF LIFE)

Sometimes the sebaceous glands within the skin become blocked. As a result, sebum stagnates and is exposed to air, drying it out. When this occurs, the sebum turns black, creating the infamous *blackhead!* To make matters worse, if that blackhead becomes infected, a *pimple* is formed (medically known as a *pustule*) usually right before your big date. Blackheads should not be squeezed because doing so can create craters at the site, not to mention interesting formations on the mirror! The best thing to do is keep those areas clean through gentle washing with soap and water and let nature take its course.

This brings us to the topic of cleaning your skin. Be careful not to wash too frequently with too hot water and/or too harsh soap, and avoid aggressive drying. This is important because excessive cleaning has the potential to dry out your skin and remove the antibacterial layer of sebum. In fact, aggressive washing with a soap that isn't pH balanced (the same acidity as your skin) can cause skin to lose its antibacterial abilities for 45 minutes after washing. As with most things in life, moderation is the key.

The collagenous and elastic fibers of this layer help your skin flex with the movements that you make. Without that ability, your skin would eventually tear from all of your moving around. In addition to flexing, these fibers allow your skin to return to its normal shape when at rest. In older people and people regularly exposed to high levels of sunlight, the skin's firmness and ability to recoil to normal decreases. To better understand this process, try this experiment. With one of your hands resting palm down, take the thumb and index finger of your other hand and gently pinch and pull up the skin on the back of your resting hand. Let go and observe how quickly the skin recoils to normal. Try this experiment with an older person and observe how much slower his or her skin returns to normal. Another example of the skin's resilience due to the collagenous and elastic fibers is when it returns to normal after an injury that caused swelling.

apocrine *(APP oh crin)*
eccrine *(EKK rin)*

There are two main types of sudiferous or sweat glands: **apocrine** and **eccrine** glands (see Figure 7–2 ■). Apocrine sweat glands secrete at the hair follicles in the

7-1 For an interactive drag-and-drop exercise on the integumentary system and the layers of skin, please go to your CD-ROM for this chapter.

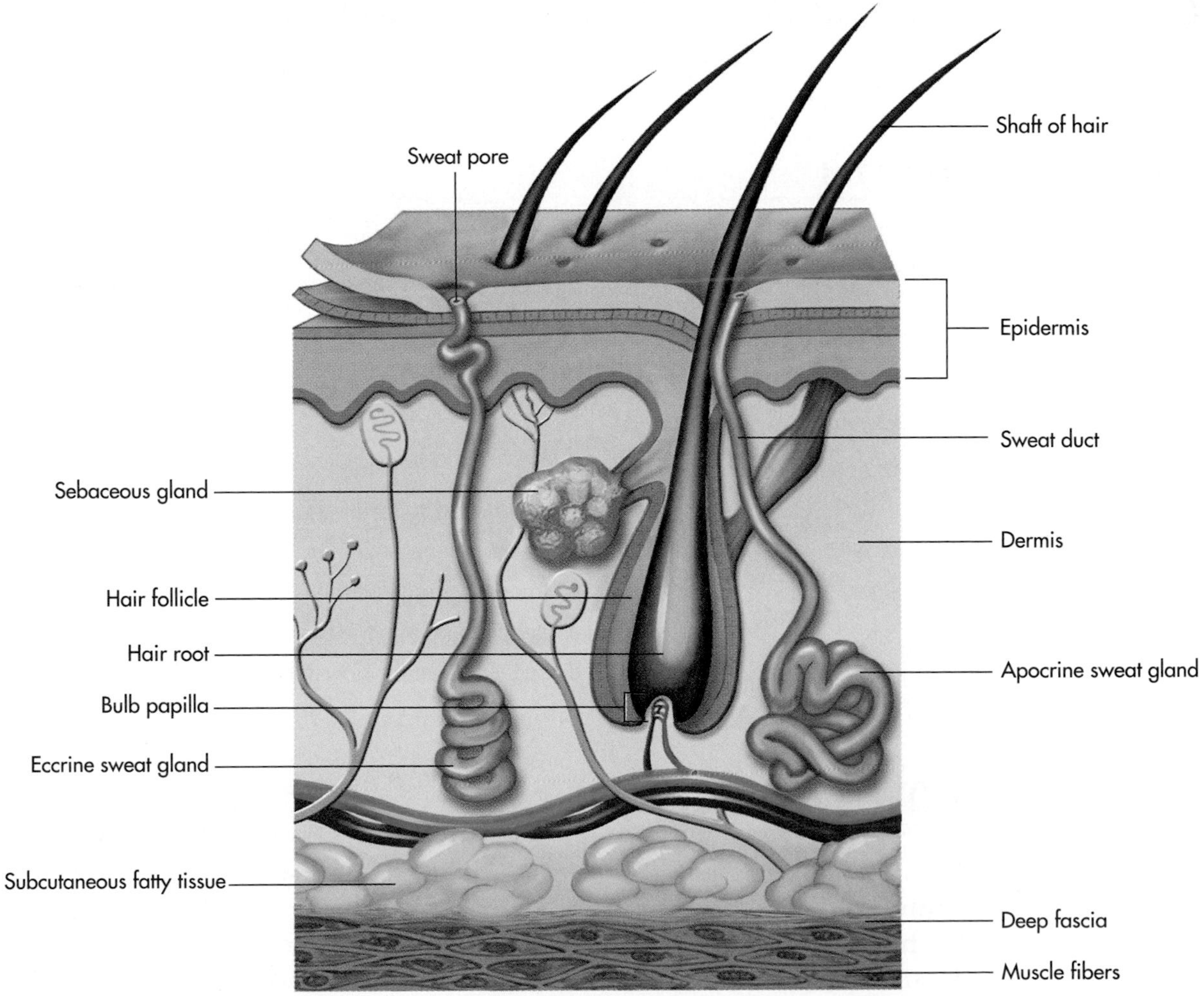

FIGURE ■ 7–2

Sweat and sebaceous glands.

groin and anal region as well as the armpits. These glands become active around puberty and are believed to act as a sexual attractant. Located all over your skin, eccrine glands are important in the regulation of body temperature. Eccrine glands are found in greater numbers on your palms, feet, forehead, and upper lip. Your body has approximately 3,000,000 sweat glands! It is interesting to note that sweat by itself does not have a strong odor. However, if it is left on the skin, bacteria degrades substances in the sweat into chemicals that give off strong smells, commonly called body odors.

Sebaceous glands play an important role by secreting oil, or sebum, that keeps the skin from drying out. Because it is somewhat acidic in nature, it also helps destroy some pathogens on the skin's surface.

SUBCUTANEOUS FASCIA

hypo = *below, under*

lipo = *fat*
cyte = *cell*

Finally, the innermost layer of skin is the subcutaneous fascia, or **hypodermis,** which is composed of elastic and fibrous connective tissue and fatty tissue. Within this layer, **lipocytes,** or fat cells, produce the fat needed to provide padding to protect the deeper tissues of the body and act as insulation for temperature regulation. Fat is also necessary as an efficient store for energy. The hypodermis is also the layer of skin that is attached to the muscles of your body.

TEST YOUR KNOWLEDGE 7-1

Complete the following:

1. List the three main layers of skin.
   a.
   b.
   c.
2. List four of the functions of your integumentary system.
   a.
   b.
   c.
   d.

Choose the best answer:

3. Which cells are responsible for your normal skin color?
   a. manocytes
   b. jandicytes
   c. eyecytes
   d. melanocytes
4. The two main types of sudiferous glands are
   a. apocrine and pelicine
   b. appeltine and eccrine
   c. eccrine and apocrine
   d. sudacrine and melocrine

HOW SKIN HEALS

Just as storms can damage homes by high winds tearing off shingles or siding, lightning burning portions of the exterior, or damage caused by ice, everyone has had a skin injury of some type. As a result, the body has developed ways to repair itself when injury threatens its first line of defense—the skin.

If skin is punctured and the wound damages blood vessels in the skin, as shown in Figure 7–3 ■, the wound fills with blood. Blood contains substances that cause it to clot. The top part of the clot that is exposed to air hardens to

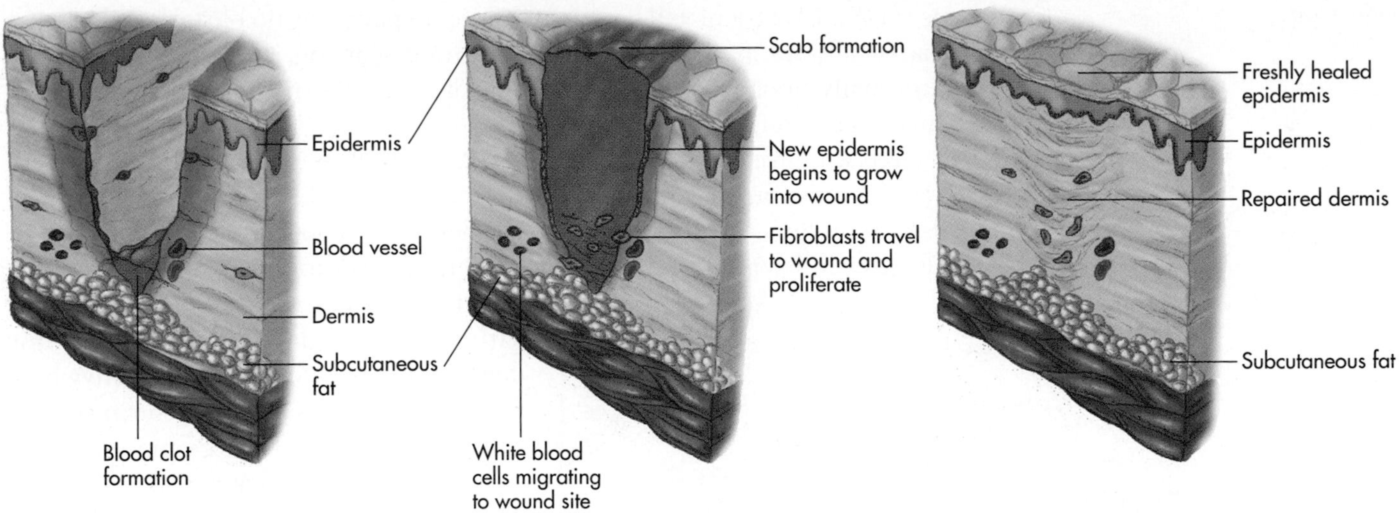

FIGURE ■ 7–3

Wound repair.

form a scab. This is nature's bandage, forming a barrier between the wound and the outer environment to prevent pathogens from entering—so don't pick your scabs.

Next, white blood cells enter to destroy any pathogens that may have entered when the wound occurred. At about the same time, cells called **fibroblasts** (cells that can develop into connective tissue) come in and begin pulling the edges of the wound together. The basal layer of the epidermis begins to hyperproduce new cells for the repair of the wound. If the wound is severe enough, a tough scar composed of collagen fibers may form. Scars usually don't contain any accessory organs of the skin or any sense of feeling. Scar production can be greatly minimized if stitches, adhesive strips, or a specialized glue are used to draw the margins of the wound together before the healing process begins.

fibro = *fibers, or fibrous tissue*
blast = *immature cellular development*

Ideally, the wound starts to heal from the *inside*, working its way to heal the wound *toward* the outside. This aids in preventing pathogens from becoming trapped between a healed surface and the deeper layers of skin where they could develop into a major pocket of infection.

> **7-2** For an animation on wound repair and the formation of scar tissues, visit the CD-ROM for this chapter.

Burns to the Skin

Burns to the skin present special problems for healing. We naturally think that burns are caused by heat, and that is true. However, burns can also be caused by chemicals, electricity, or radiation. When assessing the damage caused by burns, there are two factors to consider: the *depth* of the burn and the *size of the area damaged* by the burn.

> **WWW** Emergency medical technicians (EMTs) and paramedics often deal with burn victims as a result of structural or automobile fires. To learn more about emergency professions, please go to the companion website for information and to view a video.

The depth of a burn relates to the layer or layers of skin affected by the burn. A *first-degree burn* has damaged only the outer layer of skin, the epider-

auto = *self*

mis. In this case there will be skin redness and pain, but no blistering. The pain usually subsides in about 2 to 3 days with no scarring. The damaged layer of skin usually sloughs off in about a week or so. Sunburn is a classic example of a first-degree burn.

Second-degree burns involve the entire depth of the epidermis and a portion of the dermis. Such burns cause pain, redness, and blistering. The extent of blistering is directly proportional to the depth of the burn. Blisters continue to enlarge even after the initial burn. Excluding any additional complications such as infection, these blisters usually heal within 10 to 14 days, but burns reaching deeper into the dermis require anywhere from 4 to 14 weeks to heal. Scarring in second-degree burn cases is common.

Third-degree burns affect all three of the skin layers. Here the surface of the skin has a leathery feel to it and varies in color: black, brown, tan, red, or white. The victim will feel no pain because pain receptors are destroyed by third-degree burns. Also destroyed are the sweat and sebaceous glands, hair follicles, and blood vessels. *Fourth-degree burns* are burns that penetrate to the bone.

A clinician can estimate the extent of the area covered by the burn by using the "rule of nines." As you can see in Figure 7–4 ■, the body is divided into the following regions and given a percentage of body surface area value: head and neck, 9%; *each* upper limb, 9 percent; *each* lower limb, 18 percent; front of trunk, 18 percent; back of trunk and buttocks, 18 percent; perineum (including the anal and urogenital region), 1 percent. These regions can also be further divided for smaller burn areas, as you can see in the figure.

The clinical concerns for burn patients relate to the functions of the skin already discussed:

- bacterial infection
- fluid loss
- heat loss

Severe burns require healing steps at an intensity level that the body can't normally achieve on its own. Damaged

Clinical Application

MEDICINE DELIVERY VIA THE INTEGUMENTARY SYSTEM

A variety of medicines can be delivered via the integumentary system. Medicines can be applied to adhesive patches that are placed on the skin where it is slowly absorbed into the bloodstream. These are called transdermal patches. Nicotine (for smoking cessation), nitroglycerin (for vasodilation in the heart), birth control compounds, and pain medication, for example, can be delivered in this manner. If a more rapid response is required, the cardiac drug nitroglycerin can be placed under the tongue (*sublingually*) where it is rapidly absorbed into the bloodstream because of the high vascularization of the mucosa in that area.

Of course, the other method of injecting drugs is a little more painful but very effective. This method is used when a drug can't be taken by mouth or the digestive system may alter the desired effects of the drug. Medication can be injected utilizing a syringe and needle to deliver the medication either *subcutaneously* (under the skin) or *intradermally* (into the skin). Other routes of injection also include intramuscular, intraspinal, and intravenous (IV) routes.

7-3 To view an animation of pressure sores formation, prevention, and treatment, please go to your CD-ROM.

The nursing profession requires much interaction with the integumentary system. Nurses administer medications through all delivery routes, routinely perform wound care, and help prevent skin problems such as pressure or bed sores. This exciting profession has training in and interactions with all the body systems. Please go to the companion website for information and to view videos concerning the nursing profession.

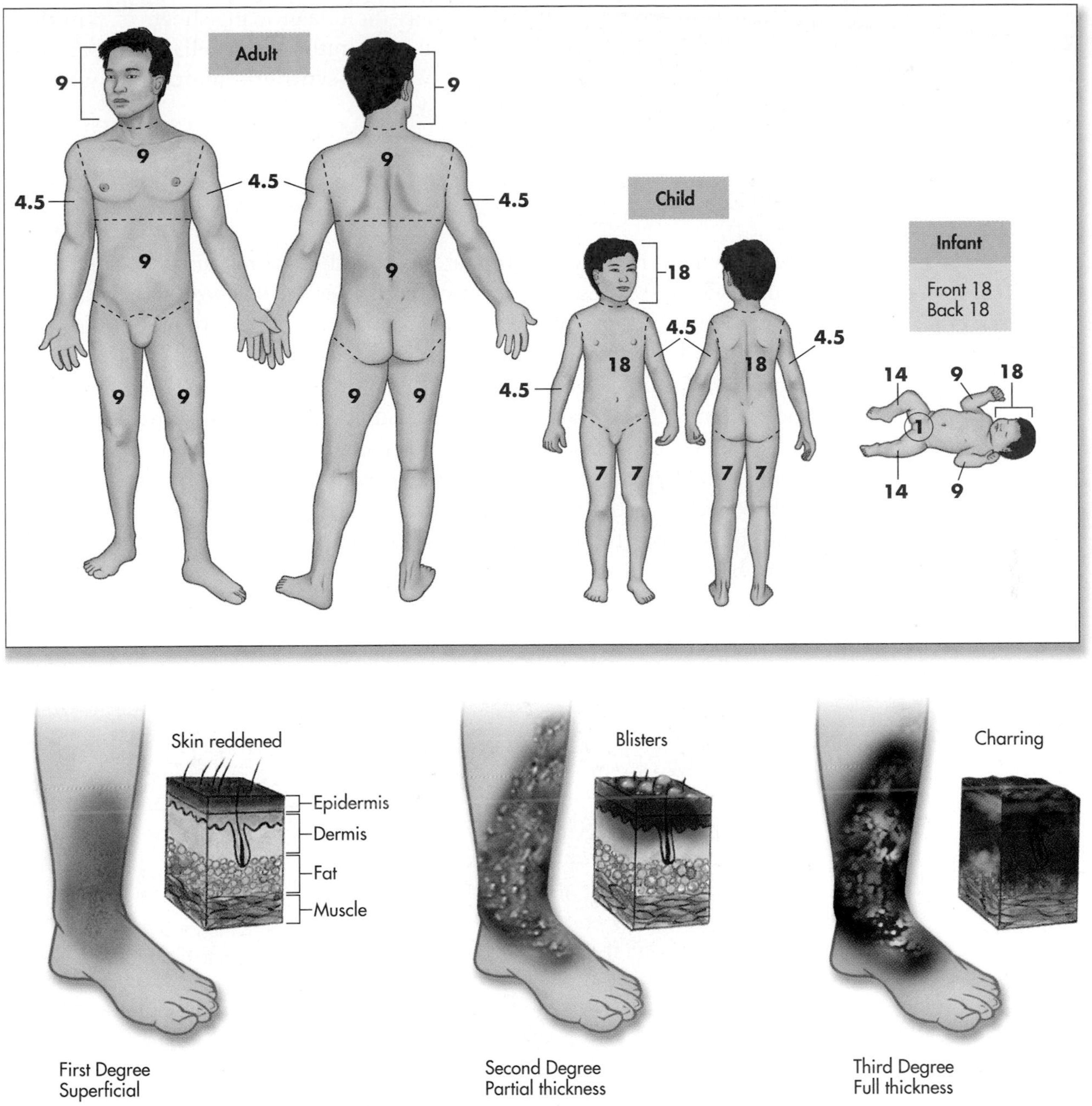

FIGURE ■ 7–4

Assessing the degree of the burn.

skin must be removed as soon as possible to allow the process of skin grafting to begin. In this process, healthy skin is placed over damaged areas so it may begin to grow. Ideally, it is best to use the patient's own skin, known as *autografting*, because it generally eliminates the chances of tissue rejection. However, the destruction may be severe enough to require tissue from a donor (heterografting). Grafting usually requires repeat surgeries because large areas cannot be done all at once, and often the grafts don't "take." Other options

7-4 To perform an interactive drag-and-drop exercise on the hair follicle, please go to your CD-ROM.

may include growing sheets of skin tissue in a laboratory from cells of the patient or utilizing synthetic materials that act as skin.

NAILS

keratinized *(KAIR ah tin ized)*
kerat/o = *hard or horny*

lunula *(LOO nyoo lah)*
luna = *moon*

Specialized epithelial cells originating from the *nail root* form your nails (see Figure 7–5 ■). As these cells grow out and over the *nail bed* (actually a part of the epidermis), they become **keratinized,** forming a substance similar to the horns on a bull that is the same protein that fills the cells of the stratum corneum. This process occurs as cells dry and shrink, are pushed to the surface, and become filled with a hard protein called keratin. The **cuticle** is a fold of tissue that covers the nail root. The portion that we see is called the *nail body*. Nails normally grow about 1 millimeter every week. The pink color of your nails comes from the vascularization of the tissue under the nails, while the white half-moon shaped area, or **lunula,** is a result of the thicker layer of cells at the base.

Clinical Application

ASSESSING PERIPHERAL PERFUSION

The pink color of the nail bed is clinically significant in that it can aid in the assessment of perfusion (blood flow) to the extremities and can be a determinant of oxygenation. If you pinch one of your fingernails straight down with the thumb and index finger of your other hand for 5 seconds and release that pinch, you will note that the nail bed went from a blanched white color back to pink in a matter of seconds. This shows good perfusion as a result of the blood rushing back into the nail bed. In cases of poor perfusion, it takes longer for the nail bed to "pink-up." Normally, it takes less than 3 seconds for the nail to return to pink from the blanched white state. If that time is greater than 3 seconds, perfusion to the extremities is considered sluggish. If the refill time is greater than 5 seconds, there is clearly an abnormal situation occurring.

Diabetes is a disease that causes a condition of reduced blood flow to the extremities known as **peripheral vascular disease** (**PVD**). PVD can cause an increase in the time required to re-perfuse the nail bed. Blood clots or vascular spasms can decrease blood flow and thereby extend refill time, as can hypothermia, which naturally constricts blood vessels in the periphery to conserve heat.

In addition, nail beds can change colors under certain condition. For example, as the level of oxygen decreases in the tissue, the nail beds become bluish in tint. Of course, one can always paint their nails different colors!

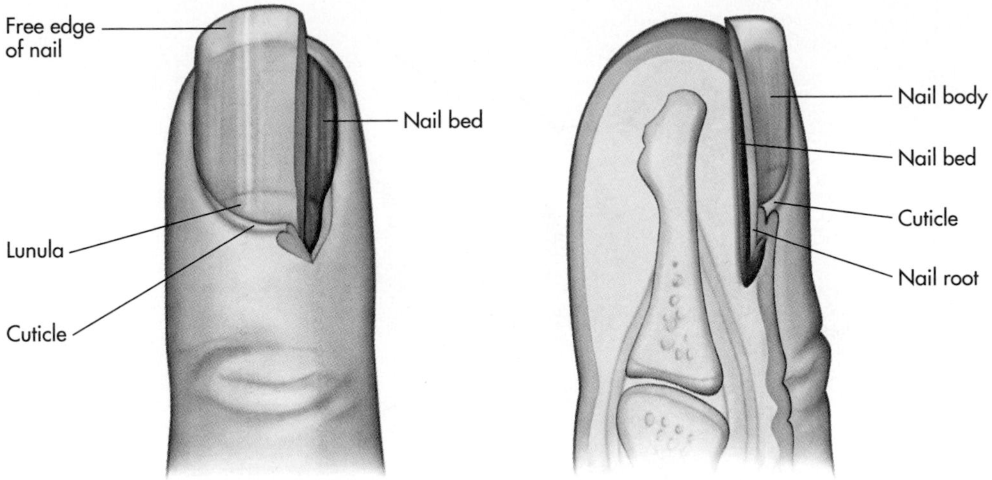

FIGURE ■ 7–5

Structures of the fingernail.

HAIR

Body hair is normal and served important purposes in our evolutionary past as well as today. Hair helps to regulate body temperature, as you will see in the next section, and it functions as a sensor to help detect things on your skin, such as bugs or cobwebs. Eyelashes help to protect our eyes from foreign objects, and hair in the nose helps to filter out gross particulate matter.

Hair is composed of a fibrous protein called **keratin** just like your fingernails and toe nails. The hair that you see is called the shaft, and the root extends down into the dermis to the **follicle** (see Figure 7–6 ■). The follicle is formed by epithelial cells, which have a rich source of blood provided by the dermal blood vessels. As a result, cells divide and grow in the base of the follicle. As new cells continually form, the older cells are crowded out and pushed upward toward the skin's surface. As these old cells are pushed away from the blood source (which provides their nourishment), they die, becoming keratinized in the process. So basically, the hair you see on the individual next to you is a bunch of dead cells. This isn't so bad considering that if your hairs were alive, your haircuts would be extremely painful with a good chance of your bleeding to death if you got more than a light trim! The old, popular belief that shaving or frequent cutting of hair makes it grow quicker or thicker is wrong. Neither shaving nor cutting does anything to effect the rate of cell growth at the base of those hair follicles.

keratin *(KAIR ah tin)*

follicle *(FALL ih kle)*

If you look at Figure 7–6, you will note that there is a **sebaceous gland** associated with the hair follicle. The sebaceous gland secretes **sebum,** an oily substance that coats the follicle and works its way to the skin's surface. Sebum is somewhat antibacterial, so it aids in decreasing infections on your skin. Although it also waterproofs and lubricates the skin and hair, sebum production decreases with age. As a result, older individuals exhibit drier skin and more brittle hair.

sebaceous gland *(see BAY shuss)*
sebo = *tallow*
sebum *(SEE bum)*

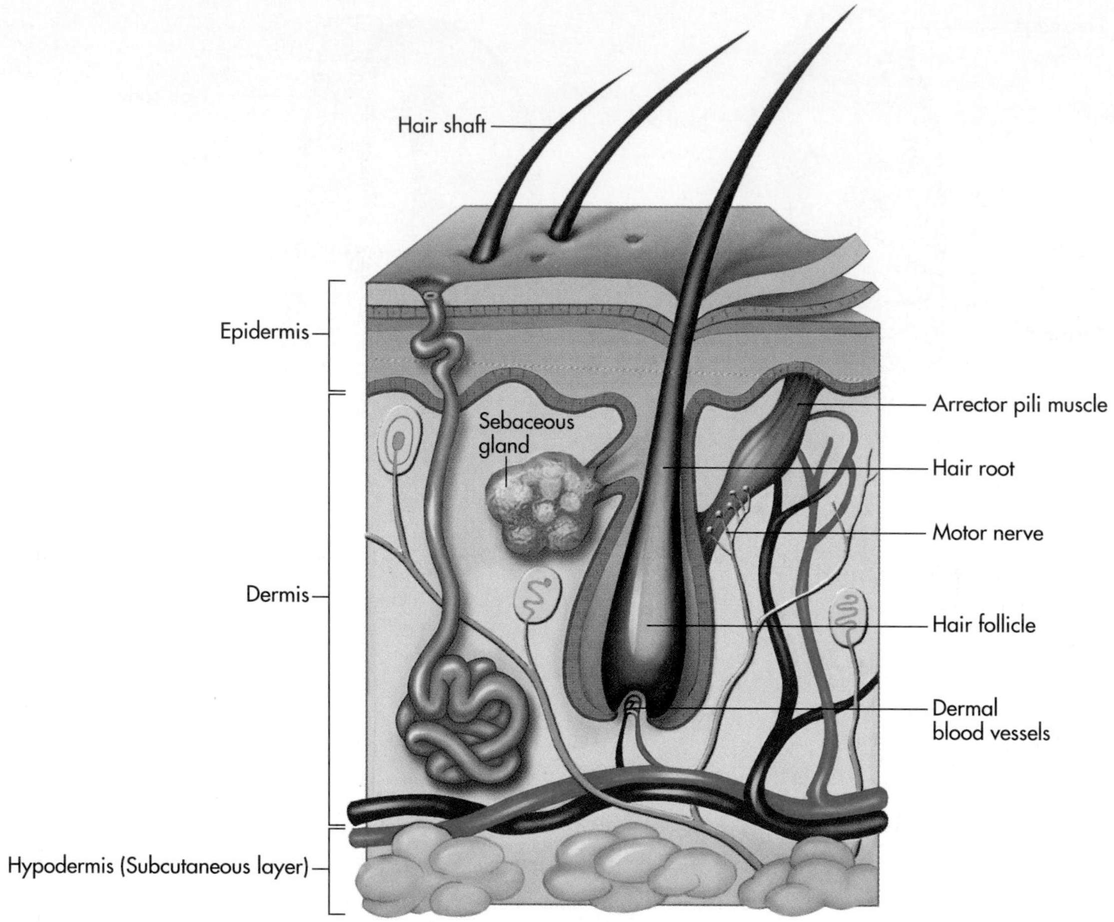

FIGURE ■ 7–6

Diagram of a hair follicle.

TEST YOUR KNOWLEDGE 7-2

Choose the best answer:

1. The blood clot that forms in a wound that is exposed to air becomes a
   a. scar
   b. scab
   c. hematoma
   d. keloid

2. When assessing the skin damage caused by a burn, the two main factors to assess are
   a. temperature and depth
   b. depth and odor
   c. area of damage and depth
   d. odor and color

3. The white, half-moon shaped area of your fingernail is called
   a. cuticle
   b. lunula
   c. keratin
   d. lingula

4. Corium is another term for
   a. epidermis
   b. contrasta
   c. corneum
   d. dermis

Like skin color, your hair color is dependent on the amount and type of melanin you produce. Generally, the more melanin, the darker the hair. White hair occurs in the absence of melanin. Red hair is a result of an altered melanin that has iron in it.

You may be extremely envious of someone with a head full of curly hair or of someone with absolutely straight hair. Don't be envious of the person—just envy his or her hair shafts! Flat hair shafts produce curly hair, while round hair shafts produce straight hair.

Applied Science

FORENSICS AND HAIR

An interesting sidelight concerning hair is its ability to tell a pathologist if an individual ingested certain drugs or other substances, such as lead or arsenic. Trace amounts of ingested substances can become part of the hair's composition. As a result, analysis of a hair sample can reveal what and how long ago something was ingested. The longer the length of hair, the longer the record of what was consumed by that individual.

The life span of hair is dependent on location. Eyelashes last around 3 to 4 months, while the hair on the scalp lasts for about 3 to 4 years. Teachers with difficult classes usually pull their hair out sooner!

TEMPERATURE REGULATION

The integumentary system plays a major role in the regulation of the body's temperature. It is amazing how we can stay in a relatively "tight" range of body temperature while we do a variety of things in a variety of environments. Of course, clothes do help tremendously, but still it is critical to have a properly functioning temperature regulator like our integumentary system. This is accomplished through a complex series of activities.

Part of temperature regulation is accomplished by changes in the size of blood vessels in your skin. As your temperature rises, your body signals the blood vessels in your skin to get larger in diameter. The correct term is **vasodilation.** This is the body's attempt to get as much "hot" blood exposed to a cooler surrounding environment so the heat radiates away from the body. In addition, sweat glands excrete water (as well as some waste products such as nitrogenous wastes and sodium chloride) onto the skin's surface. As the water evaporates, cooling occurs. As long as you stay hydrated so you can produce sweat, this system works pretty well. Hydration is especially important before and during activities to avoid feeling thirsty. Thirst indicates the body is already dehydrating. It's pretty easy to dehydrate especially when you realize that you can have up to 3,000 sweat glands on a square inch of skin on your hands and feet and you can potentially excrete up to 12 liters of sweat in a 24 hour period! The risk of dehydration can be serious.

vasodilation *(vaz oh DYE lay shun)*
vaso = *vessel*
dilation = *enlargement*

Conversely, if you were in a cold environment and needed to warm up, your blood vessels would become smaller in diameter, or **vasoconstrict.** This act forces blood away from the skin and back toward the core of the body where the heat is. The perfect visual explanation of vasoconstriction is a skinny little kid running around a pool on a chilly summer day, shivering, with blue lips. The lips are blue because of vasoconstriction. Rings have a tendency to slide off your fingers in cold weather more readily than in hot weather because of vasoconstriction.

vasoconstrict *(vaz oh kon STRIKT)*

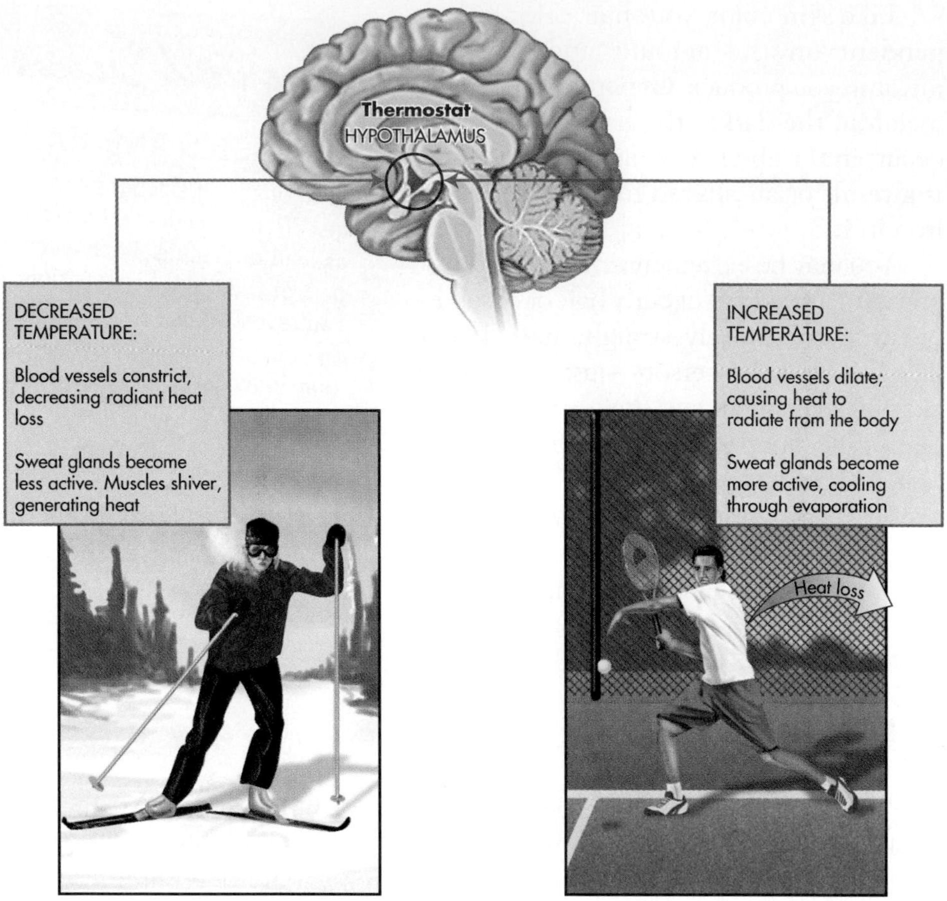

FIGURE ■ 7–7

Integumentary regulation of body temperature.

Body temperature regulation is also aided by the hairs on your skin. Muscles in your skin called *arrector pili*, or erector muscles, are attached to your hairs, and when those muscles contract, they make your hairs stand erect. The constriction of those muscles shows up as goose flesh or goose pimples when you are chilled. When the hair stands up, pockets of still air are formed right above the skin, creating a dead air space that insulates the skin from the cooler surrounding environment. This is also how goose down (feathers) clothing works in protecting against winter's cold. Interestingly, older homes built before the now common and effective practice of placing insulation in the walls and ceilings, actually insulated the homes through the creation of dead air (nonmoving) spaces between the outer and inner walls. See Figure 7–7 ■, which illustrates how your integumentary system regulates body temperature with the aid of your nervous system.

COMMON DISORDERS OF THE INTEGUMENTARY SYSTEM

There are whole sections of medical libraries dedicated to diseases of the skin. This section will provide you with some basic terms and diseases related to the integumentary system.

A **lesion** is a pathologically altered piece of tissue that can include a wound or injury or a single infected patch of skin. The color of a lesion is usually different than that of normal skin. Figure 7–8 ■ shows a variety of lesion types.

> **7-5** Please go to the CD-ROM for this chapter to view short videos on diseases of the skin, such as decubitus ulcers, eczema, and skin cancer.

In addition to several types of skin lesions, there are many common pathologic conditions of the integumentary system. Table 7–1 describes some of these conditions. Please see Figure 7–9 ■ to view various photos on types of integumentary conditions.

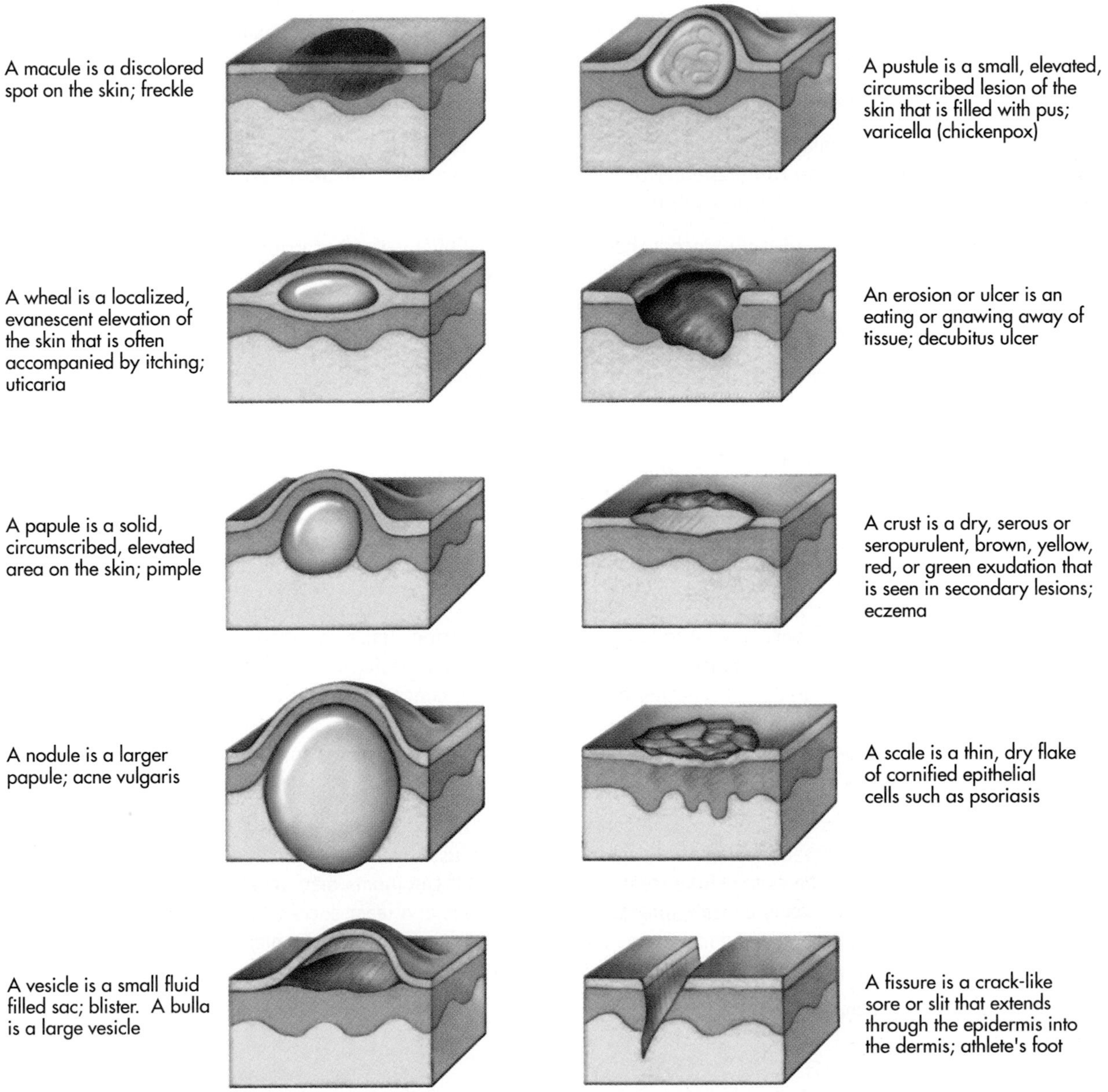

A macule is a discolored spot on the skin; freckle
A pustule is a small, elevated, circumscribed lesion of the skin that is filled with pus; varicella (chickenpox)
A wheal is a localized, evanescent elevation of the skin that is often accompanied by itching; uticaria
An erosion or ulcer is an eating or gnawing away of tissue; decubitus ulcer
A papule is a solid, circumscribed, elevated area on the skin; pimple
A crust is a dry, serous or seropurulent, brown, yellow, red, or green exudation that is seen in secondary lesions; eczema
A nodule is a larger papule; acne vulgaris
A scale is a thin, dry flake of cornified epithelial cells such as psoriasis
A vesicle is a small fluid filled sac; blister. A bulla is a large vesicle
A fissure is a crack-like sore or slit that extends through the epidermis into the dermis; athlete's foot

FIGURE ■ 7–8

Various types of skin lesions.

TABLE 7–1 Common Pathological Conditions of the Integumentary System

NAME OF CONDITION	DESCRIPTION
Abrasion	A condition that results from mechanically scraping away a portion of the skin's layer(s). This may be a result of injury or a deliberate clinical procedure.
Acne	Sebaceous glands oversecrete sebum which, along with the dead keratinized cells, clog the hair follicle. If the blocked follicle becomes infected with bacteria, pimples develop.
Athlete's foot	This is a common fungal infection that occurs in areas of continuous moisture, such as between the toes, or on palms or fingers. Jock itch is a fungal infection of the groin area.
Bed sores (decubitus or pressure ulcers)	These sores are a result of a lack of blood flow to skin that has had pressure applied to a bony prominence. This often occurs in bedridden patients who aren't turned often enough. Often called decubitus (dee KYOO bih tus) ulcers.
Boil (furuncle)	Also known as a furuncle (FOO rung kle), this is an acute inflammatory* process involving either the subcutaneous layer of skin, a hair follicle, or a gland.
Cold Sore	Often called a fever blister, these watery vesicles are caused by the herpes simplex virus.
Contusion	A traumatic skin injury in which the skin is not broken but an injury still occurs. A contusion can present with pain, discoloration due to breakage of small blood vessels (capillaries), and swelling.
Dermatitis	An inflammatory process that can be caused by a variety of irritants such as from plants or chemical sources. Patients with dermatitis can exhibit erythema (redness), papules, vesicles, and crusty scabbing. Touching poison ivy or poison oak can lead to the condition called contact dermatitis.
Eczema	A superficial form of dermatitis that exhibits redness, papules, vesicles, and crusting.
Hives (urticaria)	This disorder is a result of an allergic reaction and produces reddened patches (wheals) and itching (pruritis), which can be severe.
Psoriasis	From the Greek word meaning "to itch," psoriasis is a chronic, inflammatory skin condition that exhibits red, dry, crusty papules, which form circular borders over the affected areas.
Scabies	An infectious and contagious disease caused by egg-laying mites, usually seen in children; causes severe itching.
Shingles	This is a very painful inflammatory skin condition that also involves the nervous system. Shingles presents itself in the form of patches of vesicles mainly on the trunk of the body, but can be found on other body regions. This condition is caused by the virus herpes zoster. *Zoster* is from the Greek word meaning "belt" and relates to the distribution of those patches around the trunk. The pain often remains for some time after the vesicles have healed.
Skin cancer	There are a variety of skin cancers. Squamous cell carcinoma and basal cell carcinoma are the two most common. Basal cell carcinoma usually spreads locally and therefore can usually be successfully treated. Squamous cell carcinoma may develop deeper into tissue, but it usually doesn't spread. The most serious and least successfully treated skin cancer is malignant melanoma. This is a cancer that initially affects the melanocytes, which produce skin pigments. This cancer can spread throughout the body to various organs.

*Inflammation literally means to "flame within." The inflammatory response is tissue's reaction to injury where there is pain, heat, redness, and swelling.

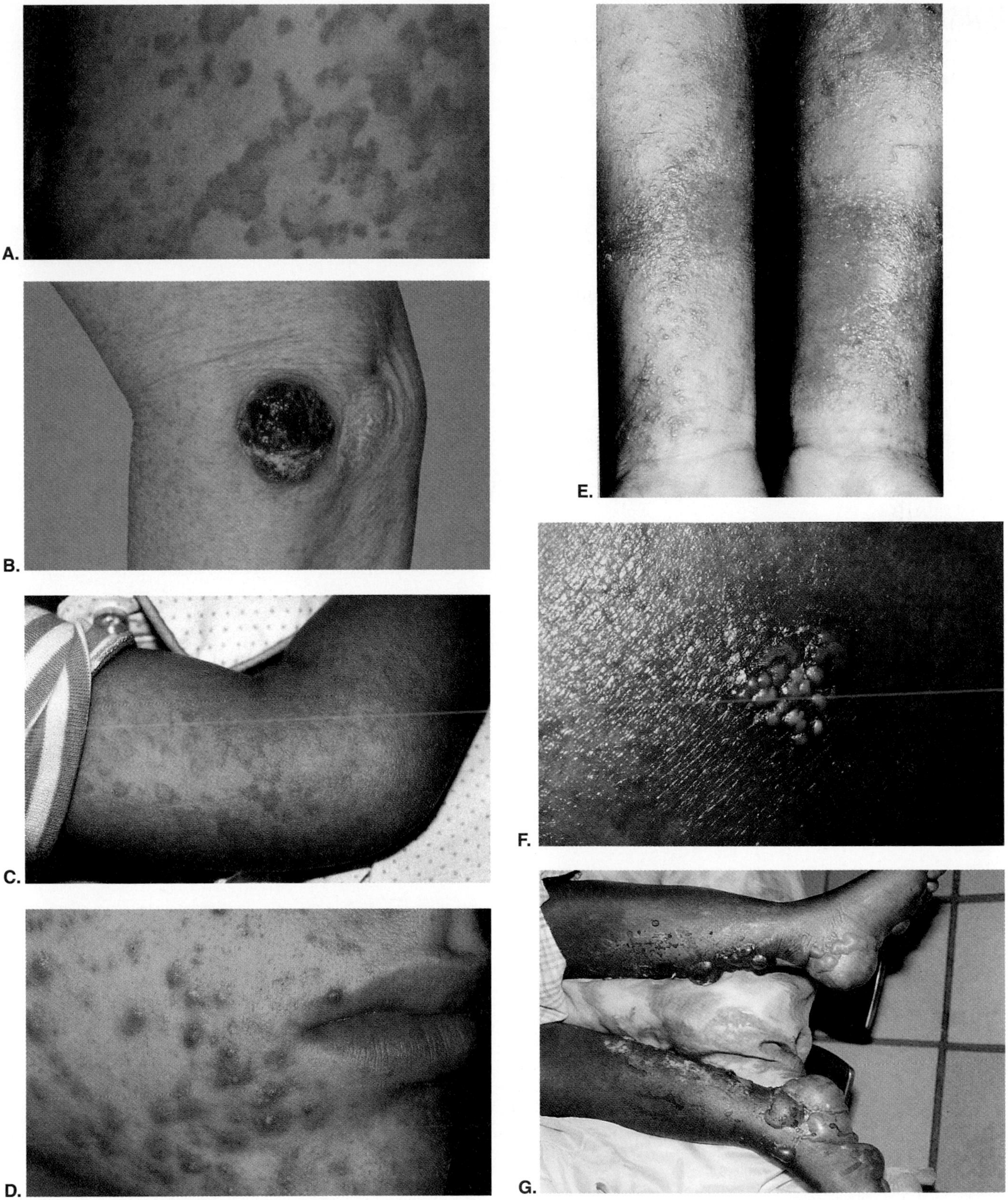

FIGURE ■ 7–9

Various types of integumentary conditions. (a) Urticaria (hives). (Courtesy of Jason L. Smith, MD.) (b) Malignant melanoma. (Source: Biophoto Associates/Photo Researchers, Inc.) (c) Erythema infectiosum (fifth disease). (Courtesy of Jason L. Smith, MD.) (d) Acne. (Courtesy of Jason L. Smith, MD.) (e) Poison ivy (dermatitis). (Courtesy of Jason L. Smith, MD.) (f) Herpes simplex. (Courtesy of Jason L. Smith, MD.) (g) Burn, second degree. (Courtesy of Jason L. Smith, MD.)

SUMMARY

Snapshots from the Journey

- Your skin is your largest organ.
- Your skin is an amazing organ that does the following:
  a. Acts as a barrier to infection both as a physical shield and through secretion of an antibacterial substance
  b. Acts as a physical barrier to injury
  c. Helps to keep the body from dehydrating
  d. Stores fat (yes, you do need some fat!)
  e. Synthesizes and secretes vitamin D with the help of sunshine
  f. Regulates body temperature
  g. Provides a minor excretory function in the elimination of water, salts, and urea
  h. Provides sensory input
- The skin is composed of three layers: epidermis, dermis, and subcutaneous fascia.
- Skin is not static; it constantly recreates itself.
- Various glands in the skin help moisturize, waterproof, and control body temperature as well as excrete some waste products.
- The severity of burns to the skin is evaluated by the depth of the burn and the area that the burn covers.
- Nails are protective devices composed of dead material.
- Hair (also dead material) aids in controlling body temperature.

Case Study

A 27-year-old female presents to her doctor's office with complaints of red, itching, and oozing skin for the past two days. Physical examination and history reveal the following: a well-nourished white female who is in otherwise good health, no known allergies, normal vital signs, pupils normal and reactive, reflexes good, breath sounds normal, liquid-filled vesicles and scabbing on both legs from the top of her sock lines to the bottom of her shorts, new vesicles have formed around her eyes. The patient stated that she returned from a primitive camping and hiking vacation in Virginia two days ago.

Based on this information, what do you think is the diagnosis?

What caused the vesicles to begin to form around her eyes?

REVIEW QUESTIONS

Multiple Choice

1. The substance that is mainly responsible for skin color is
   a. melanin
   b. pigmentin
   c. carrots
   d. luna

2. Whether you have naturally curly or straight hair is dependent on the shape of your
   a. hair follicle
   b. hair shaft
   c. sebum
   d. melanin

3. The fibrous protein that makes up your hair and nails and fills your epidermal cells is called
   a. carotene
   b. myelin
   c. keratin
   d. dermasene

4. In a cold environment, in order to maintain a core body temperature, peripheral blood vessels
   a. vasodilate
   b. venospasm
   c. shiver
   d. vasoconstrict

5. The hair on your scalp can last
   a. 3 to 4 months
   b. until your 40s
   c. 3 to 4 years
   d. until you have kids

Fill in the Blanks

1. The three main layers of skin are the ____________________, ____________________, and ____________________.

2. The two main types of sweat glands are the ____________________ and the ____________________ glands.

3. Sebaceous glands secrete an oily substance called ____________________.

4. For some individuals, melanin locates in small patches called ____________________.

5. Yellow jaundice, a condition associated with liver disease, occurs as a result of the build-up of ____________________.

Short Answer

1. Discuss three functions of the integumentary system.

2. Discuss the functions of sebum.

3. Why is there an increased production of melanin when there is an increased sun exposure?

4. How does the integumentary system assist in the regulation of body temperature?

Suggested Activities

1. Contact a local dermatologist to speak to your class on diagnosing and treating skin diseases.

2. Research the variety of medications used to treat acne and focus on the mode of action, benefits, and side effects.

7-6 Now that you have completed your journey through this chapter, please go to the CD-ROM for interactive games and puzzles concerning the medical terms and concepts contained in this chapter. By playing the games you will reinforce your learning of medical terminology in a fun way.

Greetings from THE NERVOUS System

The Body's Control Center, PART ONE

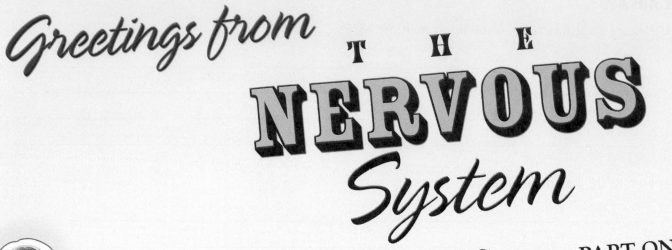

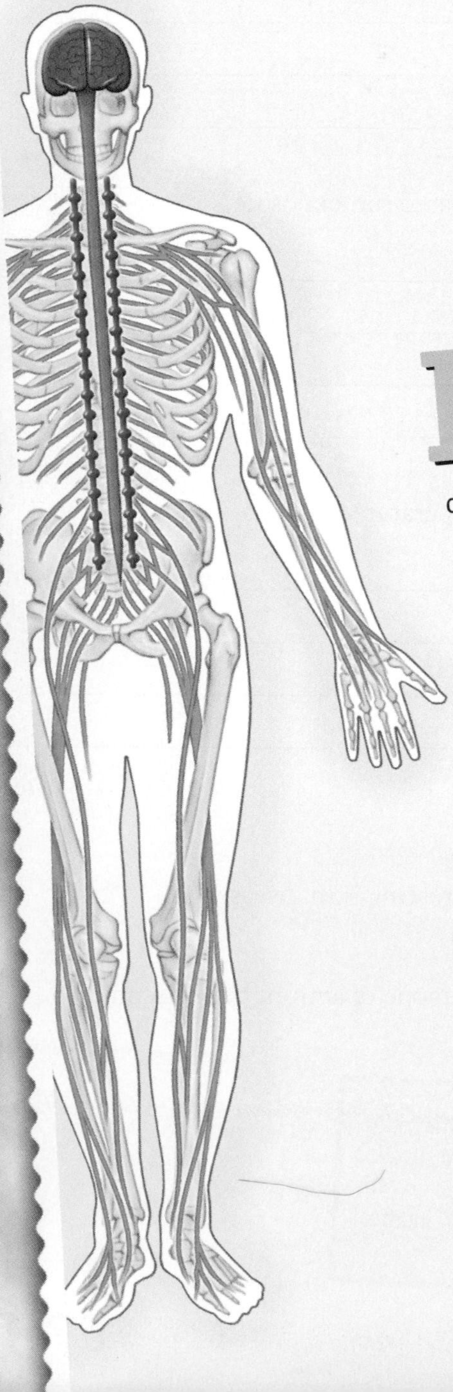

It's often a good idea to take an interesting novel along when we travel. The nervous system, due to its complexity and importance, is our novel for this journey! Don't be dismayed by the length of this novel, because the related control system Chapters (10 and 11) will be the "short stories" by comparison. So far on our journey, we have seen infrastructure, the building blocks and support systems of the city. Soon we will visit transportation, protection, and energy delivery systems. Like any good city, the body must have a control system, a system to monitor conditions, take corrective action when necessary, and keep everything running smoothly. Imagine what would happen if a traffic light network in a city were to suddenly fail. The control systems of the body are the nervous and endocrine systems, which receive help from your special senses. Like any control system, they have a large, complex job that is sometimes difficult to understand. They must keep track of everything that is happening in the body. Therefore, the nervous and endocrine systems are perhaps the most complex and vital systems we will visit. To make the trip more manageable, we have subdivided the nervous system into two separate chapters. In this chapter (Part I), we start at the bottom of the control hierarchy, the cells and the spinal cord. In Chapter 9, Part II, we focus on the higher level control at the brain.

Chapter 8

LEARNING OBJECTIVES

Upon completion of your journey through this chapter, you will be able to:

- List and describe the components and basic operation of the nervous system
- Contrast the central and peripheral nervous systems
- Explain the relationship of the sensory system to the nervous system
- Define the parts and functions of the nervous tissue
- Describe the process of neuromuscular transmission
- Discuss the anatomy and physiology of the spinal cord
- List and describe various nervous system disorders of the nerves and spinal cord

MULTIMEDIA APPLICATIONS

CD-ROM Interactive Exercises

- Animation of multiple sclerosis, 8-1
- Animation of neurochemical synaptic transmission, 8-2
- Animation of neuromuscular contraction, 8-3
- Videos of epidural placement, 8-4
- 3-D animation of brachial and lumbosacral plexus and spinal cord, 8-5
- Animation of cervical spine injuries, 8-6
- Animation of neuroreflex arc, 8-7
- Video of carpal tunnel syndrome (CTS), 8-8
- Interactive games and puzzles, 8-9

www.prenhall.com/colbert

- Professional Profile: END; Electroneurodiagnostician
- Related Internet Links
- Additional Review Questions

Pronunciation Guide

Correct pronunciation is important in any journey so that you and others are completely understood. Here is a "see and say" Pronunciation Guide for the more difficult terms to pronounce in this chapter.

arachnoid mater (ah RAK noyd MAY ter)
astrocytes (ASS troh SITES)
axon (AK son)
cerebrospinal fluid (ser eh broh SPY nal FLOO id)
chemical synapse (KEH mih cull SIH naps)
commissures (KAH mih sures)
dendrites (DEN drights)
dorsal root ganglion (DOR sal ROOT GANG lee on)
dura mater (DOO ra MAY ter)
ependymal cells (ep PEN deh mall)
epidural space (eh pih DURE all)
ganglia (GANG lee ah)
glial Cells (GLEE all sells)
gyri (JIE rie)
meninges (men IN jeez)
microglia (mie crow GLEE ah)
myelin (MY eh lin)
neuroglia (glial cells) (noo ROH glee ah)
nodes of Ranvier (ron vee AYE)
oligodendrocytes (AH li go DEN droe site)
pia mater (PEE ah MAY ter)
plexus (PLECK sus)
Schwann cells (SHWAN sells)
somatic nervous system (so MAT ick)
subarachnoid space (SUB ah RACK noyd)
subdural space (sub DOO ral)
sulcus (SULL cuss)
vesicles (VESS ih klz)

ORGANIZATION

We begin this journey with an overview of the entire system to show how all the components are interrelated. Let's start with the basic operations.

The Parts and Basic Operation of the Nervous System

The organization of the nervous system can be compared to a computer. Information is inputted to the computer by various means ("senses"): keyboard, mouse, microphone, internet connection, and so on. The main components of the computer's "brain" are the hard drive ("long-term memory"), random access memory ("short-term memory"), and central processing unit ("thinking" and "decision making"). The computer's output—its "interaction with the world"—exits via ports and cables to printers, displays, speakers, and other devices.

Typically, we refer to the brain and spinal cord as the **central nervous system (CNS)** and everything outside of the brain and spinal cord, which represent the input and output pathways, as the **peripheral nervous system (PNS)**. Figure 8–1 ■ is a schematic of the organization of the branches of the nervous system.

The nervous system's "input devices" comprise the **sensory system.** Your senses sample the environment and bring the information to the nervous system, as explored further in Chapter 11. Everything that can possibly be measured about your body and the world around you is measured by your sensory system. The sensory information goes into the nervous system where it is handled by the brain and spinal cord. The brain and spinal cord (the hard drive, random access memory, and processor) combine the input with other kinds of information, compare it to information from past experiences, and make decisions about how to respond to the information. Once the brain and spinal cord decide what response is required

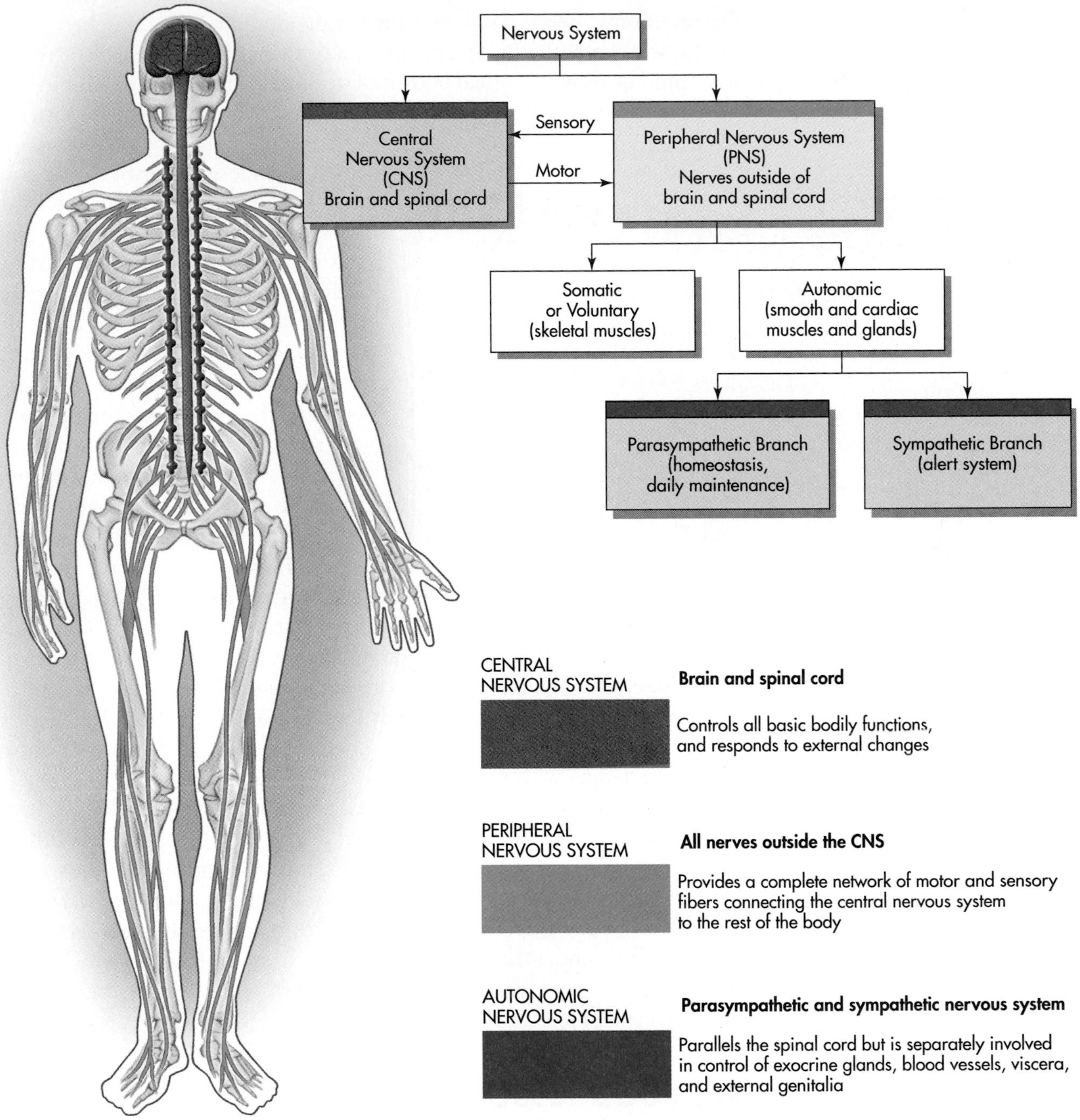

FIGURE ■ 8–1

Organization of the nervous system.

to deal with the new information, the output side is activated. The output side carries out the orders from the brain and spinal cord. The output side, often called the **motor system,** carries orders to all three types of muscles and to the body's glands, telling them how to respond to the new information. The motor system is divided into two different branches: the **somatic nervous system,** which controls skeletal muscle and usually voluntary movements, and the **autonomic nervous system,** which controls smooth and cardiac muscle in your organs and also

moto = *movement*

somatic nervous system
(so MAT ick)

several glands. Autonomic output is involuntary and not under conscious control. The autonomic nervous system is further divided into two branches: **parasympathetic** and **sympathetic.** The parasympathetic branch, often called "resting and digesting," deals with normal body functioning, while the sympathetic branch is the body's alert system, commonly known as the "fight-or-flight" response system.

The organization of the nervous system is easier to understand if we look at a real-life event. You drive over to your friend's house. As you step onto her walkway, a large dog bounds down the front steps barking and snarling at you. Your sensory system gathers the following information about the new stimulus: a large unfriendly dog; you are far from the protection of the car; nobody is coming to help. The information goes into your spinal cord and brain, and several decisions are made. You are in danger, something must be done. Your brain and spinal cord send directions via your autonomic nervous system to your organs to gear up for action. Your heart rate, blood pressure, and respiration rate rise. You begin to sweat. More blood is delivered to your skeletal muscles and heart in order to get you fully ready to respond. This is all involuntary, meaning you cannot consciously control it. Your nervous system readies your skeletal muscles to get you out of there. This fight-or-flight response is discussed later in further depth. If you can control your fear, you back slowly away from the situation. If you are scared witless, you run from the yard as fast as you can. Either way, you can hopefully escape the danger with your skin and your pride intact.

Amazing Body Facts

FASTER THAN A SPEEDING BULLET

Well, not literally! Your nervous system must respond very quickly to stimuli. Think about how fast you pull your hand away from a hot stove or step on the brake when something runs in front of your car. Nerve impulses can move very quickly. Some neurons have speeds as fast as 100 meters per second. That's in the neighborhood of 200 miles per hour. Bullets, on the other hand, can travel 3,000 miles per hour!

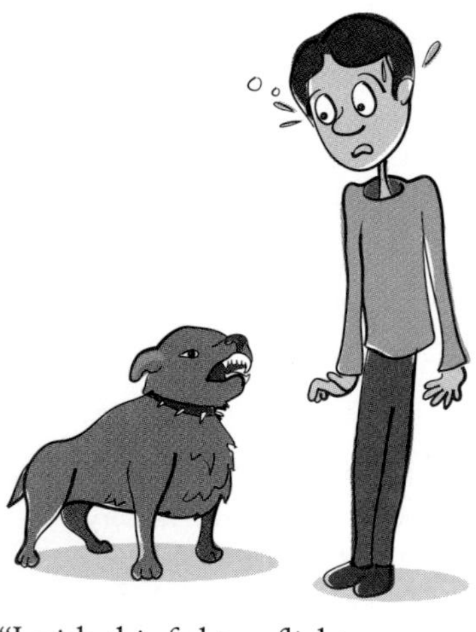

"I wish this fight or flight response would allow me to actually grow wings to fly away!!"

Each part of the nervous system has separate but unmistakably connected roles to play in assessing a situation and responding to it. The nervous system is active 24 hours a day, seven days a week, for your entire life. Some situations, like the unfriendly dog, or a sudden drop in blood pressure, or a terrible car accident, may be life-threatening. Others, like an ant crawling across your foot or a pencil rolling under the desk just out of reach, are simply annoying. Everything that happens in your world is monitored and responded to by your nervous system. It's a truly Herculean task!

NERVOUS TISSUE

Like all organs, the components of the nervous system are made up of tissue. But unlike other systems, the nervous system contains no epithelium, connective tissue, or muscle tissue. Nervous tissue is made up of two different types of cells: neurons and neuroglia.

neuroglia *(noo ROH glee ah)*
glial cells *(GLEE all sells)*

astrocytes *(ASS tre SITES)*
astro = *star*
cyte = *cell*
microglia *(mie crow GLEE ah)*
ependymal cells *(ep PEN deh mall)*
oligodendrocytes *(AH li go DEN droe sites)*
oligo = *few*
dendro = *branches*
myelin *(MY eh lin)*

Neuroglia

The **neuroglia** or **glial cells** are specialized cells in nervous tissue that allow it to perform nervous system functions. In the CNS, there are four types of glial cells. **Astrocytes** are metabolic and structural support cells. **Microglia** remove debris. **Ependymal cells** do the job of epithelial cells, covering and lining cavities. **Oligodendrocytes** make a lipid insulation called **myelin,** described in more

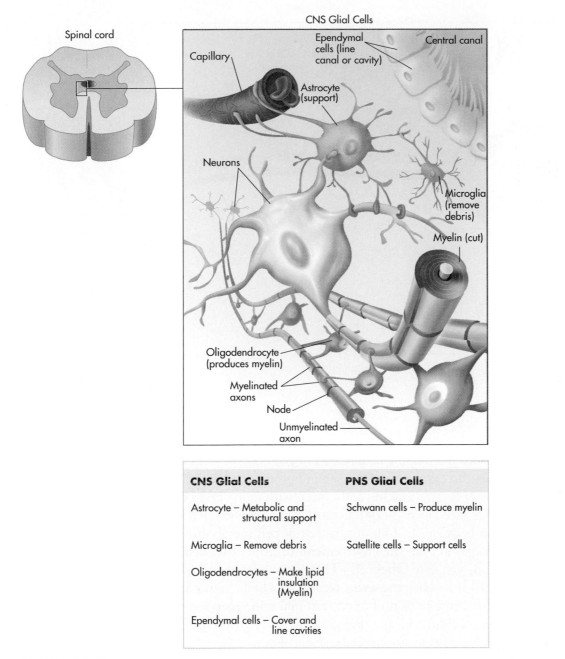

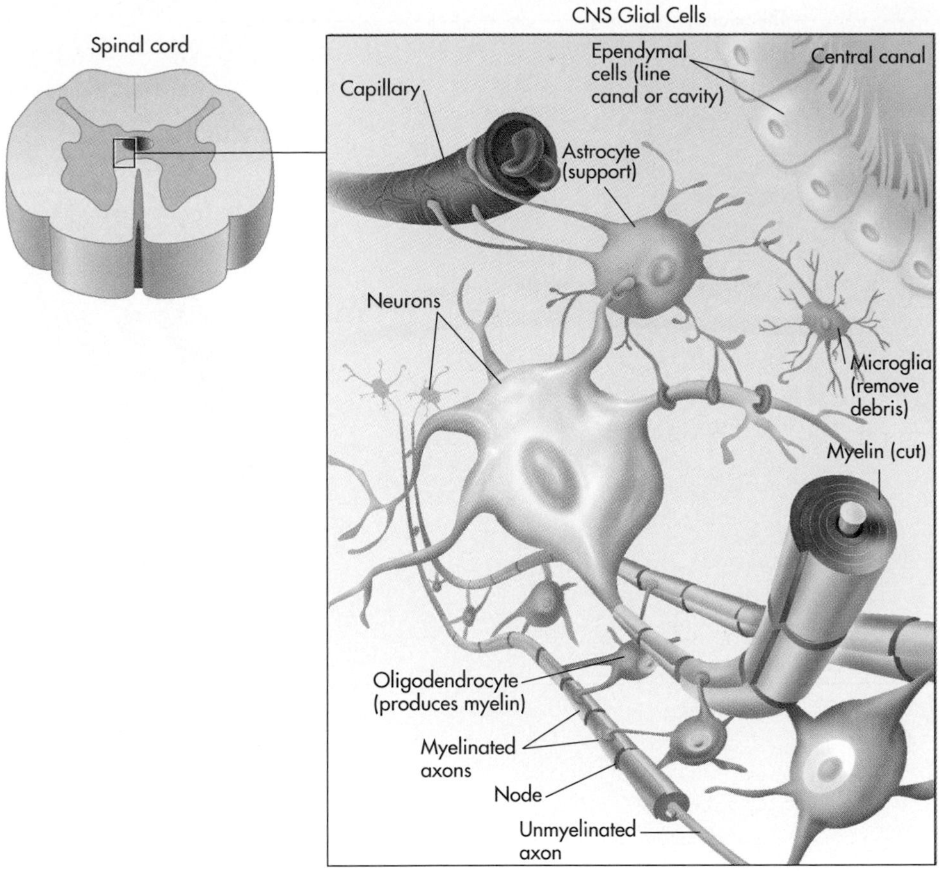

CNS Glial Cells	PNS Glial Cells
Astrocyte – Metabolic and structural support	Schwann cells – Produce myelin
Microglia – Remove debris	Satellite cells – Support cells
Oligodendrocytes – Make lipid insulation (Myelin)	
Ependymal cells – Cover and line cavities	

FIGURE ■ 8–2

Glial cells and their functions.

detail a bit later. In the PNS, there are only two types of glial cells: **Schwann cells,** which make myelin for the PNS, and **satellite cells,** which are support cells. Please see Figure 8–2 ■ which shows a cutaway view of the spinal cord of the CNS showing the four types of neuroglial cells found there.

Schwann cells *(SHWAN sells)*

Neurons

The glial cells do all the support activities for the nervous system, such as lining and covering cavities and supporting and protecting structures. None of the glial cells, however, are capable of measuring the environment, making de-

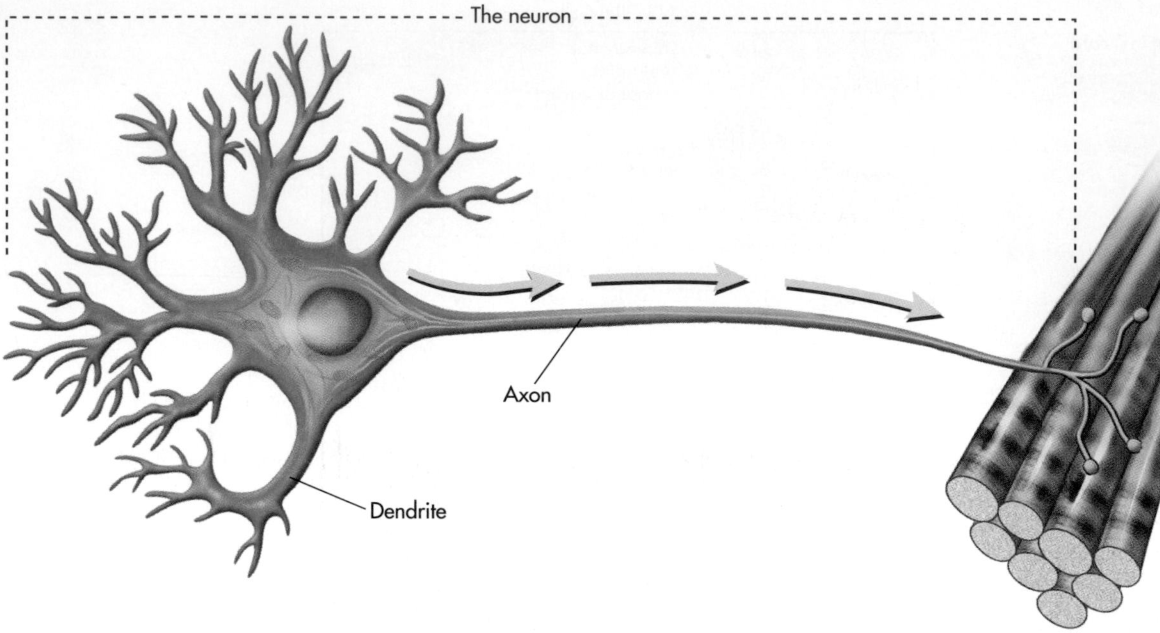

FIGURE ■ 8–3

A neuron connecting to a skeletal muscle.

cisions, or sending orders. All of the control functions of the nervous system must be carried out by a second group of cells called **neurons.** Neurons are rather bizarre-looking cells, often with many branches and what appears to be a tail (see Figure 8–3 ■). Each part of a neuron has a specific function. The neuron body's main function is that of cell metabolism. Its **dendrites** receive information from the environment or from other cells. The **axon** generates and sends signals to other cells. Those signals leave the cell and travel down the axon until it reaches the **axon terminal,** which then connects to a receiving cell. This combination of axon terminal and receiving cell is called a **synapse.** If the receiving cell is a skeletal muscle cell, then this particular synapse is called the *neuromuscular synapse* or *junction*.

dendrites *(DEN drights)*
axon *(AK son)*
synapse *(SIH naps)*

Neurons can be classified by how they look (structure) or what they do (function). From a structural point of view, neurons can have either one axon and one dendrite (bipolar), one axon and many dendrites (multipolar), or one process that splits into a central and a peripheral projection (unipolar). Classified by function, input neurons are known as **sensory neurons** and output neurons are known as **motor neurons.** Neurons that carry information between neurons are called **interneurons** (*inter* means between) or **association neurons.**

interneurons (association neurons) *(in ter Noo rons)*

TEST YOUR KNOWLEDGE 8-1

Choose the best answer:

1. Which cells are the support cells in the nervous system?
   a. neurons
   b. neuroglia
   c. epithelium
   d. all of the above

2. The output side of your nervous system is called
   a. sensory
   b. motor
   c. central
   d. exit

3. The part of the nervous system that integrates and processes information is known as the
   a. PNS
   b. PBS
   c. CNS
   d. CIA

4. The lipid insulation of nervous tissue is called:
   a. glia
   b. myelin
   c. Schwann cells
   d. astrocytes

HOW NEURONS WORK

Now that we know the basic structure of neurons, let's look closer at how they function.

Excitable Cells

A neuron is a kind of cell called an *excitable cell.* An excitable cell carries a small electrical charge when stimulated. Each time charged particles flow across a cell membrane, a tiny electrical current is generated. (Electricity is just the movement of charges from one place to the other.) All three types of muscle cells are excitable cells, as are many gland cells. Because neurons are excitable cells, it makes sense that the way neurons send and receive signals is via tiny electrical currents. (This is also one of the reasons electrocution can cause nervous system damage. It literally shorts out the electrical pathways in the neurons.)

How, you might ask, can cells carry electricity? It seems hard to believe, but cells are like miniature batteries, able to generate tiny currents simply by changing the permeability of their membranes. Perhaps the plot of the *Matrix* movies in which humans are used by machines as batteries is not so far-fetched.

Action Potentials

A cell that is not stimulated or excited is called a resting cell and is said to be *polarized*. It has a difference in charge across its membrane such that it is more negative on the inside than on the outside. When that cell gets stimulated (excited), gates in the cell membrane spring open. When these gates, called sodium gates, open, they allow sodium ions (Na^+) to travel across the cell membrane. These sodium bits are positively charged, so when they go into the cell, the cell becomes more positive. A cell that is more positive than resting is called **depolarized.** In less than a millisecond, the gates on the sodium channels shut, just like the automatic doors at the supermarket shut by themselves. Then other gates open for potassium channels. Potassium (K^+), which is also positive, leaves the cell, taking its positive charges with it. The inside of the cell becomes more negative again, eventually returning to rest. This is **repolarization** (see Figure 8–4 ■). Sometimes a cell overshoots and becomes more negative than when it is at rest. Then the cell is **hyperpolarized.** Eventually the cell will return to resting. It should be noted that the cell is unable to accept another stimulus until it repolarizes (returns to its resting state), and this time period during which it cannot accept another stimulus is called the **refractory period.** This whole series of permeability changes within the cell and the resultant changes of the in-

> *Applied Science*
>
> **FUGU**
>
> The puffer fish, fugu, is considered a delicacy in Japan because if you eat it, you could die! Fugu can be served only by specially certified chefs trained to prepare the fish so it is safe to eat. Puffer fish contain a poison, tetrodotoxin (TTX), in their tissues that blocks sodium channels, preventing sodium from entering cells. Cells exposed to TTX cannot depolarize. Thus, neurons cannot fire action potentials. People who consume improperly prepared fugu become paralyzed. Symptoms develop as ascending paralysis within 15 minutes to 20 hours post ingestion. If untreated, death can result in 4 to 6 hours.

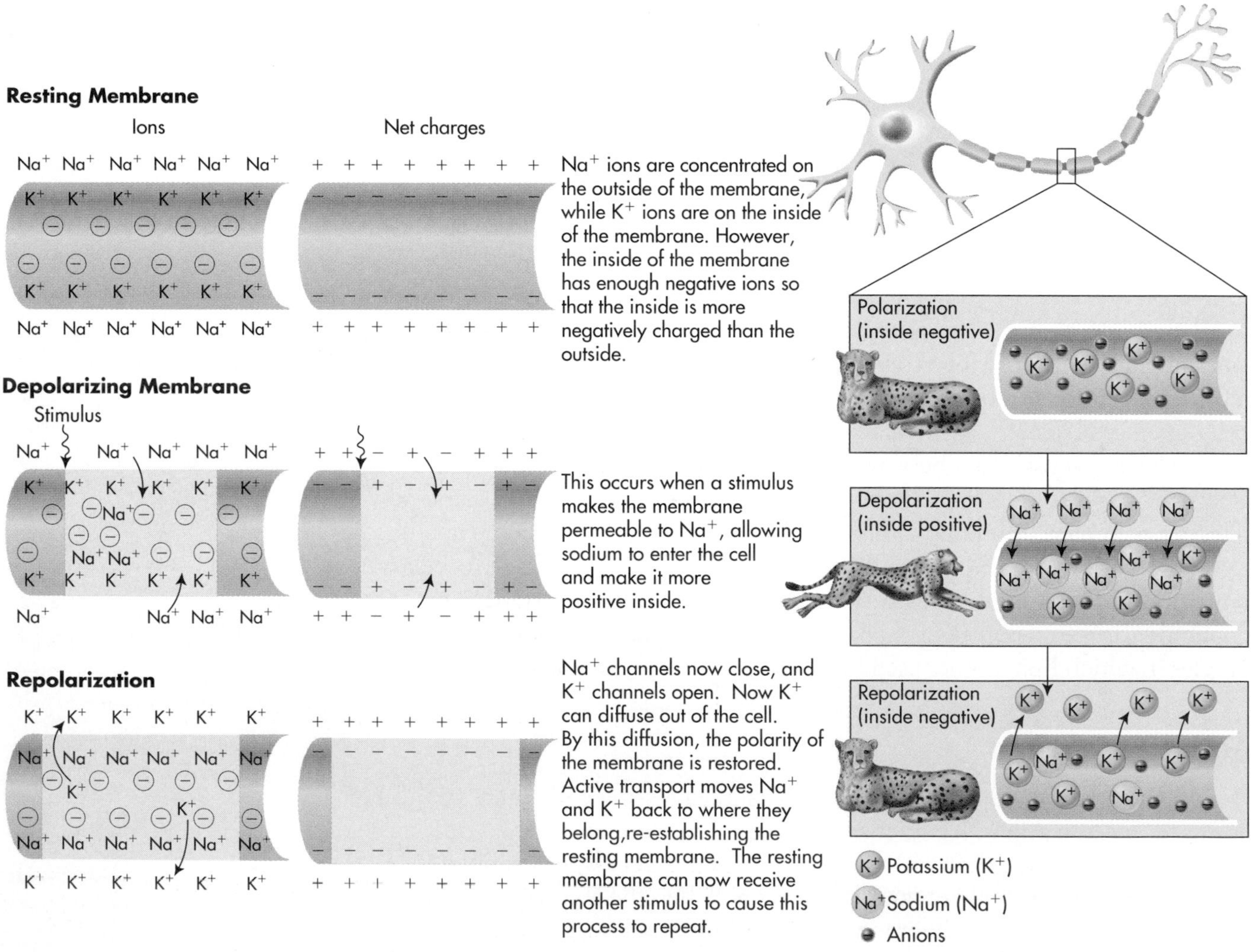

Resting Membrane
Ions
Net charges
Na+ ions are concentrated on the outside of the membrane, while K+ ions are on the inside of the membrane. However, the inside of the membrane has enough negative ions so that the inside is more negatively charged than the outside.
Depolarizing Membrane
Stimulus
This occurs when a stimulus makes the membrane permeable to Na+, allowing sodium to enter the cell and make it more positive inside.
Repolarization
Na+ channels now close, and K+ channels open. Now K+ can diffuse out of the cell. By this diffusion, the polarity of the membrane is restored. Active transport moves Na+ and K+ back to where they belong, re-establishing the resting membrane. The resting membrane can now receive another stimulus to cause this process to repeat.
Polarization (inside negative)
Depolarization (inside positive)
Repolarization (inside negative)
Potassium (K+)
Sodium (Na+)
Anions

FIGURE ■ 8–4

Depolarization and repolarization.

ternal and external charges to carry the impulse down the axon is called the **action potential.**

Local Potentials

Neurons can use their ability to generate electricity to send, receive, and interpret signals. Let's look at an example of how this works. You are hammering a picture hanger into the wall of your newly painted bedroom, and you hit your thumb. The blow from the hammer stimulates the dendrites in your thumb, and sodium gates open. Sodium flows into the dendrites, which become depolarized. If you hit your thumb softly, the cell is stimulated only a little, only a few gates open, and the cell does not depolarize very much. (The pain isn't too bad, either.) If you hit your thumb really hard, more gates open and the cell depolarizes much more. (It hurts a lot more, too!) This phenomenon is known as a **local potential.** In a local potential, the size of the stimulus determines the excitement of the cell. A big stimulus causes a bigger depolarization than a small stimulus. Many sensory cells work via local potentials. That's often how your CNS tells the size of the environmental change.

The dendrites carry the depolarization to the sensory neuron cell body. The cell body takes that information and generates an action potential, if the stimulus is big enough. One difference between action potentials and local potentials is that action potentials are "all-or-none," which means that the action potential, once it starts, will always finish and will always be the same size. You either have one or you don't. There are no small action potentials or big ones as there are with local potentials. Action potentials are always the same. Once an action potential is formed, it travels down the axon from the cell body to the terminal. This movement is called *impulse conduction*.

Impulse Conduction

The speed of impulse conduction along an axon is determined by two characteristics: the presence of myelin and the diameter of the axon. Myelin is a lipid insulation or sheath formed by the oligodendrocytes in the CNS and the Schwann cells in the PNS. In preserved brains, the myelinated axons look white. Unmyelinated parts of the CNS, like cell bodies, look gray. Therefore, what we call "white matter" is typically made of axons, and what we call "gray matter" is made of cell bodies. The cell membranes of oligodendrocytes or Schwann cells are wrapped around an axon like a bandage. Between adjacent glial cells are tiny bare spots called **nodes of Ranvier** (see Figure 8–5 ■). When an axon is wrapped in myelin, we call the axon myelinated. Myelin

Clinical Application

MULTIPLE SCLEROSIS

Multiple sclerosis (MS) is a disorder of the myelin in the CNS. Patients with multiple sclerosis have many areas where the myelin has been destroyed. In areas without myelin, impulse conduction is slow or impossible. Imagine an electrical wire with many bare spots or with no insulation. These bare or exposed parts can "short out" and prevent the current from passing further down the wire. Symptoms of multiple sclerosis differ from patient to patient depending on where the myelin damage occurs. Patients may have disturbances in vision, balance, speech, or movement. MS is more common in women than in men and is diagnosed most often in people under the age of fifty.

8-1 For more information on multiple sclerosis and to view an animation showing the destruction of the myelin sheath and subsequent pathophysiologic changes, please go to the CD-ROM for this chapter.

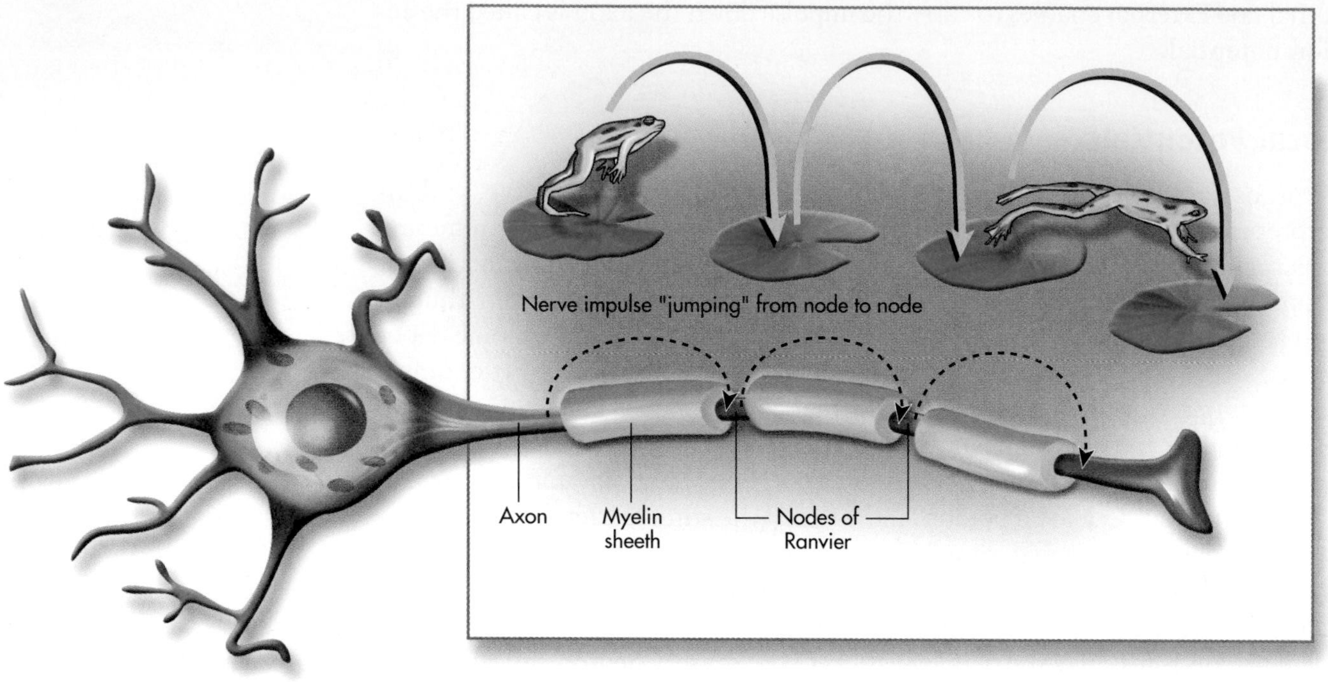

FIGURE ■ 8–5

Impulse conduction via myelinated axon.

is essential for the speedy flow of action potentials down axons. In an unmyelinated axon, the action potential can only flow down the axon by depolarizing each and every millimeter of the axon. Every single sodium channel must open, and every single potassium channel must open. It is a relatively slow process. In a myelinated axon, only the channels at the nodes must open for the action potential to flow down the axon. Myelin prevents ions from passing through channels, because ions are water soluble and myelin is a lipid. (Remember, charged particles cannot get through lipids.) The action potential therefore "skips" down the axon from node to node (nodal transmission) rather than creeping along the entire length of the axon. It works the same way as if you try to walk across the floor heel to toe, never missing a spot and then skip across the floor in large leaps. Which is faster?

The diameter of the axon also affects the speed of action potential flow. Think about moving through two different pipes, say on a playground or obstacle course. One pipe is one-half meter in diameter (less than 2 ft). To move through the pipe, you must crawl. The other pipe is 2 meters in diameter (more than 6 ft). Most of you can stand in this pipe with room to spare. Which trip would be faster? Obviously, it's the one through the larger diameter pipe. You don't have to crawl, you don't get hung up on the side. Heck, you could even run through the big pipe! For ions, the axon is essentially a pipe. The wider the axon, the faster the ions flow. The combination of myelination and large diameter makes a huge difference in speed. Small, unmyelinated axons have speeds as low as 0.5 meters per second, while large-diameter, myelinated axons may be as fast as 100 meters per second. That's 200 times faster!

How Synapses Work

In order for neurons to communicate, there must be some way for a message to be sent from one neuron to the other. This communication occurs at the synapse. An action potential is generated and flows toward the axon terminal.

CHEMICAL SYNAPSES

When an impulse arrives at the axon terminal, the terminal depolarizes and calcium gates open. Calcium flows into the cell. When calcium flows in, it triggers a change in the terminal. There are tiny sacs in the terminal called **vesicles,** which release their contents from the cell via exocytosis when calcium flows in. These vesicles are filled with molecules called **neurotransmitters.**

vesicles *(VESS ih klz)*

neurotransmitter *(noo roh TRANS mit ter)*

These neurotransmitters are used to send the signal from the neuron across the synapse to the next cell in line. The neurotransmitter binds to the cell receiving the signal and causes gates to open or close. Some neurotransmitters excite the receiving cell and some calm it down. In the case of the hammered thumb, the neurotransmitter would be released in your spinal cord and would excite a pain neuron. The receiving neuron would be stimulated and take the information about your thumb to your brain, where you would register the pain.

The last step in the transfer of information is clean-up. The neurotransmitter must be taken away from the synapse or it will continually bind to the receiving cell. This clean-up is accomplished through an inactivator. For example, if the neurotransmitter chemical is acetylcholine (ACh), it will be inactivated by acetylcholinesterase, an enzyme that breaks down ACh. This type of information flow, using neurotransmitters, is called a **chemical synapse,** because chemicals (neurotransmitters) are used to carry the information from one cell to another. See Figure 8–6 ■ for the steps in chemical synaptic transmission.

ase = *to break down*

chemical synapse *(KEH mih cull SIH naps)*

Our understanding of chemical synapses has led to several breakthroughs for treating mental illness. Many medications on the market today are designed to modify synapses. Selective serotonin reuptake inhibitors (SSRI) are good examples. These medications prevent the clean-up of the neurotransmitter serotonin from synapses, thereby increasing the effects of serotonin on the receiving cell. Many antidepressants and anti-anxiety medications are SSRIs. Table 8–1 contains other examples of clinically important neurotransmitters.

ELECTRICAL SYNAPSES

> **8-2** Because the concept of neurochemical transmission at the synapse is sometimes hard to grasp, go to your CD-ROM to view an animation of this process.

Some cells do not need chemicals to transmit information from one cell to another. These synapses are called **electrical synapses.** The cells in an electrical synapse can transfer information freely because they have special connections called **gap junctions.** Such connections can exist between many types of excitable cells. They are found, for example, in the intercalated disks between cardiac muscle fibers.

THE NEUROMUSCULAR JUNCTION

One chemical synapse, the **neuromuscular junction,** is particularly important to the function of your motor system, as we mentioned briefly in Chapter 6, The Muscular System. The neuromuscular junction is a specialized synapse between somatic (voluntary) motor neurons and the skeletal muscles they in-

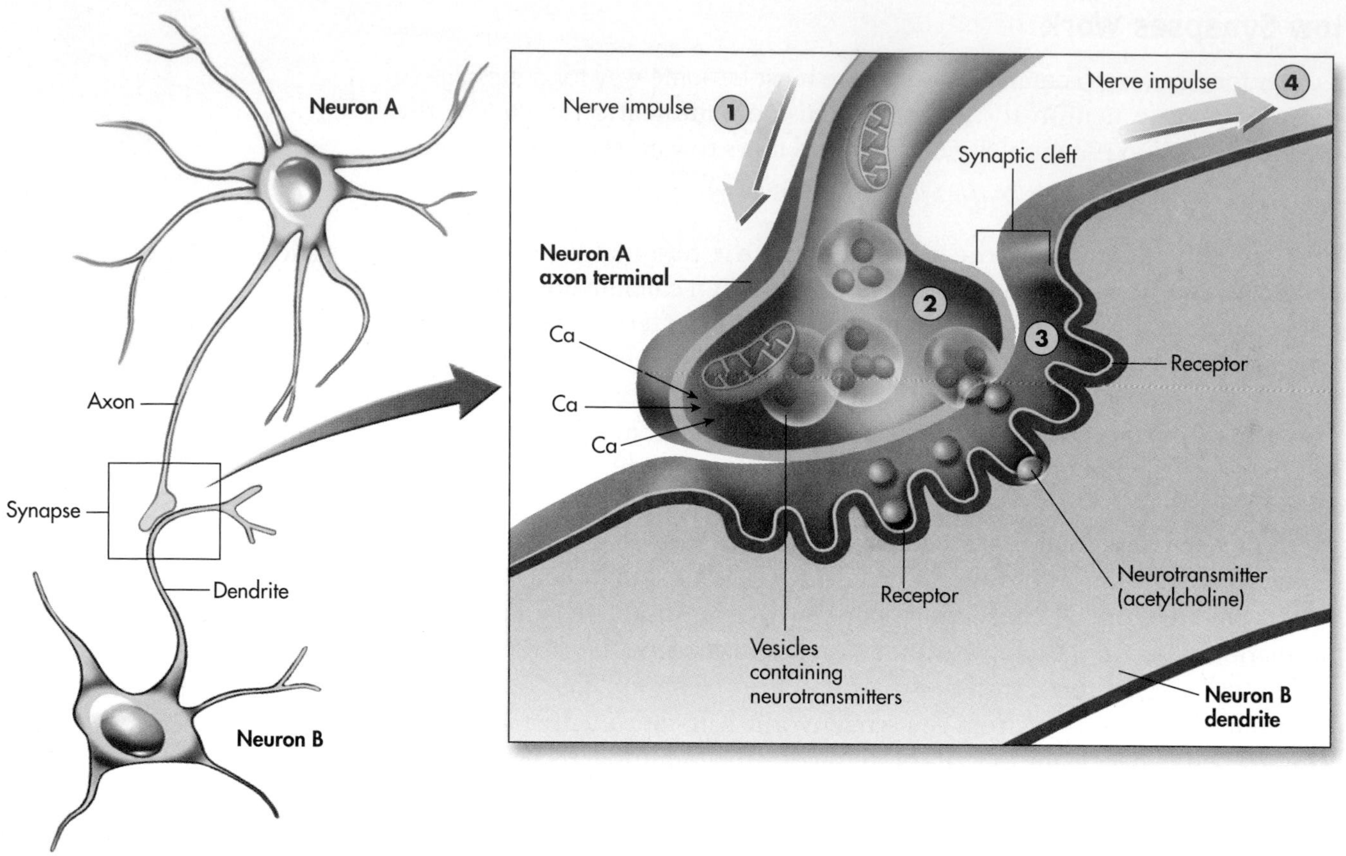

FIGURE ■ 8–6

The Chemical Synapse. Step 1: the impulse travels down the axon. Step 2: vesicles are stimulated to release neurotransmitter (exocytosis). Step 3: the neurotransmitter travels across the synapse and binds with the receptor site of post synaptic cell. Step 4: the impulse continues down the dendrite.

TABLE 8–1 Selected Common Neurotransmitters

NEUROTRANSMITTER	LOCATION	FUNCTION	COMMENTS
Acetylcholine	CNS* and PNS*	Generally excitatory but is inhibitory to some visceral effectors	Found in skeletal neuromuscular junctions and in many ANS* synapses
Norepinephrine	CNS and PNS	May be excitatory or inhibitory depending on the receptors	Found in visceral and cardiac muscle
Epinephrine	CNS and PNS	May be excitatory or inhibitory depending on the receptors	Found in pathways concerned with behavior and mood
Serotonin	CNS	Generally inhibitory	Found in pathways that regulate temperature, sensory perception, mood, onset of sleep
Endorphins	CNS	Generally inhibitory	Inhibit release of sensory pain neurotransmitters

*CNS = central nervous system; PNS = peripheral nervous system; ANS = autonomic nervous system.

nervate. The surface of the muscle is studded with sodium channels that are ligand gated. A ligand-gated channel opens or closes when a molecule binds to a receptor that is part of the channel, like a key fitting into a lock. In the case of skeletal muscles, the ligand, or key, is the neurotransmitter acetylcholine. Acetylcholine is released from the terminal of a motor neuron and binds to the surface of skeletal muscle, opening sodium channels and causing the skeletal muscle to be depolarized. This depolarization leads to the changes described in Chapter 6, and the muscle contracts. Like all chemical synapses, the neuromuscular junction must be cleaned up at the end of transmission. The enzyme responsible for cleaning up the synapse is called acetylcholinesterase.

Clinical Application

BIOTERRORISM

If acetylcholinesterase activity is prevented, acetylcholine continually stimulates the muscle eventually, paralyzing it. Some insecticides and the nerve gas Sarin, which killed several hundred people during a terrorist attack in a Tokyo subway tunnel in 1995, are acetylcholinesterase inhibitors. They kill by causing paralysis of skeletal muscles, including the diaphragm, the most important respiratory muscle. Victims of Sarin or overexposure to organophosphate insecticides may die from respiratory arrest.

8-3 Go to your CD-ROM or the companion website to see how the neuromuscular junction functions to cause a muscular contraction.

The electroneurodiagnostician (END) is involved in assessing and testing patients with potential neurological diseases to aid the physician in an accurate diagnosis. To view a video on this health care career, please go to the companion website for this chapter.

TEST YOUR KNOWLEDGE 8-2

Choose the best answer:

1. Which ions move *into* neurons during the action potential?
   a. potassium
   b. calcium
   c. sodium
   d. acetylcholine

2. Which of the following is all-or-none?
   a. local potential
   b. action potential
   c. chemical synapse
   d. impulse conduction

3. The molecules used to send signals across synapses are called
   a. hormones
   b. ions
   c. neurotransmitters
   d. messengers

4. When you hit your thumb with a hammer, what happens next in your nervous system?
   a. synaptic transmission
   b. a local potential
   c. an action potential
   d. resting potential

5. What is another name for myelinated axons?
   a. gray matter
   b. dura mater
   c. white matter
   d. duzitmater

SPINAL CORD AND SPINAL NERVES

So far we've discussed the nervous system at the cellular and tissue level. In addition, we've described how impulses are transmitted in the nervous system. Now let's focus on the main highway that these impulses travel.

> **Learning Hint**
>
> **DIRECTIONAL TERMS**
>
> In the spinal cord, directional terms—anterior, posterior, dorsal, and ventral—are very important because function is linked to location. It is easy to get confused by the use of anterior and posterior for some structures and dorsal and ventral for others. Just keep in mind that in humans, anterior is ventral and posterior is dorsal. The names are interchangeable for all the structures except the spinal roots. The spinal roots are *always* called dorsal and ventral.

External Anatomy

The **spinal cord** is located in a hollow tube running inside the vertebral column from the *foramen magnum* to the second lumbar (L2) vertebrae. You can think of your spinal cord as a very sophisticated neural information superhighway. It is divided into 31 segments, each with a pair of **spinal nerves.** The spinal cord segments

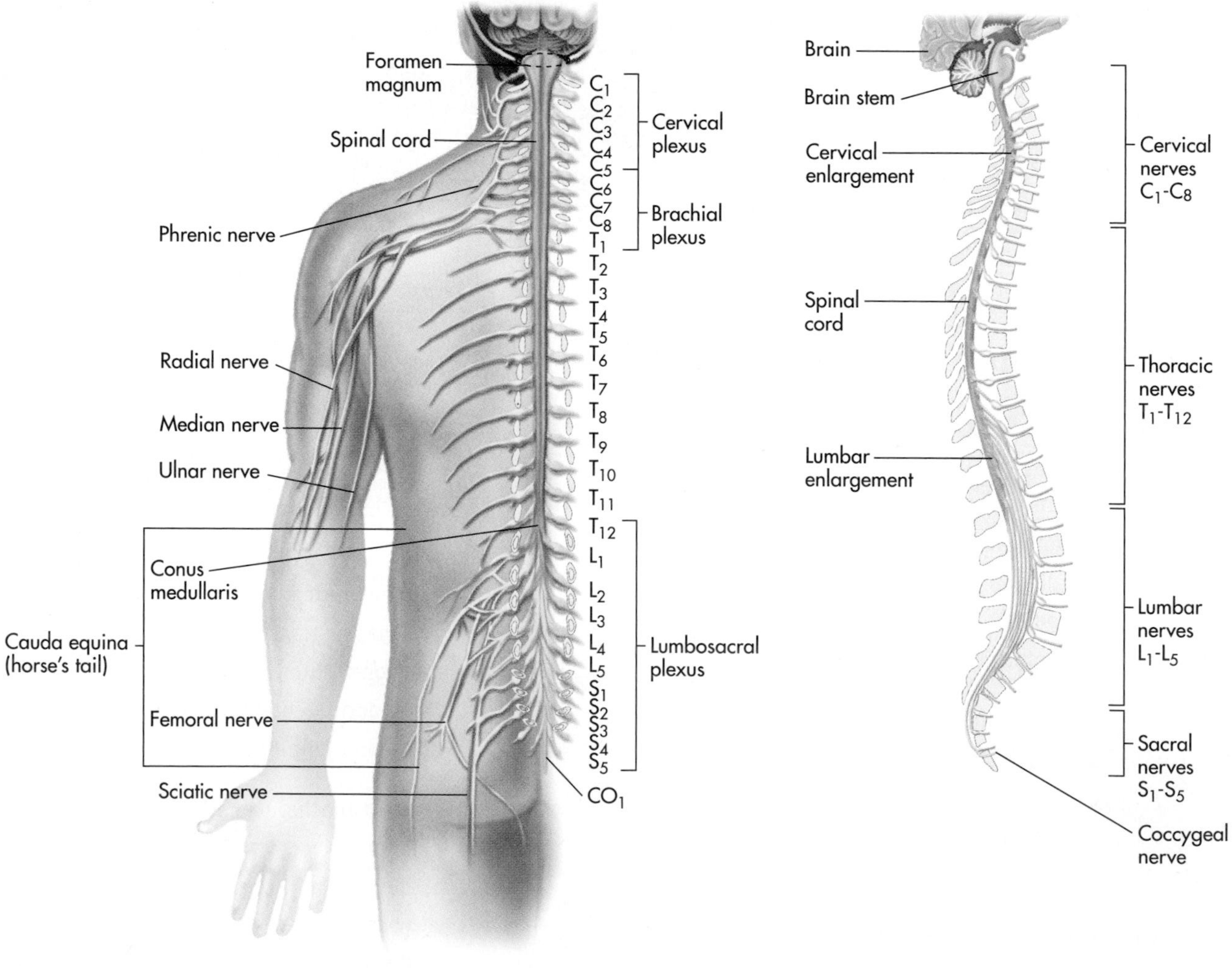

FIGURE ■ 8–7

The spinal cord.

and the spinal nerves are named for their corresponding vertebrae. The spinal cord ends at L2 in a pointed structure called the *conus medullaris*. Hanging from the conus medullaris is the *cauda equina* (literally "horses tail"). The cauda equina is the bunch of spinal nerves L2 through the coccygeal (Co) nerves dangling loosely in a bath of **cerebrospinal fluid** (CSF). The spinal cord has two widened areas, the cervical and lumbar enlargements, which contain the neurons for the limbs. See Figure 8–7 ■.

cauda = *tail*
equina = *horse*
cerebrospinal fluid *(ser eh broh SPY nal FLOO id)*

MENINGES

The CNS, both brain and spinal cord, are surrounded by a series of protective membranes called the **meninges.** The purpose of the meninges is to cover the delicate structures of the brain and spinal cord. In essence, they help to set up layers that act as cushioning and shock absorbers for the brain and spinal cord. The meninges form three distinct layers. The outer layer of thick, fibrous tissue is called the **dura mater.** The middle layer, a wispy, delicate layer resembling spider webs, is the **arachnoid mater.** This layer, which is composed of collagen and elastic fibers, contains cerebrospinal fluid and acts as a shock absorber. In addition, it can also transport dissolved gases and nutrients as well as chemical messengers and waste products. The third, innermost layer, which is fused to the neural tissue of the CNS, is the **pia mater.** This layer contains blood vessels that serve the brain and spinal cord.

Clinical Application

EPIDURAL ANESTHESIA

Often, during labor or in preparation for a Cesarean section, a woman receives an *epidural.* An epidural is an injection of local anesthetic into the epidural space. The anesthetic is usually delivered via a catheter (a small tube). Ideally, epidural anesthesia allows a woman to continue to participate actively in the birth without severe labor pains. Epidural injections of steroids are sometimes prescribed for patients with chronic lower back injuries to relieve pain and inflammation.

dura mater *(DOO ra MAY ter)*
arachnoid mater *(ah RAK noyd MAY ter)*
mater = *mother; the three layers formed by the meninges literally mean "hard mother" (dura mater), "soft mother" (pia mater), and "spider mother" (arachnoid layer)*
pia mater *(PEE ah MAY ter)*

A series of spaces are associated with the meninges. Between the dura and the vertebral column is a space filled with fat and blood vessels called the **epidural space.** Between the dura mater and the arachnoid mater is the **subdural space,** which is filled with a tiny bit of fluid. Between the arachnoid mater and the pia mater is the large **subarachnoid space,** filled with cerebrospinal fluid, acting as a fluid cushion for the CNS. These three membranes and their fluid-filled spaces, together with the bones of the skull and vertebral column, form a strong protection system against CNS injury. Please see Figure 8–8 ■.

epidural space *(eh pih DURE all)*
epi = *on top*
subarachnoid space *(SUB ah RACK noyd)*
subdural space *(sub DOO ral)*
sub = *under*

8-4 To see videos of actual epidural procedures on patients, please go to your CD-ROM for this chapter.

Internal Anatomy of the Spinal Cord

The spinal cord is divided in half by a ventral median fissure and a dorsal median sulcus. A **fissure** is a deep groove on the CNS surface while a **sulcus** is a shallow groove on the CNS surface. Please see Figure 8–9 ■. The interior of the spinal cord is then divided into a series of sections of white matter **columns** and gray matter **horns.** There are three types of horns. The dorsal horn is involved in sensory functions, the ventral horn in motor functions, and the lateral horn in autonomic functions. The horns are the regions where the neurons have their cell bodies.

fissure *(FISH er)*
sulcus *(SULL cuss)*

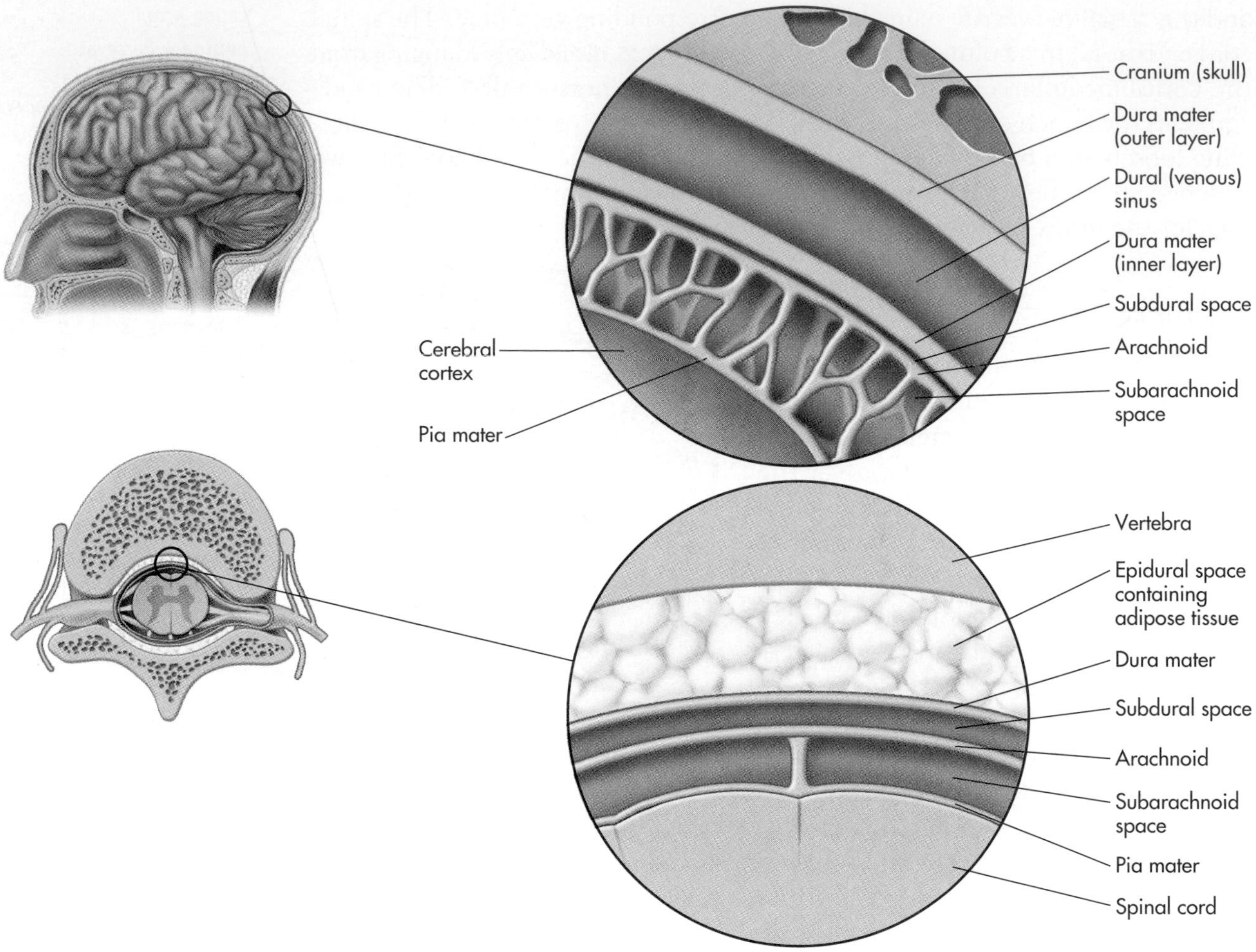

FIGURE ■ 8–8

The meninges of the brain and spinal cord.

The columns also have a ventral, dorsal, and lateral aspect. These columns act as nerve tracts, pathways, or axons, running up and down the spinal cord to and from the brain. Think of the columns as communication wires, part of a vast network of wires, transporting information to the appropriate parts of the system. This is the neural information superhighway. (We discuss the functions of these regions later in the chapter.)

commissures *(KAH mih sures)*

In addition, the spinal cord has several other features. The **commissures,** gray and white, connect left and right halves of the cord so the two sides of the CNS can communicate. (So the right hand does usually know what the left hand is doing even if it doesn't always seem like it!) The central canal is a cavity in the center of the spinal cord that is filled with cerebrospinal fluid. The **spinal roots,** projecting from both sides of the spinal cord in pairs, fuse to form spinal nerves. (The roots are the on-ramps and off-ramps of the neural superhighway.) The dorsal root, with the embedded **dorsal root ganglion,** a collection of sensory neurons, carries sensory information, while the **ventral root** carries motor information. Refer to Figure 8–9.

ganglion *(GANG lee on)*

SPINAL NERVES

Nerves are the connection between the CNS (brain and spinal cord) and the world outside the CNS. Nerves are therefore part of the PNS. Isn't it amazing that the brain,

> **8-5** For a 3-D animation of the spinal cord, brachial plexus, and lumbosacral plexus, please go to this chapter on your CD-ROM.

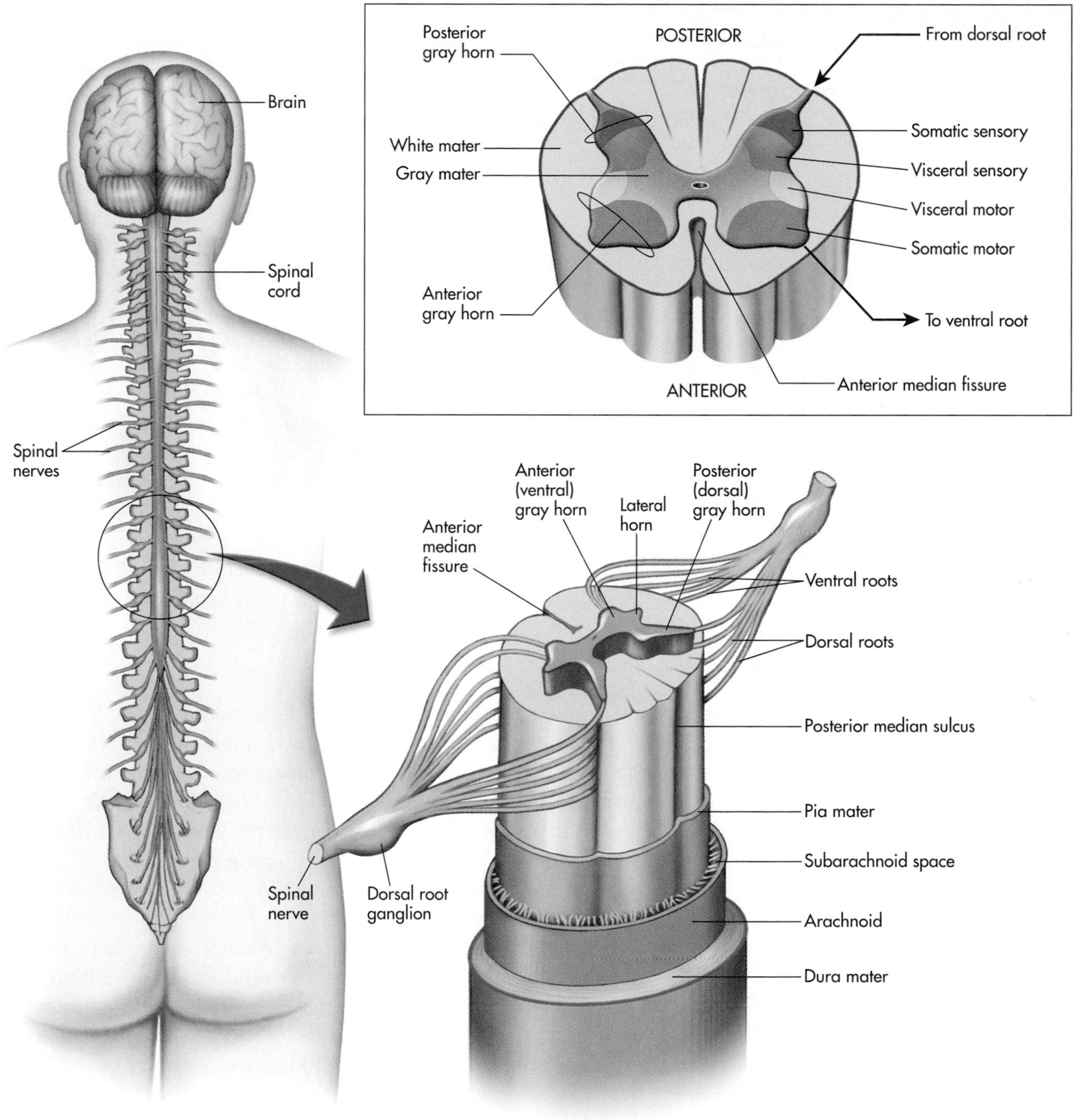

FIGURE ■ 8–9

Internal Anatomy of the Spinal Cord.

which is totally encased in darkness, can receive and interpret the nerve messages from the PNS to allow us to see the wonderful world around us? All nerves consist of bundles of axons, blood vessels, and connective tissue. Nerves run between the CNS and organs or tissues, carrying information into and out of the CNS. The nerves connected to the spinal cord are called *spinal nerves*. There are 31 pairs of spinal nerves, each named for the spinal cord segment to which they are attached. Since each spinal nerve is a fusion of dorsal and ventral roots, spinal nerves carry both sensory and motor information. A nerve that carries both types of information is called a **mixed nerve.** All spinal nerves are mixed. When spinal nerves leave the vertebral column, they can go through a number of different pathways to reach the peripheral tissues. Spinal nerves from the thoracic spinal column project directly to the thoracic body wall without branching. Spinal nerves from the cervical, lumbar, and sacral regions of the spinal cord go through complex branching patterns, recombining with nerves from other spinal cord segments before projecting to peripheral structures. These complex branching patterns are called **plexuses.** See Figure 8–10 ■.

8-6 To view an animation on cervical spine injuries and immobilizations, please go to your CD-ROM for this chapter.

Clinical Application

A MATTER OF CENTIMETERS

Did you know that the difference between being able to breathe on your own after a spinal cord injury and being dependent on a ventilator is literally a matter of centimeters? It's true. One of the nerves that projects from the cervical plexus is called the phrenic nerve. This nerve is the motor nerve for your diaphragm, your main breathing muscle. If the spinal cord is damaged below the cervical plexus, say in the high thoracic region, the phrenic nerve can receive signals from the brain and send them to the diaphragm and the injured person is able to breathe. However, if the damage to the spinal cord is between the brain and the cervical plexus, the path from the brain to the phrenic nerve is blocked and the signals can't get to the diaphragm from the brain. The diaphragm is paralyzed, and the person cannot breathe on his or her own. The difference is a matter of a few centimeters.

REFLEXES

Reflexes are the simplest form of motor output. Reflexes are generally protective, keeping you from harm. They are involuntary, and usually the response is proportionate to the stimulus. Some familiar reflexes are the *withdrawal* reflex, activated for example, when you pound your thumb with a hammer or touch a hot stove; the *vestibular* reflex, which keeps you vertical; and the *startle* reflex, which causes you to jump at loud sounds. The amazing thing about reflexes is that they can often occur without your brain being involved. For many reflexes, only the spinal cord is necessary.

The most common example of a reflex is the patellar tendon (knee-jerk) reflex. You may have experienced this reflex at the doctor's office. The doctor taps your knee with a hammer and your leg kicks, seemingly against your will. What exactly is going on? When the doctor taps your knee, the hammer gently tugs on a tendon that is connected to your quadriceps muscles. The quads are gently tugged. This causes them to lengthen slightly. This length change is received by a sensory neuron and transmitted back to the

8-7 For an animation of the neural-reflex arc, please go to your CD-ROM.

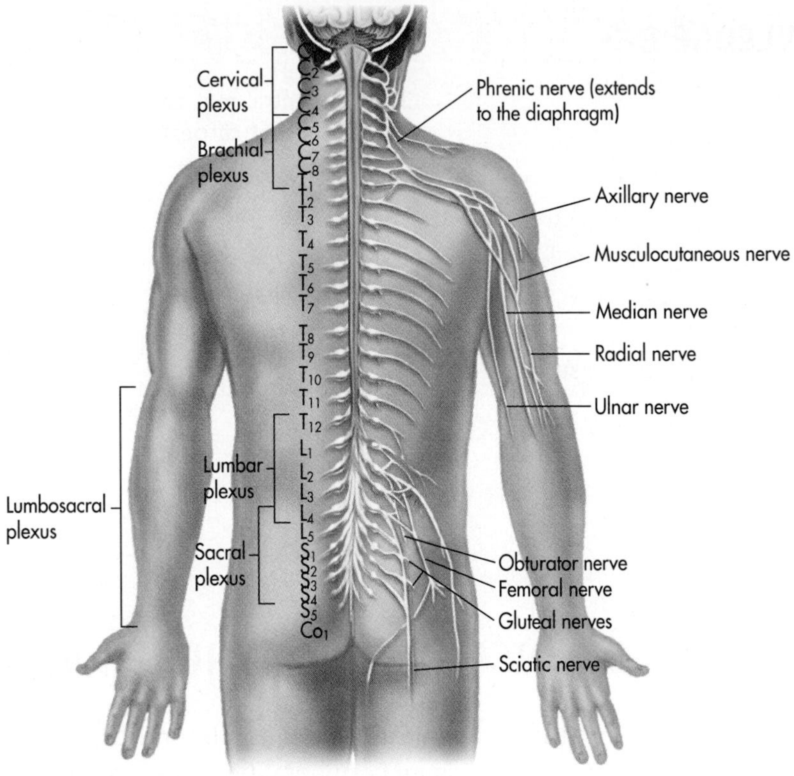

SPINAL NERVE PLEXUSES

PLEXUS	LOCATION	SPINAL NERVES INVOLVED	REGION SUPPLIED	MAJOR NERVES LEAVING PLEXUS
Cervical	Deep in the neck, under the sternocleidomastoid muscle	C_1-C_4	Skin and muscles of neck and shoulder; diaphragm	Phrenic (Diaphragm)
Brachial	Deep to the clavivle, between the neck and the axilla	C_5-C_8, T_1	Skin and muscles of upper extremity	Musculocutaneous Ulnar Median Radial Axillary
Lumbosacral	Lumbar region of the back	T_{12}, L_1-L_5, S_1-S_4	Skin and muscles of lower abdominal wall, lower extremity, buttocks, external genitalia	Obturator Femoral Sciatic Pudendal

FIGURE ■ 8–10

Spinal cord plexuses.

spinal cord. The sensory neuron synapses with a motor neuron in the ventral horn. The motor neuron sends a signal to the quadriceps to stop the stretch. How do the quads stop the stretch? They shorten (contract). When a muscle shortens, it causes a movement. The shortening of the quadriceps muscles extends your knee, causing your leg to kick.

This action is totally reflexive (no pun intended). You can't stop yourself from kicking, even if you try. You do not have to think about kicking. The action happens without your brain. Only the spinal cord is necessary.

TEST YOUR KNOWLEDGE 8-3

Choose the best answer:

1. The segments of the spinal cord are named for
   a. the bones of the skull
   b. the vertebrae
   c. their function
   d. none of the above

2. This layer of the meninges is fused to the surface of the CNS.
   a. dura mater
   b. pia mater
   c. arachnoid mater
   d. whatsa mater

3. The ventral root carries _____ information, and the dorsal root carries _____ information.
   a. motor, motor
   b. motor, sensory
   c. sensory, sensory
   d. sensory, motor

4. What is the term for axon pathways carrying information up and down the spinal cord?
   a. horns
   b. roots
   c. columns
   d. ganglia

COMMON DISORDERS OF THE NERVOUS SYSTEM

Peripheral neuropathy encompasses a number of disorders involving damage to peripheral nerves. Because peripheral nerves are involved in sensory, motor, and autonomic function, the symptoms of peripheral neuropathy vary greatly among patients. Symptoms include muscle weakness and decreased reflexes, numbness, tingling, paralysis, pain, difficulty controlling blood pressure, abnormal sweating, and digestive abnormalities. Nongenetic neuropathy can be grouped into three broad categories: systemic disease, trauma, and infection or autoimmune disorders. Trauma, such as falls or automobile accidents, causes mechanical injury to nerves. Nerves may be severed, crushed, or bruised. Systemic disorders that cause peripheral neuropathy include kidney disorders, hormonal imbalance, alcoholism, vascular damage, repetitive stress (like carpal tunnel), chronic inflammation, diabetes, toxins, and tumors. Infections such as shingles, Epstein-Barr virus, herpes, HIV, Lyme disease, and polio cause peripheral neuropathy. Guillain-Barré syndrome is an acute form of peripheral neuropathy. Some forms of neuropathy are inherited.

Even though the spinal cord is well protected by the bones and meninges, trauma can cause damage to the delicate neural tissue. The spinal cord may be partially or completely severed, crushed, or bruised. Bruises to the spinal cord may resolve with time and rehabilitation, but a severed or crushed spinal cord is usually a permanent injury. Spinal cord injury usually results in paralysis and sensory loss below the injury, and the extent of the paralysis is related to the location of the spinal cord injury. Patients with injuries to the cervical spinal cord are quadriplegics, paralyzed in all four limbs. Some quadriplegics, with damage very high in the cervical spinal cord, have paralyzed diaphragms and cannot breathe on their own. Patients with injuries in the thoracic spinal cord and lower have paraplegia. They can move their arms but their legs are paralyzed.

Guillain-Barré syndrome (GBS) is a paralysis caused by inflammation of peripheral nerves. Patients develop, over variable periods of time, weakness and ascending paralysis of the limbs, face, and diaphragm. Some patients may have a mild form of Guillain-Barré syndrome, but those with severe disease must be kept on a ventilator until the paralysis resolves. The cause of the disease is not known, though many patients develop Guillain-Barré syndrome after a viral infection. Other evidence suggests that autoimmune attack of peripheral myelin may be to blame. There is no effective treatment except supportive care. Fortunately, the disorder is usually temporary. Many patients need rehabilitation after their PNS recovers.

Myasthenia gravis is an autoimmune disorder in which the immune system attacks and destroys acetylcholine receptors at the neuromuscular junction. Motor neurons continue to release acetylcholine, but the receptor number is reduced, so motor neurons cannot communicate with skeletal muscles. Eye muscles are typically the first muscles affected, but some patients initially experience difficulty chewing, swallowing, or talking. The disorder, like most autoimmune disorders, is progressive, though the course of the disease varies widely among patients. Treatment for myasthenia gravis includes acetylcholinesterase inhibitors, corticosteroids, immunosuppressant drugs, and plasma exchange. In a few patients, the disease disappears spontaneously.

Botulism is a form of paralysis caused by toxins produced by the bacterium *Clostridium botulinum*. Botulism can be caused by ingesting the toxin in food and can result from wound infections. The bacteria grow most commonly in improperly prepared canned food, especially home-canned food. The toxin keeps neurotransmitters from being released at the neuromuscular junction, causing paralysis. Initial symptoms include vision disturbances, slurred speech, dry mouth, and muscle weakness. If left untreated, paralysis will spread to limbs and respiratory muscles. Botulism can be treated by administration of antitoxin and supportive care. Botulism is a rare disorder. Only 169 cases were reported in the United States in 2001.

> **Learning Hint**
>
> Often on a journey, you cannot see or appreciate the big picture. For example, if you are in a portion of the Grand Canyon, it can be quite impressive, but when you stand on top at the rim of the Grand Canyon, the "whole picture" becomes clear and spectacular. This chapter on the nervous system has given you a picture of the nervous tissue and how nervous transmission occurs. In addition, this chapter has begun to develop the role of the spinal cord. The next chapter focuses on the brain and then pulls everything together so you can see the big picture.

Meningitis is an infection, usually from viruses or bacteria, of the meninges, the lining of the brain and spinal cord. Bacterial meningitis is a potentially fatal infection. The bacteria first infect the upper respiratory tract and then travel to the meninges. High-risk groups include the elderly, people with suppressed immune systems, very young children, and college students who live in dorms. Patients who survive bacterial meningitis often have severe neurological impairment, including deafness and severe brain damage. Viral meningitis is a much milder disease caused by viruses that enter the mouth and travel to the meninges.

The relationship between the muscular system and nervous system can be seen in the condition of carpal tunnel syndrome (CTS), which occurs with an inflammation and swelling of the tendon sheaths surrounding the flexor tendon of the palm. This is a result of repetitive motion such as typing on a keyboard. As a result of this inflammation and swelling, the median nerve is compressed, producing a tingling sensation or numbness of the palm and first three fingers.

> **8-8** to view a video on carpal tunnel syndrome, please go to your CD-ROM for this chapter.

SUMMARY

Snapshots from the Journey

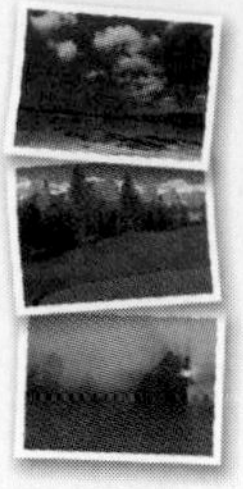

- The nervous system is the body's computer. It has a sensory (input) system, an integration center, the CNS, and a motor (output) system. The input and output nerves are in the PNS, and the brain and spinal cord are the CNS.
- The tissue of the nervous system is made up of two types of cells: neurons, which send, receive, and process information; and neuroglia, which support the neurons.
- Neurons are excitable cells. They do their jobs by carrying tiny electrical currents caused by changes in cell permeability to certain ions.
- These tiny electrical currents can be all-or-none (action potentials), can change depending on the size of the stimulus (local potentials), can travel down axons (impulse conduction), or can be used to transmit information from one cell to another (synapses).
- The CNS is composed of the brain and spinal cord.
- The cavities in your brain are known as ventricles, and the spinal cord cavity is the central canal. These cavities are part of an elaborate protection system for your CNS and are filled with cerebrospinal fluid.
- Your CNS is surrounded by a three-layered membrane system: dura mater, arachnoid mater, and pia mater, collectively known as the meninges. Cerebrospinal fluid is also contained in the space between the arachnoid and pia maters.
- The spinal cord has 31 segments, each with a pair of spinal nerves. The spinal nerves are a part of the peripheral nervous system.
- The spinal nerves are made of a pair of spinal roots. The ventral root is integral to motor function, and the dorsal root is integral to sensory function. Spinal nerves are mixed: they carry both sensory and motor information.
- A series of tracts run up and down the spinal cord to and from the brain. The tracts going toward the brain carry sensory information to the brain. The tracts coming from the brain toward the spinal cord carry motor information from the brain.

Case Study

During the biggest game of his high school football career, Bill, the best wide receiver in the league, leaps high into the air in the end zone to score the game-winning touchdown. A player for the other teams hits him hard, knocking him into the goal post. Bill crumples to the ground, unmoving. When the EMTs get to him, Bill is paralyzed on both sides of his body and in respiratory arrest.

Where is Bill's most likely injury? How can you tell?

REVIEW QUESTIONS

Multiple Choice

1. The input side of your nervous system is known as
   a. motor
   b. sensory
   c. association
   d. all of the above

2. Neurons with a central and peripheral projection are known as
   a. unipolar
   b. bipolar
   c. multipolar
   d. northpolar

3. During depolarization, _____________ ions move _____________ a neuron.
   a. K^+, out of
   b. K^+, into
   c. Na^+, out of
   d. Na^+, into

4. The ventral root of the spinal cord is
   a. sensory
   b. motor
   c. association
   d. none of the above

5. Spinal nerves carry what kind of information?
   a. sensory
   b. motor
   c. mixed
   d. vertebral

Fill in the Blank

1. The speed of impulse conduction is determined by _____________ and _____________.

2. _____________ potentials are all-or-none.

3. The spinal cord has white matter _____________ and gray matter _____________.

4. _____________ fluid is contained in the _____________ space between the arachnoid mater and pia mater.

5. A _____________ is an involuntary, protective movement that is sometimes generated without the brain.

Short Answer

1. Explain the changes in a neuron during an action potential.

____

____

____

____

2. List the steps in chemical synaptic transmission.

____
____
____
____

3. List the layers of protection around the CNS.

____
____
____
____

4. List the types of neuroglia and their functions.

____
____
____
____

Suggested Activities

1. With a partner, test your knee-jerk reflexes using reflex hammers. Try to control the reflex. Can you? Try it with your eyes closed. What does that say about reflexes?

2. Grab a friend and explain the action potential and chemical synapse to her or him. Can you do it?

8-9 Now that you have completed your journey through this chapter, please go to the CD-ROM for interactive games and puzzles concerning the medical terms and concepts contained in this chapter. By playing the games you will reinforce your learning of medical terminology in a fun way.

Greetings from THE NERVOUS System

The Body's Control Center, PART TWO

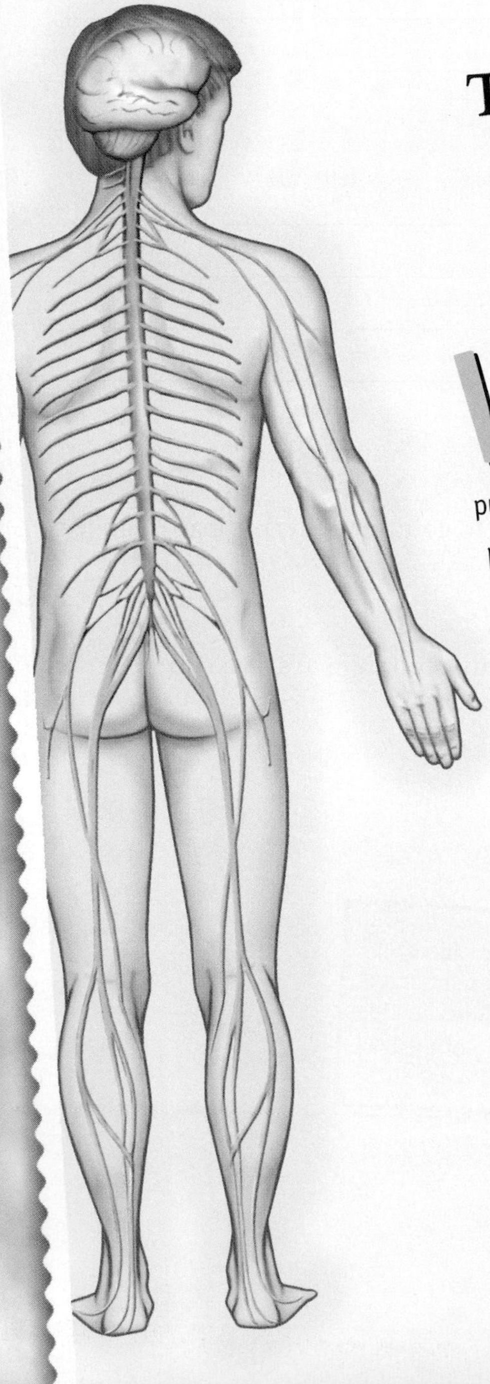

Welcome to the final leg of your trip through the nervous system. In this chapter, we focus on the main controller of the nervous system, the brain. Then we pull everything together to see how all the pieces of the puzzle form the big picture. Staying with our journey analogy, the previous chapter presented the roadways we travel. There are all kinds of roads that lead to all kinds of places. However, the flow of traffic must be precisely controlled, or chaos and wrecks would occur. The control system of the roadways includes such things as traffic signs and lights, toll booths and draw bridges. The brain is the control system of the nervous system superhighway, attempting to keep everything running smoothly. Let's hope this journey is not as "nerve wracking" as some of the highways you may have been on.

Chapter 9

LEARNING OBJECTIVES

Upon completion of your journey through this chapter, you will be able to:

- Organize the hierarchy of the nervous system
- Locate and define the external structures and their corresponding functions of the brain
- Locate and define the internal structures and their corresponding functions of the brain
- Describe the sensory functions of the brain with related structures
- Describe the motor functions of the brain with related structures
- Contrast the parasympathetic and sympathetic branches of the autonomic nervous system
- Discuss some representative diseases of the nervous system

MULTIMEDIA APPLICATIONS

CD-ROM Interactive Exercises

- Positron emission tomography (PET) scan of the brain, 9-1
- Drag-and-drop exercise: brainstem and arachnoid space, 9-2
- Video on Parkinson disease, 9-3
- Videos of related nervous system disorders, 9-4
- Interactive games and puzzles, 9-5

www.prenhall.com/colbert

- Professional Profile
  - Pharmacy
- Related Internet Links
- Additional Review Questions

Pronunciation Guide

Correct pronunciation is important in any journey so that you and others are completely understood. Here is a "see and say" Pronunciation Guide for the more difficult terms to pronounce in this chapter.

anterior commissure (an TEE ree or KAH mih sure)
basal nuclei (BAY sal noo KLEE ie)
cerebellum (ser eh BELL um)
cerebrum (ser EE brum)
corpus callosum (KOR pus kah LOH sum)
corticobulbar tract (KOR ti coe BUL bar)
corticospinal tract (KOR ti coe SPY nal)
diencephalon (dye en SEFF ah lon)
fornix (FOR niks)
gyri (JIE rie)
hypothalamus (high poh THAL ah mus)
limbic system (LIM bick)
medulla oblongata (meh DULL lah ob long GA ta)
occipital lobe (ok SIP eh tal)
parietal lobe (pah RYE eh tal)
pineal body (pih NEE al)
spinocerebellar tract (SPY no ser eh BELL ar)
spinothalamic tract (SPY no thol AH mic)
subarachnoid space (sub ah RAK noyd)
sulcus (SULL cuss)
thalamus (THAL ah mus)

THE BRAIN AND CRANIAL NERVES

The brain and cranial nerves represent the major control system of the nervous system. The brain acts as the main processor and director of the entire system. The cranial nerves leave the brain and go to specific body areas where they receive information and send it back to the brain (sensory), and the brain sends back instructions as to the appropriate response (motor). Let's again begin with an overview and then get more specific.

OVERALL ORGANIZATION

At the top of the spinal cord, beginning at the level of the foramen magnum and filling the cranial cavity, is the brain. Just like a grocery store needs to be organized into sections such as produce, meats, and deli, the brain can be divided into several anatomical and functional sections. We will talk about each section separately and then describe the interactions between the brain parts and the spinal cord.

Note

The scarecrow on *The Wizard of Oz* "thought" he needed a brain. As you work through this chapter, can you "think" of several reasons why you knew all along he had a brain?

The Brain's External Anatomy

Let's start our journey looking at the outside of the brain, and then we will zoom in on the internal structures. From the outside, you can see that the brain consists of a **cerebrum, cerebellum,** and **brain stem.** Please see Figure 9–1 ■.

cerebrum *(ser EE brum)*
cerebellum *(ser eh BELL um)*

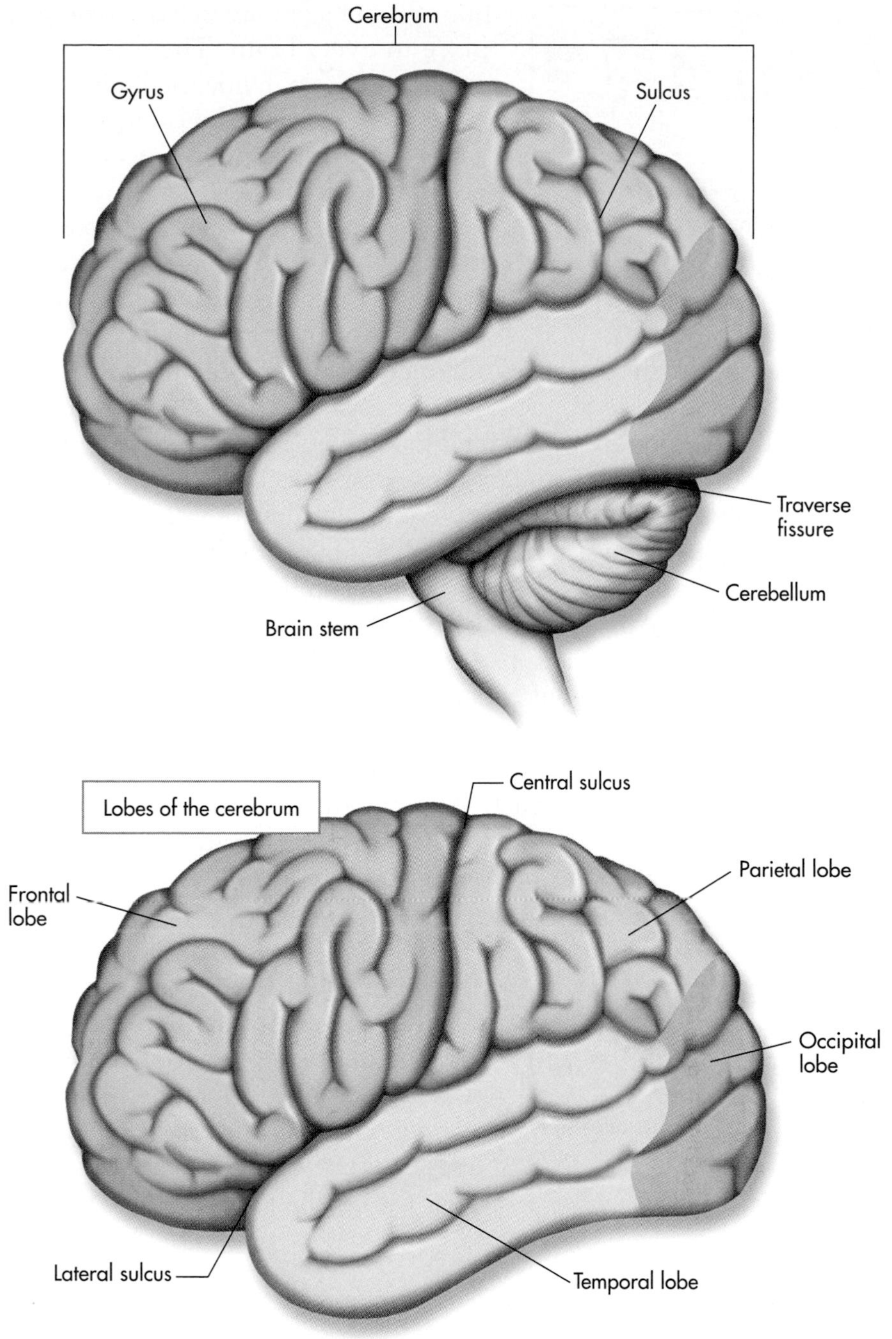

FIGURE ■ 9–1

External brain anatomy and lobes.

CEREBRUM

The cerebrum, which is the largest part of the brain, is divided into two **hemispheres,** a right and left, by the longitudinal fissure, and divided from the cerebellum ("little brain") by the transverse fissure. The surface of the cerebrum is not smooth, but broken by ridges (**gyri**) and grooves (**sulci**) collectively known as *convolutions*. These convolutions serve a very important purpose by increasing the surface area of the brain, yet allowing it to be "folded" into a smaller space. Most of the sulci are extremely variable in their locations among

gyri *(JIE rie)*
sulci *(SULL kie)*

Amazing Body Facts

WHY NOT A SMOOTH BRAIN?

The surface of the brain is folded and rippled into a series of convolutions. These convolutions allow lots of brain surface area to fit into a very small space. If you could lay the convolutions flat, they would be the size of a pillow case. Talk about your big heads!

humans, but a few are in basically the same place in every brain. These less variable sulci are used to divide the brain into four large sections called **lobes,** much like the major departments in a grocery store are separated by aisles.

The lobes (see Table 9–1) are named for the skull bones that cover them, and they occur in pairs, one in each hemisphere. The most anterior lobes, separated from the rest of the brain by the central sulci, are the **frontal lobes.** The frontal lobes are responsible for motor activities, conscious thought, and speech. Posterior to the frontal lobe are the parietal lobes. The **parietal lobes** are involved with body sense perception, primary taste, and speech. Posterior to the parietal lobes are the **occipital lobes,** which are responsible for vision. (There is no obvious dividing line between the parietal and occipital lobes, and these represent the most posterior lobes at the back of the skull.) The most inferior lobes, separated by the lateral fissures, are the **temporal lobes,** which are involved in hearing and integration of emotions. Again, please see Figure 9–1 which shows the lobes of the brain and the sulci that separate them. There is a section of the brain, the **insula,** deep inside the temporal lobes, which is often listed as a fifth lobe, but it is not visible on the surface of the cerebrum. The insula helps coordinate autonomic functions. Much of the information coming into your brain is *contralateral.* That is, the left side of the body is controlled by the right side of your cerebrum, and the right side of the body is controlled by your left brain.

parietal lobe *(pah RYE eh tal)*

occipital lobe *(ok SIP eh tal)*

contra = *against, opposite*
lateral = *side*

Note

Does contralateral control mean that if the left brain controls the right hand, and the right brain controls the left hand, then only left-handed people are in their right minds?

CEREBELLUM

The cerebellum is posterior to the brain stem and plays an important role in sensory and motor coordination and balance. Its surface is also convoluted like that of the cerebrum. From its external appearance, it is easy to see why anatomists consider the cerebellum the "little brain."

9-1 The brain can be imaged using positron emission tomography, more commonly known as PET scan. To view a video of this procedure, please refer to your CD-ROM for this chapter.

TABLE 9–1 Cerebral Lobes and Cerebellum

STRUCTURE	MAJOR FUNCTIONS
Cerebral Lobes	
frontal lobe	motor function, behavior and emotions, memory storage, thinking, smell
parietal Lobe	body sense, perception, taste, and speech
occipital	vision
temporal lobe	hearing, taste, language comprehension, integration of emotions
Cerebellum	the "little brain"; sensory and motor coordination and balance

TABLE 9–2 The Brain Stem

STRUCTURE	FUNCTION
midbrain	relays sensory and motor information
pons	relays sensory and motor information; role in breathing
medulla oblongota	regulates vital functions of heart rate, blood pressure, breathing, and reflex center for coughing, sneezing, swallowing and vomiting

THE BRAIN STEM

The brain stem (see Table 9–2) is a stalk-like structure inferior to and partially covered by the cerebrum. It is divided into three sections. The **medulla oblongata** is continuous with the spinal cord. The medulla is responsible for impulses that control heartbeat, breathing, and the cardiovascular system muscle tone and therefore blood pressure. The **pons** is just superior to the medulla oblongata and connects the medulla oblongata and the cerebellum with the upper portions of the brain. The pons plays a role in breathing. The **midbrain,** which is the most superior portion of the brain stem, acts as a two-way conduction pathway to relay visual and auditory impulses (see Figure 9–2 ■). The brain stem receives sensory information and contains control systems for vital functions such as blood pressure, heart rate, and breathing. The brain controls the vital functions of life, and patients with severe brain injuries with an intact brain stem can

medulla oblongata
(meh DULL lah ob long GA ta)

9-2 To perform an interactive drag-and-drop exercise on the brain stem, please go to your CD-ROM.

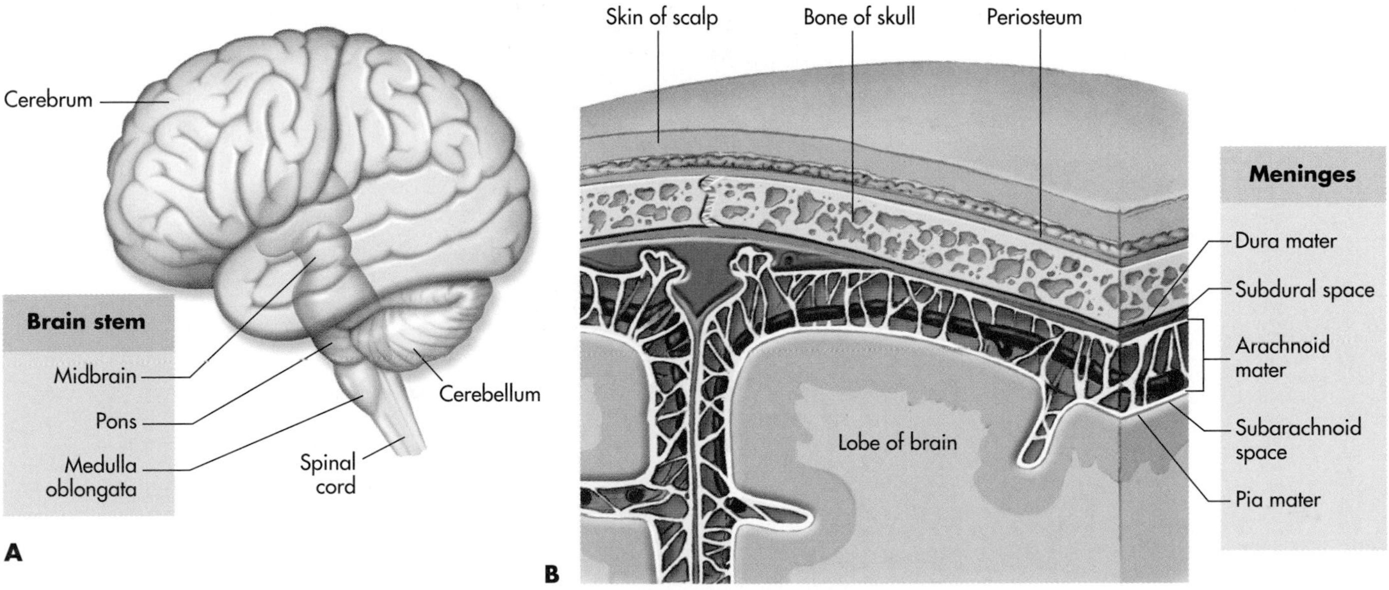

FIGURE ■ 9–2

(A) The brain stem and (B) meninges.

continue in a vegetative state as long as they are nutritionally supported. This condition is called a persistent vegetative state (PVS).

The brain, like the spinal cord, is covered with protective membranes called *meninges*. Again, please see Figure 9–2. The meninges of the brain are continuous with the spinal cord meninges. A potentially fatal condition is an infection of the meninges called **meningitis,** which can rapidly spread and affect the brain and spinal cord through this common covering.

meningitis *(men in JYE tiss)*
itis = *inflammation of*

Internal Anatomy of the Brain

The inside of the brain has, like the spinal cord, white matter and gray matter, and hollow cavities containing cerebrospinal fluid. (See! We really do have holes in our heads.) Unlike the spinal cord, however, the white matter is surrounded by the gray matter in the brain. (Remember, in the spinal cord, the white matter surrounds the gray matter.) The layer of gray matter surrounding the white matter is called the **cortex.** In the cerebrum it is called the cerebral cortex, and in the cerebellum it is called the cerebellar cortex. Throughout the brain there are deep "islands" of gray matter surrounded by white matter. These islands are called **nuclei.**

ventricles *(VEN trik lz)*
subarachnoid space *(sub ah RAK noyd)*

The fluid-filled cavities in the brain are called **ventricles,** and they are continuous with the central canal of the spinal cord and the **subarachnoid space** of both the brain and the spinal cord. These ventricles allow for the circulation of cerebrospinal fluid throughout the brain. The lateral ventricles (ventricles 1 and

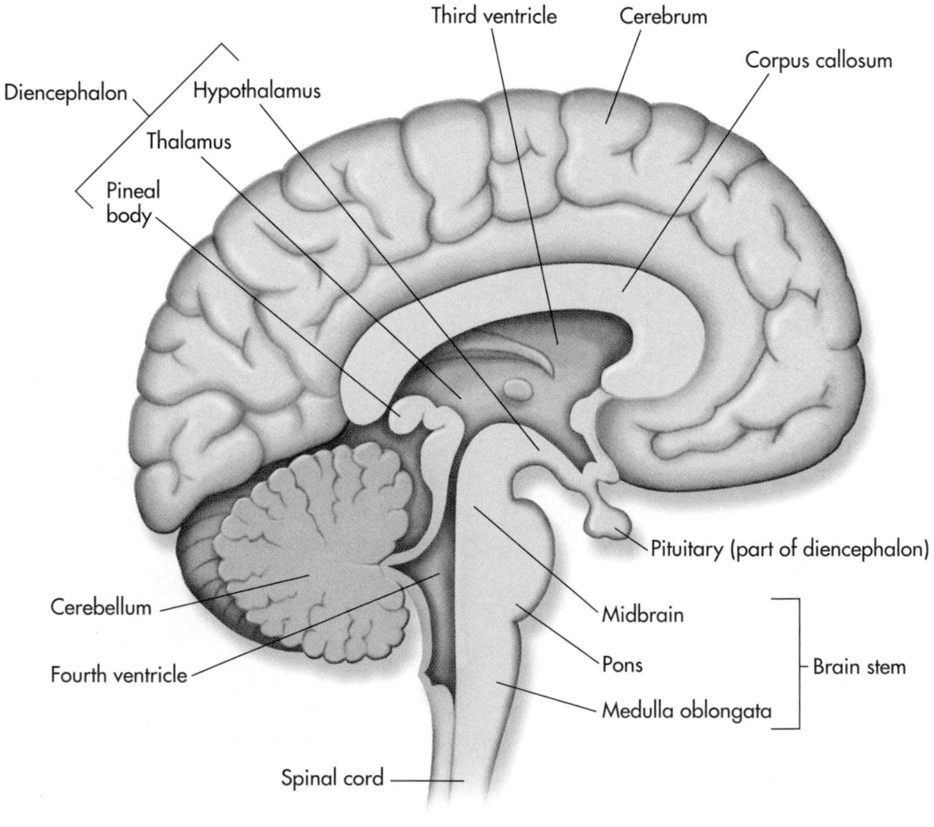

FIGURE ■ 9–3

Internal anatomy of the brain.

2) are in the cerebrum; the third ventricle is in the diencephalon, a region between the cerebrum and brain stem; and the fourth ventricle is in the inferior part of the brain between the medulla oblongata and the cerebellum (see Figure 9–3 ■).

THE CEREBRUM

The inside of the cerebrum reflects its external anatomy (see Figure 9–4 ■). The lobes—frontal, temporal, parietal, and occipital—are clearly visible. On

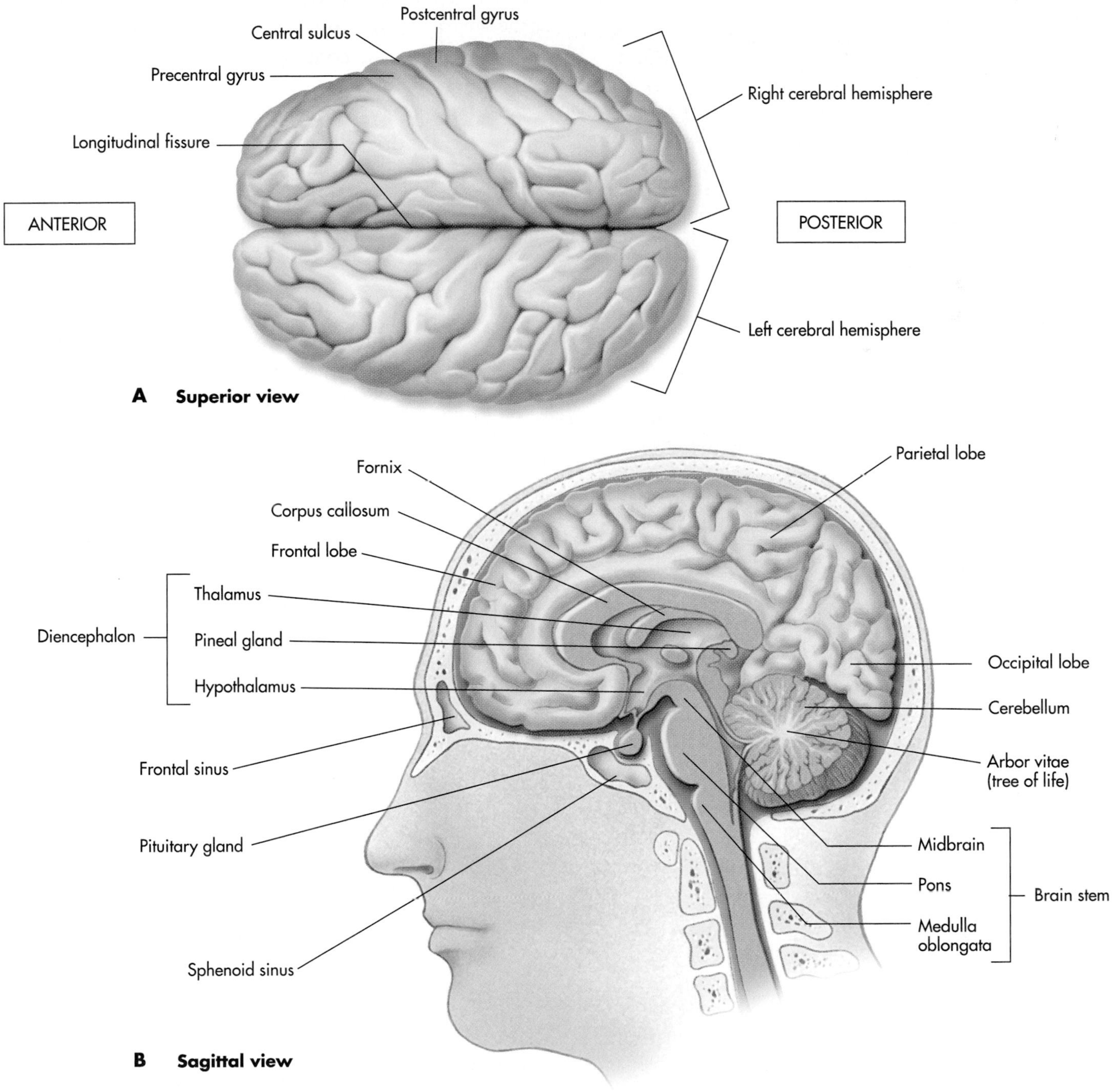

FIGURE ■ 9–4

Superior (a) and sagittal (b) views of the brain.

gyrus *(JIE rus)*

corpus callosum *(KOR pus kah LOH sum)*

either side of the central sulcus are two gyri named for their locations: the **precentral gyrus,** anterior to the central sulcus, and the **postcentral gyrus,** posterior to the central sulcus. The importance of these gyri will become obvious when we discuss function of the brain later in the chapter. The right and left hemispheres are connected by a collection of white matter surrounding the lateral ventricles, called the **corpus callosum.** This connection allows for cross-communication between the right and left sides of the brain. Many of our day-to-day activities, like walking or driving, require both sides of the body, and therefore both sides of the brain, to be well coordinated. Imagine walking if your legs were acting independently!

Clinical Application

CEREBROSPINAL FLUID CIRCULATION AND HYDROCEPHALUS

The ventricles of the brain, the central canal of the spinal cord, and the subarachnoid space, surrounding both parts of the CNS, are all filled with cerebrospinal fluid (CSF). The CSF is filtered from blood in the ventricles by tissue called choroid plexus. Produced at the rate of 750 milliliters daily, CSF made in the lateral ventricles flows through a tiny opening into the third ventricle and then through another opening into the fourth ventricle. From the fourth ventricle, CSF flows into the central canal of the spinal cord and the subarachnoid space. CSF is returned to the blood via special "ports" (the arachnoid villi) between subarachnoid space and blood spaces in the dura mater (the dural sinuses).

The balance of CSF made and CSF reabsorbed by the blood is very important. The brain is a very delicate organ captured between the liquid CSF and the bones of the skull. If there is too much CSF, pressure inside the skull rises, eventually crushing brain tissue. This condition, in which there is too much CSF, is called hydrocephalus (literally "water in the head"). Hydrocephalus can be caused by blockage of the narrow passages between the ventricles due to trauma, by birth defects or tumors, or by decreased reabsorption of CSF due to subarachnoid bleeding. Hydrocephalus may be treated by medication, but the most common treatment is insertion of a shunt, a tube that drains the extra CSF into the patient's heart or abdominal cavity.

THE DIENCEPHALON

diencephalon *(dye en SEFF ah lon)*

Inferior to the cerebrum is a section of the brain that is not visible from the exterior, called the **diencephalon.** The diencephalon consists of several parts: the **thalamus, hypothalamus, pineal body,** and the **pituitary gland** (see Table 9–3). The hypothalamus, pituitary, and pineal represent an interface with the endocrine system (the other control system), covered in Chapter 10. The diencephalon contains the third ventricle and a number of nuclei that are part of the basal nuclei and limbic system. Specific nuclei of the diencephalon are responsible for controlling hormone levels, hunger and thirst, body temperature, and sleep–wake cycles, and for coordinating the flow of information around the brain.

THE CEREBELLUM

The external similarities between the cerebellum and cerebrum are also obvious internally (see Figure 9–4). The cerebellum has a gray matter cortex and a white matter center, known as the *arbor vitae* (tree of life). The cerebellum also has nuclei that coordinate motor and sensory activity. Essentially, the cerebellum fine-tunes voluntary skeletal muscle activity and helps in the maintenance of balance.

Learning Hint

GRAY VS. WHITE MATTER

The gray matter is composed of the cell bodies of the neurons. White matter is composed of axons, which are surrounded with myelin. Remember from the previous chapter that myelin allows messages to be transmitted faster.

TABLE 9–3 Diencephalon

STRUCTURE	FUNCTION
thalamus	relays and processes information going to the cerebrum
hypothalamus	regulates hormone levels, temperature, water-balance, thirst, appetite, and some emotions (pleasure and fear); regulates the pituitary gland and controls the endocrine system
pineal body	responsible for secretion of melatonin (body clock)
pituitary gland	secretes hormones for various functions (explained in Chapter 10)

thalamus *(THAL ah mus)*

hypothalamus *(high poh THAL ah mus)*

pineal body *(pih NEE al)*

CRANIAL NERVES

In order for the CNS to function, it must be connected to the outside world via nerves of the PNS. We have already seen that the spinal cord is connected to the outside via spinal nerves. The brain also has nerves to connect it to the outside, aptly named **cranial nerves** (see Figure 9–5 ■). Cranial nerves are like spinal nerves in that they are the input and output pathways (PNS) for the brain, just as the spinal nerves are the pathways for the spinal cord. However, that is really where the similarities end. You should remember that there are 31 pairs of spinal nerves and that all of them are mixed nerves: they carry both sensory and motor information because they are formed by a combination of dorsal and ventral roots. There are far fewer cranial nerves—only 12 pairs. All but the first two pairs arise from the brain stem. Cranial nerves are not *all* mixed as are spinal nerves. Some cranial nerves are mainly sensory nerves, providing input; some are mainly motor nerves, directing activity; and some are mixed. Cranial nerves are much more specialized than spinal nerves and are named based on their specialty. Some cranial nerves carry sensory and motor information for the head, face, and neck, while others carry visual, auditory, smell, or taste sensation. (Table 9–4 lists cranial nerves and their functions.)

> **Learning Hint**
>
> **MNEMONIC DEVICES**
>
> A mnemonic device is a tool used to help you memorize long lists. It can be very useful in anatomy. To make a mnemonic device, take the first letter of each part of the list you are trying to memorize and make it into a sentence. For example, the five great lakes in order from west to east are Superior, Michigan, Huron, Erie, and Ontario. The mnemonic device used to remember the right order is **S**am **M**ade **H**arry **E**at **O**nions, much easier to remember than the lakes themselves. An example for the cranial nerves is this one: **O**n **O**ld **O**lympus **T**owering **T**ops **A** **F**inn **V**ith **G**erman **V**alked **A**nd **H**opped.

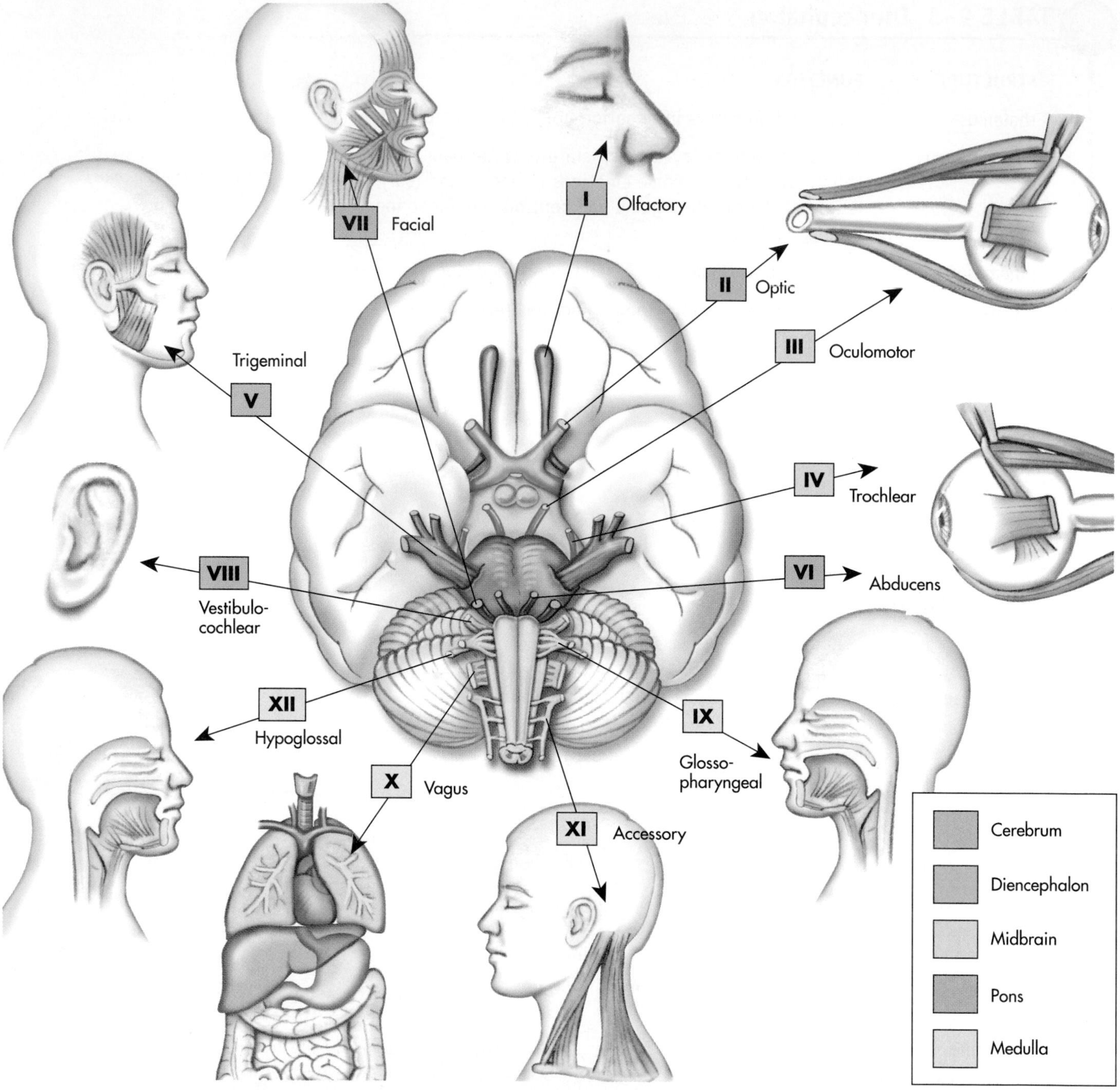

FIGURE ■ 9–5

Cranial nerves.

TABLE 9–4 Cranial Nerves and Functions

NERVE	FUNCTION
olfactory (I)	sensory (smell)
optic (II)	sensory (vision)
oculomotor (III)	mixed, chiefly motor for eye movements
trochlear (IV)	mixed, chiefly motor for eye movements
trigeminal (V)	mixed, chiefly motor for face
abducens (VI)	mixed, chiefly motor for facial muscles
facial (VII)	mixed, for lower face, throat and mouth
vestibulocochlear (VIII)	sensory, hearing, and balance
glossopharyngeal (IX)	mixed, motor for throat muscles; sensory for taste
vagus (X)	mixed, motor for autonomic heart, lungs, viscera; sensory for viscera, taste buds, and so on
accessory (XI)	mixed, chiefly motor; motor and sensory for larynx, soft palate, trapezius, and sternocleidomastoid muscles
Hypoglossal (XII)	mixed, chiefly motor for tongue muscles; sensory, same as motor

TEST YOUR KNOWLEDGE 9-1

Choose the best answer:

1. Which of the following is *not* part of the brainstem?
   a. pons
   b. medulla oblongata
   c. midbrain
   d. diencephalon

2. Deep islands of gray matter are known as
   a. hemispheres
   b. gyri
   c. nuclei
   d. nerves

3. Which of the following is *not* found in the diencephalon?
   a. thalamus
   b. pineal
   c. postcentral gyrus
   d. hypothalamus

4. This lobe contains the primary visual cortex.
   a. frontal
   b. temporal
   c. occipital
   d. parietal

5. The cerebrum is divided into right and left hemispheres by the
   a. central sulcus
   b. transverse fissure
   c. corpus callosum
   d. none of the above

THE BIG PICTURE: INTEGRATION OF BRAIN, SPINAL CORD, AND PNS

So how does the brain work with the spinal cord and peripherial nervous system? Let's begin to put the pieces together by revisiting the overall organizational chart of the nervous system. To serve as our guide or GPS to keep our location clear. See Figure 9–6 ■ to show our current location.

The Somatic Sensory System

The **Somatic sensory system** provides sensory input for your nervous system. We have already mentioned the parts of your brain that are dedicated to your special senses: vision (occipital lobe), hearing (temporal and parietal lobes), taste (frontal), and smell (frontal). We have not yet talked about the sense of touch, called **somatic sensation.** Somatic sensation allows you to feel the world around you. Somatic sensation includes not just fine touch, which allows you to tell the difference between a peach and a nectarine or a golf ball and a ping pong ball, but also crude touch, vibration, pain, temperature, and body position. While your special senses are all carried on cranial nerves, information for somatic sensation comes into *both* the brain and the spinal cord. Ultimately, for you to attach meaning to the sensation, the sensory information must get to your brain.

somatic *(soh MAHT ik)*

Let's start with the spinal cord. When we talked about reflexes, we saw somatic sensory information come into the spinal cord via the dorsal root and synapse with a motor neuron in the ventral horn. Let's say you place your hand on a hot iron. The sensory neuron carries pain information to your spinal cord. The motor neuron then activates the muscle, allowing you to respond to the stimulus *immediately* and pull your hand away to minimize injury. The same axon that carries information to the motor neuron further carries the sensory

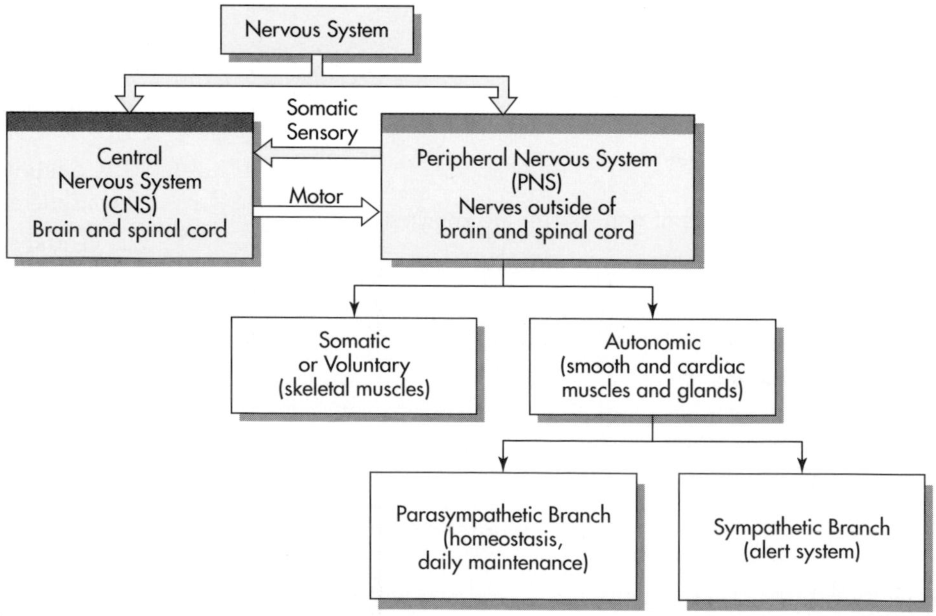

FIGURE ■ 9–6

Nervous system flow chart highlighting the areas thus far explained.

information to your brain via tracts in the white matter of the spinal cord, so you feel the pain associated with your action and wonder why the heck you ever put your hand on the hot iron in the first place.

Because there are so many variations of "touch" information that must come in from all parts of the body, different neural highways are needed to more effectively take that information to the brain. Three pathways, the **dorsal column tract,** the **spinothalamic tract,** and the **spinocerebellar tract,** carry somatic sensory information to the spinal cord and then to your brain from all parts of the skin, joints, and tendons.

spinothalamic tract
(SPY no THAL ah mic)
spinocerebellar tract
(SPY no ser eh BELL ar)

- The dorsal column tract carries fine-touch and vibration information to the cerebral cortex.
- The spinothalamic tract carries temperature, pain, and crude touch information to the cerebral cortex.
- The spinocerebellar tract carries information about posture and position to the cerebellum.

See Table 9–5 for a description of spinal cord pathways.

The sensory information coming into the brain must come to a specific area for processing. As you can see from Table 9–5, the dorsal column and spinothalamic tracts both transport sensory information from your skin and joints to a portion of the cerebrum known as the primary somatic sensory cortex located in the postcentral gyrus of the parietal lobe.

The axons transport information to specific parts of the somatic sensory cortex that correspond to parts of the body. This route can be mapped out, as in Figure 9–7 ■. The neurons in the somatic sensory cortex are the neurons that allow conscious sensation. You feel an insect crawling on your arm because the "arm" neurons in your somatic sensory cortex are stimulated by the insect.

SOMATIC SENSORY ASSOCIATION AREA: HOW DO WE INTERPRET TOUCH?

There is another area of the cerebral cortex that allows *understanding* and *interpretation* of somatic sensory information. It is located in the parietal lobe just posterior to somatic sensory cortex and is known as the somatic sensory association area.

The somatic sensory system works on a kind of hierarchy, with the sensory neurons in the spinal cord and brain stem (brain stem neurons transport information in the same fashion as the spinal sensory neurons, but without going to

TABLE 9–5 Spinal Cord Pathways for Sensory Information

PATHWAY	INFORMATION	FROM	TO
spinothalamic		skin	somatic sensory cortex
lateral	pain; temperature		
anterior	itch; pressure; tickle		
dorsal column	fine touch; limb position	skin; joints	somatic sensory cortex; cerebellum
spinocerebellar	posture	joints; tendons	cerebellum

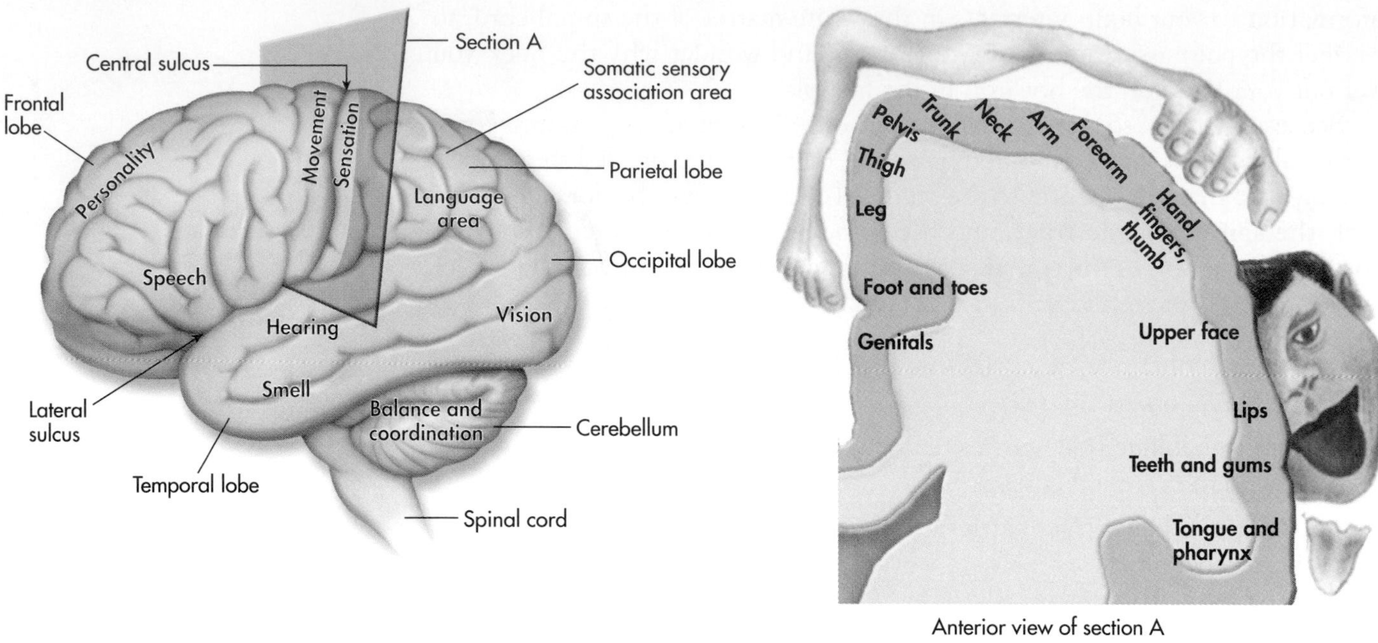

FIGURE ■ 9–7

Primary somatic sensory area. Notice the size of the body parts are proportional to the amount of the sensory input provided. For example, the hands provide much more sensory input due to touch than your neck would and as a result the area devoted to the neck is much smaller. Remember that the map is contralateral.

the spinal cord first) collecting information and passing it to areas in the thalamus, cerebellum, and cerebral cortex for processing. The *actual* understanding of complex sensory input happens only *after* the information is passed to somatic sensory cortex and somatic sensory association area.

Let's go back to hitting your thumb with a hammer. The pain neurons, with bodies in the dorsal root ganglion, are depolarized and send signals to the spinal cord via the spinal nerve and dorsal root. The neurons synapse with motor neurons, causing you to pull your hand away from the stimulus. These same pain neurons join the spinothalamic tract in your spinal cord and simultaneously send a pain signal to your brain. The signal goes first to the thalamus and other parts of the diencephalon, causing physiological symptoms, like sweating and increased heart rate. The pain then continues along the pathway to your somatic sensory cortex. There, the exact location of the pain becomes apparent to you. Now you know *where* the pain is but still may not recognize it as pain. The *understanding* occurs when the information is integrated with sensation in the somatic sensory association area. Now you know that you have hurt yourself! All this receiving of information and processing and associated actions happen almost instantaneously.

THE BIG PICTURE: THE MOTOR SYSTEM

The motor system is also a hierarchy, working in parallel with the somatic sensory system. However, now information is moving in the opposite direction, from brain to spinal cord. See Figure 9–8 ■ to show our current progress on the nervous system organizational chart.

The somatic motor system controls voluntary movements under orders from the cerebral cortex. In the frontal lobe are the premotor and prefrontal areas,

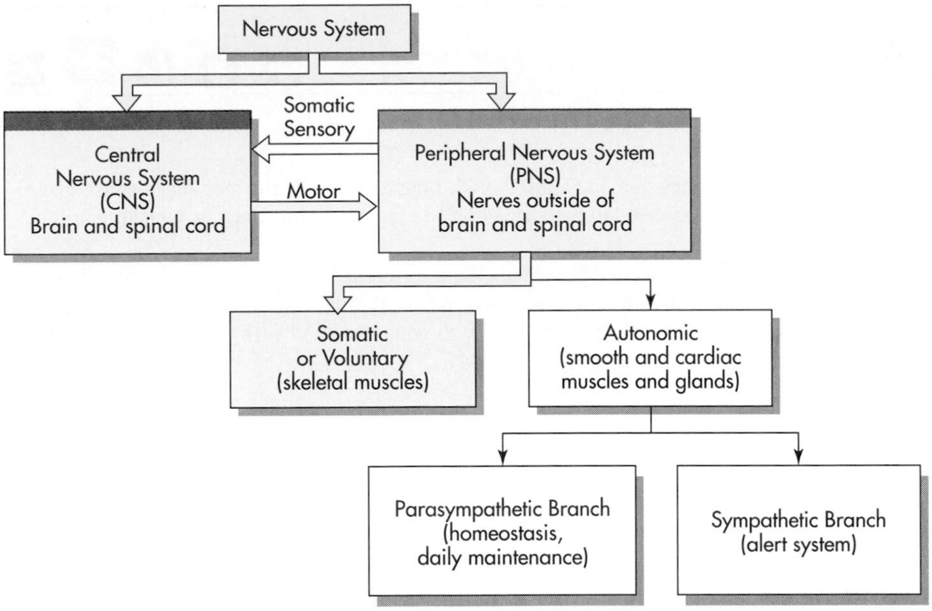

FIGURE ■ 9–8

Progress thus far on the nervous system flow chart.

which *plan* movements. The plan from these two areas is sent to the primary motor cortex. The primary motor cortex is located in the precentral gyrus, in the frontal lobe, just anterior to the somatic sensory cortex just discussed. The primary motor cortex should seem familiar. Just like the somatic sensory cortex, the motor cortex has a map of the body. The size of the map in the motor cortex is proportional to the amount of movement control. Therefore, the hands and tongue have larger maps than the trunk or forearms.

Subcortical Structures

Deep in the cerebrum are several areas of gray matter, which are surrounded by white matter and are known as **nuclei.** The nuclei in the cerebrum can be part of the **basal nuclei,** which is a motor coordination system, or part of the **limbic system,** which controls emotion and mood. We are concerned with motor neurons now, so basal nuclei is our focus.

basal nuclei *(BAY sal noo KLEE ie)*
limbic system *(LIM bick)*

The plan for movement leaves the motor cortex and connects with neurons in the thalamus, which is located in the diencephalon. The thalamus, basal nuclei, and cerebellum are part of a complicated *motor coordination loop*. Here, the movement must be fine-tuned, posture and limb positions are taken into account, other movements are turned off, and movement and senses are integrated. This loop is fundamental. Without the coordination loop among the subcortical structures (subcortical: "under the cortex"), movements would be at the very least jerky and inaccurate. Some movements would be impossible. Patients with parkinsonism have a disorder of one of the basal nuclei and are unable to start new movements or turn off other movements. Patients have difficulty walking and swallowing and usually have an uncontrollable tremor when sitting still.

9-3 For more information on Parkinson disease, see your CD-ROM for this chapter.

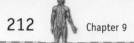

Amazing Body Facts

SIZE MATTERS

Check out the size of the primary motor cortex dedicated to each body part in Figure 9–9 ■. Does the size of the map make sense given the size of the body parts? Not really: the hands, lips, and head have very large maps, while the legs and arms have very small maps compared to each body part's size.

What determines map size? What do the hand and lips have in common that makes them different from the arms and legs? They are required to perform more finely coordinated movements, such as speaking and handwriting (or typing), and therefore have more motor output. If you aren't convinced, think about how much harder it would be to type with your feet than with your hands. This map can be drawn as a homunculus (little man) with huge hands, lips, and head (see Figure 9–9).

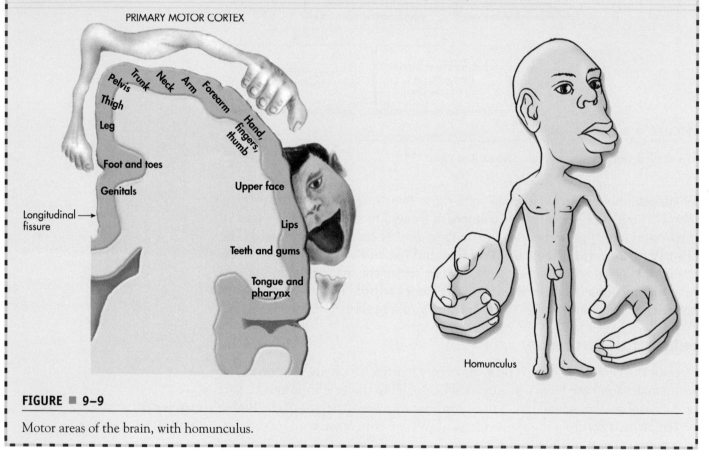

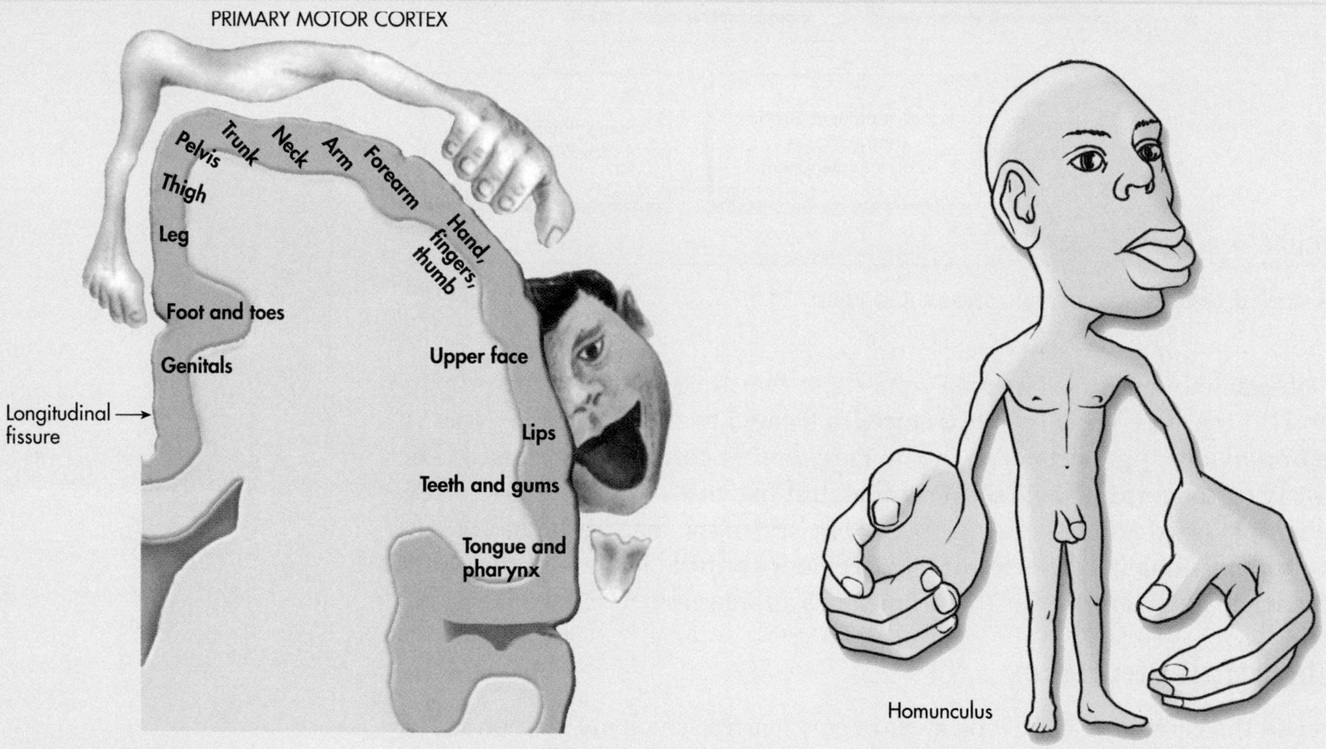

FIGURE ■ 9–9

Motor areas of the brain, with homunculus.

Spinal Cord Pathways

corticospinal tract
(KOR ti coe SPY nal)
corticobulbar tract
(KOR ti coe BUL bar)

After the movement information is processed by the thalamus basal nuclei and cerebellum, it moves to the spinal cord and brain stem via the **corticospinal** and **corticobulbar tracts** and several other tracts. The corticospinal and corticobulbar tracts from your motor cortex are direct pathways, while others coming from subcortical structures are considered indirect pathways. The axons from all pathways synapse on motor neurons in the ventral horn. These motor neurons connect to skeletal muscles via the cranial nerves (in brain stem) or the ventral roots and spinal nerves (spinal cord), sending orders to the skeletal muscles to carry out the planned movement or coordinating ongoing movements (Remember, these neurons communicate with the muscles via the neuromuscular junction and therefore release the neurotransmitter acetylcholine across the synapse.)

A second function of the motor tracts is fine-tuning of reflexes. These tracts inhibit reflexes, making them softer than they would be if they had no influence from the brain.

Let's go back again to hitting your thumb with the hammer. After you hit your thumb, the first motor activity is a withdrawal reflex. You pull your thumb away from the painful stimulus. As we mentioned before, this is not a voluntary movement. It isn't planned. Only your spinal cord motor neurons are necessary for withdrawal. However, after the initial withdrawal, some jumping up and down and perhaps some cursing, you stop and think. What do you do next? You look at your thumb. That is a planned movement. It requires coordination between your motor system, to uncover your thumb and move it into you visual field, and your visual system to look at your thumb. You walk to the kitchen, open the freezer, get out the ice, and make an ice pack. Then you grab a cold soda from the fridge and walk back into the living room, nursing your wounds. All of this activity requires motor planning and coordination. You must reach for the freezer door and open it accurately. You must stay upright with respect to gravity. You must open a plastic bag and put ice in it. None of this happens without careful motor planning and coordination.

The Role of the Cerebellum

We have really glossed over the important function of the cerebellum. The cerebellum has both motor and sensory inputs and outputs from the cerebral cortex, the thalamus, the basal nuclei, and the spinal cord. The cerebellum gets information about the *planned* movement and the *actual* movement and *compares* the plan to the actual. If the plan and the actual do not match, the cerebellum can adjust the actual movement to fit the plan. The function of the cerebellum is subtle and still a bit of a mystery, but without the cerebellum, movements would be inaccurate at best.

TEST YOUR KNOWLEDGE 9-2

Choose the best answer:

1. The size of the map for a particular body part in the precentral gyrus is determined by
   a. the amount of fine motor control
   b. the size of the body part
   c. the importance of the body part
   d. all of the above

2. The cerebellum compares
   a. shapes of objects
   b. planned movement to actual movement
   c. textures
   d. position of objects in space

3. Which of the following spinal cord pathways carries pain and temperature information?
   a. dorsal column
   b. spinothalamic
   c. corticospinal
   d. thermostatic

4. The _____ sends direct messages to ventral horn motor neurons, while the _____ are involved in indirect pathways.
   a. thalamus, basal nuclei
   b. primary sensory cortex, thalamus
   c. cerebellum, primary motor cortex
   d. primary motor cortex, basal nuclei

THE AUTONOMIC NERVOUS SYSTEM

The peripheral nervous system is divided into two systems: the somatic system, which controls skeletal muscles, and the autonomic system, which controls involuntary muscles. These muscles are the smooth muscles found in structures such as the blood vessels and airways and cardiac muscle found in the heart. Glands are also controlled by this system. The autonomic system, then, controls physiological characteristics such as blood pressure, heart rate, respiration rate, digestion, and sweating.

The neurons for the autonomic system, like the somatic motor neurons, are located in the spinal cord and brain stem, and release the neurotransmitter acetylcholine. This is where the similarity ends. The autonomic motor neurons are all located in the lateral horn rather than the ventral horns, and unlike the somatic motor neurons, autonomic neurons do not connect directly to muscles. Instead, they make a synapse in a ganglion outside of the CNS. A **ganglion** is group of nerve cell bodies outside of the CNS. You can think of this as a junction box where the signal can be passed on to the next part of the circuit. Then a second motor neuron, called a *postganglionic neuron*, connects to the smooth muscle or gland.

ganglion *(GANG lee on)*

The Sympathetic Branch

The autonomic nervous system is divided into two subdivisions: the **sympathetic** and the **parasympathetic** divisions. Please see Figure 9–10 ■. The sympathetic division controls the flight-or-fight response. It is charged with getting your body ready to expend energy. Sympathetic effects include increased heart rate, increased blood pressure, sweating, and dry mouth, all the symptoms of an adrenaline rush. This part of the autonomic system was responsible for your racing heart, rapid breathing, and intense sweating when confronted with the snarling dog. Your heart pumped more blood to your muscles, and your lungs took in more oxygen, both of which got you "up" to either fight or, most likely, flee. Another sympathetic response is dilation of your pupils to help you see the situation at hand much better. Sympathetic output is pretty strong when you hit your thumb with the hammer, too.

para = *near or around*

The *preganglionic neurons* for the sympathetic system are located in the thoracic and first two lumbar segments of the spinal cord. They are *thoracolumbar*. The preganglionic neurons, which secrete acetylcholine, synapse with the postganglionic neurons in the sympathetic ganglia. The ganglia for the sympathetic division form a pair of chainlike structures that run parallel to the spinal cord. These are called *paravertebral ganglia*. The postganglionic neurons release the neurontransmitter *norepinephrine*. One of the most important effects of the sympathetic system is its stimulation of the adrenal gland to release the hormone *epinephrine* (adrenaline), the chemical that causes that familiar adrenaline rush by circulating in the blood stream.

The Parasympathetic Branch

If you have a gas pedal, you also need a brake. The parasympathetic division is often called "resting and digesting" because it has the opposite effect of the sympathetic division. The parasympathetic division is responsible for mainte-

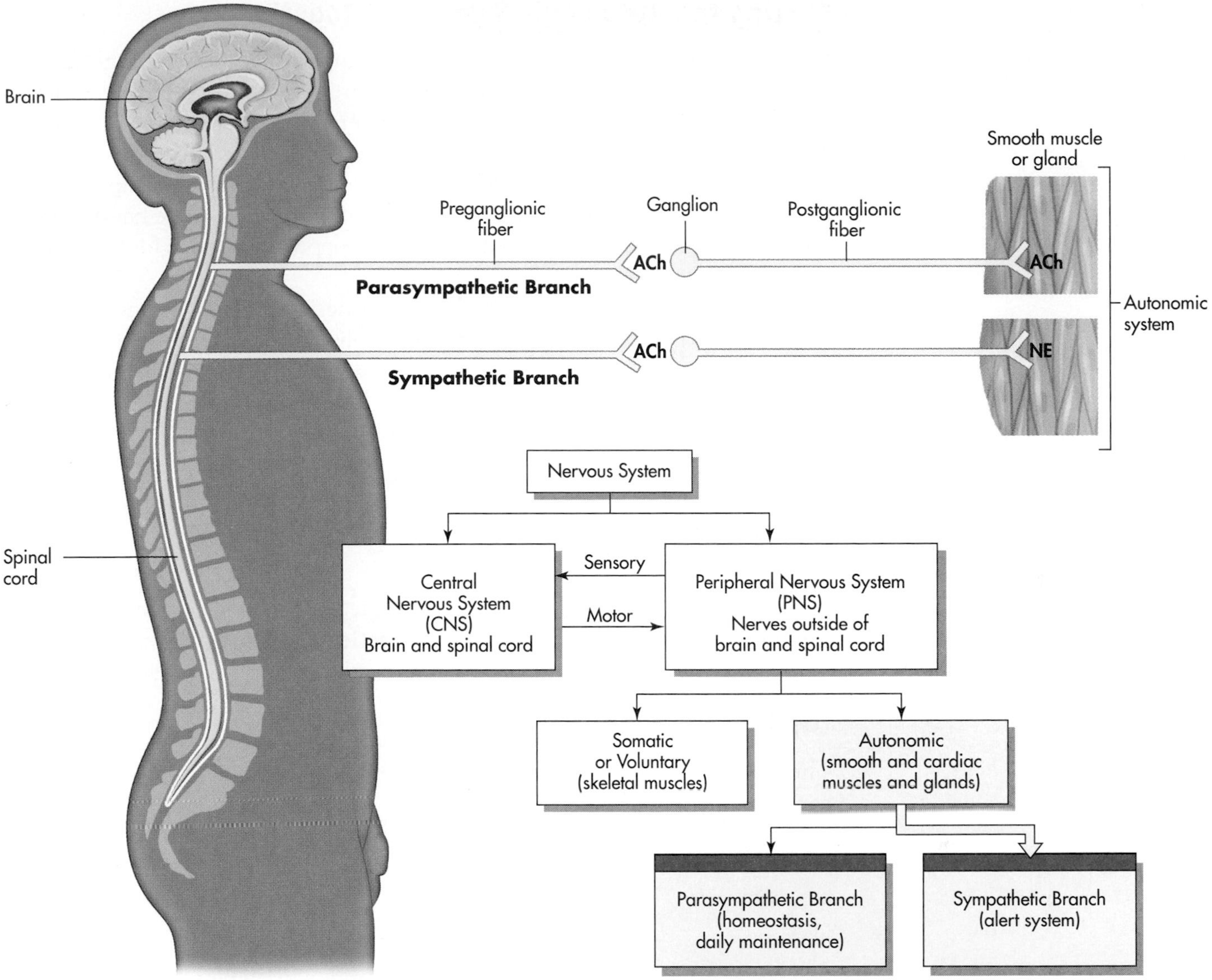

FIGURE ■ 9–10

General representation of autonomic nervous system. ACh = acetylcholine and NE = norepinephrine.

nance of everyday activities. It also helps bring you back down to normal from a sympathetic response. Parasympathetic effects include decreased heart rate, respiration, and blood pressure and increased digestive activity, including salivation and even stomach rumbling. The parasympathetic system allows you to calm down after you get the ice pack on your thumb or the dog is safely locked inside its cage.

The neurons of the parasympathetic system are in the brain stem and the sacral spinal cord and thus are called *craniosacral*. They, too, release acetylcholine. The preganglionic neurons synapse with postganglionic neurons in the parasympathetic ganglia. Parasympathetic ganglia are located near the organs. Postganglionic neurons release the neurotransmitter acetylcholine. (Remember, acetylcholine excites skeletal muscle but inhibits smooth and cardiac muscle.)

Putting the Autonomic System All Together

Let's revisit the snarling dog. When you encounter him, the sympathetic nervous system is stimulated and the impulses are sent from the thoracolumbar region of the spinal cord to preganglionic fibers, which release the neurotransmitter acetylcholine. Acetylcholine combines with receptors on the postganglionic neurons which generate an action potential and carry the impulse to the target area where norepinephrine is released. If this occurs at the heart (cardiac muscle), the rate and force of contraction will supply more blood for the fight-or-flight response.

Once the emergency is over, the sympathetic pathway will not be as active, and the norepinephrine will be metabolized so you don't remain in that stimulated state. The parasympathetic system now takes over to slow your system down to normal. This is another example of homeostasis in which normal heart rate is regulated by a balance between these two systems.

OTHER SYSTEMS

Two other systems that do not have a single, specific location but are found throughout the brain are the limbic and recticular systems.

The Limbic System

The limbic system is a series of nuclei in the cerebrum, diencephalon, and superior brain stem. These nuclei are involved in mood, emotion, and memory. One nucleus helps attach emotion to movement. Another coordinates emotion and your sense of smell. Still another is responsible for storing and retrieving memories.

The Reticular System

The reticular system is a diffuse network of nuclei in the brain stem that is responsible for "waking up" your cerebral cortex. The reticular system activity is vital for the maintenance of conscious awareness of your surroundings. When your alarm clock wakes you in the morning, your reticular system is responsible for nudging your cortex out of slumber. General anesthesia inhibits the reticular system, rendering surgery patients unconscious. Injury due to ischemia, mechanical damage, or drugs can damage the reticular system and lead to coma.

COMMON DISORDERS OF THE NERVOUS SYSTEM

Paralysis is the inability to control voluntary movements. Paralysis can be *spastic* or *flaccid*. Spastic paralysis is characterized by muscle rigidity or increased muscle tone (*hypertonia*) and overactive reflexes (*hyperreflexia*). In spastic paralysis, the muscles are rigid and the reflexes overactive because of decreased communication from the brain to the ventral horn motor neurons in the spinal cord.

Muscles contract randomly, and reflexes do not have any control signals from the brain. Stroke, head injuries, and spinal cord injuries can cause spastic paralysis.

9-4 Due to the complexity of the nervous system, there are a host of diseases we could cover. For a representative sampling of diseases not discussed in this chapter but that you may have heard about, we have included additional information on your CD-ROM. To view videos on autism, bipolar disorders, dissociative identity disorders, obsessive compulsive disorder (OCD), schizophrenia, Alzheimer disease, epilepsy, and seizures disorders, go to your CD-ROM for this chapter.

Flaccid paralysis is characterized by floppy muscles (decreased muscle tone, or *hypotonia*) and decreased reflexes (*hyporeflexia*). In flaccid paralysis, the damage is to the spinal nerves. Impulses cannot get to the muscles from the motor neurons. Therefore, the muscles are floppy and reflexes are absent. Flaccid paralysis can be caused by peripheral injury or disorders like polio and Guillain-Barré syndrome.

Cerebral palsy is a collection of movement disorders that are not progressive and that occur in young children. Patients with cerebral palsy exhibit signs of classic spastic paralysis. The disorder is caused by improper development of or damage to the motor system of the brain. Symptoms of cerebral palsy can range from minor motor loss to significant motor deficits, including the inability to walk or speak. Patients with cerebral palsy may have significant developmental delays or blindness or may have average or above-average intelligence.

The condition known as a stroke, or cerebral vascular accident (CVA), is caused by the disruption of blood flow to a portion of the brain due to either hemorrhage or blood clot. If the oxygen is disrupted for long enough, brain tissue will die. The symptoms of stroke vary depending on the location of the stroke. Muscle weakness, paralysis, or the lack of sensation due to stroke is contralateral (remember, the right hemisphere controls the left side of the body). Strokes can also rob patients of the ability to speak and can cause blindness and destroy memory. Symptoms of stroke appear suddenly. Some patients have a series of minor strokes (almost like tiny earthquakes before the big one) with minor, temporary symptoms before they have a major stroke. These ministrokes are called *transient ischemic accidents*, or TIAs.

WWW Numerous drugs are used to treat nervous system disorders. There are various career opportunities and levels within the pharmaceutical profession. To learn more about it and view a video on the profession of pharmacy, please go to the Web site for this chapter.

A subdural hematoma is a pool of blood between the dura mater and arachnoid mater, in the subdural space. Subdural hematomas are usually caused by head injuries. A blow to the head ruptures tiny blood vessels in the skull, causing them to bleed into the space. If the hematoma is large, or growing, the condition can cause irreversible brain damage and death. Hematomas cause damage by increasing pressure inside the skull. As the blood collects in the subdural space, pressure increases. The skull cannot expand and blood cannot be compressed as pressure rises, so the increasing pressure can cause severe damage to the delicate brain tissue. Some subdural hematomas resolve themselves, and some can be treated with medication. However, large or rapidly growing subdural hematomas must be treated by surgery.

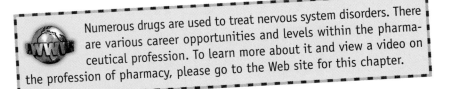

Huntington disease is a progressive genetic disorder causing deterioration of neurons in the basal nuclei and eventually of the cerebral cortex. The disease begins with mood swings and memory disturbances, writhing movements of the hands and face, or clumsiness. Eventually, the disease causes difficulty swallowing, speaking, and walking, as well as memory loss, psychosis, and loss of cognitive function. There is no cure for Huntington disease, and most patients die from accidental injuries, infections, or other complications. There is a genetic test to determine if a person carries the gene for the disease. Offspring of parents who have the disease have a 50 percent chance of inheriting the gene for Huntington disease. A carrier of the gene will eventually develop the disease.

SUMMARY

Snapshots from the Journey

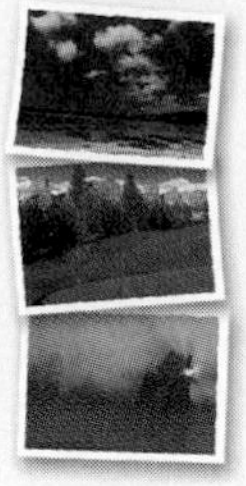

- The nervous system is your body's computer system, its information superhighway. Without the nervous system, people could not sample the environment, make decisions, or respond to stimuli. The nervous system handles millions of pieces of information every minute, making sure that every system in the body is working properly and correcting any problem that occurs.
- The brain is a hierarchical organ. It is is divided into compartments (lobes), each with very specific functions. The brain also has nerves attached to it, called cranial nerves. There are 12 pairs of cranial nerves, and they can be sensory, motor, or mixed.
- The cerebrum controls your conscious movement and sensation. Beneath the cerebrum are the diencephalon, brain stem, and cerebellum. Each part plays important roles in coordinating sensory and motor information for the cerebrum. Other parts of the brain, called association areas, allow you to make connections between different types of sensory information and to compare current experience to memories.
- The somatic sensory cortex is in the postcentral gyrus of the parietal lobe. Sensory information from the spinal cord tracts eventually ends up in this part of the cortex. When the information arrives there, you become aware of your sense of touch.
- There are motor and sensory maps of the body in the cerebral cortex. Orders for voluntary movements originate in the primary motor cortex in the precentral gyrus of the frontal lobe and travel down the spinal cord via direct spinal cord tracts. Subcortical structures coordinate this information via indirect tracts.
- The nervous system also controls involuntary movement via a part of the system known as the autonomic nervous system. The sympathetic division controls the flight-or-fight response, and the parasympathetic division controls day-to-day activities.

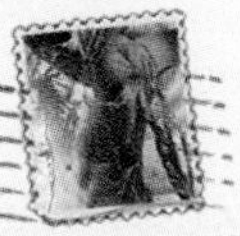

Case Study

A young woman finds her elderly father lying at the bottom of the basement stairs. He is semiconscious. He is paralyzed on his right side, but he seems to be able to feel that side of his body. At the hospital, he is diagnosed with a stroke.

What part of his brain is damaged? How can you tell?

REVIEW QUESTIONS

Multiple Choice

1. One of the following brain parts is *not* subcortical. Which one?
   a. hypothalamus
   b. medulla oblongata
   c. precentral gyrus
   d. pineal body

2. This cranial nerve controls the abdominal visceral.
   a. olfactory (I)
   b. trigeminal (V)
   c. vestibulocochlear (VII)
   d. vagus (X)

3. The size of the map of each body part in the postcentral gyrus is determined by the
   a. sensitivity of the body part
   b. size of the body part
   c. importance of the body part
   d. fine motor control of the body part

4. The sympathetic nervous system
   a. causes decreased heart rate
   b. has ganglia near the organs
   c. has ganglia near the spinal cord
   d. all of the above

5. This part of the brain contains the body's set-points and controls most of its physiology, including blood pressure and hunger level.
   a. thalamus
   b. hypothalamus
   c. amygdale
   d. hippocampus

Fill in the Blank

1. The ______________ are nuclei that coordinate motor output.

2. The occipital lobe is responsible for this sensation: ______________.

3. The white matter of the spinal cord contains ______________ tracts, which are motor, and ______________ tracts, which are sensory.

4. Emotion, mood, and memory are controlled by this collection of nuclei: ______________.

5. This portion of the brainstem has vital nuclei for respiration and the cardiovascular system: ______________.

Short Answers

1. List the differences between cranial and spinal nerves.

2. List the differences between the sympathetic and parasympathetic nervous systems.

3. Explain how the cerebral cortex and subcortical structures interact to produce motor output.

Suggested Activities

1. Find the parts of the brain on a preserved brain, diagram, or model.

2. Select a partner and play nervous system jeopardy. Can you identify the function of all of the parts of the nervous system?

9-5

Now that you have completed your journey through this chapter, please go to the CD-ROM for interactive games and puzzles concerning the medical terms and concepts contained in this chapter. By playing the games you will reinforce your learning of medical terminology in a fun way.

Greetings from THE ENDOCRINE System

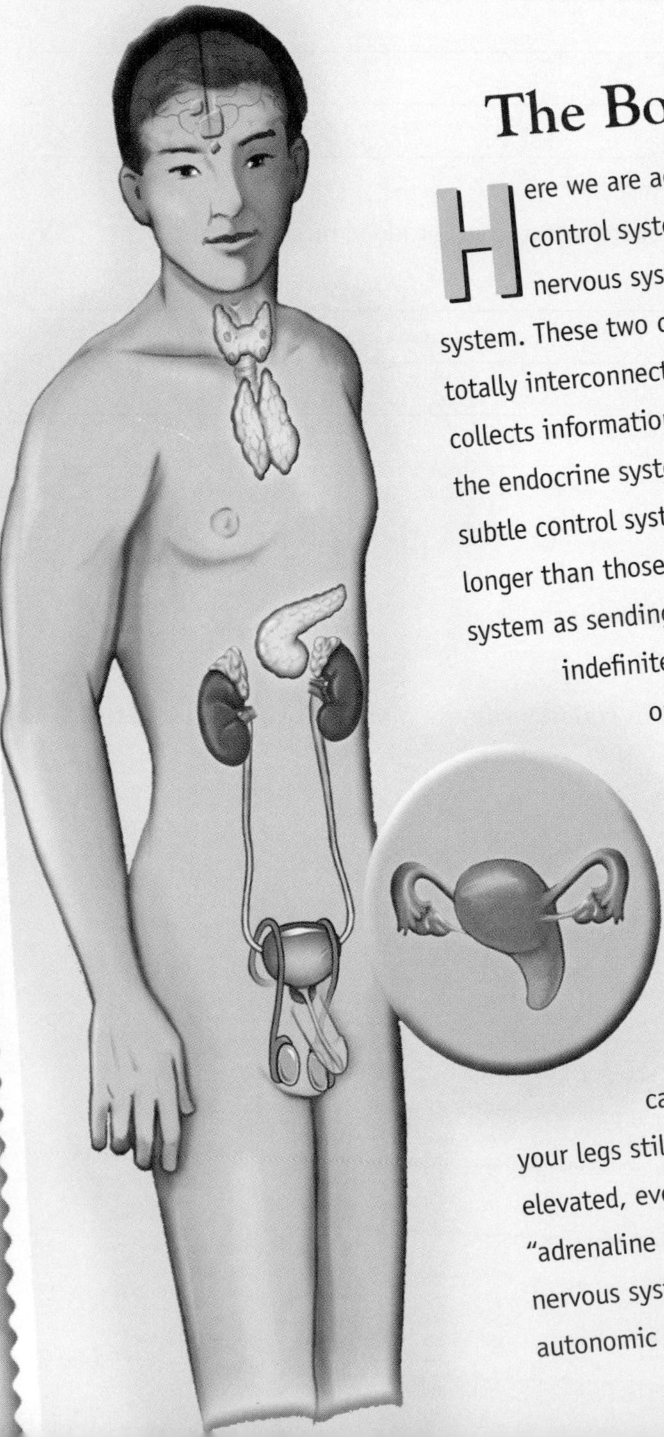

The Body's Other Control Center

Here we are again, talking about control. We have already visited one of the control systems: the complex structure of cells and connections known as the nervous system. Now we visit yet another control system, the endocrine system. These two control systems may seem like separate systems, but they are totally interconnected and always monitor each other's activities. The nervous system collects information and sends orders with a speed that is truly mind boggling. While the endocrine system also collects information and sends orders, it's a slower, more subtle control system. The endocrine system's orders to the body also last much longer than those made by the nervous system. You might think of the endocrine system as sending "standing orders," which are orders meant to be obeyed indefinitely unless changed by another set of orders. The orders change subtly on a regular basis, but their intention is constant. The nervous system, on the other hand, issues orders that are to be obeyed instantaneously but are used for short-term situations. The endocrine system demands organs to "carry on" while the nervous system expects them to respond immediately.

On our journey suppose we stop at an amusement park to ride a roller coaster. Afterward, enroute to our next destination, we are forced off the road because of a near miss with a truck. In both cases—when the roller coaster ride is over and the truck is long gone—your legs still shake, your heart continues to race, and your blood pressure remains elevated, even though you are no longer in danger. We call such lingering effects the "adrenaline rush." These lingering effects are not due to continued activity of the nervous system, but rather to endocrine activity deliberately triggered by the autonomic nervous system.

Chapter 10

LEARNING OBJECTIVES

At the completion of your journey through this chapter, you will be able to:

- Discuss the functions of the various endocrine glands
- Describe the purpose and effects of hormones within the body
- Discuss the process of homeostatic control
- Differentiate between hormonal and humoral control
- Explain common diseases of the endocrine system

MULTIMEDIA APPLICATIONS

CD-ROM Interactive Exercises

- Animation and video spotlighting the pathology of diabetes, 10-1
- Interactive games and puzzles, 10-2

www.prenhall.com/colbert

- Professional Profiles
  - Phlebotomy
  - Dietician

Pronunciation Guide

Correct pronunciation is important in any journey so that you and others are completely understood. Here is a "see and say" Pronunciation Guide for the more difficult terms to pronounce in this chapter.

adrenal cortex (ad REE nal KOR teks)
adrenal medulla (ad REE nal meh DULL lah)
endocrine (EHN doh krin)
epinephrine (EP ih NEFF rinn)
homeostasis (hoh mee oh STAY siss)
hypothalamus (high poh THAL ah mus)
norepinephrine (NOR ep ih NEFF rinn)
oxytocin (AHK see TOH sin)
parathyroid gland (PAIR ah THIGH royd)
pineal gland (pih NEE al)
pituitary (pih TOO ih tair ee)
prolactin (proh LAK tinn)
testes (TESS teez)
thymus (THIGH muss)

ORGANIZATION OF THE ENDROCRINE SYSTEM

The endocrine system has many organs that secrete a variety of chemical substances. Let's begin by looking at the basic organization of the system.

Endocrine Organs

endocrine *(EHN doh krin)*
endo = *into*
crine = *to secrete*

The **endocrine** system is a series of organs and glands (see Figure 10–1 ■) in your body that secrete chemical messengers called hormones *into* your bloodstream. (There are also glands that secrete *outside* the body, like sweat glands [*exocrine* glands], but they are not part of the *endo*crine system because their secretions leave the body.)

We have already discussed some of the endocrine glands, such as the hypothalamus, pituitary, and pineal glands, because they are part of the nervous system and provide a link *between* the two control systems. We visit some of the other endocrine organs later when we journey through the urinary, reproductive, and digestive systems. Many of these glands, like the hypothalamus and pancreas, have multiple functions.

It may seem like an overwhelming task to learn all the endocrine glands and their associated hormones, and therefore we will begin our discussion with a concise overview to lay a foundation upon which to build. As we journey through this chapter, these concepts are reinforced and expanded. For now, see Table 10–1, which lists the wide variety of functions of endocrine organs. (The hypothalamus and pituitary warrant more in-depth discussion under "The Major Endocrine Organs" later in this chapter.)

Amazing Body Facts

LESSER KNOWN ENDOCRINE GLANDS

Did you know that many organs, such as the heart, small intestines, stomach, and placenta, can also secrete hormones? These and many other organs are not listed as endocrine organs because their primary jobs are focused on other tasks, like pumping blood, storing and digesting food, or nourishing an embryo. But the hormones secreted by other organs are still an important part of the body's control systems. We will learn more about them when we discuss the body's other systems.

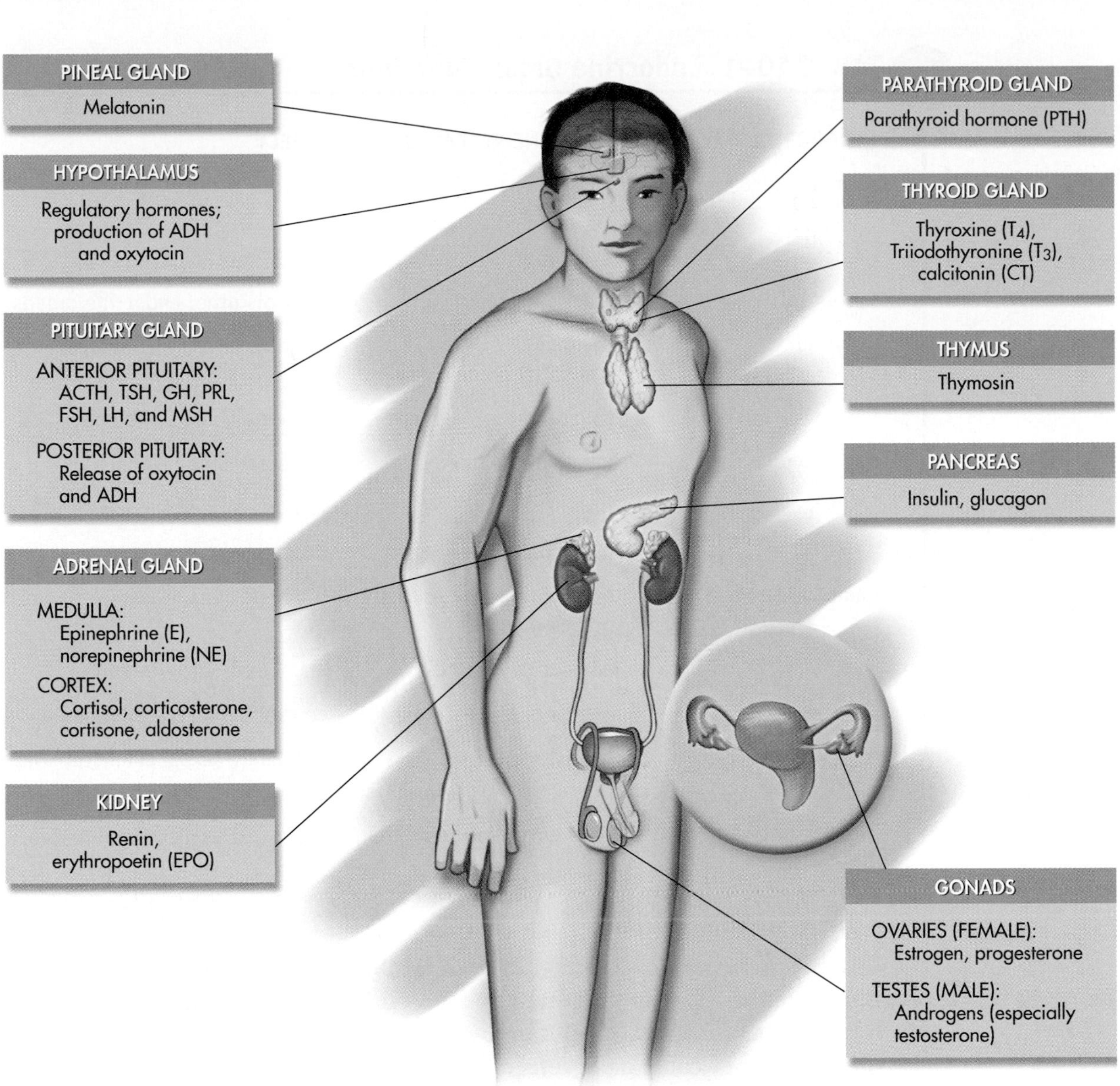

FIGURE ■ 10–1

The endocrine glands and their hormones.

Hormones

hormone *(HOR moan)*

The chemical messengers released by endocrine glands are called **hormones.** We have already seen one type of chemical messenger, the neurotransmitter. Neurotransmitters are released by neurons at chemical synapses. They diffuse across the synapse, a very tiny space, to a cell on the other side and bind to that cell. They are cleaned up quickly, so their effects are localized and short lived. Hormones, on the other hand, are released into the bloodstream and travel all over your body. Some hormones can affect millions of cells simultaneously. Their effects last for minutes or even hours or days. Many hormones are secreted constantly, and the amount secreted changes as needed. To help clarify the simi-

TABLE 10–1 Endocrine Organ Functions

ENDOCRINE ORGAN	HORMONE RELEASED	EFFECT
hypothalamus	(see Table 10–3)	controls pituitary hormone levels
pineal	melatonin	believed to regulate sleep
pituitary	(see Table 10–3)	controls other endocrine organs
thyroid	thyroxine, triiodothyronine	controls cellular metabolism
	calcitonin	decreases blood calcium
parathyroid glands	parathyroid hormone	increases blood calcium
pancreas	insulin	lowers blood sugar
	glucagon	raises blood sugar
adrenal glands	epinephrine, norepinephrine	flight-or-fight response
	adrenocorticosteroids	many different effects
ovaries/testes	estrogen, progesterone	control sexual reproduction and
	testosterone	secondary sexual characteristics

larities and differences between a neurotransmitter and hormone, please see Table 10–2.

HOW HORMONES WORK

Like neurotransmitters, hormones work by binding to receptors on target cells. But hormones may bind not only to sites on the outside of the cell, like neurotransmitters, but also to sites inside the cell. If hormones bind to the outside of the cell, they can have several different effects, either changing cellular permeability or sending the target cell a message that changes enzyme activity in-

TABLE 10–2 Comparison of Neurotransmitters and Hormones

NEUROTRANSMITTERS	HORMONES
chemical messengers	chemical messengers
bind to receiving cell	bind to receiving cell
control cell excitation	control cell activities
released by neurons	released by neurons, glands, or organs
released at chemical synapse	released into bloodstream
intended target very close	travel to distant target
effects happen quickly (less than a second)	effects take time (seconds or minutes)
effects wear off quickly (few seconds)	effects long lasting (minutes or hours)
affect single cell	can affect many cells

side the cell. Thus, the target cell changes what it has been doing, usually by making a new protein or turning off a protein it has been making.

One special class of hormones, **steroids,** is particularly powerful because steroids can bind to sites inside cells. Steroids are lipid molecules that can pass easily through the target cell membrane. These hormones, then, can interact directly with the cell's DNA, the genetic material, to change cell activity. These hormones are carefully regulated by the body because of their ability, even in very small amounts, to control target cells. See the section "The Adrenal Glands" for further discussion of steroid hormones and the dangers of taking steroids.

TEST YOUR KNOWLEDGE 10-1

Choose the best answer:

1. What chemical, when secreted into the bloodstream, controls the metabolic processes of target cells?
   a. neurotransmitter
   b. secretion
   c. hormone
   d. ligand

2. Steroid hormones are very powerful because they
   a. are hormones
   b. are medicine
   c. interact directly with DNA
   d. are secreted outside the body

3. Which of the following is true of hormones?
   a. They last a short time.
   b. They are fast acting.
   c. They affect distant targets.
   d. They leave the body.

CONTROL OF ENDOCRINE ACTIVITY

Many endocrine organs are active all the time. The amount of hormone they secrete changes as the situation demands, but unlike neurons, the cells in the endocrine organs often secrete hormones continuously. How is the activity controlled? How do the organs know how much hormone to secrete?

Homeostasis and Negative Feedback

In order to understand how the endocrine system is controlled, we first have to revisit the concept of **homeostasis** discussed at the beginning of our journey in Chapter 1 (see Figure 10–2 ■). Recall that many of the chemical and physical characteristics of the body have a standard level, or **setpoint,** that is the ideal level for that particular value. Blood pressure, blood oxygen, heart rate, and blood sugar, for example, all have "normal" ranges. Your control systems, nervous and endocrine, work to keep the levels at or near ideal. There is a way for your body to measure the variable, a place where the "ideal" level is stored, and a way for the body to correct levels that are not near ideal. For example, neurons measure your body temperature. The hypothalamus stores the setpoint. If your temperature falls below the setpoint temperature, the hypothalamus causes

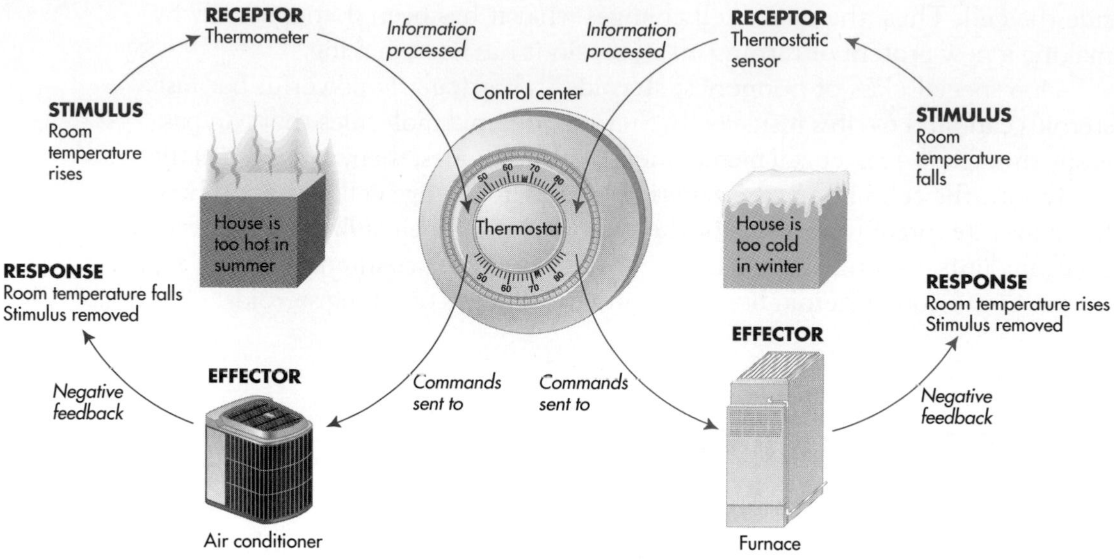

FIGURE ■ 10–2

Homeostasis is analogous to regulation of temperature via a thermostat.

shivering to produce additional heat. If body temperature rises above the setpoint, the hypothalamus causes sweating.

If any of the body's dozens of homeostatic values become seriously disrupted, the control systems work to bring them back to setpoint. This process is called **negative feedback** (see Figure 10–3 ■). Most of you are familiar with negative feedback in real life. When you pump gas, there is a sensor in the nozzle that turns *off* the flow of gas when the tank is full. That is negative feedback. The gas is flowing, the tank is filling, and when the goal is reached, the gas stops flowing. (A "timeout" for a toddler who has misbehaved is also negative feedback. The timeout is designed to turn *off* the naughty behavior.) In the body, negative feedback counteracts a change. As blood pressure rises, for example, your body works to bring it down to "normal," the setpoint. If blood pressure falls, your body works to raise it back to setpoint. Hormones work the same way. If hormone levels rise, negative feedback turns off the endocrine organ that is secreting the hormone.

> *Amazing Body Facts*
>
> **FEVER**
>
> When you get an infection, sometimes your body temperature rises above normal (setpoint). We call this "running a fever." The medical term for a patient with a fever is *febrile.* A fever is the deliberate raising of your body temperature setpoint by your hypothalamus. In an attempt to make things too hot for the germs that have invaded your body, the hypothalamus resets your body temperature setpoint to a higher level. Initially, the new setpoint is higher than your normal temperature. Your body thinks you are cold and takes steps to raise your body temperature to the new setpoint. Now you have a fever. Your head aches as blood vessels expand, your heart rate and blood pressure rise. You feel miserable, and you have your hypothalamus to blame! (Actually it's the fault of the invading bacteria or virus the hypothalamus is trying to defeat.)

The body is also capable of **positive feedback,** which increases the magnitude of a change. The flow of sodium into a neuron during depolarization is a real-life example we have already visited. The more depolarized a neuron becomes, the more sodium flows in, so it becomes more depolarized, so more flows in, and so on. Such a process is also known as a vicious cycle. Therefore, positive feedback is not a way to regulate your body because it increases a change

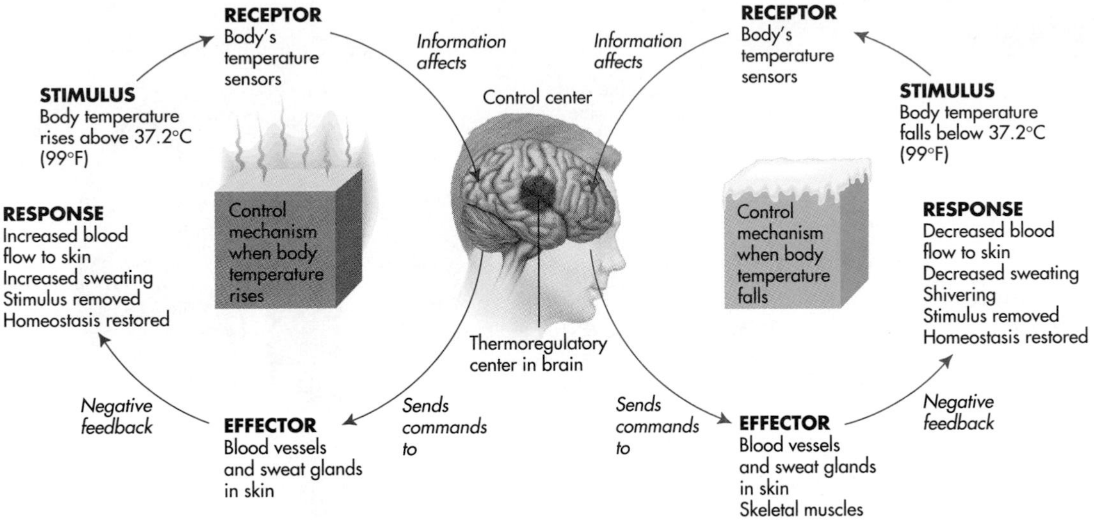

FIGURE ■ 10–3

Homeostasis and negative feedback as related to control of body temperature.

away from setpoint. What if instead of shivering when you got cold, to raise your body temperature, you got colder and colder and colder?

Sources of Control of Hormone Levels

Hormone levels can be controlled by the nervous system (neural control), by other hormones (hormonal control), or by body fluids such as the blood (humoral control).

NEURAL CONTROL

There are three basic ways in which endocrine organs function to maintain hormone levels and body function. Some hormones are directly controlled by the nervous system. For example, the adrenal glands receive signals from the sympathetic nervous system. When the sympathetic nervous system is active (remember the near-wreck), it sends signals to the adrenal glands to release epinephrine and norephinephrine as hormones, prolonging the effects of sympathetic activity (see Figure 10–4 ■).

> *Clinical Application*
>
> **CHILD BIRTH AND POSITIVE FEEDBACK**
>
> Often, positive feedback is harmful if the vicious cycle cannot be broken, but sometimes positive feedback is necessary for a process to run to completion. A good example of necessary positive feedback is the continued contraction of the uterus during childbirth. When a baby is ready to be born, a signal, not well understood at this time, tells the hypothalamus to release the hormone **oxytocin** from the posterior pituitary. Oxytocin increases the intensity of uterine contractions. As the uterus contracts, the pressure inside the uterus caused by the baby moving down the birth canal increases the signal to the hypothalamus: more oxytocin is released and the uterus contracts harder. As pressure gets higher inside the uterus, the hypothalamus is signaled to release more oxytocin, and the uterus contracts even harder. This cycle of ever-increasing uterine contractions due to ever-increasing release of oxytocin from the hypothalamus continues until the pressure inside the uterus decreases—that is, when the baby is born.

HORMONAL CONTROL

Other hormones are part of a hierarchy of hormonal control in which one gland is controlled by the release of hormones from another gland higher in the chain, which is controlled by another gland's release of hormones yet

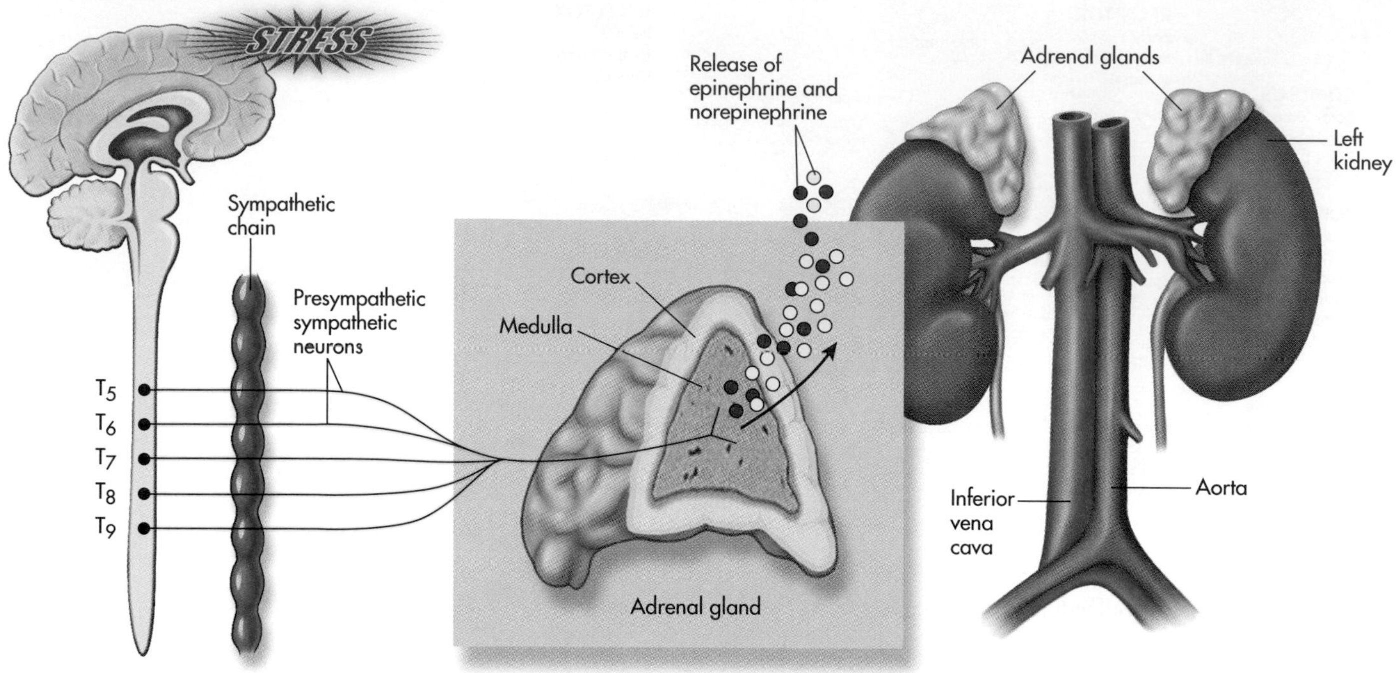

FIGURE ■ 10–4

Sympathetic control of adrenal gland.

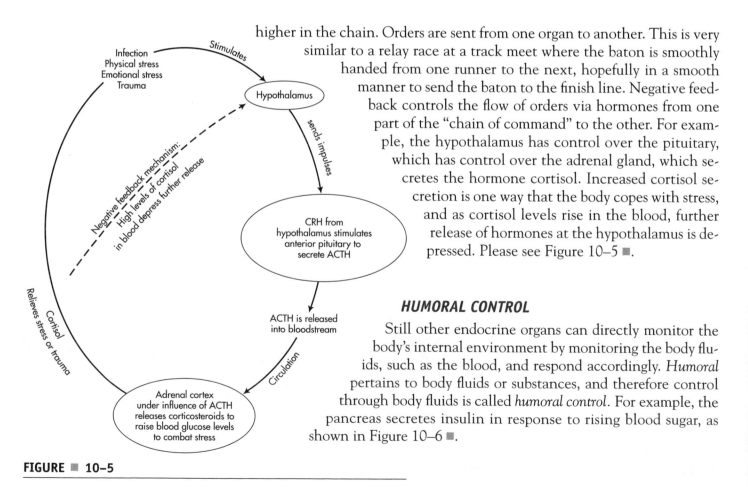

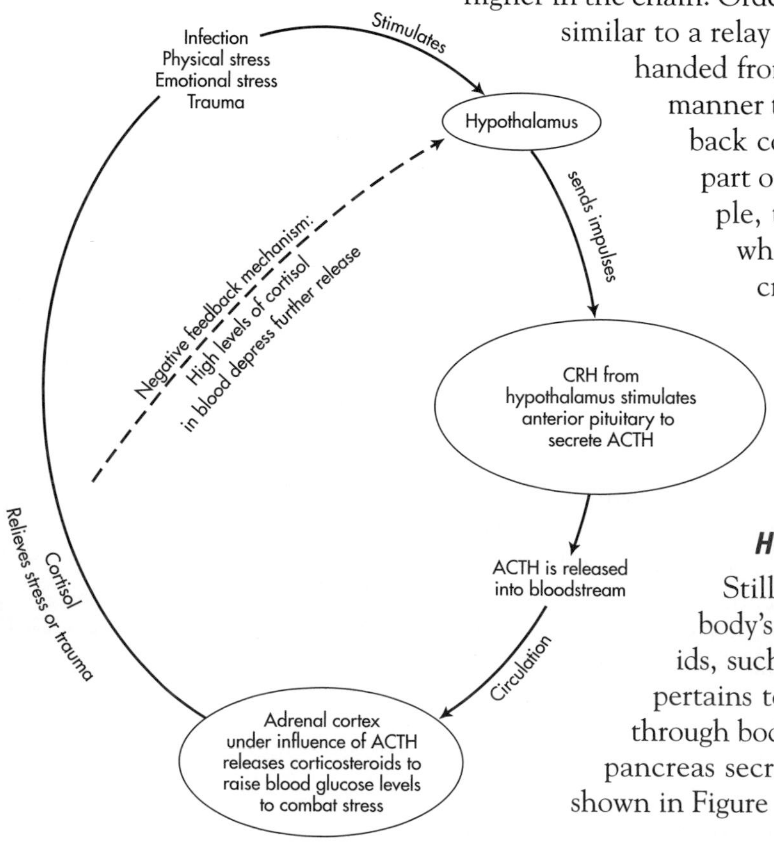

FIGURE ■ 10–5

Hormonal control of adrenal gland.

higher in the chain. Orders are sent from one organ to another. This is very similar to a relay race at a track meet where the baton is smoothly handed from one runner to the next, hopefully in a smooth manner to send the baton to the finish line. Negative feedback controls the flow of orders via hormones from one part of the "chain of command" to the other. For example, the hypothalamus has control over the pituitary, which has control over the adrenal gland, which secretes the hormone cortisol. Increased cortisol secretion is one way that the body copes with stress, and as cortisol levels rise in the blood, further release of hormones at the hypothalamus is depressed. Please see Figure 10–5 ■.

HUMORAL CONTROL

Still other endocrine organs can directly monitor the body's internal environment by monitoring the body fluids, such as the blood, and respond accordingly. *Humoral* pertains to body fluids or substances, and therefore control through body fluids is called *humoral control*. For example, the pancreas secretes insulin in response to rising blood sugar, as shown in Figure 10–6 ■.

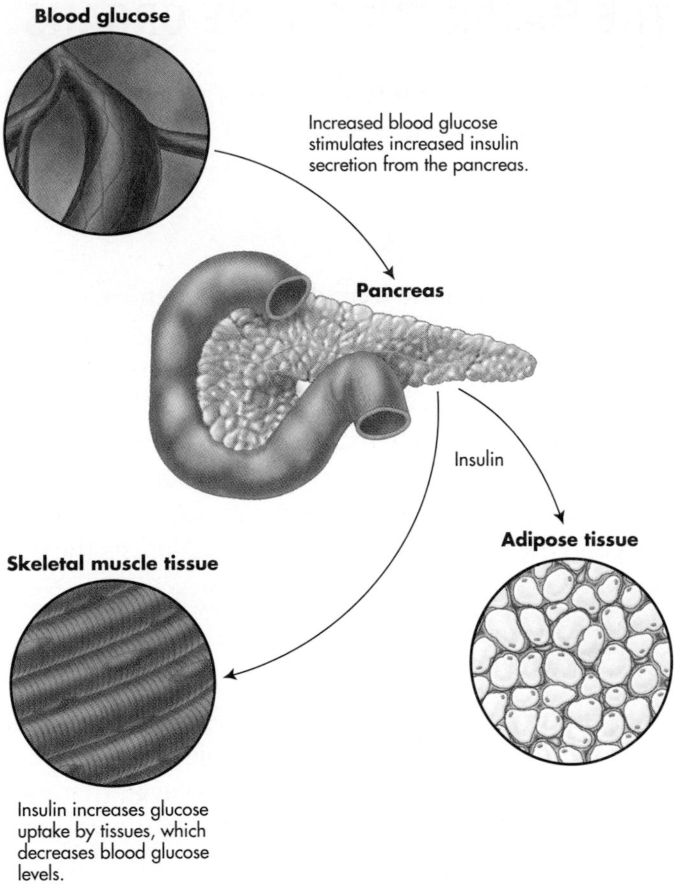
Blood glucose
Increased blood glucose stimulates increased insulin secretion from the pancreas.
Pancreas
Insulin
Adipose tissue
Skeletal muscle tissue
Insulin increases glucose uptake by tissues, which decreases blood glucose levels.

FIGURE 10–6

Humoral control of blood sugar levels.

TEST YOUR KNOWLEDGE 10-2

Choose the best answer:

1. Which of the following is *not* a way that hormone levels are regulated?
   a. negative feedback
   b. chain of command
   c. positive feedback
   d. direct control by nervous system

2. The "ideal" value for a body characteristic is called the
   a. setpoint
   b. average
   c. goal
   d. feedback point

3. __________ feedback enhances a change in body chemistry
   a. negative
   b. positive
   c. regular
   d. cyclic

THE MAJOR ENDOCRINE ORGANS

The endocrine system has several organs, and each has specific tasks within the body. The messages to carry out these tasks are related to the hormones they release.

The Hypothalamus

hypothalamus *(high poh THAL ah mus)*

We already visited the **hypothalamus** when we stopped at the central nervous system. Located in the diencephalon, this gland is an important link between the two control systems, nervous and endocrine (please see Figure 10–7 ■). The hypothalamus controls much of the body's physiology, including hunger, thirst, fluid balance, and body temperature, to name only a few of its functions. The hypothalamus is also, in part, the "commander-in-chief" of the endocrine system, because it controls the pituitary gland and therefore most of the other glands in the endocrine system. Table 10–3 lists the hypothalamic and pituitary hormones.

lactin = *milk*

The Pituitary

pituitary *(pih TOO ih tair ee)*

The **pituitary,** also a part of the diencephalon, is commonly known as the "master gland," indicating its important role in control of other endocrine glands. However, that name is misleading because the pituitary gland rarely acts on its own. The pituitary acts only under orders from the hypothalamus. If the hypothalamus is the "commander-in-chief," the pituitary is a high-ranking soldier who carries out the orders.

> **Learning Hint**
>
> **HORMONE NAMES**
>
> Most hormones are named according to where they are secreted or what they do. If you learn the meanings of their names, you can usually tell something about the hormone. For example, growth hormone stimulates cells to grow. Prolactin increases milk production. Even a complicated hormone name like adrenocorticotropic hormone can be picked apart fairly easily. Adreno refers to the adrenal gland, cortico refers to the cortex, and tropic means change. Therefore, adrenocorticotropic hormone is a hormone that changes the activity (in this case increases) of the adrenal cortex. Also keep in mind that most hormones are known by their abbreviations, for obvious reasons. Adrenocorticotropic hormone, for example, is abbreviated ACTH, which is much easier to say and write.

THE POSTERIOR PITUITARY (OR NEUROHYPOPHYSIS)

The pituitary is split into two segments: the *posterior* pituitary and the *anterior* pituitary. The posterior pituitary is an extension of the hypothalamus. Hypothalamic neurons, specialized to secrete hormones instead of neurotransmitters, extend their axons through a stalk to the posterior pituitary. Using the posterior pituitary as a sort of launch pad, these neurons secrete two hormones: **antidiuretic hormone (ADH)** (also called vasopressin) and **oxytocin.** Both of these hormones are secreted from the posterior pituitary, but they are made by the hypothalamus.

antidiuretic hormone *(AN tye dye yoo RET ik)*
oxytocin *(AHK see TOH sin)*

ADH does exactly what its name suggests. A diuretic is a chemical that increases urination, so an antidiuretic decreases urination. The effect of ADH, then, is to decrease fluid lost due to urination, increasing body fluid volume. ADH is secreted when the hypothalamus senses decreased blood volume or increased blood osmolarity (more solids suspended in blood). ADH circulates through the bloodstream and targets the kidneys specifically, causing them to

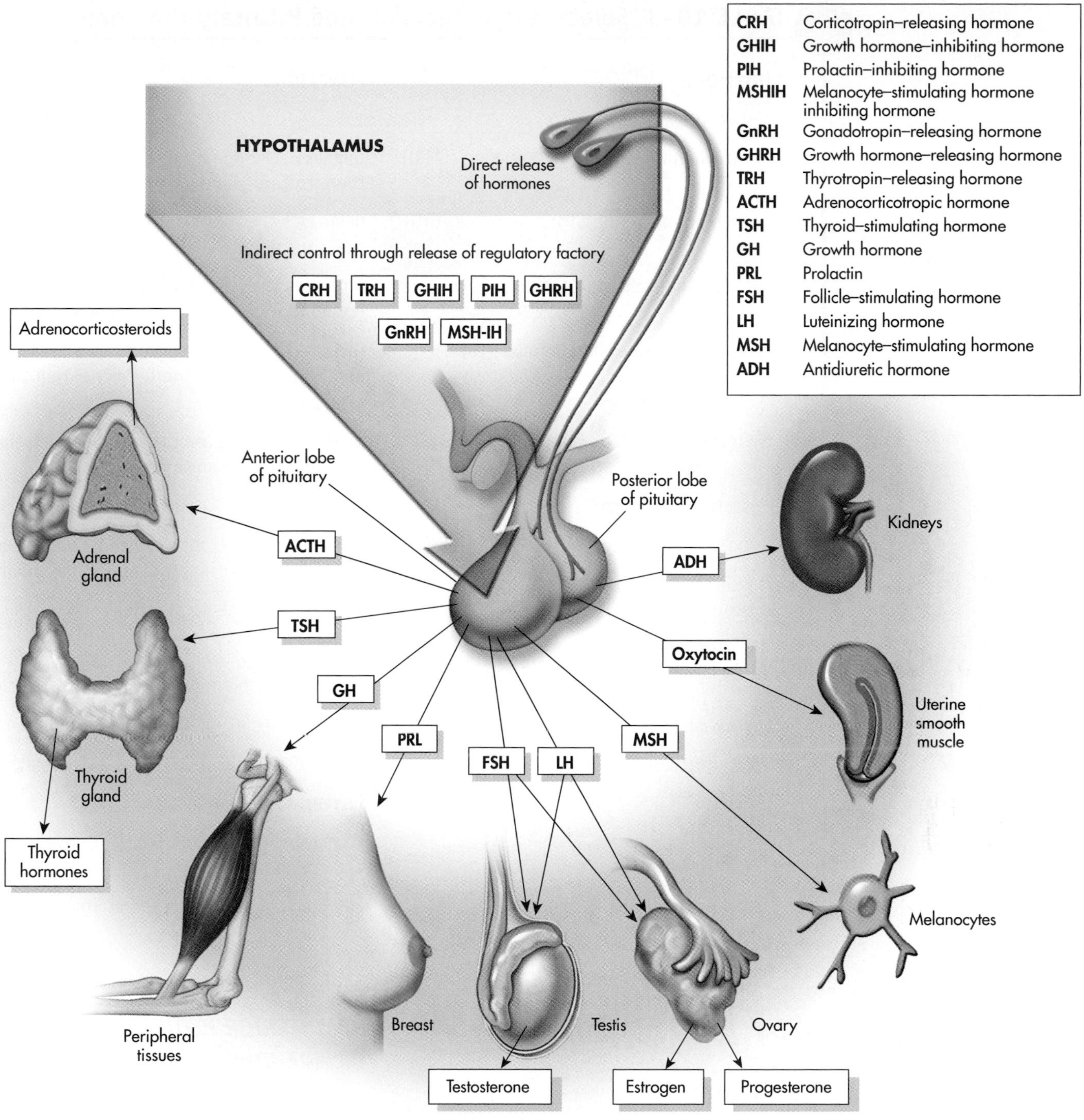

FIGURE ■ 10–7

The hypothalamus, anterior and posterior pituitary glands, and their targets and associated hormones.

absorb more water. It is very important in long-term control of blood pressure, especially during dehydration. (For more information on ADH, see Chapter 16 The Urinary System).

The second hypothalamic hormone released from the posterior pituitary is oxytocin. Oxytocin is important in maintaining uterine contractions during labor in women and is involved in milk ejection in nursing mothers. Oxytocin's function in males is unknown.

prolactin *(proh LAK tinn)*
pro = *for*

TABLE 10–3 Selected Hypothalamic and Pituitary Hormones

HORMONE	FUNCTION
Hypothalamus	
growth hormone–releasing hormone (GHRH)	increases the release of growth hormone from the pituitary gland
growth hormone–inhibiting hormone (GHIH)	decreases the release of growth hormone from the pituitary gland
corticotropin-releasing hormone (CRH)	increases the release of adrenocorticotropic hormone from the pituitary gland
gonadotropin-releasing hormone (GRH)	increases the release of luteinizing hormone and follicle-stimulating hormone from the pituitary gland
thyrotropin-releasing hormone (TRH)	increases the release of thyroid-stimulating hormone from pituitary gland
Posterior Pituitary	
antidiuretic hormone (ADH)	dilutes blood and increases fluid volume by increasing water reabsorption in the kidney
oxytocin	increases uterine contractions
Anterior Pituitary	
growth hormone (GH)	increases tissue growth
thyroid-stimulating hormone (TSH)	increases secretion of thyroid hormones
adrenocorticotropic hormone (ACTH)	increases steroid secretion from adrenal gland
prolactin	increases milk production
luteinizing hormone (LH)	stimulates ovaries and testes for ovulation and sperm production
follicle-stimulating hormone (FSH)	estrogen secretion and sperm production

Amazing Body Facts

ADH, ALCOHOL, AND COFFEE

Drinking too much alcohol can lead to several unpleasant consequences, not the least of which is the development of a hangover. The symptoms of a hangover are due to many side effects from alcohol consumption, but the most important may be that alcohol turns off ADH. The more alcohol you drink, the less ADH you secrete and the more dehydrated you become. That makes you thirsty, so you drink some more beer, and you secrete even less ADH and become even more dehydrated. (This is another example of a vicious cycle.) The more beer you drink, the more you urinate and the more dehydrated you are. This is part of the reason why consuming too much alcohol on Friday night can make you miserable on Saturday morning. The caffeine in coffee also has the same effect in inhibiting ADH. That's why you make frequent trips to the bathroom if you pull an "all-nighter" studying for your A&P tests using coffee (caffeine) to stay awake. Too much caffeine will even make you feel pretty miserable.

THE ANTERIOR PITUITARY (OR ADENOHYPOPHYSIS)

The anterior pituitary is also controlled by the hypothalamus but is an endocrine gland in its own right. The anterior pituitary makes and secretes a number of hormones, under hormonal control of the hypothalamus, that control other endocrine glands. (Growth hormone and prolactin are exceptions to this rule.) Refer back to Table 10–3 and Figure 10–7 for a list of hypothalamic and pituitary hormones. We discussed this relationship previously when we talked about hormonal control. The hypothalamus secretes a hormone that controls hormone secretion by the anterior pituitary, which usually controls the secretion of hormones by another endocrine gland. The hormone levels are controlled by negative feedback to both the pituitary and the hypothalamus.

Clinical Application

STATURE DISORDERS

Stature disorders are those disorders that result in *well*-below-average height (called dwarfism) or well-above-normal height (called giantism or gigantism). Some of these disorders are caused by abnormalities in skeletal development or nutritional deficiencies. However, growth hormone (GH) problems are often implicated. If GH secretion is insufficient during childhood, children do not grow to "standard" height. This type of dwarfism results in stunted adult height. However, if GH deficiency is diagnosed before closure of the growth zones of the long bones, it can be treated with GH injections. Children treated with GH injection attain full height. On the other end of the spectrum are those who secrete too much GH. If the oversecretion happens during childhood, people get extremely tall. (Robert Wadlow, the tallest man ever to live according to *Guinness Book of World Records,* was more than 8 feet tall. We're not talking NBA stars here!) Gigantism causes many health problems. The body gets so big that it cannot support itself. Surgery and medication are the only treatments for this type of gigantism. If GH oversecretion begins after a person has stopped growing (bone closure), he or she does not get any taller, but the tissues of the hands, feet, face, and many internal organs continue to grow out of control, causing pain and organ dysfunction. Most oversecretion of GH is caused by noncancerous pituitary tumors.

TEST YOUR KNOWLEDGE 10-3

Choose the best answer:

1. Oxytocin
   a. is secreted by the anterior pituitary
   b. decreases uterine contractions
   c. is released by the posterior pituitary
   d. is a way to get more oxygen to your toes

2. The _____ is controlled by hormones from the hypothalamus, while the _____ actually secretes hypothalamic hormones.
   a. posterior pituitary, posterior pituitary
   b. anterior pituitary, anterior pituitary
   c. anterior pituitary, posterior pituitary
   d. posterior pituitary, anterior pituitary

3. This gland, under orders from the hypothalamus, releases hormones that control other endocrine glands.
   a. adrenal gland
   b. anterior pituitary
   c. thyroid gland
   d. pancreas

4. Which gland does ACTH control?
   a. adrenal gland
   b. anterior pituitary
   c. thyroid gland
   d. pancreas

The Thyroid gland

thyroid *(THIGH royd)*

The **thyroid** gland, located in the anterior portion of your neck, is a butterfly-shaped organ. It is responsible for secreting the hormones thyroxine (T_4) and triiodothyronine (T_3), under orders from the pituitary gland (see Figure 10–8 ■). Thyroxine and triiodothyronine contain iodine and control cell metabolism and growth. The thyroid gland also secretes a third hormone, calcitonin, which decreases blood calcium by stimulating bone-building cells. Thyroxine and triiodothyronine are generally referred to as "thyroid hormones" and are of great clinical importance. Overproduction (hyperthyroidism) or underproduction (hypothyroidism) can cause a variety of clinical symptoms, because the level of these hormones is essential in controlling growth and metabolism of body tissues, particularly in the nervous system. The importance of these hormones is so great that table salt contains added iodine to ensure that people get enough iodine in their diets to make thyroid hormones.

> *Clinical Application*
>
> **HYPERTHYROIDISM**
>
> Jenny was a healthy 25-year-old school teacher starting her first job when she began to have strange symptoms. Her heart sometimes beat so fast it frightened her, she would sweat copiously, and she was always hungry. Initially, she ignored these changes, attributing them to the stress of moving away from home for the first time, but then more alarming symptoms appeared. Typically rather laid back, Jenny became irritable and restless. She began to have trouble sleeping and couldn't concentrate. Soon she could barely focus long enough to read the newspaper or get through a half-hour sitcom. Her thoughts became so scattered she thought she might be losing her mind. Frightened, she made an appointment to see her physician. Testing confirmed that she did have a problem, but she was not losing her mind. Jenny had Graves' disease, a disorder that causes the thyroid gland to secrete too much thyroid hormone.

parathyroid *(PAIR ah THIGH royd)*

The thyroid gland has two small pairs of glands embedded in its posterior surface. These glands are called the **parathyroid glands,** and they produce **parathyroid hormone (PTH)** which regulates the levels of calcium in the bloodstream. If calcium levels get too low, the parathyroid glands are stimulated to release PTH, which stimulates bone-dissolving cells and thereby releases needed calcium in the bloodstream. Again, see Figure 10–8.

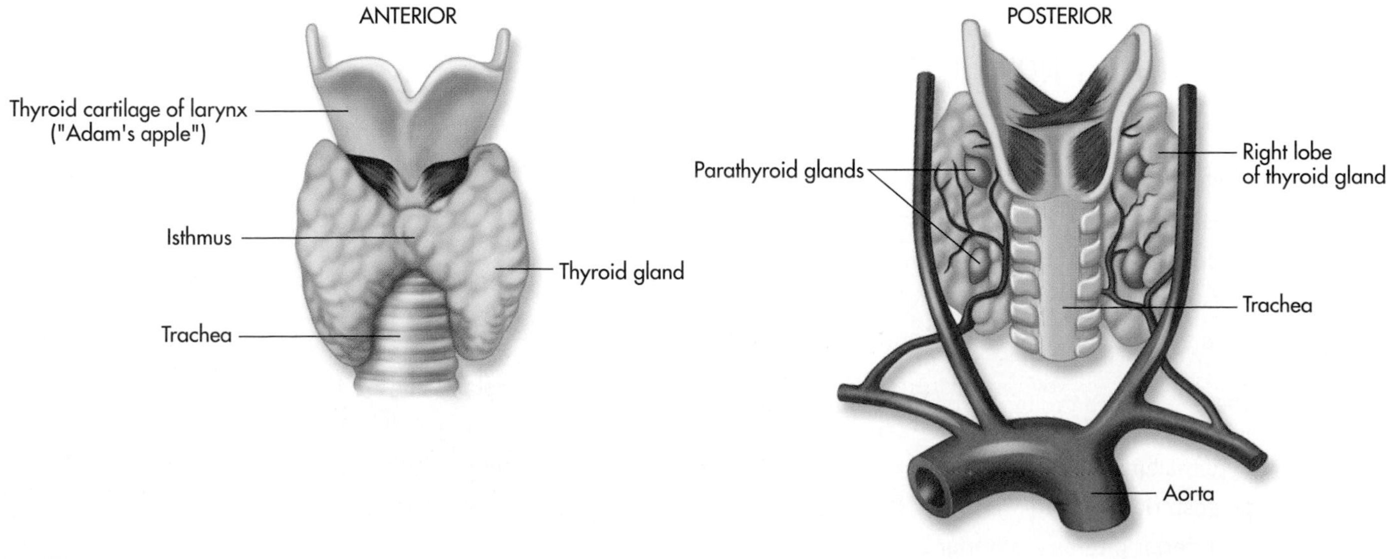

FIGURE ■ 10–8

The thyroid and parathyroid glands.

The Thymus Gland

The **thymus gland** is located in the upper thorax and plays an important function in the immune system. It produces a hormone called thymosin, which helps with the maturation of white blood cells during childhood to fight infections. This gland is further discussed in Chapter 14, The Lymphatic and Immune System.

thymus *(THIGH muss)*

The Pineal Gland

The tiny **pineal gland** is found in the brain, and its full function still remains unknown. However, it has been shown to produce the hormone **melatonin,** which rises and falls during the waking and sleeping hours. It is believed this hormone is what triggers our sleep by peaking at night and causing drowsiness.

pineal gland *(pih NEE al)*
melatonin *(MELL ah TOH ninn)*

The Pancreas

The **pancreas** is largely responsible for maintaining blood sugar (glucose) levels at or near a setpoint. The normal clinical range for blood glucose levels is 70 to 105 mg/dL (milligrams per deciliter). The pancreas can measure blood sugar, and if the blood glucose is high or low, the pancreas releases a hormone to correct the level. To understand the importance of the pancreas, let's go back in your journey to the chapter on cells. Why does it matter how much glucose is in your blood? Why devote an organ, and a pretty big one at that, to controlling blood sugar? There are two reasons why blood glucose is important. Too much glucose floating around in your blood causes many problems with the fluid balance of your cells. Recall that if the concentration of the fluid outside a cell is high in solids, the cell will lose water to the surroundings. If the solids are low outside the cell, the cell will fill with water and eventually can even explode! Obviously, that's a serious problem. It does not matter if the solids are salts or glucose, the result is the same. Blood glucose must therefore be maintained at a certain level for cells to neither gain nor lose water. Why else is glucose important? Glucose is vital for cellular respiration. Cellular respiration is needed to get energy, by making adenosine triphosphate (ATP) so cells need to have enough glucose that they can make sufficient ATP to carry out their daily activities.

pancreas *(PAN kree ass)*

10-1 For videos spotlighting the pathology of diabetes, please go to your CD-ROM.

Clinical Application

DIABETES MELLITUS

Diabetes mellitus is a condition characterized by abnormally high blood glucose (hyperglycemia). Insulin-dependent diabetes mellitus (IDDM, type 1, juvenile onset) is caused by the destruction of the insulin-producing cells of the pancreas. Patients with IDDM do not produce enough insulin. They are always dependent on daily insulin injections. Noninsulin-dependent diabetes mellitus (NIDDM, type 2, late onset) is caused by insensitivity of the body's tissues to insulin. Patients with NIDDM can often be treated with a carefully controlled diet and weight-loss regimen. In both types of diabetes, abnormally high blood glucose must be resolved. If blood glucose remains high, the kidneys work overtime to secrete the excess sugar. Increased urination and dehydration are the most obvious symptoms. But the stress of trying to get rid of the excess blood sugar eventually causes kidney damage. In addition, if insulin is not effective, glucose cannot get into cells. Cells must have glucose in order to make ATP. If cells can't get glucose and can't make ATP, they will look for other sources of energy. Untreated diabetics often lose weight as their body searches for other energy sources. Often, their blood becomes increasingly acidic as waste products from abnormal cell metabolism accumulate in the bloodstream. The changes in blood chemistry lead to tissue and organ damage. Left untreated, diabetes mellitus may lead to coma and death.

The pancreas makes two hormones that control blood glucose: *insulin*, which most of you have heard of before, and *glucagon*. Insulin, the hormone that is missing or ineffective in diabetes, removes glucose from the blood by directing the liver to store excess glucose and by helping glucose to get inside the cells so it can be used to make ATP. (Remember that glucose, a carbohydrate, is pretty big and very water soluble, so it cannot get into cells by itself.) When would insulin be secreted by the pancreas: when blood glucose is high or when blood glucose is low? Because insulin removes glucose from the blood, it lowers blood sugar, so it is released when blood sugar is high (hyperglycemia), like right after a meal.

It is critically important to monitor blood glucose levels and maintain an appropriate diet for patients with diabetes. Phlebotomists are specially trained allied health professionals who draw and test blood samples. Dieticians are intensively involved in the design of specialized diets for diabetes and many other illnesses. To learn more about these important allied health professions, please go to the companion Web site for this chapter.

Glucagon does the opposite of insulin. Glucagon puts glucose into the bloodstream mainly by directing the liver to release stored glucose in the form of glycogen. Glucagon is released typically several hours after a meal to prevent blood glucose from dropping too low (hypoglycemia). These two hormones control blood glucose very tightly in healthy humans (see Figure 10–9 ■). Other hormones, like the adrenal hormone cortisol, also aid in the control of blood sugar.

adrenal *(ad REE nal)*
adrenal cortex *(ad REE nal KOR teks)*
adrenal medulla *(ad REE nal meh DULL lah)*
epinephrine *(EP ih NEFF rinn)*
norepinephrine *(NOR ep ih NEFF rinn)*

The Adrenal Glands

The **adrenal** glands are a pair of small glands that sit on top of your kidneys like baseball hats. The adrenal glands are split into two regions: the **adrenal cortex,** an outer layer, and the **adrenal medulla,** the middle of the gland. (Note that it is best to be specific when talking about the adrenal cortex, since your cerebrum has a cortex, too.)

THE ADRENAL MEDULLA

The adrenal medulla releases two hormones: **epinephrine** (also known as adrenalin) and **norepinephrine.** These hormones increase the duration of the effects of your sympathetic nervous system. (Remember your friend's snarling dog.) Cells of the adrenal medulla receive the neurotransmitter norepinephrine (it is both a hormone and a neurotransmitter, depending on where it is released) from the sympathetic nervous system. The neurotransmitter triggers the release of norepinephrine and epinephrine into the bloodstream, increasing heart rate, blood pressure, and respiration rate, and giving you sweaty palms and dry mouth. (Not a great combination!) Again, the effects of the hormones last much longer than effects of the neurotransmitter.

Clinical Application

PREDNISONE

Prednisone (hydrocortisone) is clinically important in the treatment of inflammation, organ transplant rejection, and immune disorders, but prescription steroids are a double-edged sword. These medications are so powerful that they can cause dangerous side effects, such as bone density loss, weight gain, hair growth, fat deposits, and delayed wound healing. These drugs, even when taken for a short time, cannot be discontinued suddenly. Patients must be weaned off their medication slowly. Why? When a patient takes a steroid medication, the adrenal gland decreases steroid production in response. (Remember negative feedback: as hormone levels rise, hormone secretion decreases.) Therefore, if the medication is removed suddenly, patients are left with a severe hormone deficiency, which could be fatal. Their adrenal gland must be given some time to "gear up" to secrete hormones at the appropriate level. It is no surprise, then, that taking steroid medications for the purpose of increasing athletic performance is prohibited by amateur and professional sports organizations.

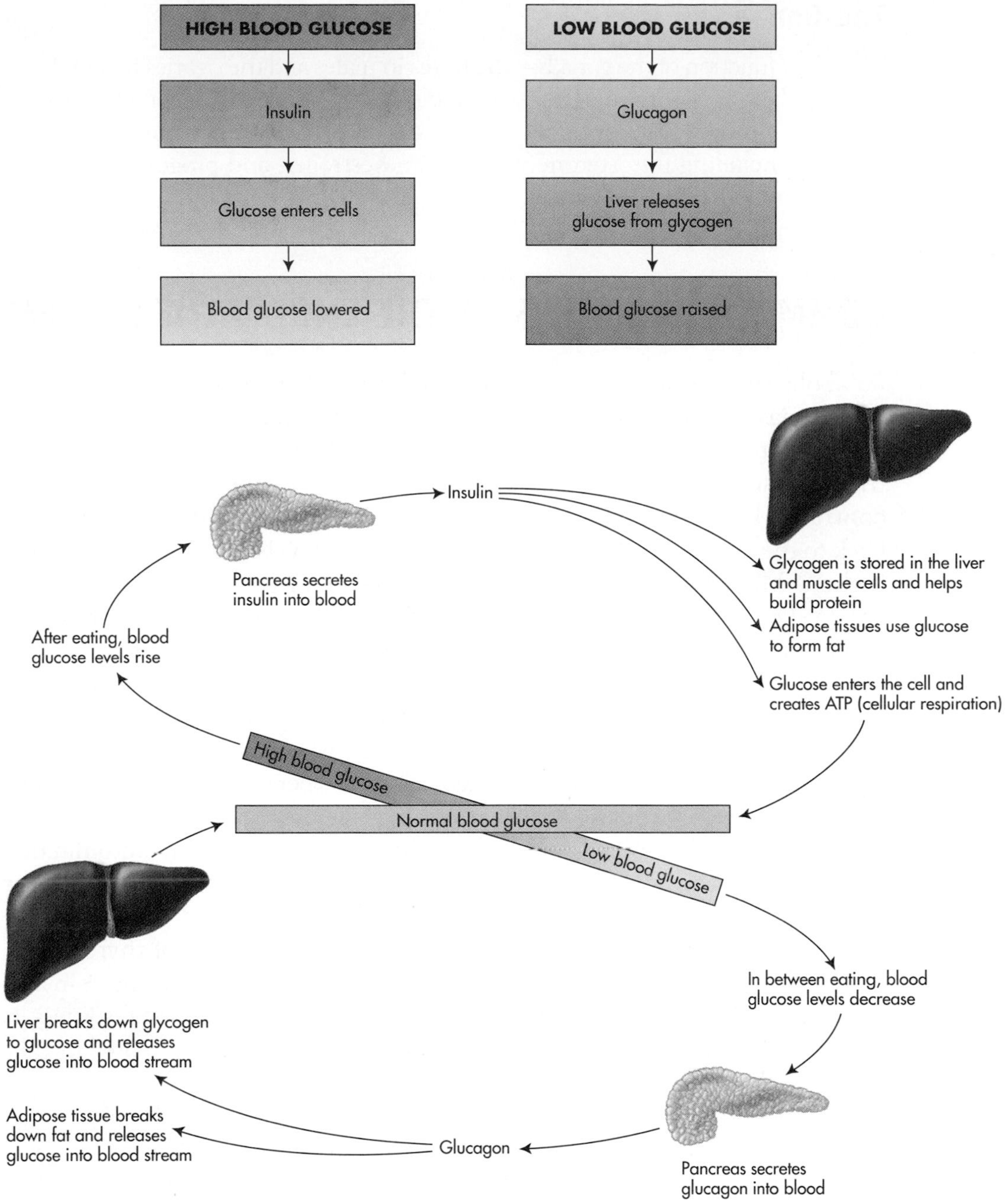

FIGURE ■ 10–9

Control of blood glucose by pancreatic hormones.

THE ADRENAL CORTEX

The adrenal cortex, on the other hand, makes dozens of steroid hormones known collectively as *adrenocorticosteroids* (steroids in the adrenal cortex). The adrenal cortex releases steroid hormones under the direction of the anterior pituitary. Many of these steroid hormones are so important that a decrease in their production could be fatal relatively quickly. Some of these hormones regulate electrolyte (salt) and fluid balance, others regulate blood sugar, others are responsible for regulation of reproduction and secondary sexual characteristics, and still others control cell metabolism, growth, and immune system function.

The Gonads

The chief function of the gonads—the testes in males and the ovaries in females—is to produce and store gametes, eggs, and sperm. However, the gonads also produce a number of sex hormones that control reproduction in both males and females, including testosterone in males and estrogen and progesterone in females. For more details on the hormones produced by the gonads, see Chapter 17.

COMMON DISORDERS OF THE ENDOCRINE SYSTEM

Anabolic steroids are a class of steroid molecules that cause large increases in muscle mass when compared to working out without steroids. Some athletes use anabolic steroids to enhance performance or to get big muscles much faster than they would without steroids. Because steroid hormone levels are so tightly controlled by the body, anabolic steroids have a number of side effects. (Think back to the discussion of prednisone at therapeutic levels; abuse levels are much higher.) Men abusing steroids may experience changes in sperm production, enlarged breasts, and shrinking of their testicles. Women may experience deepening of the voice, decreased breast size, and excessive body hair growth. Steroid abuse may lead to cardiovascular diseases and increased cholesterol levels. Many steroids suppress immune function, and because steroid use is illegal, many abusers expose themselves to hepatitis B and HIV when sharing needles. Steroid abuse has also been linked to increased aggressive behavior. All major professional and amateur athletic organizations ban the use of steroids.

Hashimoto's disease is a form of hypothyroidism caused by an autoimmune attack on your thyroid gland. For unknown reasons, the immune system begins to attack the cells in the thyroid, causing inflammation and damage to the gland. This damage eventually leads to decreased production of thyroid hormones—hypothyroidism. In addition, the thyroid may swell, causing pain and difficulty swallowing. Hashimoto's disease, like many autoimmune disorders, is most common in women between 30 and 50 years old. It can be treated by taking thyroid hormones daily.

Graves' disease is also an immune disorder that affects the thyroid, but in this case the immune system stimulates the thyroid, resulting in hyperthyroidism and bulging eyes. Treatment for Graves' disease involves decreasing the activity of the thyroid with medication. If medication does not work, the thyroid may be removed, and the patient must take thyroid hormones.

A *pheochromocytoma* is a tumor of the adrenal gland that causes the gland to secrete excess epinephrine. The symptoms of these tumors are what you might expect: an adrenaline rush. Patients experience severe headaches, excessive sweating, racing heart, anxiety, abdominal pain, heat intolerance, and weight loss. Pheochromocytomas are not generally cancerous, but they must be removed or the effects of excess epinephrine will be fatal.

Addison's disease is caused by insufficient production of the adrenocorticosteroid cortisol. The deficiency causes weight loss, muscle weakness, fatigue, low blood pressure, and excessive skin pigmentation. Aldosterone may also be deficient. Many cases of Addison's disease are autoimmune. Addison's disease is treated with hormone replacement.

Cushing's syndrome is caused by oversecretion of cortisol. Symptoms include upper body obesity, round face, easy bruising, weakened bones, fatigue, high blood pressure, and high blood sugar. Women may have excess facial hair and irregular periods; men may have decreased fertility and decreased sex drive. Cushing's syndrome may be a side effect of medical use of steroids, like prednisone, or may be due to pituitary tumors, lung tumors, adrenal tumors, or one of several genetic disorders. Treatment depends on the underlying cause of the disorder. Typically, the cause of the excess production must be removed, and patients generally must take hormone replacement. Figure 10–10 ■ shows examples of some common endocrine disorders.

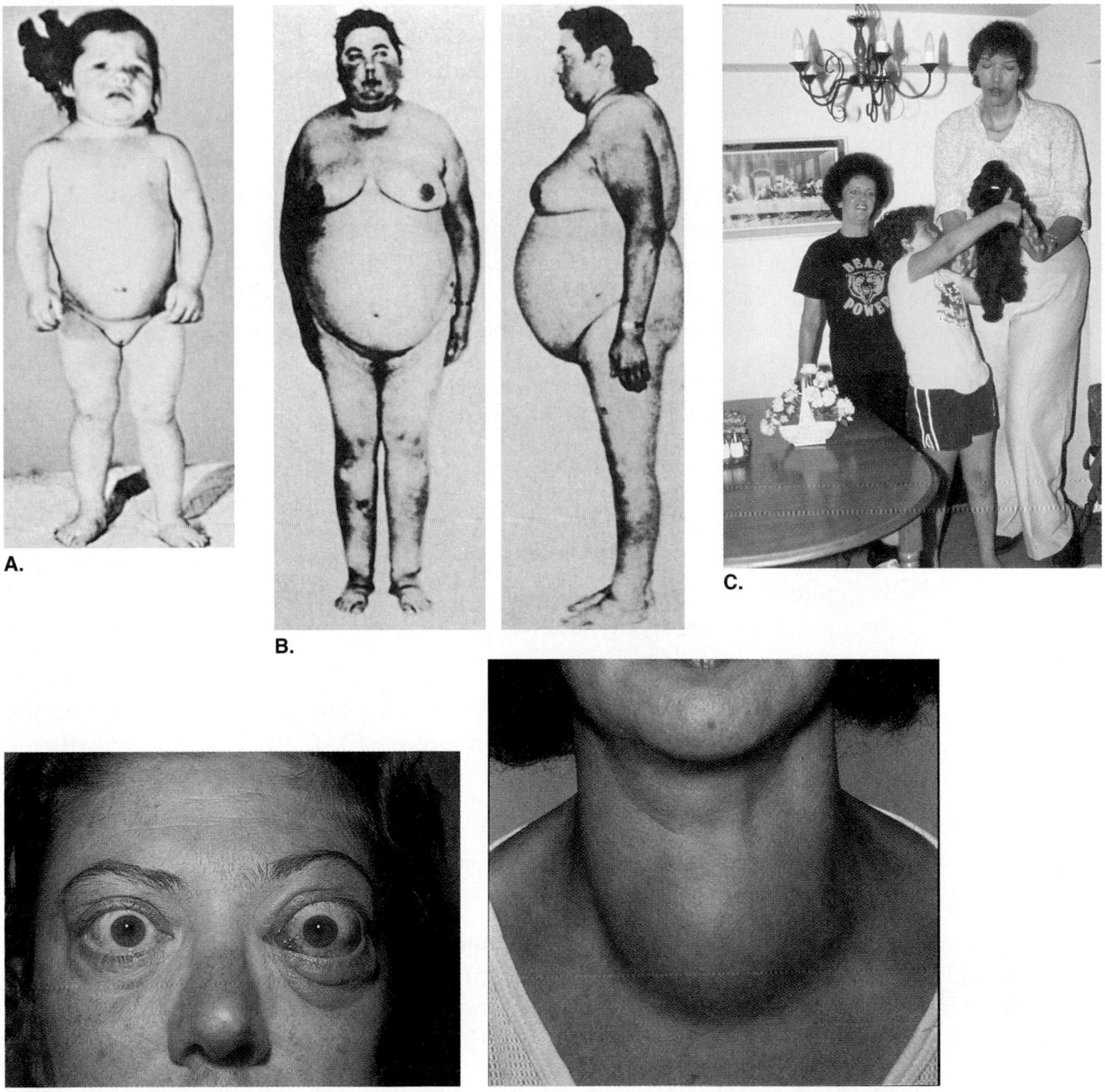

A. B. C. D. E.

FIGURE ■ 10–10

Examples of Endocrine Disorders. a) A 6-year-old child with congenital hypothyroidism. b) a patient with Cushing's syndrome. c) a patient with gigantism. (Source: Bettina Cirrone/Photo researchers, Inc.) d) a patient with exophthalmos, a symptom of hyperthyroidism (Graves' disease). (Source: Custom Medical Stock Photo, Inc.) e) a patient with a goiter. (Source: Custom Medical Stock Photo, Inc.)

SUMMARY

Snapshots from the Journey

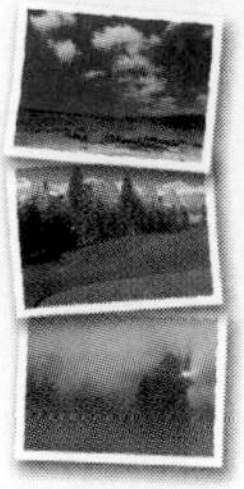

- The endocrine system works together with the nervous system to regulate the activities of all the body systems. The endocrine system is linked to the nervous system but works very differently. The endocrine system secretes hormones that act very slowly on distant targets. Their effects are long lasting.
- Some organs, like the pancreas and the thyroid gland, function mainly to release hormones. However, many other organs, like the heart and stomach, can also release hormones. They aren't considered endocrine glands because hormone release isn't their primary role.
- Most hormones act on cells by binding to external receptors, causing changes in enzyme activity inside the target cell. Steroids, however, can enter cells and interact directly with DNA, which makes steroids very powerful.
- Hormone levels are controlled largely by negative feedback. When hormone levels rise, signals are transmitted to the endocrine organ releasing the hormone, telling the organ to decrease the amount of hormone released. Hormone levels will then decrease. The optimal level of the hormone is called the setpoint. If the signal brings a hormone back to setpoint, the action is called negative feedback. If the signal causes the hormone to get further away from setpoint, the action is positive feedback.
- Hormone levels can be regulated by three mechanisms: changes in the body's internal environment, control by hormones release by another endocrine gland, and direct control by the nervous system.
- The hypothalamus, a part of the diencephalon, controls much of the endocrine system by controlling the pituitary gland. The pituitary gland has two parts: the posterior pituitary, which is part of the hypothalamus and actually secretes hypothalamic hormones (ADH and oxytocin), and the anterior pituitary, which secretes several different hormones under the influence of hormones from the hypothalamus. The hormones secreted by the anterior pituitary typically control other endocrine glands (growth hormone is an exception).
- Several other endocrine glands have important control functions. The thyroid gland secretes the iodine-containing hormones triiodothyronine (T_3) and thyroxine (T_4), which control growth and cellular metabolism.
- The pancreas secretes two hormones: insulin, which lowers blood sugar, and glucagon, which raises blood sugar. Diabetes is caused by a decrease in insulin secretion or decreased sensitivity to insulin. Very high blood sugar is the result.
- The adrenal glands are split into two parts. The adrenal medulla is an extension of the sympathetic nervous system, releasing epinephrine and norepinephrine as hormones during fight-or-flight response. The adrenal cortex releases many different adrenocorticosteroid hormones, which control reproduction, inflammation, tissue growth, and immunity.

Case Study

A 40-year-old patient presents in the emergency department with the following symptoms:

- recent weight loss
- generalized weakness
- excessive thirst and urination

Portions of his laboratory values show a blood glucose level of 150 mg/dL and an acidic urine and blood. He has a family history of diabetes, but this is the first time he presented with these symptoms.

What type of diabetes does he have?

What organs will be affected if he is not properly diagnosed and treated?

What treatment and life style suggestions would you give?

REVIEW QUESTIONS

Matching

1. Match the hormone or neurotransmitter on the left with the description on the right.

_____ ADH	A. decreases blood sugar
_____ insulin	B. increases thyroid hormone secretion
_____ glucagon	C. regulates cell metabolism
_____ oxytocin	D. increases steroid release
_____ epinephrine	E. increases uterine contractions
_____ thyroxine	F. decreases urination
_____ prolactin	G. prolongs sympathetic response
_____ ACTH (adrenocorticotropic hormone	H. stimulates tissue growth
_____ TSH	I. increases blood sugar
_____ growth hormone	J. increases milk production in females

Multiple Choice

1. ADH stands for
   a. antidiuretic hormone
   b. androdoginin hormone
   c. american department of health
   d. all-diglyceride hormone

2. The “master gland” is the
   a. adrenals
   b. pituitary
   c. Graves’
   d. pancreas

3. The thymus gland’s main function is for
   a. reproduction
   b. growth
   c. immunity
   d. RBC levels

4. The pineal gland is located in/on the
   a. kidneys
   b. brain
   c. thorax
   d. abdomen

5. Glucagon performs the opposite action of
   a. glucose
   b. insulin
   c. ATP
   d. WBCs

Short Answers

1. Compare and contrast neurotransmitters and hormones.

2. List the sources of control of hormone levels.

3. Explain negative feedback and its role in controlling hormone levels.

4. Discuss why the use of anabolic steroids should be outlawed for performance enhancement.

5. What is the difference between neural control and humoral control of endocrine glands?

Suggested Activitities

1. Review the hormones secreted by each endocrine organ and their functions. Make up 3 × 5 cards with the endocrine gland on front and the hormones it produces on back. Pick a partner and quiz each other. Once you and your partner can match the gland to the hormones, make up another set of cards with the hormone on front and its activity or function on back, and again quiz each other.

2. Review the endocrine diseases listed in this chapter. Make up 3 × 5 cards with the signs and symptoms on the front and the actual disease printed on the back. In a small group or with a partner, try to stump each other in determining the correct disease diagnosis.

10-2 Now that you have completed your journey through this chapter, please go to the CD-ROM for interactive games and puzzles concerning the medical terms and concepts contained in this chapter. By playing the games you will reinforce your learning of medical terminology in a fun way.

Greetings from THE SPECIAL Senses

The Sights and Sounds

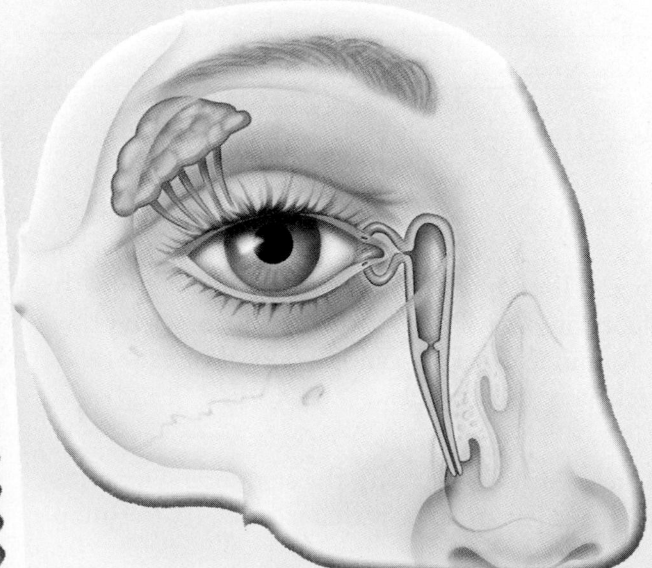

As we stroll through the city on our journey, we take in many sights, sounds, and smells. As you look around you may see many different buildings and types of people. The city is also noisy, full of car horns honking, brakes squealing and people talking. You will smell delicious food wafting out restaurant windows or the stench of garbage overflowing dumpsters. Our special senses receive all of this input and send it to the brain for interpretation so we can understand and appreciate what is happening around us. These special senses are highly integrated with the nervous system, enabling us to respond quickly and thereby protecting us from harm. For example, we need to *see* that oncoming speeding car as we step away from the curb and *hear* the blaring horn in order to respond by quickly stepping back to the safe confines of the sidewalk. See how sensory input can determine motor response?

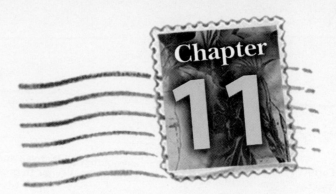

Chapter 11

LEARNING OBJECTIVES

At the end of your journey through this chapter, you will be able to:

- Differentiate general and special senses
- Describe the internal and external anatomy and functions of the eye
- Describe the internal and external anatomy and functions of the ear
- Discuss the process involved with the senses of taste, smell, and touch
- Contrast the types of pain and the pain response
- Explain several common disorders of the eye and ear

MULTIMEDIA APPLICATIONS

CD-ROM Interactive Exercises

- Video on opthalamic medications and their delivery, 11-1
- Interactive drag-and-drop exercise of the eye structures and 3-D animation of the eye, 11-2
- Video on tympanic membrane thermometer measurements, 11-3
- Animation of the workings of the middle ear, 11-4
- Interactive drag-and-drop exercise of the ear structures, 3-D animation of the ear, and animations of the child and adolescent ear, 11-5
- Video on heat and cold therapy procedures, 11-6
- Pathophysiologic spotlights on eye disorders such as cataracts and conjunctivitis, 11-7
- Pathophysiologic spotlights on ear disorders such as otitis media, 11-8
- Interactive games and puzzles, 11-9

www.prenhall.com/colbert

- Professional Profiles:
  - Ophthalmology and Opticians
  - Audiologist
- Related Internet Links
- Additional Review Questions

Pronunciation Guide

Correct pronunciation is important in any journey so that you and others are completely understood. Here is a "see and say" Pronunciation Guide for the more difficult terms to pronounce in this chapter.

amblyopia (am blee OH pee ah)
aqueous humor (AY kwee uss HYOO mer)
auricle (AW rih kl)
cataract (KAT ah rakt)
cerumen (seh ROO men)
ceruminous glands (seh ROO men us)
choroid (KOH royd)
ciliary muscles (SILL ee air ee)
cochlea (KOHK lee ah)
conjunctiva (kon JUNK tih vah)
endolymph (EN doe limf)
eustachian tubes (yoo STAY she ehn)
external auditory meatus (AW dih tor ee mee AY tuss)
glaucoma (glaw KOH mah)
gustatory sense (GUSS ta tore ee)
hyperopia (HIGH per OH pee ah)
incus (ING kuss)
labyrinth (LAB ih rinth)
lacrimal apparatus (LAK rim al app ah RA tuss)
malleus (MALL ee us)
Meniere's disease (MEN yerz)
myopia (my OH pee ah)
ossicle (AH sih kel)
otitis media (oh TYE tiss MEH dee ah)
perilymph (per ih LIMF)
pinna (PINN ah)
presbyopia (PRESS bee OH pee ah)
sclera (SKLAIR ah)
stapes (STAY peez)
tactile corpuscles (KOR puss el)
tinnitus (tinn EYE tuss)
tympanic membrane (tihm PAN ik)
vestibule chamber (VESS tih byool)
vitreous humor (VITT ree uss HYOO mer)

THE DIFFERENT SENSES

Our body senses allow us to experience all aspects of our journey. They are truly remarkable sensors through which we see, hear, smell, taste, and feel the world around us.

Our senses monitor and detect changes in the environment and send this information from the receptor to the brain via sensory or afferent neurons. The brain interprets the information and in many circumstances makes the appropriate motor or efferent response.

Traditionally, we are taught that we possess five senses: vision, hearing, smell, taste, and touch. However, there are more areas of sensory input into the brain. What about pain and pressure sensations? How do we "feel" hot and cold? How does our body sense position and balance (equilibrium)? What about feelings of hunger and thirst? These, too, are senses that are very important to our survival.

The senses of sight (eyes), sound and equilibrium (ears), taste (tongue), and smell (nose) are referred to as our *special senses*. These senses are found in a well-defined region of the body. However, other senses, called *general senses*, are scattered throughout various regions of the body. These include the sensations of heat, cold, pain, nausea, hunger, thirst, and pressure or touch.

The senses can be further broken down. For example, the receptors of the skin are called the *cutaneous senses* and include touch, heat, cold, and pain. The *visceral senses* include nausea, hunger, thirst, and the need to urinate and defecate.

Note

While it may not be an actual sense, have you ever heard of common sense? What do you think of the statement that "common sense is not all that common nowadays"?

cutaneo = *skin*
visceral = *pertaining to organs*

Before finishing this discussion of the various senses, we should also mention a final, more controversial sense. By "reading your mind," we see you already identified it as extrasensory perception or ESP. Notice that this means senses outside the normal sensory perceptions. While there is still debate over whether this phenomenon exists, we just "know" this chapter will be an "eye-opening" experience for you. We hope the puns aren't stimulating your visceral senses and making you nauseous.

SENSE OF SIGHT

While on our journey, we see many amazing sites. To record these sites for later viewing, we may take along a camera and film. The eye has many similarities to a camera. The light rays from the images photographed with a camera pass through the small opening (comparable to the pupil) and through the transparent lens (lens of the eye) where the rays are then focused on a photoreceptive film (retina). The shutter of a camera opens and closes at various speeds to adjust the amount of light exposure on the film. The shutter (iris) must allow just the right amount of light to enter and focus properly on the film for a clear image. A camera may be packed away in a suitcase or thrown in a car and therefore needs protection from being dropped or exposed to a harsh environment. You will soon see how the external structures of the eye help protect it from injury, much like a camera case protects a camera. In addition, the camera lens must be kept clean to insure a clear picture. The lacrimal glands that secrete tears help to perform this function. Now that you have this analogy to "give you the big picture," let's explore the specific structures and functions of the eye.

The External Structures of the Eye

The **orbit** is a cone-shaped cavity formed by the skull that houses and protects the eyeball. This cavity is padded with fatty tissue that cushions and protects the eye from injury and has several openings through which nerves and blood vessels can pass. The eyeball is connected to the orbital cavity with six short muscles that provide support and allow rotary movement so you can see in all directions. Also protecting the eye is a pair of movable folds of skin, commonly called eyelids, which contain eyelashes to help prevent gross particles from entering. The eyelashes act as sensors to cause rapid closure as a foreign object approaches the eyeball. The eyelids close over the eye much like the lens cover of a camera to protect it from intense light, foreign particles, or impact injuries. The eyelids also contain sebaceous glands that secrete the oily substance *sebum* onto the eyelids to keep them soft, pliable, and a little sticky to trap particles.

A protective membrane called the **conjunctiva** lines the exposed surface of the eyeball and acts as a protective covering for the exposed eye surface. Each eye has a **lacrimal apparatus** that produces and stores tears. The lacrimal apparatus includes the **lacrimal gland** and its corresponding ducts or passageways that transport the tears. The lacrimal glands (exocrine because their secretion of tears go outside the body) produce the tears needed for constant cleansing

conjunctiva *(kon JUNK tih vah)*

lacrimal apparatus *(LAK rim al app ah RA tuss)*

and lubrication which are spread over the eye surfaces by blinking. Our eyes are constantly tearing, but they do not overflow because excess tears drain into the nose via two small holes in the inner corner of the eye. However, when we cry, the excess runs down our cheeks and more drains into our nose, causing it to run. The tears also act as an **antiseptic** to keep the eyeballs free of germs. Please see Figure 11–1 ■ for the structures involved with tearing.

The Internal Structures of the Eye

aqueous humor *(AY kwee uss HYOO mer)*

vitreous humor *(VITT ree uss HYOO mer)*

sclera *(SKLAIR ah)*

choroid *(KOH royd)*

retina *(RETT in ah)*

The globe-shaped eyeball is the organ of vision and is separated into two chambers of fluid that help to protect the eye. These "fluids of the eye" are called *humors*. The **aqueous humor** ("watery" humor) bathes the iris, pupil, and lens and fills the anterior and posterior chambers of the eye. The second humor is called the **vitreous humor** and is a clear, jellylike fluid that occupies the entire eye cavity behind the lens.

The eyeball has three layers. Please see Figure 11–2 ■ for the layers and internal structures of the eye. These layers are the **sclera, choroid,** and **retina.** The sclera is the outermost layer and is a tough, fibrous tissue that serves as the protective shield we commonly call the "whites of the eye." The sclera contains a specialized portion called the **cornea,** which is transpar-

> **11-1** Drugs can be given through the eyes as eye drops or opthalamic medication. To see a video on this topic and procedure, please go to you CD-ROM

opthalm/o = *eye*

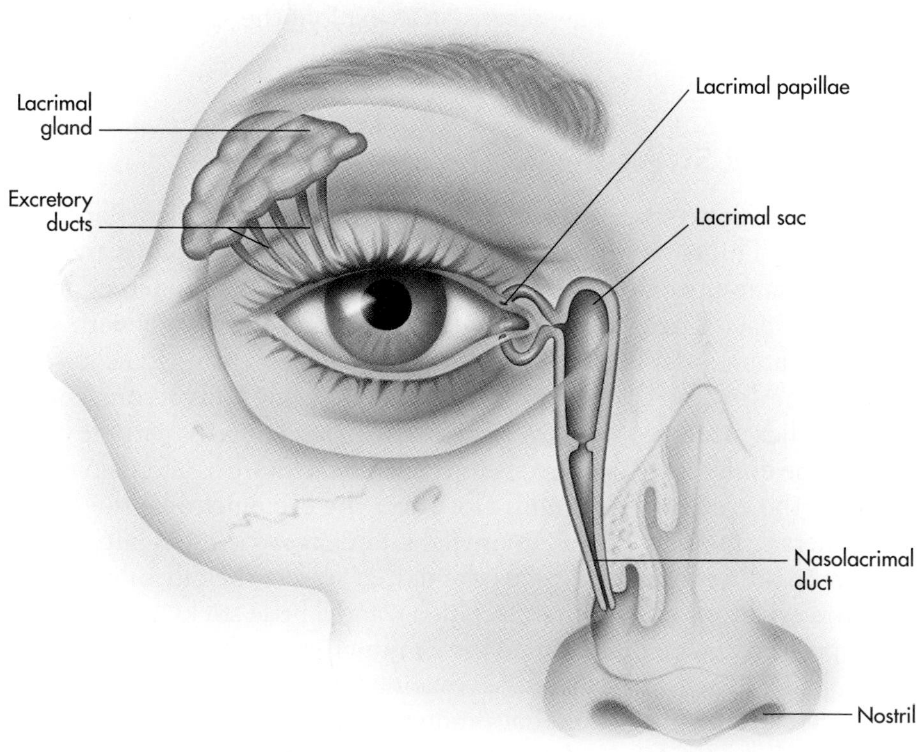

FIGURE ■ 11–1

Lacrimal structures of the eye.

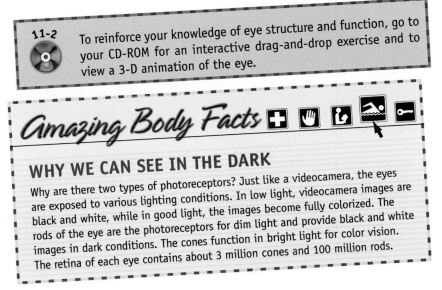

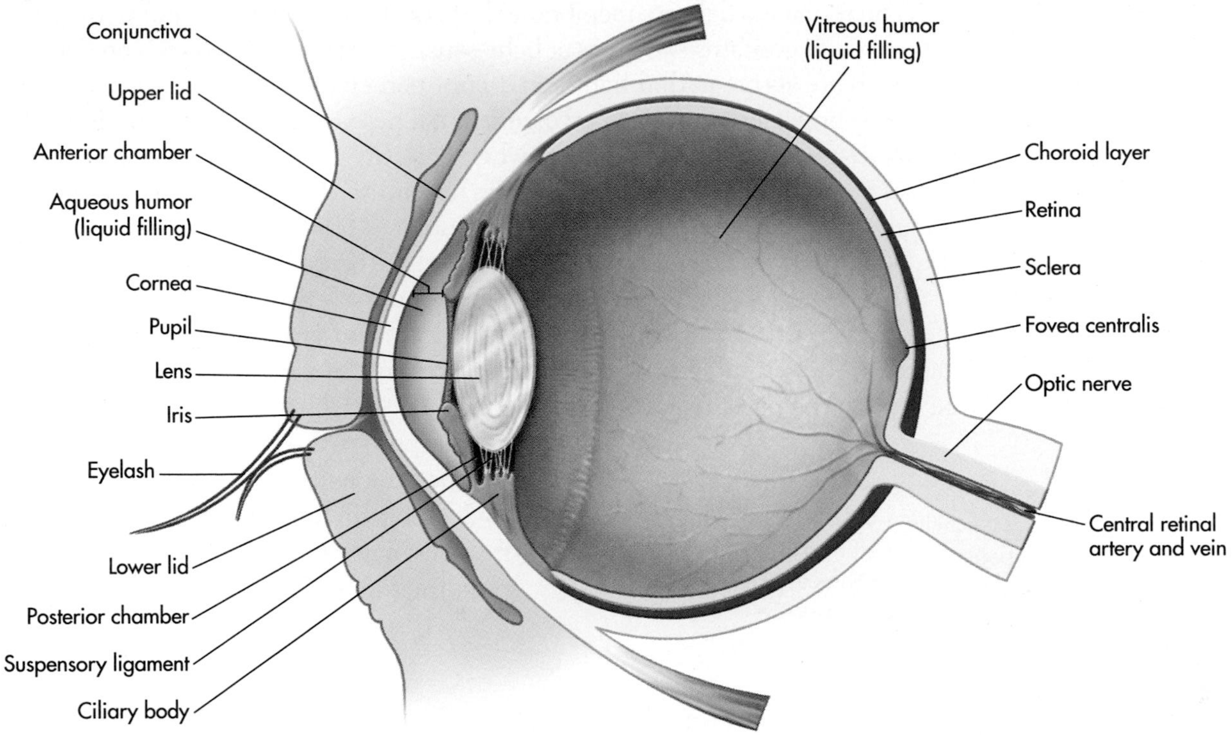

FIGURE ■ 11–2

Internal structures of the eye.

ent to allow light rays to pass into the eye. The cornea has a curved surface that allows it to bend the entering light waves to focus them on the surface of the retina.

The middle layer, or choroid, is a highly vascularized (rich blood supply) and pigmented region that provides nourishment to the eye. This layer also contains the **iris** and the **pupil.** The iris is the colored portion of the eye that controls the size of the opening (pupil) where light passes into the eye. The iris is a sphincter, which means it can relax or contract, thereby making the center opening, or pupil, larger or smaller depending on light conditions. In low light, the iris relaxes, causing the pupil to dilate and thereby allowing more light into the eye for a better image.

iris *(EYE riss)*
pupil *(PYOO pill)*

ciliary muscles *(SILL ee air ee)*

The third and innermost layer is the retina. This area contains the nerve endings that receive and interpret the rays of light into images. Located behind the pupil is the **lens,** which is surrounded by **ciliary muscles.** These muscles can alter the shape of the lens, making it thinner or thicker to allow the incoming light rays to focus on the retinal area. This process is called *accommodation*, which basically combines changes in the size of the pupil and the lens curvature to make sure the image converges in the same place on the retina and therefore is properly focused.

11-2 To reinforce your knowledge of eye structure and function, go to your CD-ROM for an interactive drag-and-drop exercise and to view a 3-D animation of the eye.

Amazing Body Facts

WHY WE CAN SEE IN THE DARK

Why are there two types of photoreceptors? Just like a videocamera, the eyes are exposed to various lighting conditions. In low light, videocamera images are black and white, while in good light, the images become fully colorized. The rods of the eye are the photoreceptors for dim light and provide black and white images in dark conditions. The cones function in bright light for color vision. The retina of each eye contains about 3 million cones and 100 million rods.

optic = *pertaining to the eye*

photopigments *(FOE toe pig Ment)*

The retina is a delicate membrane that continues posteriorly and joins to the *optic nerve*. It contains two types of light-sensing receptors called **rods** and **cones.** The rods are active in dim light and do not perceive color, while the cones are active in bright light and do perceive color. These receptors contain **photopigments** that cause a chemical change when light hits them. This chemical change causes an impulse to be sent to the optic nerve and then to the brain where the impulse is interpreted, and we "see" the object. This interpretation occurs in the visual part of the cerebral cortex located in the occipital lobe.

In summation, light rays enter the eye and pass through the conjunctival membrane, cornea, aqueous humor, pupil, lens, and vitreous humor and are focused on the retina. Here the photoreceptors in the retina cause an impulse to be sent to the optic nerve, (Cranial Nerve II) which carries it to the brain for the interpretation we call vision. See if you can trace the pathway light takes in Figure 11–2. Refer to Table 11–1, which summarizes the major structures and their corresponding functions of the eye.

An optician specializes in making optical products and accessories. To learn more about this allied health profession and the field of ophthalmology, please visit the companion Web site.

TABLE 11–1 Structures and Functions of the Eye

ORGAN OR STRUCTURE	PRIMARY FUNCTION
orbit	cone-shaped cavity that contains the eyeball; padded with fatty tissues, the orbit has several openings for nerves and blood vessels to pass through
eye muscles	six short muscles that provide support and rotary movement
eyelids	moveable folds of skin containing eyelashes to protect eye from intense light, foreign particles, and impact injuries
conjunctiva	protective membrane that lines the exposed surface of eyeball
lacrimal apparatus	includes the lacrimal gland that produces tears that lubricate and cleanse the eye and the corresponding ducts or passageways to transport the tears
eyeball	globe-shaped organ of vision
sclera	outermost layer known as the "white" of the eye; contains the transparent curved cornea, which bends outside light rays to focus them on the surface of the retina
choroid	the middle layer that has rich blood vessels and pigmentation to prevent internal reflection of light rays; also contains the iris and pupil
iris	colored portion of eye that controls the size of the opening (pupil) where light passes into the eye
pupil	the opening through which light passes into the eye
retina	innermost layer that contains the nerve endings that receive and interpret the rays of light for vision
lens	located behind the pupil, the lens is controlled by ciliary muscles that shape the lens by thinning or thickening the lens to allow light to focus on the retinal surface; this process, called accommodation, combines changes in pupil size and the lens curvature to insure the light rays focus properly on the retina

TEST YOUR KNOWLEDGE 11-1

Choose the best answer:

1. Which of the following is *not* a layer of the eye?
   a. photo optic
   b. sclera
   c. choroid
   d. retina

2. Which layer of the eye contains the iris and the pupil?
   a. cornea
   b. sclera
   c. choroid
   d. retina

3. The _____ is the colored portion of the eye that controls the opening, or _____, where light passes through.
   a. retina, pupil
   b. pupil, iris
   c. sclera, pupil
   d. iris, pupil

THE SENSE OF HEARING

On our journey, we hear many interesting sounds. Without our ears, we would miss all the pleasant noises, and the not-so-pleasant ones, that add to the appreciation of the journey. Also, on our journey, we may walk over some rough and uneven terrain. Our ears are also responsible for our sense of balance so we don't fall and get hurt. We can "hear" your heart pounding with anticipation, so let's explore the specific structures and functions of the ear.

> *Applied Science*
>
> **SOUND CONDUCTION**
>
> Many people are under the false impression that sound travels best through air because this is the medium we are immersed in. However, sound is transmitted due to molecular collisions and is better transmitted where the molecules are closer together, such as in a liquid or solid medium. This is why whales can talk to each other up to two miles apart under water. This is also why trapped underground miners tap on the wall instead of shouting for help.

Structures of the Ear

The ear is responsible for hearing and maintaining our equilibrium, or sense of balance. We hear by receiving sound vibrations usually via the air (unless we are under water) and translating them into an interpretable sound via the eighth cranial nerve. The ear can be separated into three divisions: the **external ear,** the **middle ear** or **tympanic cavity,** and the **inner ear** (also called the **labyrinth.**) See Figure 11–3 ■ for the structures of the ear.

tympanic *(tihm PAN ik)*
labyrinth *(LAB ih rinth)*

THE EXTERNAL EAR

The external ear is the outer projection, the part we can see. It comes in all shapes and sizes (see Dumbo the Elephant). It also includes the canal (where we put cotton swabs despite the warning label) leading into the middle ear. The projecting part is called the **pinna** or **auricle,** which collects and directs sound waves into the **auditory canal** or **external auditory meatus.** The canal contains earwax, called **cerumen,** which is secreted by the **ceruminous glands** to lubricate and protect the ear. At the end of the canal is the **eardrum,** or **tympanic membrane,** where the external ear ends and the middle ear begins.

pinna *(PINN ah)*
auricle *(AW rih kl)*
external auditory meatus *(AW dih tor ee mee AY tuss)*
ceruminous glands *(seh ROO men us)*
cerumen *(seh ROO men)*
tympanic membrane *(tihm PAN ik)*
tympanon = *Greek word for drum*

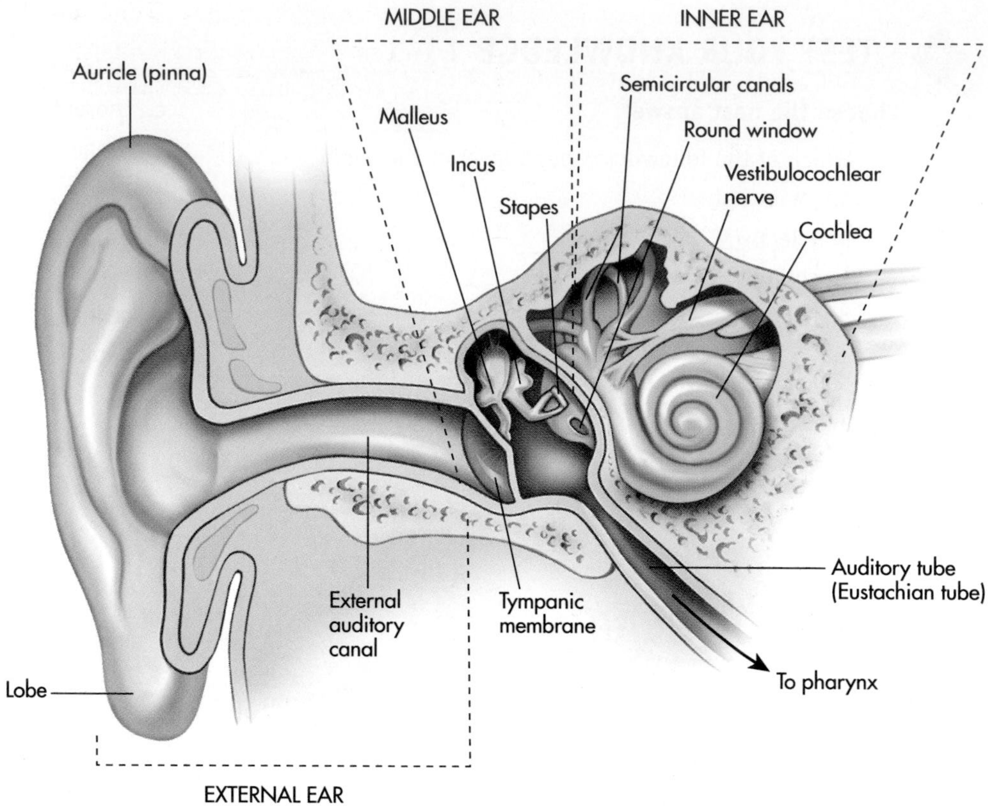

FIGURE ■ 11–3

Structures of the ear.

Don't you wish there were just ONE term everyone agreed upon for these structures!

THE MIDDLE EAR

ossicle *(AH sih kel)*

The middle ear, or tympanic cavity, is basically a space that contains the three smallest bones of your body. The three bones, or **ossicles,** are joined so they can amplify the sound waves the tympanic membrane receives from the external ear (sound travels best through a solid). Once amplified, the sound waves are transmitted to the *fluid* contained in the internal ear. Once again, this is another example of sound waves being transmitted more efficiently though a liquid medium than in air.

> **11-3** Body temperature can be quickly and accurately measured by use of a tympanic thermometer. To view a video of this procedure, you can go to your CD-ROM for this chapter.

malleus *(MALL ee us)*
incus *(ING kuss)*
stapes *(STAY peez)*

The bones of the ears are named according to their shapes. The first ossicle attached to the tympanic membrane is the **hammer,** or **malleus.** The **anvil,** or **incus,** is attached to the hammer. Finally, the **stirrup,** or **stapes,** connects to a membrane called the **oval window.** The oval window begins the internal ear and carries the amplified vibrations from the tympanic ossicles. During transmission, the sound or vibrations can be amplified as much as 22 times their original level.

Also contained within the middle ear are the **eustachian tubes.** These tubes allow for air pressure on either side of the eardrum to be equalized. The tubes connect the nose and throat to the middle ear. Therefore, they transmit both the outside atmospheric pressure through the nose and throat opening and the inner ear pressure where they are located to allow for an equalization of pressure between the atmosphere and the middle ear.

eustachian tubes
(yoo STAY she ehn)

This equalizing of pressure between the middle ear and external atmosphere allows the eardrum to freely vibrate with incoming sound waves. Sudden pressure changes, such as caused by flying in an airplane, can affect this area. This is why, when flying, you are instructed to chew gum or swallow so the inner ear can better sense and adjust to the rapidly changing outside atmosphere via the eustachian tubes.

11-4 The middle ear is critical for hearing and maintaining proper ear pressure. Go to your CD-ROM to view an animation of the middle ear at work.

THE INNER EAR

The oval window membrane is the portal into the inner ear or labyrinth. This area comprises three separate, hollow, bony spaces that form a complex maze of winding and twisting channels. Since another name for a maze is labyrinth, this area can also be called the bony labyrinth. The three areas are the **cochlea;** the **vestibule chamber,** which houses the internal ear; and the **semicircular canals.**

cochlea
(KOHK lee ah) Latin for snail shell

vestibule chamber *(VESS tih byool)*

The cochlea is the bony spiral or snail shell–shaped entrance to the internal ear connected to the oval window membrane (see Figure 11–4 ■). The cochlea contains fluid called **perilymph,** which helps to transmit the sound through this area. The sound is then transmitted to the back of the maze, which contains another fluid called **endolymph.** Here the sound is carried to tiny hairlike receptors that are stimulated and conduct the signal to the brain via the **acoustic** or **vestibulocochlear nerve** (**cranial nerve VIII**). Table 11–2 lists the major structures and functions of the ear.

perilymph *(per ih LIMF)*

endolymph *(EN doe limf)*

vestibulocochlear
(VESS tih byool o KOHK lee are)

In summary, sound waves enter the external canal and vibrate the eardrum or tympanic membrane in a process called *sound conduction*. The middle ear then amplifies the sound through the respective ossicles. This process is called *bone conduction* of sound. The last ossicle (stapes) vibrates and causes a gentle pumping against the oval window membrane. This causes cochlear fluid to vibrate small hairlike nerves found in an area called the *Organ of Corti*. As a result of the vibrating sensory cells (hairlike nerves), a nerve impulse is sent to the temporal lobe of the brain where it is interpreted as sound, a process called *sensorineural conduction*.

Low-intensity sound waves, similar to a clock ticking, send vibrations that cause the sensory cells to move in waves that are interpreted by the brain as that "tick tock" sound. In extreme cases where intense sound waves are produced, such as from a gun blast, it is believed that the vibrations are so great that they may knock over the hairlike cells much like an earthquake knocks over tall trees. Repeated assaults can lead to permanent hearing damage. Therefore, it is a "sound" investment to wear proper hearing protection around loud noises.

The ear is also responsible for your sense of balance or equilibrium. The semicircular canals process sensory input related to equilibrium. They contain nerve endings or receptors in the form of hair cells. The semicircular canals are

TABLE 11–2 Structures and Functions of the Ear

ORGAN OR STRUCTURE	FUNCTION
External Ear	
auricle, or pinna	cartilagenous projection that collects and directs sound waves into the auditory canal much like a satellite dish collects transmissions from space
auditory canal, or external auditory meatus	canal that contains earwax, or cerumen, secreted by the ceruminous glands that lubricate and trap foreign particles
eardrum, or tympanic membrane	membrane that separates the external and middle ear
Middle Ear	
ossicles	three small bones (hammer-, anvil-, and stirrup-shaped) that help amplify and transmit sound
eustachian tubes	allows for equalization of external (atmospheric) and internal (within the middle ear) pressure on the tympanic membrane so the eardrum can freely vibrate with incoming sound
Inner Ear, or Labyrinth	
cochlea	bony, snail-shaped entrance to the internal ear containing perilymph fluid, which helps to transmit sound
semicircular canals	three canals containing endolymph fluid, which transmits positional changes to tiny, hairlike receptors that are stimulated and conduct the signal to the brain via the acoustic or vestibulocochlear nerve (eighth cranial nerve) to help maintain balance

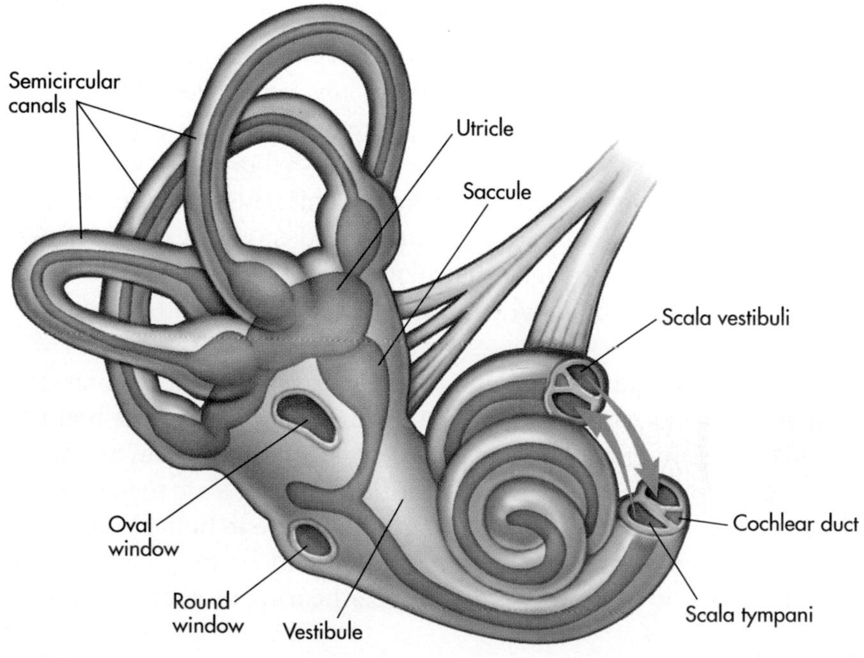

FIGURE ■ 11–4

The internal structure of the cochlea.

three loops within the inner ear that help to maintain balance. Like the cochlea, they are filled with endolymph fluid, and each canal duct contains a sensory receptor. This fluid moves when you change body position. The movement is picked up by the sensory receptor, which triggers a nerve impulse to travel to the brain stem and the cerebellum. Here the impulse is interpreted as body position to help maintain muscle coordination and body equilibrium.

11-5 To reinforce your knowledge of ear structure and function, go to your CD-ROM to perform an interactive drag-and-drop exercise on ear structures and to view several 3-D animations of the ear.

TEST YOUR KNOWLEDGE 11-2

Choose the best answer:

1. The structure that marks the end of the external ear and the beginning of the middle ear is called the
   a. pinna
   b. hammer
   c. tympanic membrane
   d. labyrinth
2. The structure of the ear that is important for balance are the
   a. ceruminous glands
   b. incus, mallus and stapes
   c. semicircular canals
   d. eustachian tubes

Provide the synonymous terms for each of the following:

3. auricle ______________________________
4. earwax ______________________________
5. malleus ______________________________
6. anvil ______________________________
7. stirrups ______________________________

OTHER SENSES

Other senses also help us to interpret the world around us. These include the senses of taste, smell, and touch.

Taste

The sense of taste is referred to as the **gustatory** sense. Taste receptors are located in the tongue and are called **taste buds.** Notice in Figure 11–5 ■ that the four tastes of *sweet*, *sour*, *salty*, and *bitter* are located in different regions of our tongue. Recently, a fifth taste, *umami*, has been included with the traditional four because it is the distinct taste of glutamates, which cannot be duplicated by the combination of any of the other four tastes. Quite often, taste preferences change with the body's need, which is why, for example, pregnant women may crave a variety of food throughout their pregnancy. The refinement of food taste is primarily dependent on the sense of smell.

gustatory sense *(GUSS ta tore ee)*

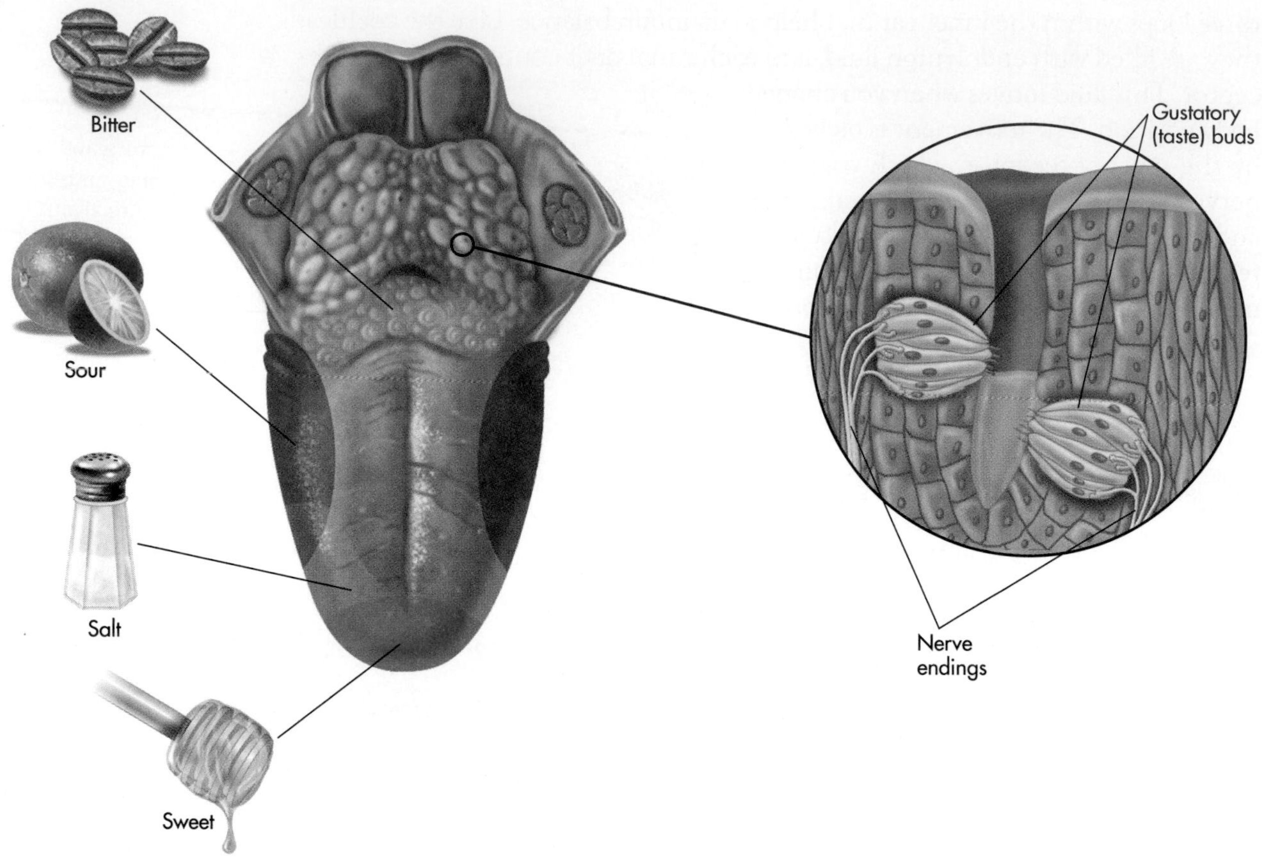

FIGURE ■ 11–5

The sense of taste.

Smell

The sense of smell arises from the receptors located in the olfactory region or the upper part of the nasal cavity (see Figure 11–6 ■). We "sniff" in order to bring smells up to this area, where they can be interpreted. Remember taste and smell are closely related, which is why we can't taste foods when we have a severe head cold. Pleasant food odors also initiate digestive enzymes, so when you smell that cinnamon apple pie baking, your mouth really may water in anticipation.

Touch

tactile corpuscles *(TAK tle KOR puss els)*

Touch receptors are small, rounded bodies called **tactile corpuscles** located in skin and especially concentrated in the fingertips. They are also located on the tip of the tongue. It is interesting to note that even when a patient is anesthetized and there are no pain sensations, patients are still conscious of pressure through these deep touch sensors.

11-6 To view a video on heat and cold therapy procedures, please go to your CD-ROM.

Temperature sensors are also found in the skin. The body has separate heat and cold receptors. These receptors may cause an interesting phenomena called **adaptation** to occur. Continued sensory stimulation causes the sensors to desensitize or

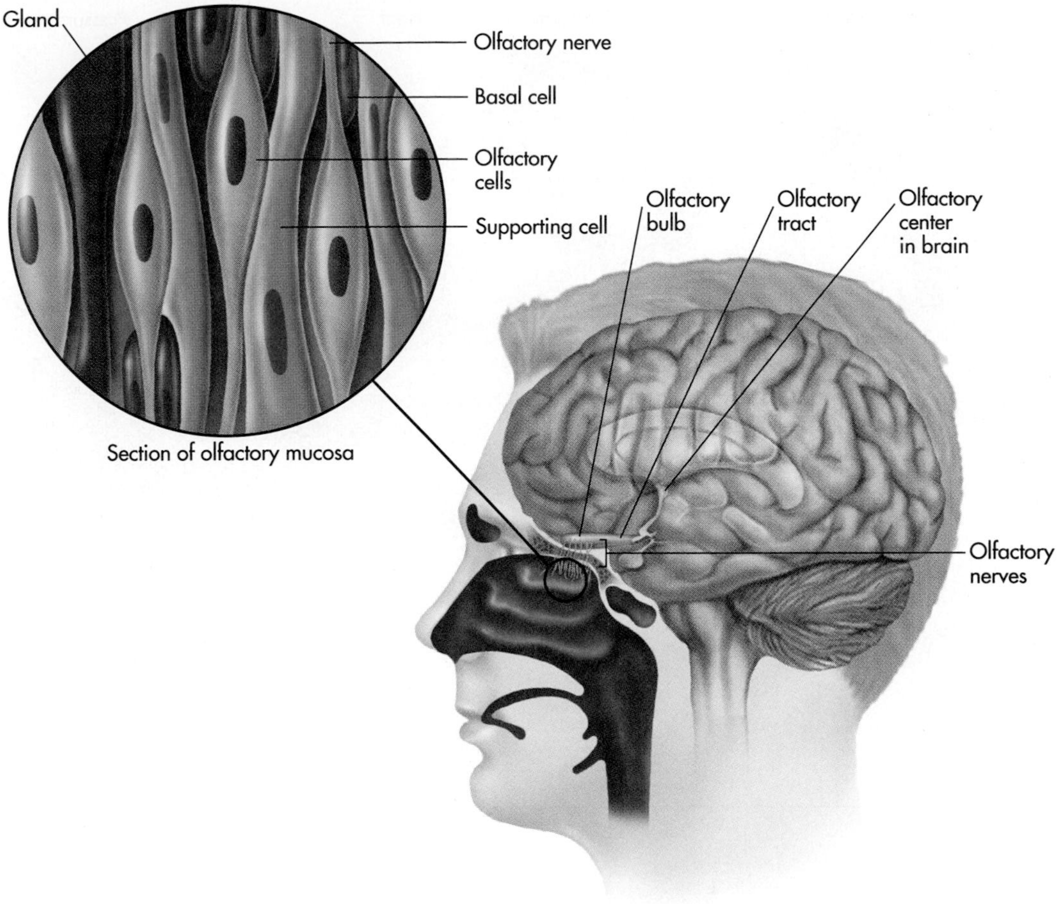

FIGURE ■ 11–6

The sense of smell.

adapt. For example, if you are continually exposed to the cold, the receptors adjust so you won't feel so cold. That is why an outside temperature of 50 degrees seems warm after a long cold winter, but that same temperature seems cold after a long hot summer. Another example is when you first enter a hot bath, it may feel extremely hot. After a few seconds, it doesn't feel so hot, yet the actual temperature of the water has not yet changed.

> *Clinical Application*
>
> **HEAT AND COLD THERAPY**
>
> Heat and cold therapy are used for a variety of injuries. They rely on physiologic changes in the body in response to either heat or cold. For example, heat relaxes muscles and dilates vessels, thereby bringing more blood flow to the site of injury. Cold therapy constricts blood vessels and minimizes the amount of blood and swelling at a site.

Pain is a very important protective sense. It is the body's way of drawing attention to a particular danger, such as the "hitting your finger with a hammer" example used earlier in the book. Pain is the most widely distributed sense, found in skin, muscle, joints, and internal organs. Pain receptors are merely branches of nerve fibers called *free nerve endings*.

There are even different types of pain. *Referred pain* originates in an internal organ yet is felt in another region of the skin. For example, liver and gallbladder

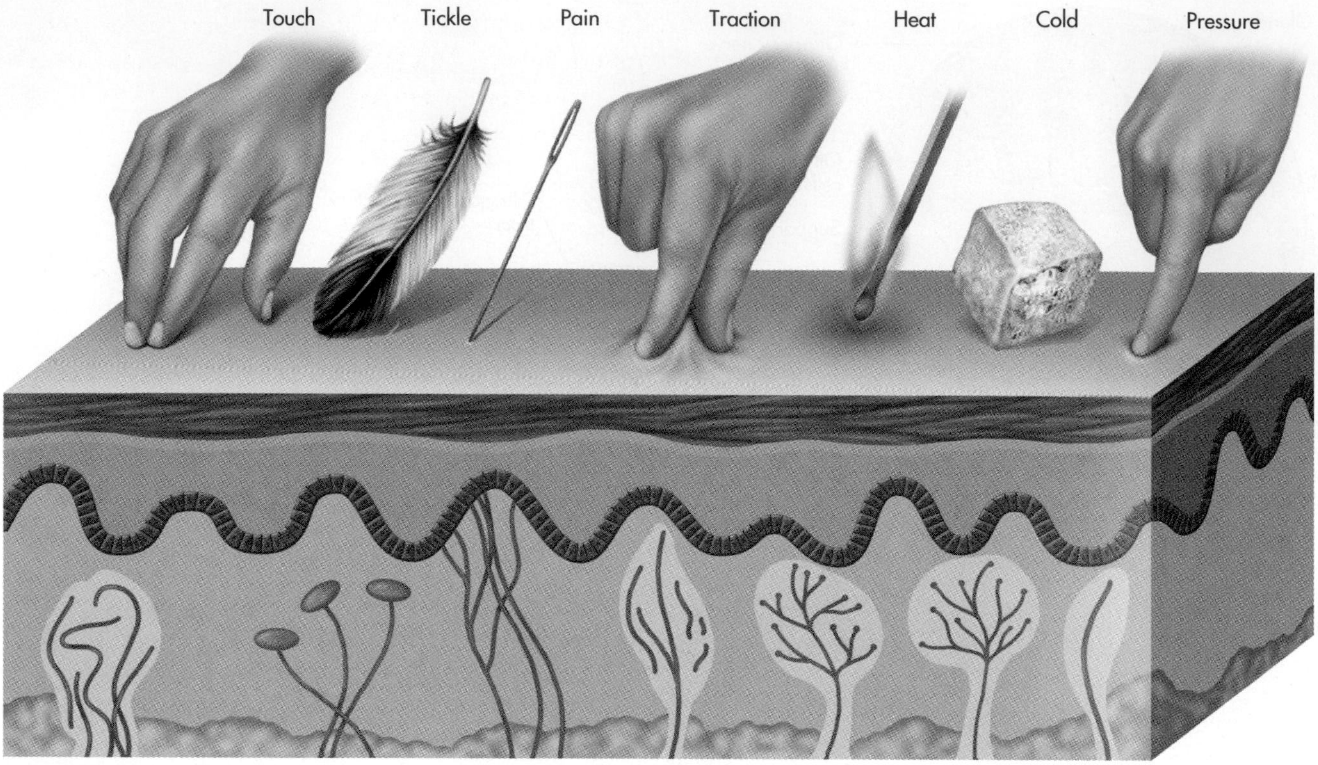

FIGURE ■ 11–7

The sense of touch.

disease often cause pain in the right shoulder. *Phantom pain* can result from an amputated limb: an individual can feel pain in an arm or leg he or she no longer has.

anesthesia *(an ess THEE zee ah)*
an = *without*
estheia = *feeling*

Pain receptors do not adapt as heat and cold receptors do. Pain is felt for as long as the stimulus is there that is causing it or unless a person is under **anesthesia.** An interesting debate is whether or not some people have higher or lower thresholds of pain. See Figure 11–7 ■ for the senses of touch.

COMMON DISORDERS OF THE EYE AND EAR

conjunctivitis *(kon JUNK tih VYE tiss)*

Conjunctivitis is an inflammation of the membrane that lines the eye. This condition can either be acute or chronic and is caused by a variety of irritants and pathogens. The acute phase is commonly called *pinkeye* and is a highly contagious form caused by a bacteria.

cataract *(KAT ah rakt)*

A **cataract** is a condition in which the lens loses its flexibility and transparency and light cannot easily pass through the clouded lens. It has been shown that increased exposure to sunlight may speed up the development of cataracts. Untreated, this condition can lead to blindness. It is interesting to note that cataract surgery was one of the earliest recorded surgical procedures, dating back to ancient Greece.

11-7 To view videos on eye disorders such as cataracts and conjunctivitis, please see your CD-ROM.

Glaucoma can also lead to blindness. It is caused by increased pressure in the fluid of the eye, which interferes with optic nerve functioning. Glaucoma occurs in 20 percent of adults over 40 and accounts for 15 percent of the cases of blindness in America. This is a tragic loss because glaucoma can be readily diagnosed and treated.

glaucoma *(glaw KOH mah)*

The eye can have several defects that impair vision. The eyes may have difficulty focusing on near or far objects because the light rays are not focusing properly on the retina. **Hyperopia** (farsightedness) occurs when the eye cannot focus properly on nearby objects. As the cilliary muscles age, they weaken and pupil size is decreased, reducing the amount of light coming into the retina. **Presbyopia** is farsightedness that occurs with age, usually between 40 and 45 years. The lens becomes stiff and yellowish. Such age-related changes make it difficult for older adults to focus and make them more sensitive to glare which can impair their nighttime driving abilities. **Myopia** (nearsightedness) causes objects at a distance to appear blurred. **Amblyopia,** or lazy eye, usually occurs in childhood. Here poor vision in one eye is caused by the abnormal dominance of the other eye, which does most of the work. Most people have a dominant eye. To find yours, look at a small, distant object with both eyes open. Extend both arms with both palms facing that object. Slowly bring your hands together so there is a small opening formed in the space between the thumbs and the index figure. Now locate your distant object in that opening with both eyes open. Now alternately close each eye to determine which eye still sees that object. This is your dominant eye. Generally speaking, right-handed people have right-dominant eyes.

hyperopia *(HIGH per OH pee ah)*

presbyopia *(PRESS bee OH pee ah)*
presby = *old*
opia = *refers to vision*

myopia *(my OH pee ah)*

amblyopia *(am blee OH pee ah)*

11-8 To view pathophysiologic spotlights on the ear such as otitis media, please go to your CD-ROM.

To learn more about the exciting profession of audiology, please visit the book's companion Web site.

In addition, the eyes can be used to help diagnose a variety of nonvisual diseases. For example, a yellow tint to the conjunctiva (jaundice) may indicate a liver disease. A neurological assessment called PERLA, which stands for *pupils equal, reactive to light and accommodation*, can be used to assess brain injury. The **rapid eye movement,** or REM, stage of sleep is measured during sleep studies and helps to diagnose sleep disorders.

Otitis media is an infection of the middle ear, usually caused by a bacteria or virus, and is frequently found in infants and young children. It is commonly associated with an **upper respiratory infection,** or **URI,** such as a cold. By examining the structure of the ear, can you see how a sinus infection can spread to an ear infection and vice versa?

otitis media
(oh TYE tiss MEE dee ah)
oto = *ear*
itis = *inflammation*
media = *middle*

Labyrinthitis is an inflammation of the inner ear and usually is caused by high fevers. Labyrinthitis can cause **vertigo,** which is a feeling of dizziness or whirling in space. If you are not sure what vertigo is, watch the Alfred Hitchcock classic movie of the same name. Not only does it clearly demonstrate vertigo, but it is a great mystery movie. **Meniere's disease** is a chronic condition that affects the labyrinth and leads to progressive hearing loss and vertigo.

labyrinthitis *(LAB ih rinn THYE tiss)*

Meniere's disease *(MEN yerz)*

Deafness can be either partial or complete and is caused by a variety of conditions, ranging from inflammation and scarring of the tympanic membrane to auditory nerve and brain damage. Finally, **tinnitus** is a ringing sound in the

tinnitus *(tinn EYE tuss)*

ears, which according to superstition, means someone is talking about you. Clinically, it can occur as a result of chronic exposure to loud noises, Meniere's disease, some medications, wax build-up or various disturbances to the auditory nerve. Figure 11-8 ■ shows some common eye disorders.

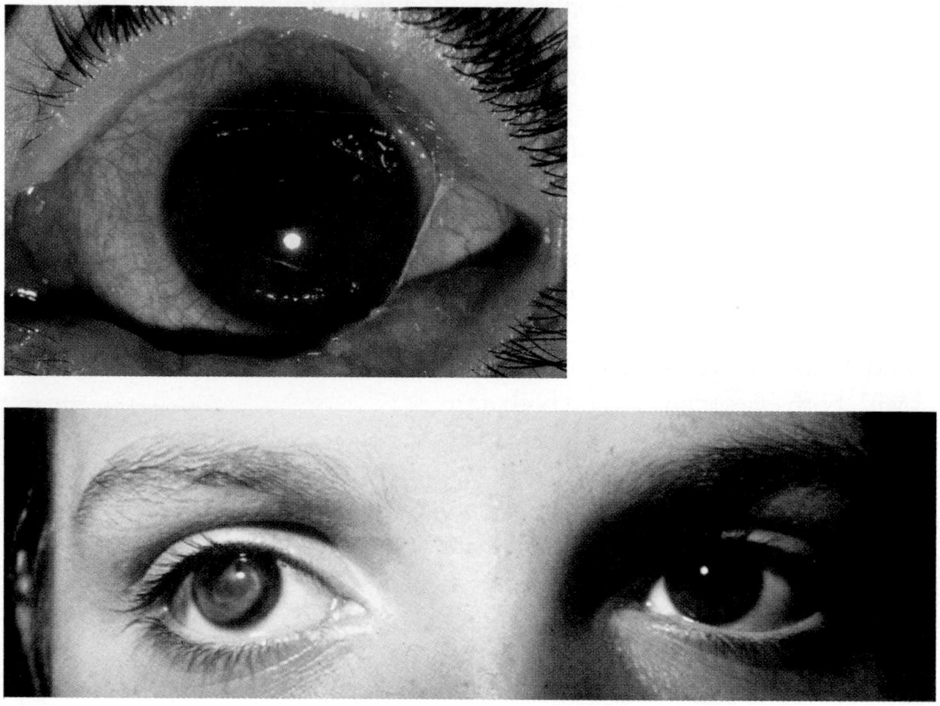

FIGURE ■ 11–8

Some common eye disorders. a) Conjunctivitis ("pink eye") (Source: Buddy Crofton/ Medical Images, Inc.) b) Cataract of right eye.

SUMMARY

Snapshots from the Journey

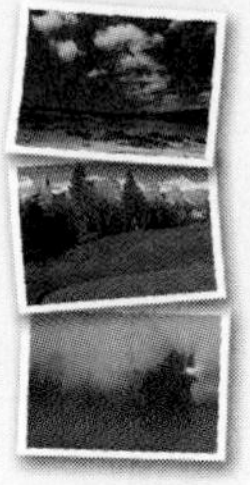

- The senses of sight (eyes), sound and equilibrium (ears), taste (tongue), and smell (nose) are called special senses. The body feels other sensations, such as touch, heat, cold, and pain, which are called general senses.
- The eye is very similar to a camera, with lens cover (eyelids), opening (pupils), shutter (iris), lens (eye lens), and photoreceptive film (retina).
- Light rays enter the eye and pass through the conjunctival membrane, cornea, aqueous humor, pupil, lens, and vitreous humor, and are focused on the retina. The photoreceptors in the retina cause a chemical impulse to be sent to the optic nerve, which carries it to the brain for the interpretation we call vision.
- The ear has three major divisions: the external, middle, and inner ear. The ear is the organ for hearing and maintaining our sense of balance.
- Sound waves enter the external canal and vibrate the eardrum, or tympanic membrane. The middle ear then amplifies the sound through the respective tiny bones, or ossicles. The last ossicle (stapes) vibrates and causes a gentle pumping against the oval window membrane. This causes cochlear fluid (perilymph) to move and vibrates tiny, hairlike neurons, which transmit an impulse to the hearing centers in the brain where the sound is interpreted.
- The semicircular canals are responsible for maintaining body balance.
- Our sense of taste, or gustatory sense, has traditionally been thought to consist of sweet, sour, salty, and bitter, a fifth taste, umami, has recently been distinguished as its own category. The sense of taste originates on taste buds on the tongue and is closely associated with the sense of smell.
- The sense of smell arises from the olfactory region of the nose.
- The sense of touch allows perceptions of pain, temperature, pressure, traction, and the sensation of being "tickled."

Case Study

A 40-year-old male patient presents with complaints of tinnitus and vertigo. He complains that his hearing is getting progressively worse and he is having dizzy spells and nausea.

Describe the patient's complaints in your own words.

What possible disease is present?

What part of the ear is affected and why?

REVIEW QUESTIONS

Multiple Choice

1. The part of the eye that allows for varying amounts of light onto the retina is the
   a. lens
   b. humor
   c. iris
   d. optic nerve
2. The photopigment structures responsible for the ability to see colors are
   a. cones
   b. rods
   c. iris
   d. pupil
3. The incus is found in the
   a. inner ear
   b. middle ear
   c. external ear
   d. region of South America
4. What is the correct descending order for the media through which sound travels, with the most efficient conductor of sound listed first:
   a. liquid, air, solid
   b. solid, liquid, air
   c. air, liquid, solid
   d. they are all equal
5. Another word for the sense of taste is
   a. olfactory
   b. vertigo
   c. mastication
   d. gustatory

Fill in the Blank

1. The two functions of the auditory system are ______________ and ______________.
2. The three ossicles of the ear are the ______________, ______________, and ______________.

Short Answers

1. Differentiate between special and general senses.

2. What are the four basic tastes? List the location of their receptor sites.

3. Define *adaptation* in relation to temperature sensors.

4. How does the body protect the eyes?

5. How is an eye like a camera?

Suggested Activities

1. Ask a local ophthalmologist to visit your class and explain the latest concepts and procedures in corrective vision surgery. In addition, have him or her bring an eye chart and explain 20/20 vision.

2. The sense of sight is also important to the interpretation of our sense of taste. Blindfold participants and have them identify similar products with varying tastes, such as different types of sodas or jelly beans, and see if they can correctly identify the flavor.

3. Hold this page about 15 inches from you face. Close your left eye and stare at the dot while bringing the page slowly closer to your face. While staring at the dot, you will notice the X in the periphery disappear. You have just discovered your blind spot.

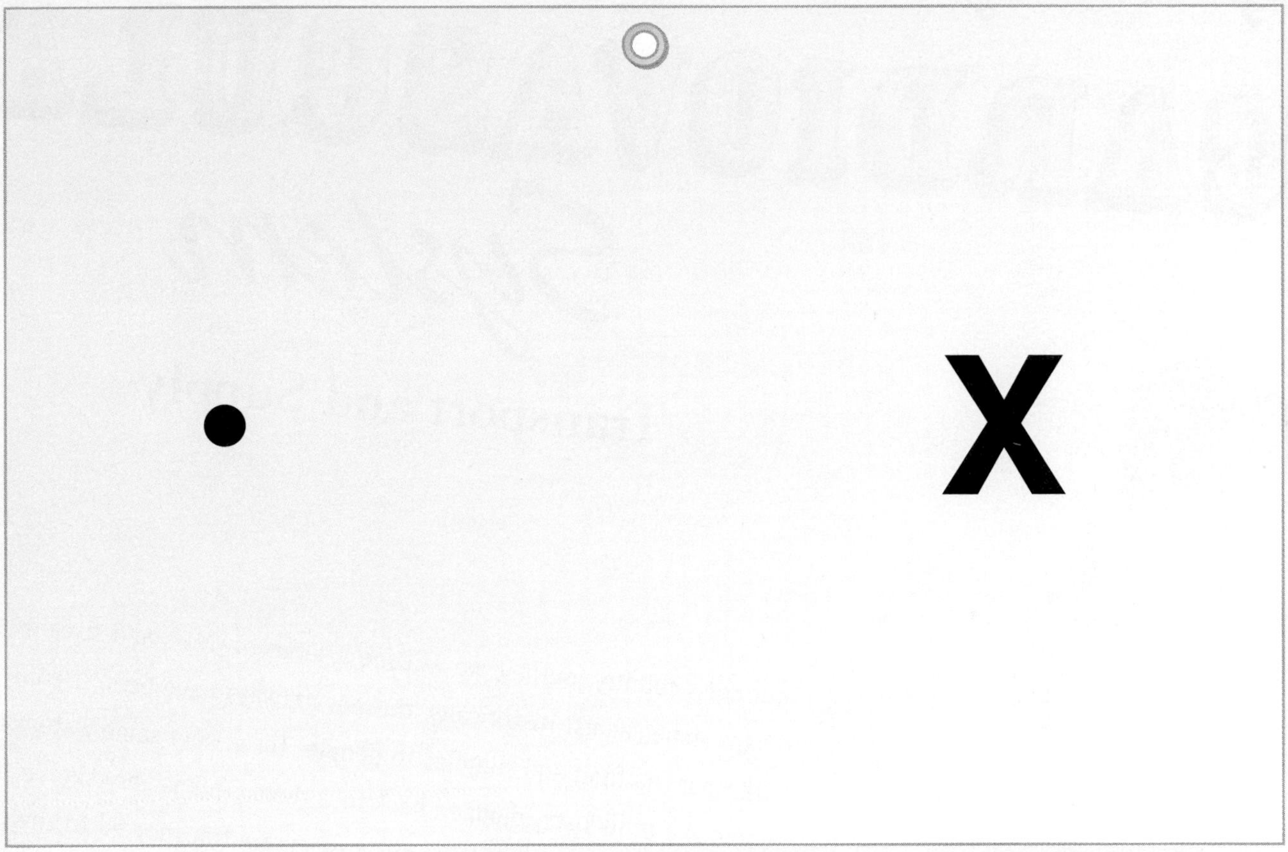

11-9 Now that you have completed your journey through this chapter, please go to the CD-ROM for interactive games and puzzles concerning the medical terms and concepts contained in this chapter. By playing the games you will reinforce your learning of medical terminology in a fun way.

Greetings from THE CARDIOVASCULAR System

Transport and Supply

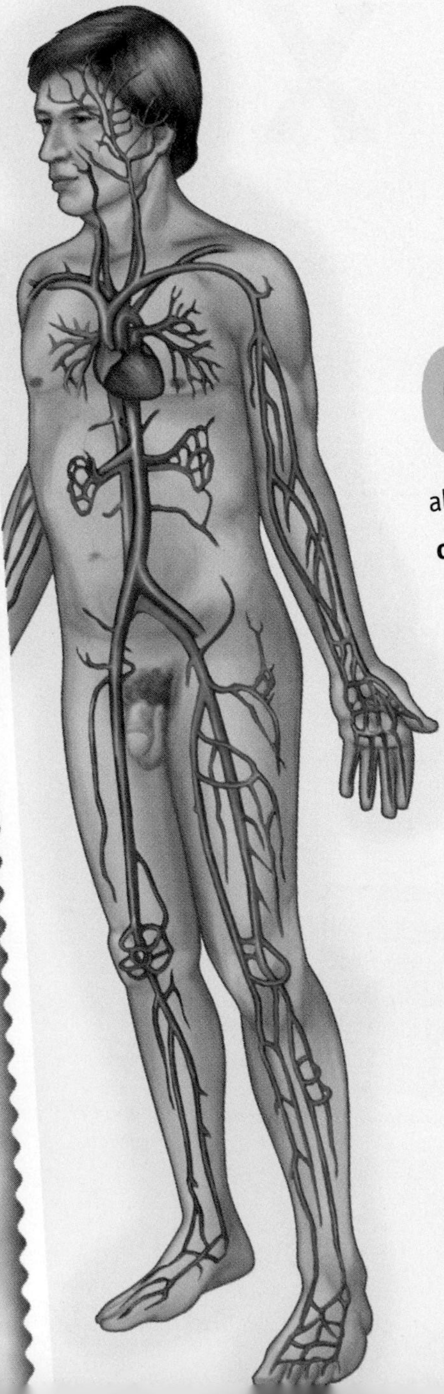

On our cross country journey, we will see a series of rivers and streams and perhaps some canals. Historically, these waterways have been used as a way of transporting food and supplies to people. These very same waterways also had byproducts of industry dumped back into them. This is very similar to the **cardiovascular system,** where nutrients and oxygen are transported to the cells in the body, and carbon dioxide and other waste products of cells' metabolism are removed.

The cardiovascular system is also a lot like a hot water heating system in your house or hotel where you are staying. The furnace has a pump (heart) to circulate the hot water (blood) through the piping system (vessels) to deliver the much needed heat to every room throughout the building. So let's get right to the "heart" of the matter.

Chapter 12

LEARNING OBJECTIVES

Upon completion of your journey through this chapter, you will be able to:

- Identify structures and functions of the cardiovascular system
- Trace the blood flow through the vessels and chambers of the heart
- Explain the coronary circulation of the heart
- Describe the contraction of the heart and the conduction system
- Differentiate between arteries, veins, and capillaries
- List the major components of blood and their functions
- Discuss the importance of blood typing
- Explain the process of blood clotting
- Describe various cardiovascular diseases

MULTIMEDIA APPLICATIONS

CD-ROM Interactive Exercises

- Animation of the chambers of the heart, 12.1
- Animation of the heart contraction and related blood flow, 12.2
- Interactive drag-and-drop exercises on labeling the various parts of the heart, 12.3
- 3-D views of the heart and blood vessels of the body, 12.4
- Interactive exercise on labeling the circulatory system, 12.5
- Animations and videos on heart attacks, dysrhythmias, coronary artery disease, angina, and shock, 12.6
- Videos and animations on sickle cell anemia and leukemia, 12.7
- Interactive puzzles and games, 12.8

www.prenhall.com/colbert

- Professional Profiles:
  - Cardiovascular Technology
- Related Internet Links
- Additional Review Questions

Pronunciation Guide

Correct pronunciation is important in any journey so that you and others are completely understood. Here is a "see and say" Pronunciation Guide for the more difficult terms to pronounce in this chapter.

agglutinate (ah GLUE tin ate)
albumin (AL byoo men)
anemia (ah NEE mee ah)
aneurysm (AN yoo rizm)
arterioles (ahr TEE ree ohls)
arteriosclerosis (ar tee ree oh skleh ROH sis)
atrioventricular node (ay tree oh vehn TRIK yoo lahr)
atrium; atria (AY tree um; AY tree ah)
autorhythmicity (aw to rith MIH sih tee)
basophils (BAY soh fills)
bundle of His (HISS)
cor pulmonale (KOR pull moh NAH lee)
diastole (dye ASS toe lee)
embolus (EM boh luss)
endocardium (ehn doh KAR dee um)
eosinophils (ee oh SIN oh fillz)
erythrocytes (eh RITH roh sights)
hemophilia (HEE moh FILL ee ah)
hemostasis (HEE moh STAY siss)
inotropism (EYE no TROPE izm)
ischemia (iss KEE mee ah)
polycythemia (pall ee sigh THEE mee ah)
prothrombin (pro THROM bin)
systole (SISS toh lee)
thrombocytes (THROM boh sights)
tunica externa (TOO nik ah ex TERN ah)
tunica interna (TOO nik ah in TERN ah)
venules (VEHN yules)

SYSTEM OVERVIEW

cardio = *heart*
vascul/o = *vessels*

arterioles = *small arteries*
venules = *small veins*

The major components of the **cardiovascular** system include the *heart* (which is the organ that pumps blood through the system), *blood* (a form of connective tissue that has a fluid component called *plasma* and a variety of cells and substances), and *blood vessels* (a network of passageways to transport the blood to and from the body's cells).

Blood vessels can be further classified. Vessels that carry blood *Away* from the heart are called *arteries*. These main vessels branch out into ever smaller vessels called **arterioles,** which eventually become *capillaries*. Capillaries are where the exchange of nutrients, gases, and waste products occurs at the cellular level. Capillaries are also the transition vessels where blood begins its trip back to the heart through ever-merging vessels, the tiniest of which are called **venules,** that form the larger *veins*. To view this transitional region along with the cardiovascular system, see Figure 12–1 ■.

In general, veins differ from arteries not only because veins bring blood back to the heart but because the blood now is *deoxygenated* (contains less than the normal arterial amount of oxygen) and has a higher level of carbon dioxide and other waste products of cellular metabolism. Veins also have thinner walls than arteries, are more numerous, and have a larger capacity to hold blood.

Applied Science

COLOR-CODED BLOOD

Notice in Figure 12–1 that blood is depicted as being blue or red depending on the area in which it is located. When the blood contains high amounts of oxygen (oxygenated), it causes a chemical change within the red blood cell. This occurs in the blood of most arteries. As a result of that change, the arterial blood turns a bright red color. As the oxygen is being delivered to the tissues in the body, the blood begins to turn darker red. This occurs mostly in the veins that have lower levels of oxygen (deoxygenated) due to their delivery or dumping of oxygen to the tissues. You can see the darker veins within your wrist or arms. However, when you cut a vein, the blood is no longer darker red because it immediately mixes with the oxygen in the atmosphere and becomes bright red.

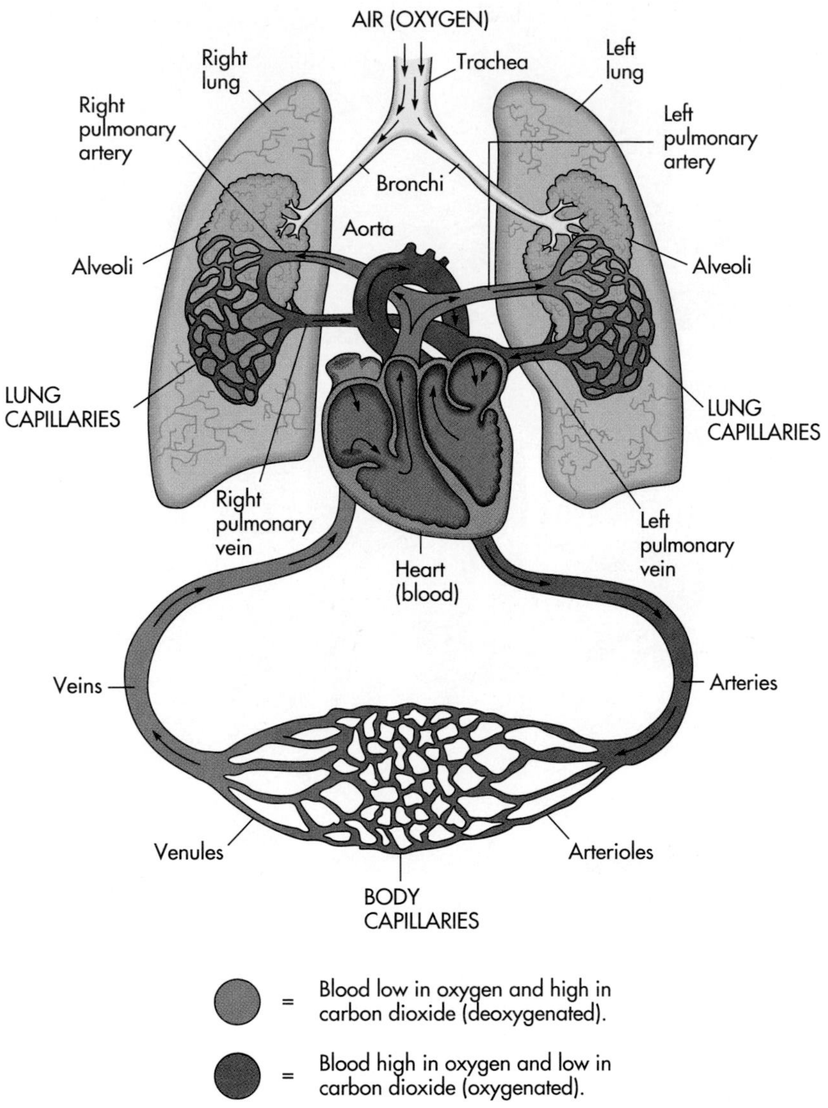

FIGURE ■ 12–1

Overview of the cardiovascular system.

INCREDIBLE PUMPS: THE HEART

Let's begin our journey with the main organ of the cardiovascular system, the heart. While it is often describe as the "pump" of the cardiovascular system, you will soon see that it is actually *two* pumps working together.

General Structure and Function

The heart is a specially shaped muscle about the size of your fist, containing a series of chambers that move blood throughout the body. The heart is surrounded by a serous membrane called the pericardium. The outer layer is a tough fibrous pericar-

> *Learning Hint*
>
> **ARTERIES OR VEINS?**
>
> Remembering what arteries and veins do can be confusing. One easy way to remember is that arteries take blood *away* from the heart. Both words start with *a*. Obviously, then, veins have to bring blood back to the heart.

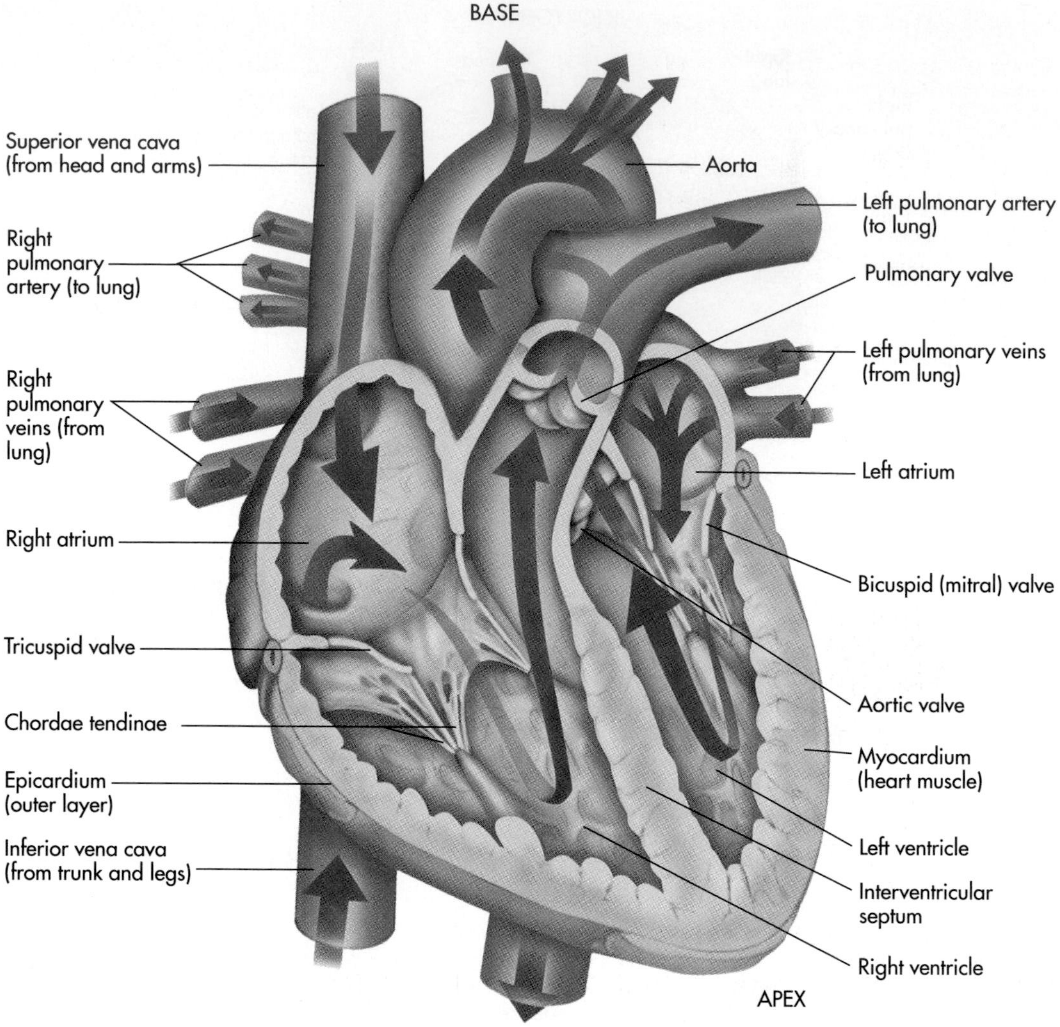

FIGURE ■ 12–2

The anatomy of the heart.

dium. Inside the fibrous pericardium is the parietal layer. The visceral layer is fused to the heart surface and there is a potential cavity between the layers called the pericardial cavity. The outer layer of the heart wall, the visceral pericardium, is also known as the epicardium. The middle layer of the heart wall, the myocardium is made of cardiac muscle. The heart is lined by epithelium, called the endocardium. See Figure 12–2 ■.

The heart's location is slightly left of the center of your chest and above your diaphragm. As strange as it may initially appear, the **base** of the heart is proximal to your head, while the **apex** of the heart is distal. Although the heart is a single organ, it is easier to understand its function if you think of it as *two separate pumps working together*. The right side of the heart is responsible for collecting blood and sending it to the lungs to pick up oxygen and get rid of carbon dioxide. The left side of the heart collects blood from the lungs and pumps it through the body. Before we explore the heart, it's important to review that blood returning to the heart travels through **veins** (thus, venous blood) and blood traveling away from the heart travels through **arteries** (thus, arterial blood).

Opening the heart reveals four chambers. The chambers of the right side of the heart are separated from the chambers of the left side of the heart, so there is no mixing of blood from one side to the other. The wall that separates the two smaller chambers is called the *interatrial* **septum;** while the wall between the two larger chambers is called the *interventricular* **septum.** When looking at Figure 12–2, you will notice the small chamber in the upper left quadrant of the picture. That is the *right* **atrium** (remember, locations are based on the *patient's* perspective). This is a collecting chamber where blood is returned to the heart after its trip through the body. The two large veins that bring the blood to the right atrium are the **superior vena cava** (blood from the head, neck, chest, and upper extremities) and **inferior vena cava** (blood from the trunk, organs, abdomen, pelvic region, and lower extremities). Once the blood is collected, it drains through a one-way valve to a larger chamber in the right side called the *right* **ventricle.** That one-way valve is called the right **atrioventricular valve,** or **AV valve.** This is also called a **tricuspid** valve because the valve is formed with three cusps.

septum = *wall (SEHP tum)*

atrium *(AY tree um)*

atrioventricular *(ay tree oh vehn TRIK yoo lahr)*
tri = *three*

Cardiac Cycle

The movements of the heart, called the cardiac cycle, can be divided into two phases called systole and diastole. Usually when discussing heart movement we refer to ventricle activity.

When the right ventricle is full of blood, the heart contracts (**systole**). Because the tricuspid valve is a one-way valve, as the right ventricular pressure increases, the valve shuts so blood doesn't squirt back into the right atrium. As the pressure increases, the blood has to go somewhere. Now the only way for the blood to travel is through the *pulmonary semilunar valve* to the pulmonary trunk, which divides into the left and right **pulmonary arteries.**

systole *(siss toh lee)*

Each pulmonary artery goes to its respective lung and branches down into ever smaller vessels to the point where they become capillaries that form a network around each air sac in the lungs. This is where the blood gives up one of the waste products of metabolism by cells (carbon dioxide) and picks up a fresh supply of oxygen from the lungs. These capillaries containing freshly oxygenated blood converge into increasingly larger vessels until they form the left and right pulmonary veins. Figure 12–3 ■ illustrates the blood flow through the heart.

The pulmonary veins meet and pour their contents into the *left* atrium. Once the left atrium is filled, blood flows through the left AV valve and into the *left* ventricle. When the left ventricle is full, the heart contracts (squeezes) again. The ventricular pressure increases, forcing the left

Learning Hint

Remember the Tricuspid valve is on the *R*ight side of the heart.

12-1 To view an animation on the chambers of the heart, please go to your CD-ROM for this chapter.

Amazing Body Facts

PULMONARY ARTERIES AND VEINS

True to what we have told you, the pulmonary arteries take blood away from the heart. What is amazing is that they are the *only* arteries in the body that carry deoxygenated blood away from the right heart to travel to the lungs to become oxygenated. The pulmonary vein collects this oxygenated blood and returns it to the left side of the heart and therefore is the only vein to carry oxygenated blood.

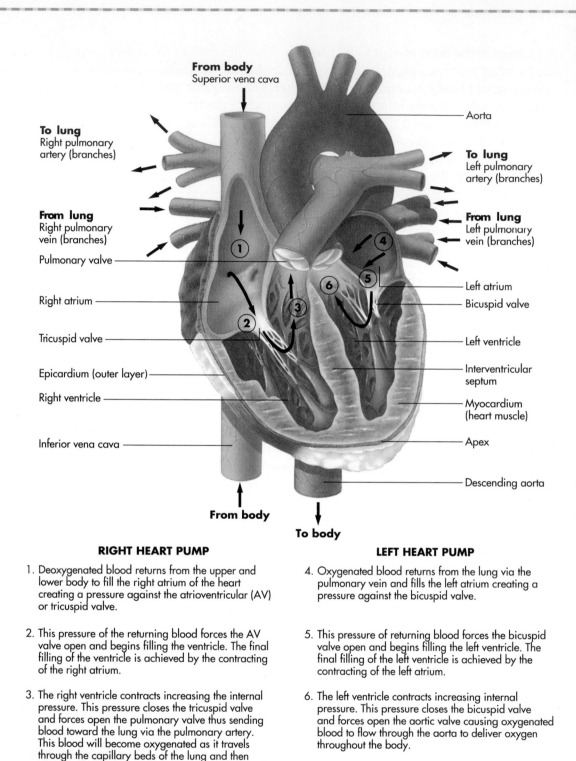

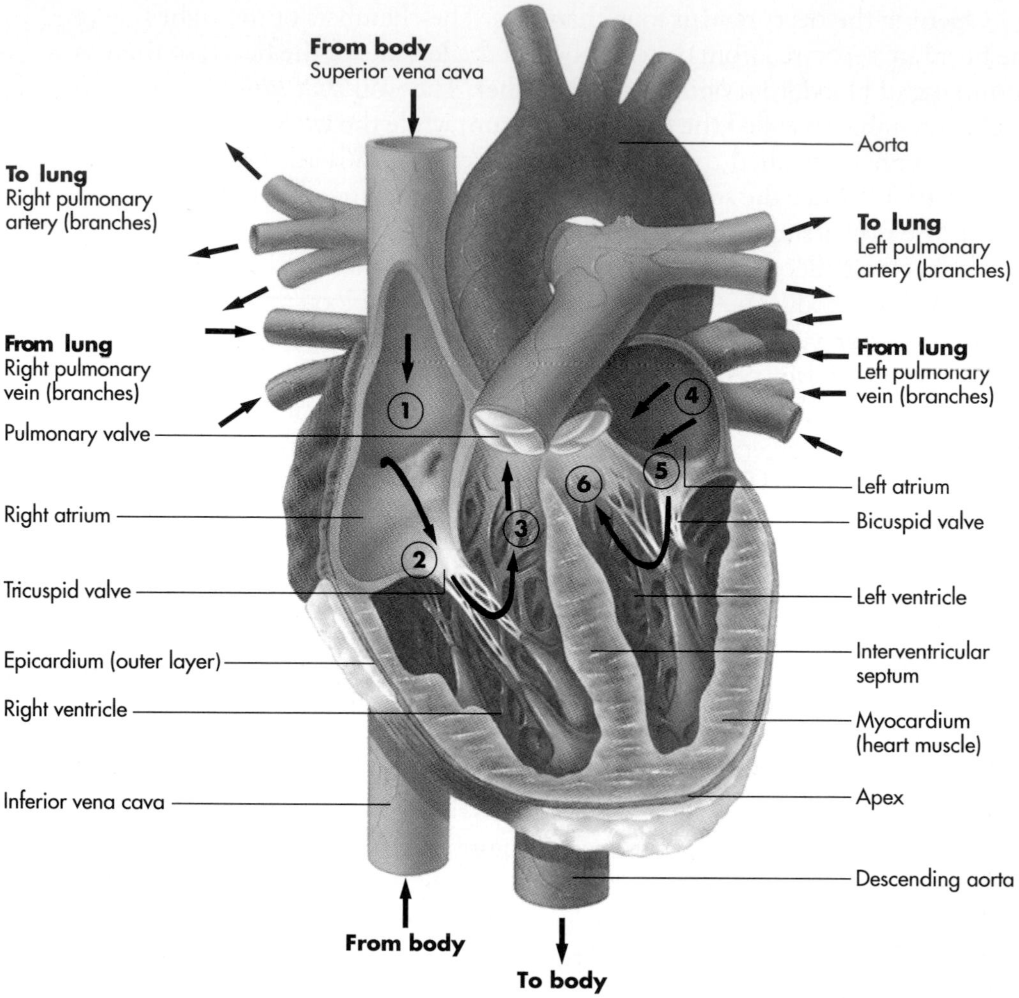

RIGHT HEART PUMP

1. Deoxygenated blood returns from the upper and lower body to fill the right atrium of the heart creating a pressure against the atrioventricular (AV) or tricuspid valve.
2. This pressure of the returning blood forces the AV valve open and begins filling the ventricle. The final filling of the ventricle is achieved by the contracting of the right atrium.
3. The right ventricle contracts increasing the internal pressure. This pressure closes the tricuspid valve and forces open the pulmonary valve thus sending blood toward the lung via the pulmonary artery. This blood will become oxygenated as it travels through the capillary beds of the lung and then return to the left side of the heart.

LEFT HEART PUMP

4. Oxygenated blood returns from the lung via the pulmonary vein and fills the left atrium creating a pressure against the bicuspid valve.
5. This pressure of returning blood forces the bicuspid valve open and begins filling the left ventricle. The final filling of the left ventricle is achieved by the contracting of the left atrium.
6. The left ventricle contracts increasing internal pressure. This pressure closes the bicuspid valve and forces open the aortic valve causing oxygenated blood to flow through the aorta to deliver oxygen throughout the body.

FIGURE ■ 12-3

The functioning of the heart valves and blood flow.

AV valve shut and ejecting the blood out of the left ventricle through the aortic semilunar valve to the ascending aorta, sending it on its way throughout the body. Two more familiar names for the left AV valve are bicuspid (formed by only two leaves or cusps) or **mitral** valves. Now the ventricles and atria can rest (**diastole**) as the atria fill with blood before they squeeze another load of blood into the ventricles. It is important to note that the chambers of the heart fill during diastole, or the relaxation phase, and eject blood during systole, or the contraction phase.

> 12-2 For a visual animation of the heart contraction and the related blood flow, please go to your CD-ROM for this chapter.

Some points to remember are that

- both atria fill at the same time.
- both ventricles fill at the same time.
- both ventricles eject blood at the same time when the heart contracts.

Do you ever get yelled at or get mad at the *other* person for squeezing the toothpaste tube in the middle? What's the big deal? When you eat a freeze pop, do you squeeze it in the middle or from the bottom and work the contents up to your mouth? These two examples are important to visualize because the heart has to contract in a certain way to make sure that all of the blood is squeezed out during each contraction. In order to do this, the contraction begins at the apex and travels upward. As you trace the flow of blood in Figure 12–3, you will see how efficient this is. You should also notice that there is a valve located at the exit of both ventricles. Since your circulatory system is a pressurized system, these valves are necessary to prevent any ejected blood from leaking back in.

Amazing Body Facts

HOW DOES IT KEEP GOING AND GOING AND GOING?

One of the amazing things about your heart is that it continues to beat day after day without your even thinking about it. Here is a neat experiment. Previously, we said that your heart is about the size of your fist. Let's pretend that your fist is your heart. To mimic the pumping action of your heart, open your fist with your fingers fully extended. Now make a tight fist. Continue this action of fully opening and tightly closing your hand for the next *60 seconds.* Chances are good that your hand will feel like it's ready to fall off of your arm! If this is how your hand feels after 60 seconds, how does your heart constantly beat approximately 100,000 times and move approximately 1,800 gallons of blood each day for decades and decades? Think back to Chapter 6 on muscles. Cardiac muscle cells have specialized connections called *intercalated discs.* These connections, along with associated pores, provide an efficient connection with adjacent muscle cells so electrical impulses, ions, and various small molecules can readily travel throughout the heart, allowing a smooth contraction from one area of the heart to another. The vasculature of the heart takes approximately 5 percent of oxygenated blood from each heartbeat to ensure there is a blood-rich environment so plenty of oxygen and nutrients are available.

If you further examine the heart illustration, you will notice that the walls of the atria are thinner than the ventricular walls. This is because higher pressures are generated in the ventricles to move blood. You should also note that the walls of the left ventricle are thicker than the walls of the right ventricle. When you think about it, this makes total sense. The right ventricle has to pump blood only a short distance through the vasculature of the lungs and back to the heart. The left ventricle, on the other hand, has to pump all of the blood throughout the body and back to the right atrium! The resistance of all those blood vessels in the body is six times greater than the resistance of the lung **vasculature** (network of blood vessels).

In the Amazing Facts box, you learned that the heart muscles have a blood-rich environment. In Figure 12–4 ■, you can see that a portion of the newly oxygen-enriched blood is diverted from the aorta by the right and left **coronary arteries.** These arteries continuously divide into smaller branches, forming a web of interconnections known as **anastomoses,** which enable the heart muscle to constantly and fairly consistently receive a rich supply of blood. It is interesting to note that regular aerobic exercise can increase the density of these blood vessels that supply the heart. The number of anastomoses also increase, as does

anastomoses *(ah NASS te MOE sis)*

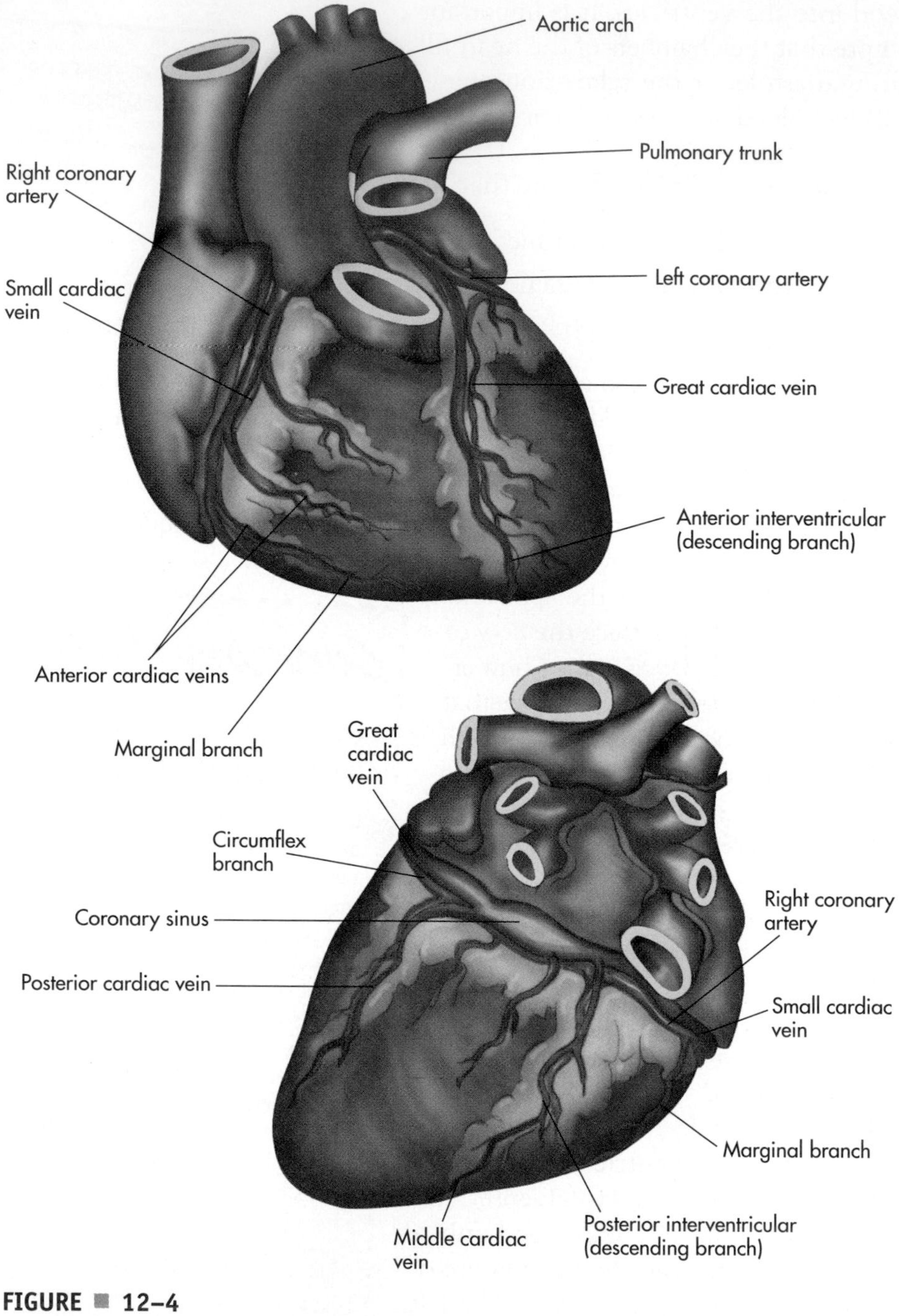

FIGURE ■ 12–4

Coronary Circulation.

> 12-3 To perform interactive drag-and-drop exercises on labeling the various parts of the heart, please go to your CD-ROM for this chapter.

their number of locations. This is important for people with blockage of a small coronary artery. They have an increased survival rate because blood now has alternate routes to travel, which help to prevent heart muscle damage.

The right coronary artery provides blood for the right ventricle, posterior portion of the interventricular septum, and inferior parts of the heart. The left coronary artery provides blood to the left lateral and anterior walls of the left ventricle and to portions of the right ventricle and interventricular septum.

TEST YOUR KNOWLEDGE 12-1

Choose the best answer:

1. Which blood vessels carry blood away from the heart?
   a. capillaries
   b. venules
   c. veins
   d. arteries

2. How many chambers are found in the human heart?
   a. one
   b. two
   c. three
   d. four

3. Which blood vessel type is involved in the exchange of oxygen and nutrients with the tissues of the body?
   a. arterioles
   b. sphincters
   c. arteries
   d. capillaries

Complete the following:

4. The chamber responsible for pumping blood to the body's various organs is the _____.

5. Which side of the heart pumps blood to the lungs? _____.

THE ELECTRIC PATHWAY

Cardiac muscles don't always rely on nerve impulses or hormones to contract. In fact, they can contract on their own. This unique ability is known as **autorhythmicity.** The problem with this ability is that uncontrolled *individual* contractions would prohibit the heart from contracting effectively. This potential problem is solved through the use of specialized cardiac cells that create and distribute an electrical current that causes a *controlled* and *directed* heart contraction. Think of this as the electric company that supplies electricity to your home and the fine educational institution you are attending.

autorhythmicity *(aw to rith MIH sih tee)*

Nodal cells (also called **pacemaker cells**) are specialized cells that not only create an electrical impulse but create these impulses at a regular interval. These cells are connected to each other and to the conducting network, which we discuss soon. Nodal cells are divided into two groups. The main group of pacemaker cells are found in the wall of the right atrium, near the entrance of the superior vena cava. This collection of pacemaker cells forms the **sinoatrial node,** or **SA node.** The SA node generates an electric impulse at approximately 70 to 80 impulses per minute. There is a second collection of pacemaker cells located at the point where the atria and the ventricles meet. This collection forms what is called the **atrioventricular node,** or **AV node.** The cells in the AV node generate an electric impulse at a rate of 40 to 60 beats per minute.

sinoatrial *(sigh noh AY tree al)*

atrioventricular *(ay tree oh vehn TRIK yoo lahr)*

So, which one dictates how fast the heart beats? Think of the SA node as the power station and the AV node as a substation that supplies electricity via an electrical grid for a small city. The SA node sends its impulse to the AV node for distribution before the AV node can send its own. However, *if* the SA node cannot generate an impulse, the AV node takes control and sends out impulses that result in a slower heartbeat, but a heartbeat nonetheless. Figure 12–5 ■ shows the conduction system of the heart.

"So, how come my heart rate isn't always 70–80 beats per minute like when I play sports or get scared?", you ask. It's true that the SA node sets the heart rate when the body is at rest, but several influences can increase or decrease heart rate. The *autonomic nervous system* (both the sympathetic and parasympathetic divisions) has direct connections to the SA and AV nodes as well as to the myocardium. The sympathetic division can release neurotransmitters that

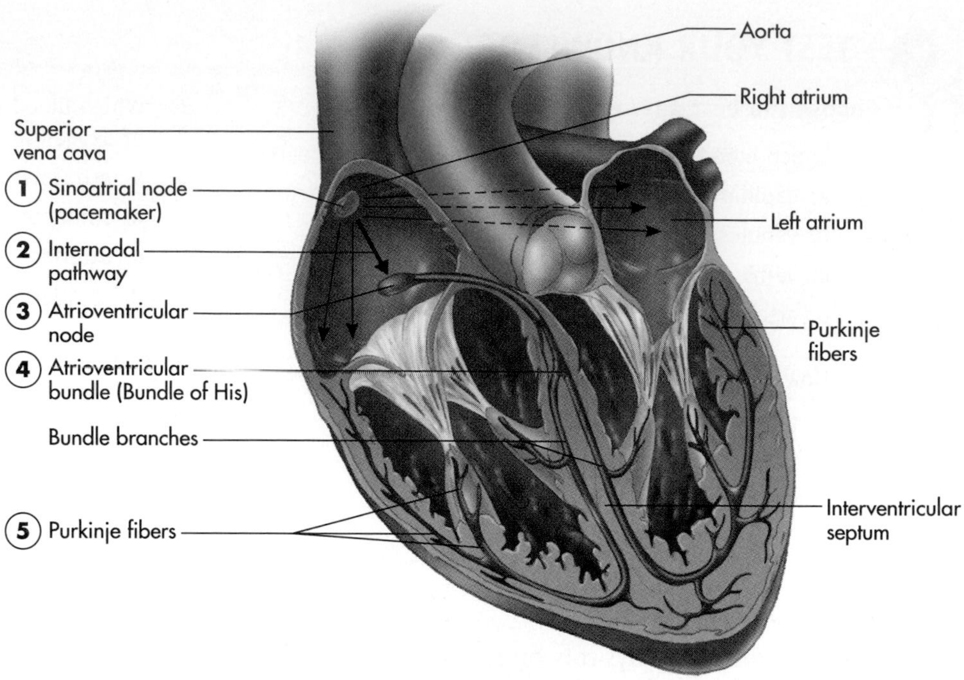

1. The sinoatrial (SA) node fires a stimulus across the walls of both left and right atria causing them to contract.
2. The stimulus arrives at the atrioventricular (AV) node.
3. The stimulus is directed to follow the AV bundle (Bundle of His).
4. The stimulus now travels through the apex of the heart through the bundle branches.
5. The Purkinje fibers distribute the stimulus across both ventricles causing ventricular contraction.

FIGURE ■ 12–5

Conduction system of the heart.

inotropism *(EYE no TROPE izm)*

increase heart rate and the force of the contraction (**inotropism**). To counteract this, the parasympathetic division, through the **vagus nerves,** releases a neurotransmitter that can decrease both the pulse and force of contraction.

In addition, ions, hormones, and body temperature can alter heart rate. For example, as body temperature increases, so does the rate and force of contractions because of the increased metabolic rate of cardiac muscle cells. Conversely, as the body cools down below normal temperature, the rate and force of cardiac contractions decrease. Epinephrine is a hormonal substance that has the same effects as the sympathetic nerves, so it increases heart rate. Electrolytes are important players, especially when there is an imbalance of too many or too few specific ones. Low sodium or potassium can alter heart activity, as can abnormal levels of calcium. Low potassium can lead to a weak heartbeat, while high levels of calcium can prolong heart muscle contractions to the point where the heart can stop beating. These are just a few examples of what can happen when electrolyte levels are outside of normal range. Age, gender, a history of exercise or lack thereof, all can impact on your heart rate. Normally, the resting heart rate for a female is 72 to 80 beats per minute, while the average resting heart rate for males is 64 to 72 beats per minute.

Clinical Application

EKG'S

Because the myocardial contraction is initiated and continues because of an electrical impulse, that charge can actually be detected on the surface of the body. This surface detection of the electric impulse traveling through the heart can be recorded by using an *electrocardiograph,* which records an *electrocardiogram* (ECG or, more commonly, the German form EKG). See Figure 12–6 ■.

The normal EKG has three distinct waves that represent specific heart activities. The *P wave* is the first wave on the EKG and represents the impulse generated by the SA node and depolarization of the atria right before they contract. The next wave is called the *QRS complex* (a combination of Q, R, and S waves). It represents the depolarization of the ventricles that occurs right before the ventricles contract. The ventricles begin contracting right after the peak of the R wave. Due to the greater muscle mass of the ventricles compared to the atria, this wave is greater in size than the P wave. The final wave is the *T wave,* which represents the repolarization of the ventricles where they are at rest before the next contraction. "Aha," you say, "where is the repolarization of the atria?" It occurs during the QRS complex but is usually overshadowed by the ventricles' activity! In the recording of a healthy heart, there are set ranges for the height, depth, and length of time for each of the waves and wave complexes. Changes in those parameters, or the addition of other abnormal types of waves, known as **cardiac arrhythmias** or **dysrhythmias,** can indicate health problems that involve the heart.

a = *without*
dys = *bad or difficult*

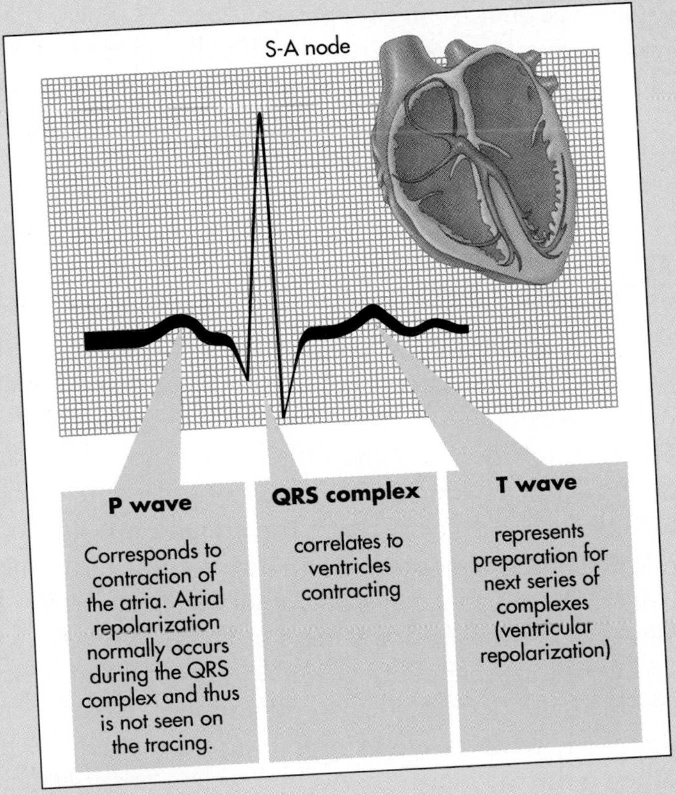
S-A node
P wave
Corresponds to contraction of the atria. Atrial repolarization normally occurs during the QRS complex and thus is not seen on the tracing.
QRS complex
correlates to ventricles contracting
T wave
represents preparation for next series of complexes (ventricular repolarization)

FIGURE ■ 12–6

Typical EKG tracing.

So far, we have our two generators and regulators of electricity. On our journey we can see how electricity is moved in the form of electric lines along the road. In the heart, the movement of the electric impulses is done by specialized *conducting* cells. This power grid of electric distribution has to be set up so the following actions can occur:

1. First, the right and left atria contract together and *before* the right and left ventricles.
2. Then, the two ventricles must contract together.
3. But the direction of the wave of ventricular contraction has to be from the *apex* to the *base* of the heart. This ensures that all of the blood is squeezed out of the ventricles (remember the tube of toothpaste?).

> Cardiovascular technicians perform EKGs and other cardiovascular tests. Please visit the companion Web site for information and to view a video about this exciting profession.

So let's retrace the electrical "wiring," as illustrated in Figure 12–5. Once an electric impulse is generated at the SA node, several pathways composed of conducting cells transmit that impulse to the AV node. A slight signal delay allows for the atria to fill with blood before contraction occurs. Once this charge reaches the AV node, it continues its journey through the **AV bundle,** also known as the **bundle of His** (which sounds like "hiss"). Traveling down the interventricular septum, the AV bundle eventually divides into the *right bundle branch* and the *left bundle branch*. These branches spread across the inner surfaces of both ventricles. Finally, another type of specialized cells called *Purkinje cells* carry the impulse to the contractile muscle cells of the ventricles. And so the contraction begins at the apex, and the wave of contraction smoothly continues up the ventricles, squeezing out all of the blood.

BLOOD

Now that we understand the pump, let's talk about what exactly the heart pumps. Blood is a fluid form of connective tissue that is responsible for three very important functions.

Blood *transports* oxygen from the lungs, nutrients and fat cells from the digestive system, and hormones from endocrine glands to the approximately 75 *trillion* cells in the body. On the return trip from those cells, blood transports carbon dioxide and other waste products that were formed from metabolic activities of the cells to the kidneys, lungs, and other organs for removal from the body.

Blood helps to *regulate* a variety of levels in the body to maintain homeostasis by ensuring that **pH** (levels of acidity or alkalinity) and **electrolyte** (ion) values are within normal parameters for proper cell functioning. Blood helps to regulate body temperature by absorbing heat generated by skeletal muscles, spreading it throughout the rest of the body. Conversely, blood can radiate excess heat out of the body through the skin. Blood can take in or give up more fluid to help regulate the fluid balance of the body.

Finally, but no less important, blood helps to *protect* us from invasion and infection by pathogens and toxins. This is done by specialized **white blood cells** (often shortened to **WBCs**) and special proteins called **antibodies.**

The amount of blood in the body depends on an individual's size and gender. Normally, the body contains between 4 and 6 liters of blood, which accounts for 7 to 9 percent of total body weight.

Blood Composition

Although we can classify blood as a connective tissue, it is important to understand all the components that make up blood. When blood is separated by a centrifuge, the *major* components are **plasma** and what we call **formed elements.** The centrifuge is a machine that spins a test tube of blood at a very fast rate. Due to the spinning force of the centrifuge, the heavier components, like the formed elements, are forced to the bottom of the tube and the lighter component (plasma) is displaced to the top of the tube (see Figure 12–7 ■).

> *Amazing Body Facts*
>
> **WHAT'S IN A DROP OF BLOOD?**
>
> In one *drop* of blood, you will find 5 *million* red blood cells; *250,000* to *500,000* platelets; and *7,500* white blood cells. Don't forget that there are a lot of other substances, such as plasma proteins, nutrients, oxygen, carbon dioxide, hormones, and electrolytes, in there too. This helps to make blood *5 times thicker* than water. With a life expectancy of approximately 120 days, new red blood cells are created to replace old ones at the rate of *2 million each second!* Even more amazing is that the total surface area of all the red blood cells in your body is greater than the surface area of a football field!

Plasma is the yellowish, straw-colored liquid that comprises about 55 percent of the blood's volume and contains about 100 different substances dissolved within. So, if your total blood volume is 5 liters, you have about 2.75 liters of plasma. While plasma is about 90 percent water; nutrients, salts, and a small amount of oxygen are also dissolved into the plasma for transport to the body's cells. Hormones and other cell activity–regulating substances are found in plasma. **Plasma proteins** are an important group of dissolved substances that include **albumin,** which aids in keeping the correct amount of water in the blood; fibrinogen, which is a substance needed for blood clotting; and globulins, which form antibodies that protect us from infection.

Albumin *(AL byoo men)*

Formed or solid elements include the following:

1. **Red blood cells** (**RBC**s) or **erythrocytes**
2. **White blood cells** (**WBCs**), or **leukocytes,** which can be further classified as basophils, eosinophils, lymphocytes, monocytes, and neutrophils
3. **Thrombocytes** (also known as **platelets**), which aid in clotting

Erythrocytes *(eh RITH roh sights)*
erythro = *red*
cytes = *cells*
leukocytes *(LOO koh sights)*
leuko = *white*
thrombocytes *(THROM boh sights)*
thrombo = *clotting*

Red Blood Cells

Lacking a nucleus, and therefore unable to divide to form new cells, red blood cells are created by the red bone marrow through a process called *hemopoiesis* and are similar in shape to a doughnut. Red blood cells perform two crucial functions. With the aid of an iron-containing red pigment called **hemoglobin,** red blood cells transport oxygen from the lungs to the cells in the body. In addition, they help to transport carbon dioxide, a byproduct of cellular metabolism, from the cells to the lungs for removal from the body.

hemopoiesis *(heme a poy EE suss)*
hemo = *blood*
poiesis (poietic) = *making or producing*

White Blood Cells

There are several types of white blood cells. Polymorphonuclear granulocytes originate from red bone marrow. Also originating from bone marrow but maturing in lymphoid and myeloid tissues (mononuclear cells), leukocytes are our guardians from invasion and infection (see Figure 12–8 ■).

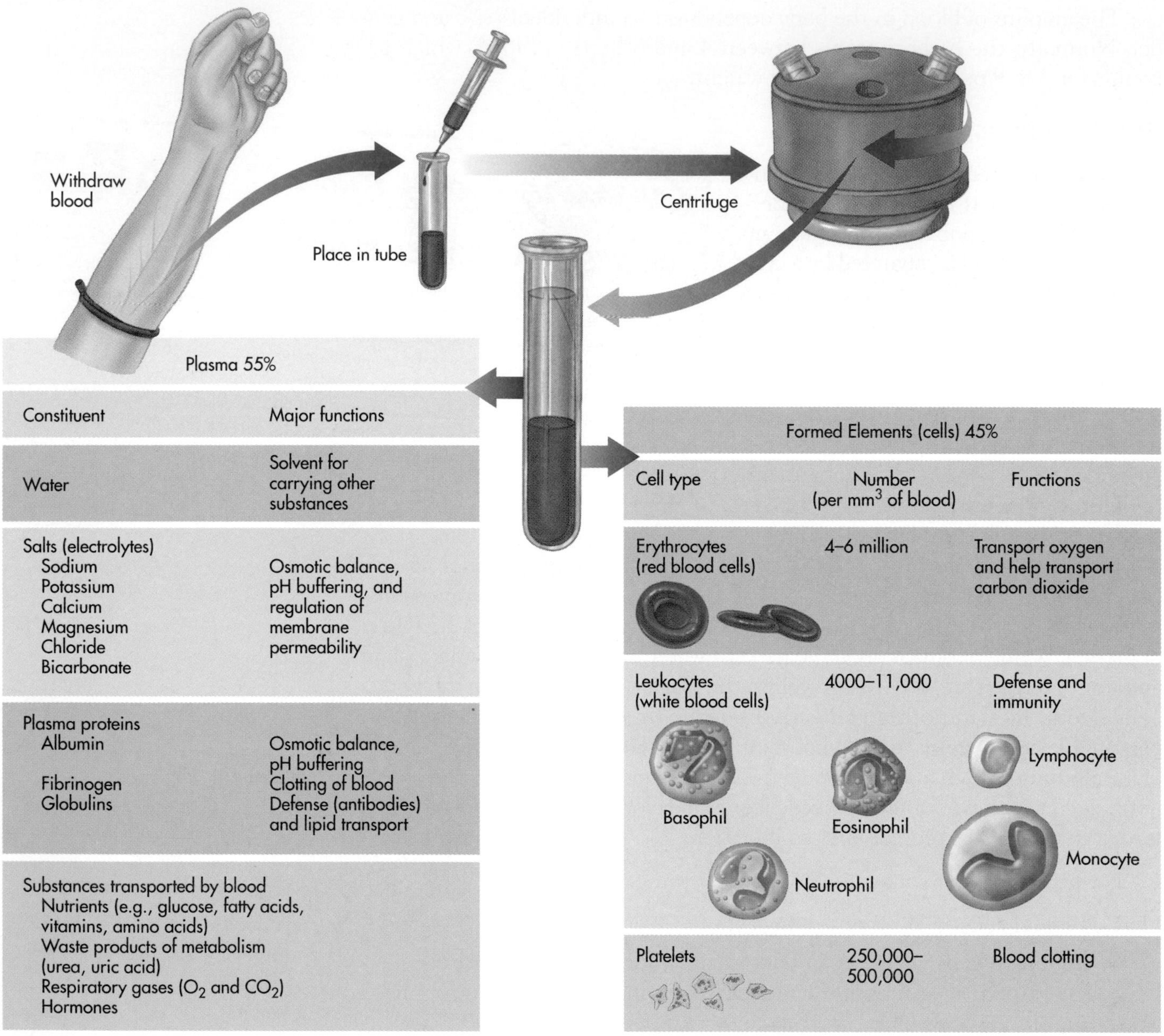

Plasma 55%	
Constituent	**Major functions**
Water	Solvent for carrying other substances
Salts (electrolytes) Sodium Potassium Calcium Magnesium Chloride Bicarbonate	Osmotic balance, pH buffering, and regulation of membrane permeability
Plasma proteins Albumin Fibrinogen Globulins	 Osmotic balance, pH buffering Clotting of blood Defense (antibodies) and lipid transport
Substances transported by blood Nutrients (e.g., glucose, fatty acids, vitamins, amino acids) Waste products of metabolism (urea, uric acid) Respiratory gases (O_2 and CO_2) Hormones	

Formed Elements (cells) 45%		
Cell type	**Number (per mm^3 of blood)**	**Functions**
Erythrocytes (red blood cells)	4–6 million	Transport oxygen and help transport carbon dioxide
Leukocytes (white blood cells)	4000–11,000	Defense and immunity
Platelets	250,000–500,000	Blood clotting

FIGURE ■ 12–7

Composition of blood.

phagocytosis *(fag oh sigh TOH siss)*
phago = *to eat*
osis = *process*
lysosomes *(LIE so soam)*
lyso = *destruction*
som(a) = *body*

The types of white blood cells that compose the polymorphonuclear granulocyte group are neutrophils, eosinophils, and basophils. Neutrophils are the most aggressive white blood cells in cases where bacteria attempt to destroy tissue. **Phagocytosis** is the process in which neutrophils surround and ingest the invader and attempt to destroy it by utilizing cell particles called **lysosomes** that release powerful enzymes. As an infection occurs, the body produces a higher than normal number of neutrophils. Eosinophils are utilized to combat parasitic invasion and a variety of body irritants that lead to allergies. Basophils are involved with allergic reactions by enhancing the body's response to irritants that cause allergies. In addition, basophils are important because they secrete the chemical **heparin,** which helps to keep blood from clotting as it courses through blood vessels.

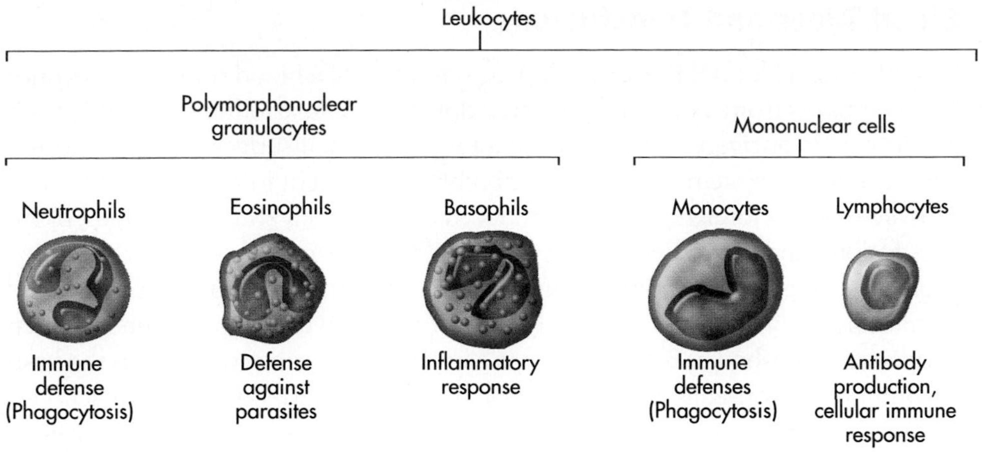

FIGURE ■ 12–8

Functions of white blood cells.

The types of white blood cells that comprise the mononuclear cell group are monocytes and lymphocytes. Monocytes are found in higher than normal amounts when a chronic (long-term) infection occurs in the body. Like neutrophils, monocytes destroy invaders through phagocytosis. Even though it takes longer for monocytes to arrive on the scene of infection, their numbers are greater than neutrophils and therefore they destroy more bacteria. Lymphocytes are unique cells that protect us from infection. Instead of utilizing phagocytosis, they are involved in a process that produces antibodies that inhibit or directly attack invaders. Fighting infection and foreign invaders is discussed, along with the lymphatic system, in Chapter 14.

Thrombocytes

Thrombocytes, also known as **blood platelets,** are the smallest of the formed elements and are responsible for the blood's ability to **clot.** In addition, thrombocytes can release a substance called *serotonin*, which can cause smooth muscle constriction and decreased blood flow.

TEST YOUR KNOWLEDGE 12-2

Choose the best answer:

1. Which cell type does not belong in this group?
   a. erythrocyte
   b. lymphocyte
   c. monocyte
   d. eosinophil

2. What substance found in red blood cells is responsible for oxygen transport?
   a. gobuloglobin
   b. hemoglobin
   c. gammaglobulin
   d. cytoplasm

3. Which portion of an EKG tracing represents ventricular depolarization?
   a. T wave
   b. QRS complex
   c. P wave
   d. SA node

Complete the following:

4. This important plasma protein helps to maintain fluid balance of your blood: _____.

5. The main pacemaker of the heart is the _____.

Blood Types and Transfusions

Not all human blood is the same. A person in need of a blood transfusion cannot be given blood from a randomly selected donor. Incompatibility of blood types is due in part to antigens. An antigen is a protein on cell surfaces that can stimulate the immune system to produce antibodies, which fight foreign invaders. Antigens are typically foreign proteins introduced into the body through wounds, blood transfusions, and so on. Because they are not "native" to the body, they are called "nonself" antigens. They differ from our own "self-antigens" that exist on the cell membrane of every cell in the body. The chain of events that occurs between antigens and antibodies is called the antigen–antibody reaction, which is the basis for immune response, as you will see in Chapter 14. Antibodies often react with the antigens that caused them to form, and the antigens stick together, or **agglutinate,** in little clumps. Although there are at least 50 different antigen types found on the surface of a red blood cell, our main focus is on the A, B, and Rh antigens.

agglutinate *(ah GLUE tin ate)*

Everybody has only *one* of the following blood types:

type A
type B
type AB
type O

Type A blood is very common. Approximately 41 percent of the American population has this type of blood. A represents a specific type of self-antigen that is found on the cell membrane of each red blood cell in the body of a person with type A blood. Since that person was born with type A blood, no antibodies were created to fight it, so there are no anti–A antibodies in his or her plasma. Interestingly, type A blood *does* contain anti–B antibodies.

Type B red blood cells possess type B self-antigens and the plasma contains anti–A antibodies. Apparently, these two blood types don't like each other!

Type AB, however, tries to get along with both A and B. Its red blood cells contain *both* of the A and B self-antigens with neither A nor B antibodies in the plasma.

Not to be out done, type O red blood cells contain *no* A or B antigens, but its plasma contains *both* A and B antibodies.

This information is important to know if there is a need to transfuse blood. If the donor's antigens and the antibodies in the blood recipient's plasma agglutinate, serious harm and even death can occur.

If a *donor* gives blood that contains no A or B antigens, agglutination by anti–A and/or anti–B antibodies in the *recipient's* blood is prevented. Since Type O doesn't have A or B antigens, it can be given to anyone, so a donor with type O blood is a **universal donor.** Since type AB doesn't contain plasma anti–A an-

Amazing Body Facts

COCONUT JUICE TRANSFUSIONS AND ARTIFICIAL BLOOD

There are reports that in the Pacific Theater during World War II, coconut juice was used on injured soldiers to bring their blood volumes up when there was a lack of real blood. The juice was supposedly sterile when taken directly from the coconut and transfused into their veins.

Currently, there is much research in the development of artificial blood or blood substitutes. The main objective is to develop a blood form that can be universally used for all humans without the need to match specific blood types. Other objectives include making a substitute that is free of blood-borne diseases, has the ability to be rapidly infused, has increased oxygen-carrying capacity, and has an extended shelf-life. Some artificial blood is made by chemically altering and refining natural blood components, and some artificial blood is synthetic in nature.

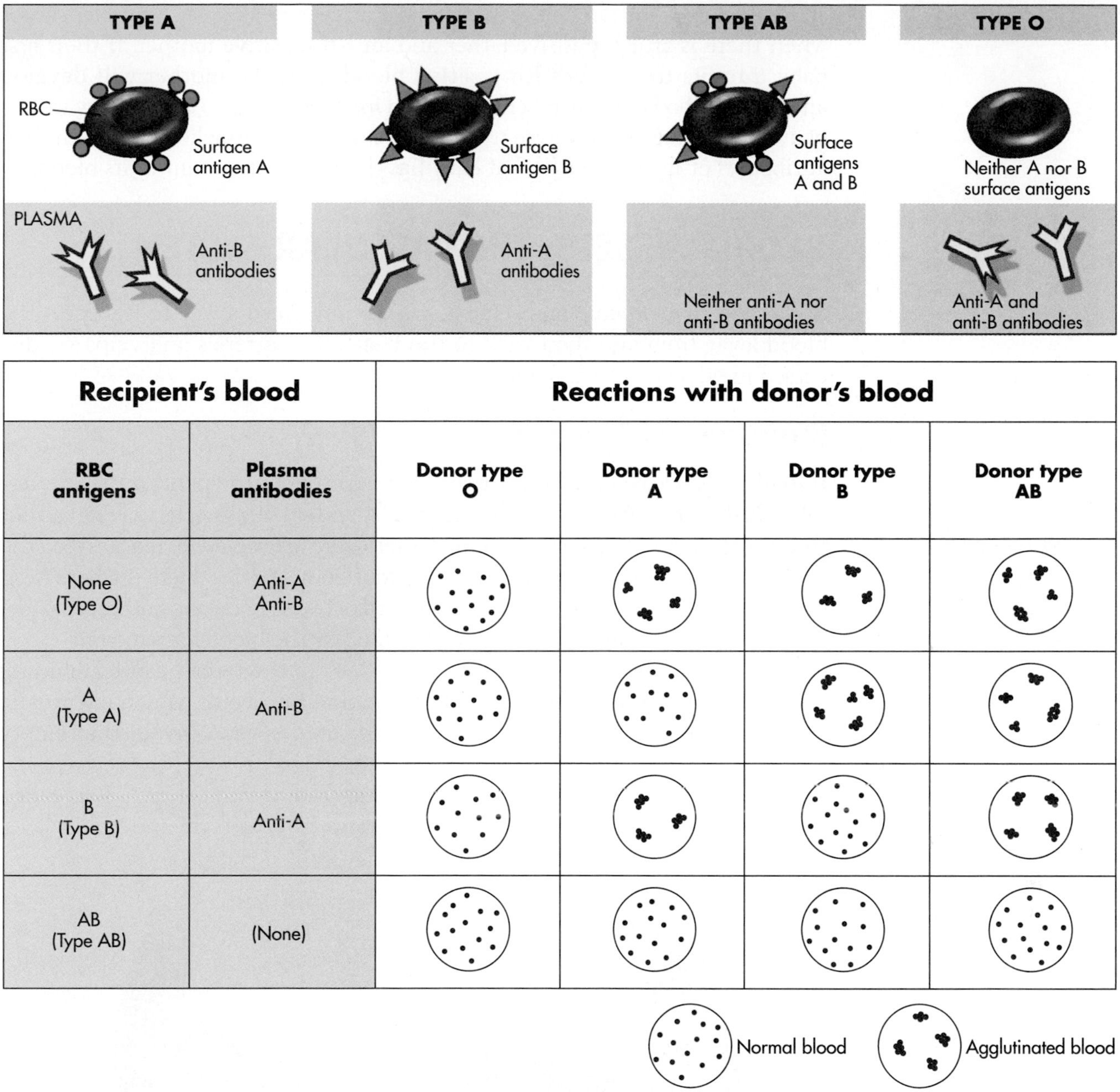

FIGURE ■ 12–9

Blood types and results of donor and recipient combinations.

tibodies or anti–B antibodies, it can't clump with any donated blood that contains A or B antigens. Because of this, a type AB person is labeled a **universal recipient.** See Figure 12–9 ■ that shows blood types with matching antigen and antibodies and which recipient blood would safely match the donor's blood.

Are you with us so far? Good. Now there is one more thing we need to add: the **Rh factor.** Based on a discovery of a special blood antigen first found in the blood of Rhesus monkeys, it was discovered that approximately 85 percent of the white and 88 percent of the African American population of the United States possess the Rh antigen in their blood. Individuals with this antigen in their blood are said to be **Rh-positive.** Conversely, those without this antigen are **Rh-negative.** When typing an individual's blood, the term, *Rh* is eliminated, so an individual would be O-positve or AB-negative, for example. A problem arises when there is an Rh-positive father and an Rh-negative mother. If their first baby inherits the father's Rh-positive blood trait, the mother will develop anti–Rh antibodies (remember the foreign invader scenario?). This baby will be okay, but any future baby born to these parents may be attacked by the anti–Rh antibodies of the mother *IF* that baby has the Rh-positive trait in its blood.

BLOOD VESSELS: THE VASCULAR SYSTEM

So far, we have a pump and some fluid. We now need a way to transport the blood away from and then back to the heart. The arteries and veins we discussed previously now come into play.

Structure and Function

arterioles *(ahr TEE ree ohls)*

tunica interna *(TOO nik ah in TERN ah)*

Initially, blood leaves the heart through the aorta, which branches into large vessels called *arteries*. Arteries divide into smaller and smaller ones as they spread out through the body. The smallest form of arteries are **arterioles.** Arterioles feed the capillaries that form the capillary beds in your body's tissues. Here is where fresh oxygen and nutrients are supplied to the cells of your body and carbon dioxide, along with other waste products, are picked up by the blood for removal.

Blood from the capillary beds begins its return trip to the heart by draining into tiny veins called venules. Venules combine into veins, which eventually combine into the great veins (superior and inferior vena cavae) that empty back into your heart.

For most blood vessels, the walls are composed of three layers, often called coats or tunics. See Figure 12–10 ■. The **tunica interna** is the innermost layer

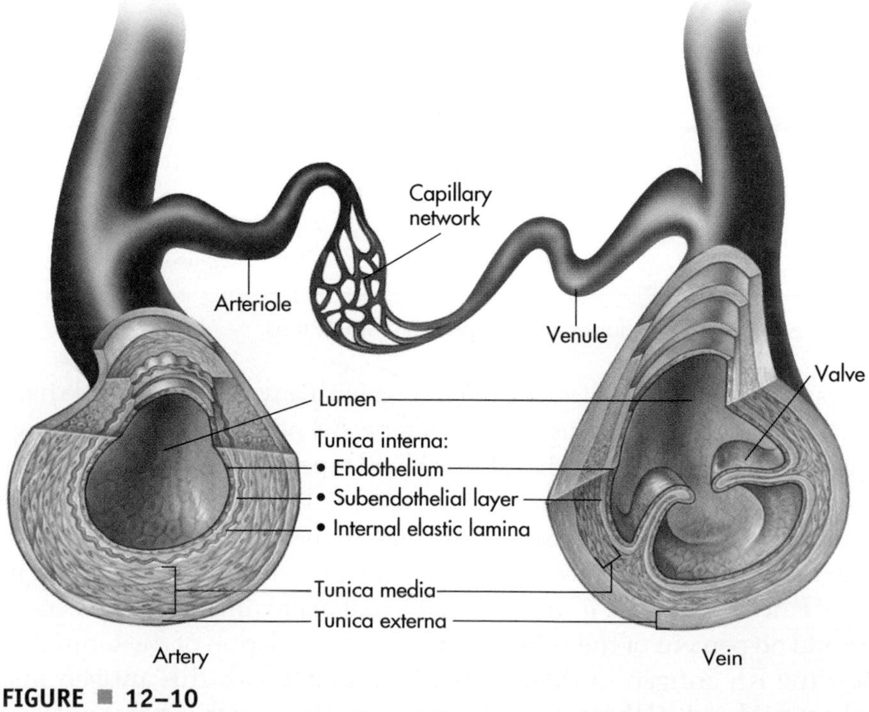

FIGURE ■ 12–10

Blood vessels and the capillary connection.

Clinical Application

TAKING A BLOOD PRESSURE

An important diagnostic test is the determination of arterial blood pressure (BP). This is done with a stethoscope and a sphygmomanometer. As shown in Figure 12–11 ■, an inflatable cuff is placed around the arm, above the elbow, so when the cuff is inflated, it squeezes the brachial artery shut. Your stethoscope is placed over the brachial artery in the proximity of the patient's elbow. The cuff can then be inflated by repeatedly squeezing the bulb while listening with the stethoscope. As you listen while you inflate the cuff, continue squeezing the bulb until you raise the pressure to about 30 millimeters of mercury (mm Hg) *beyond* the point that the pulse is no longer heard.

You can read the pressure by one of three ways, depending on the device you are using. Figure 12–11 shows a column filled with mercury (thus the pressure unit of measure mmHg) connected to the cuff via a hollow tube. Other devices use a round pressure gauge, and others use a digital readout. All of them measure pressure in units of mm Hg.

Once the pressure is 30 mm Hg above the point where pulse sound is lost, the release valve is opened *slightly* so the cuff slowly deflates as you listen to the brachial artery. As the cuff pressure decreases to slightly below systolic pressure (pressure when the heart contracts), the sound of blood being pushed through the artery by the heart can be heard. That is the peak systolic pressure, or top number of the BP reading.

As the cuff pressure decreases, the sound of the pulse decreases and then disappears. That point is where the cuff pressure is equal to the arterial pressure when the heart is at rest (diastole). This is the bottom number in the BP reading. One-twenty over eighty (120/80) has traditionally been accepted as a normal BP for healthy young adults. Recently, lower values are being considered as more in line with a healthy value. Time and continued study will tell which will be the accepted value. Please review Table 12–1 to see where various values fall within low, normal, or high ranges of BP evaluation.

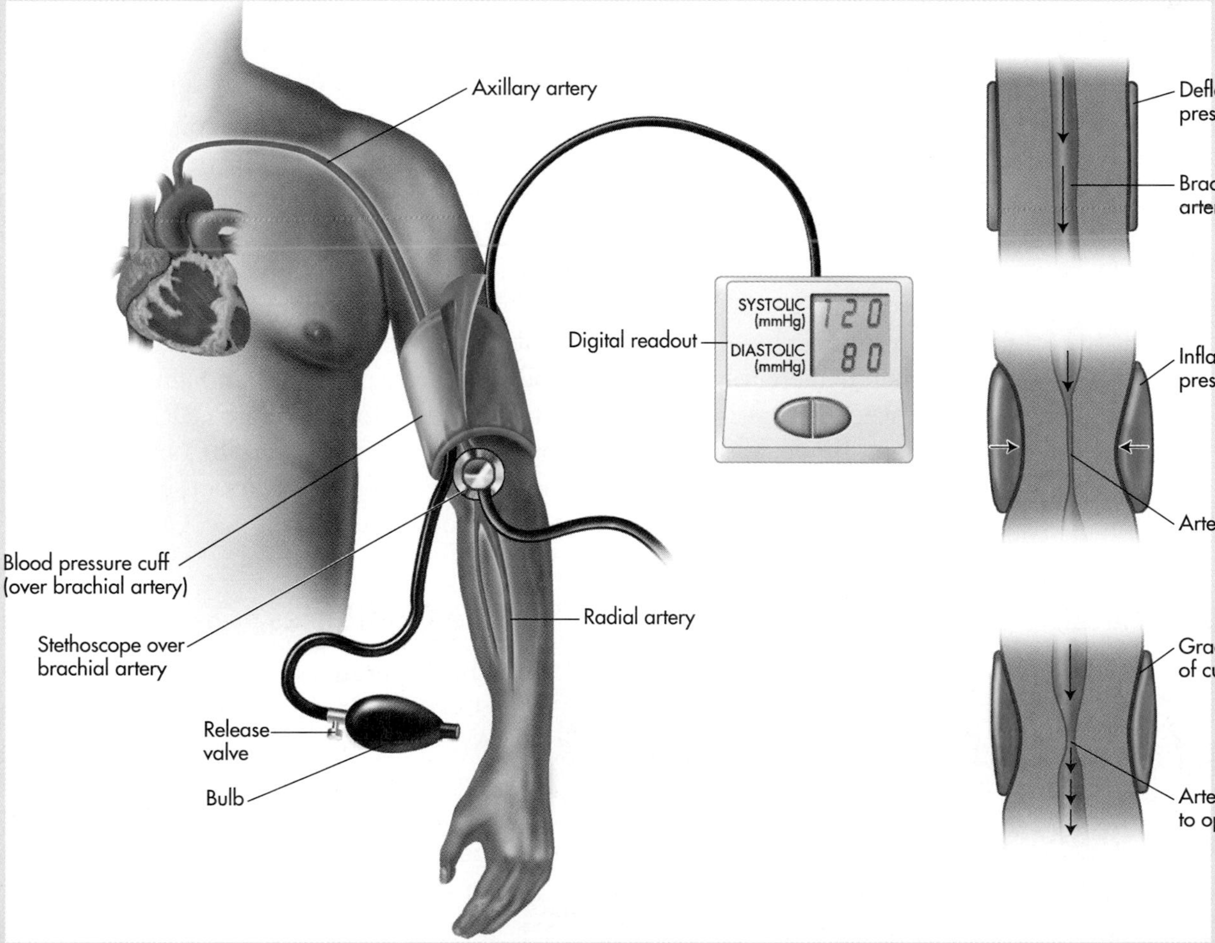

FIGURE ■ 12–11

Blood pressure measurement.

TABLE 12–1

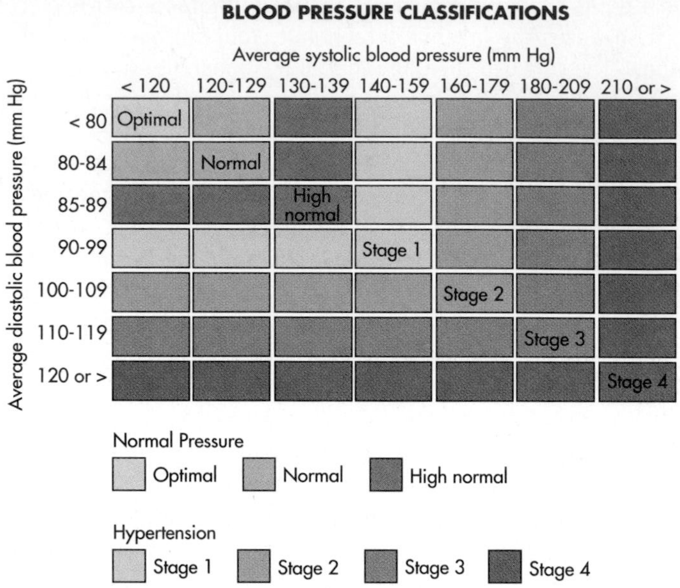
BLOOD PRESSURE CLASSIFICATIONS
Average systolic blood pressure (mm Hg)
< 120
120-129
130-139
140-159
160-179
180-209
210 or >
Average diastolic blood pressure (mm Hg)
< 80
80-84
85-89
90-99
100-109
110-119
120 or >
Optimal
Normal
High normal
Stage 1
Stage 2
Stage 3
Stage 4
Normal Pressure
Optimal
Normal
High normal
Hypertension
Stage 1
Stage 2
Stage 3
Stage 4

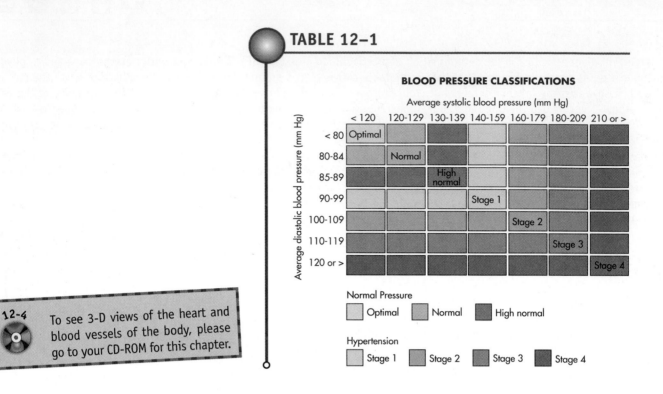

> **12-4** To see 3-D views of the heart and blood vessels of the body, please go to your CD-ROM for this chapter.

and is composed of a thin, tightly packed layer of *squamous epithelial* cells over a layer of loose connective tissue. The compacting of the epithelial cells provides a smooth surface so blood can easily pass through. The next layer is thicker and is composed mainly of smooth muscle and elastic tissue and collagen. This middle layer is called the **tunica media.** By contracting or relaxing those muscles, this layer actually controls the diameter of the vessels to meet certain blood flow needs of the body at a given time. Your sympathetic nervous system determines these needs and signals the vessels to **vasoconstrict** (decrease the inner diameter or lumen) or **vasodilate** (increase the inner diameter or lumen) as needed. This change in diameter changes blood pressure (**BP**); as the vessels dilate, BP decreases. Constriction leads to BP increases. The outermost, or external, coat is the **tunica externa.** Its job is to provide vessel support and protection, so it is composed of mostly fibrous tissue.

tunica media
(TOO nik ah mee DEE ah)

tunica externa
(TOO nik ah ex TERN ah)

hemostasis *(HEE moh STAY siss)*

> *Clinical Application*
>
> **REGULATION OF BLOOD PRESSURE**
>
> Blood pressure is controlled by both blood vessel diameter (peripheral resistance) and the amount of blood pumped by the heart (cardiac output). Cardiac output is a function of heart rate and the amount of blood pumped with each contraction (stroke volume). Stroke volume is influenced mainly by blood volume. For example, increased fluid volume, increased heart rate, and increased peripheral resistance would lead to an increased blood pressure.

The Capillaries

The differences in the structure of the blood vessels varies depending on their job. Arteries possess much thicker walls than veins. As we said earlier, this makes sense because arteries are closer to the heart and have to deal with higher pressures. In fact, larger arteries contain complete sheets of elastic tissue, *elastic laminae*, in their middle walls to help deal with increased pressure. Veins can possess thinner walls because the pressure on them is lower than in arteries, but the inside opening, known as the **lumen,** is larger than in arteries. In addition, the larger veins of the body, especially in the legs, contain valves that prevent blood from flowing backward. Remember, the venous side is lower in pressure. Another means the body has to help move venous blood toward the heart is through the use of skeletal muscle. The relaxation and contraction of skeletal muscles that surround veins help to "milk" the blood toward the heart.

Finally, we have the capillaries, which are composed of only the tunic interna. With a diameter of only 0.008 millimeters (slightly larger than the diameter of single red blood cell), this wall is only one cell in thickness so oxygen and nutrients can easily move into the tissue cells while carbon dioxide and wastes can move into the blood. This is important because even at rest, metabolizing tissue cells require approximately 250 milliliters of oxygen while producing almost 200 milliliters of carbon dioxide *every minute!* Dozens of capillaries form a web, or network, of vessels called a **capillary bed.** As you can see in Figure 12–11, capillary beds are composed of two types of blood vessels: a **vascular shunt,** which is a main road connecting the arteriole to the venule, and **true capillaries,** which make the actual exchanges with tissue cells. True capillaries can be considered the on-ramps and off-ramps to and from the vascular shunt. In Figure 12–12 ■, you will notice a group of structures called **precapillary sphincters.** These structures are composed of smooth muscle and act as toll booths either allowing blood to flow through or stopping blood flow when they contract. If the blood flows through, it travels through the true capillaries and to cells of the tissue. If the blood is stopped at the precapillary sphincters, then the blood travels through the vascular shunt.

Blood Clotting

As we have discussed, the cardiovascular system is a closed and pressurized system. Imagine what could happen if a leak or a break in the system occured. You have probably seen cars along the road with blown radiator hoses. The steam shoots out and the car goes nowhere. A similar condition can occur in your body; no steam shoots out of your blood vessels, of course, but if enough blood is lost, you won't go anywhere and will die. Thanks to several substances in your blood, some leaks or breaks that occur can be stopped. **Hemostasis** (the stoppage of blood) is accomplish through a chain of events shown in Figure 12–13 ■.

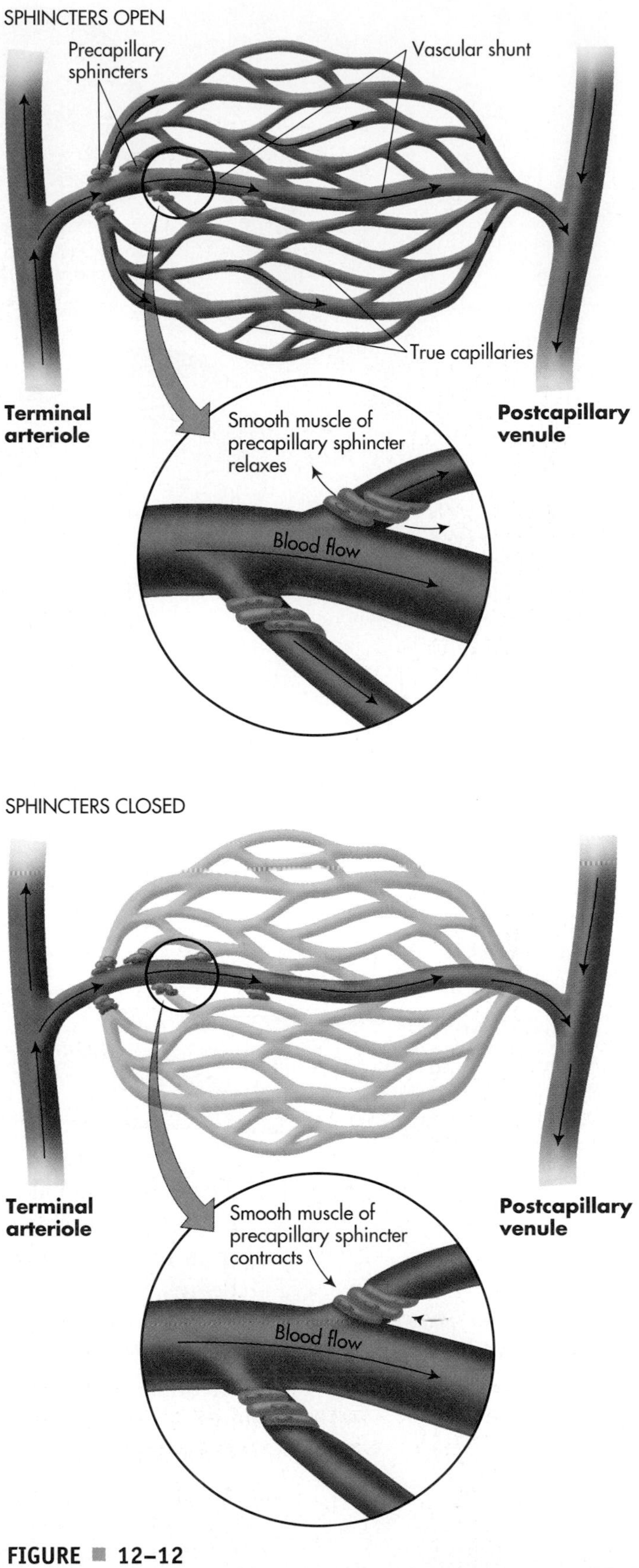

FIGURE ■ 12–12

Capillary beds and sphincters.

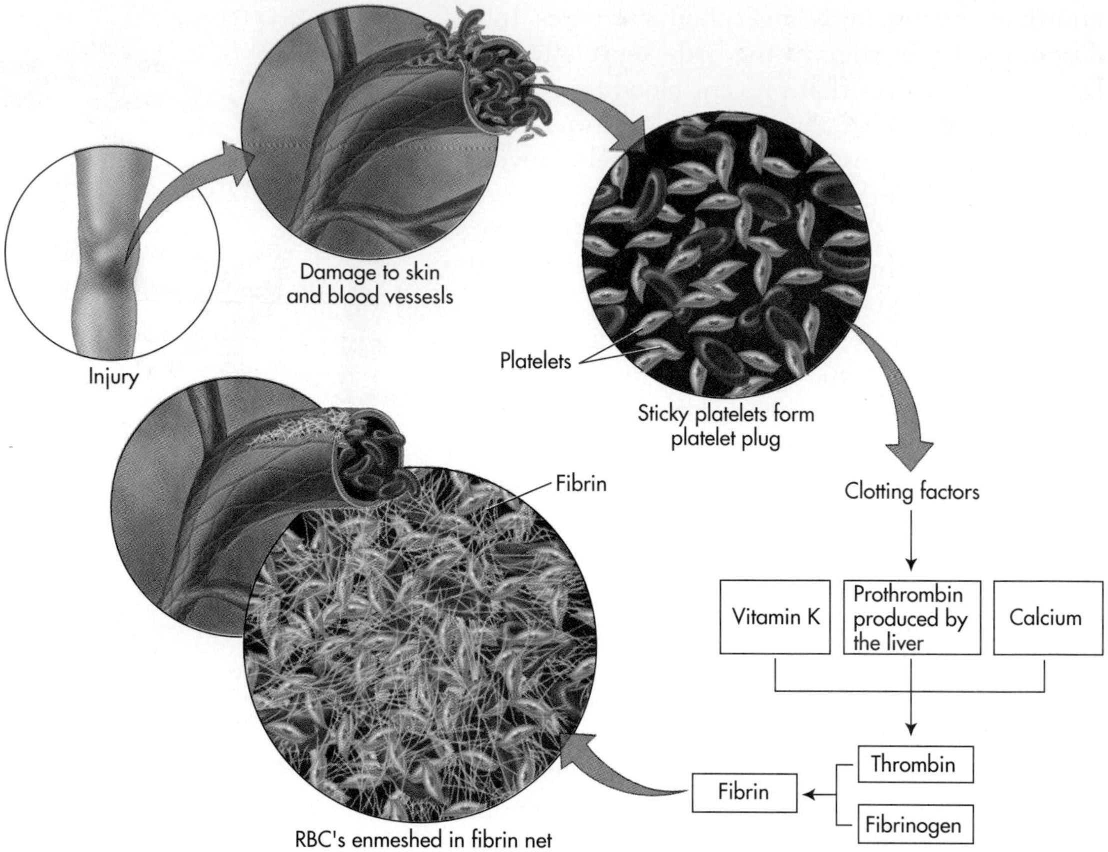

FIGURE ■ 12–13

The clotting process.

> **12-5** To perform an interactive exercise on labeling the circulatory system, please go to your CD-ROM for this chapter.

Damage to the innermost wall of a vessel exposes the underlying collagen fibers. Platelets that are floating around in the blood begin attaching to the rough, damaged site. The attached platelets release several chemicals that draw more platelets to that site, creating a *platelet plug*. These platelets also release *serotonin*, which causes blood vessels to spasm, thereby decreasing blood flow to that area. Within approximately 15 seconds from the time of the initial injury, the actual **coagulation** (clotting) of blood begins. With the help of calcium ions and 11 different plasma proteins (clotting factors), a chain reaction starts. One of the clotting proteins, **prothrombin,** which is produced by the liver with the help of vitamin K, converts to **thrombin.** Thrombin transforms **fibrinogen,** which is dissolved in the blood, into its insoluble, hairlike form called **fibrin.** Fibrin forms a netlike patch at the injury site and snags more blood cells and platelets, and within 3 to 6 minutes, a clot is created. Once the clot is formed, it eventually begins to retract, and as a result, pulls the damaged edges of the blood vessel together. This allows the edges to regenerate the necessary epithelial tissue to make a permanent repair over time. Once the clot has outlived its usefulness, it is dissolved. Again, please see Figure 12–13.

prothrombin *(pro THROM bin)*
thrombin *(THROM bin)*
fibrinogen *(fye BRINN oh jenn)*

thrombus *(THROM buss)*

Clinical Application

CLOTTING GONE BAD

The chain reaction that causes a clot must be stopped when it has accomplished its purpose, or else clotting would continue throughout the vascular system. However, there are times when unwanted clotting occurs. A rough surface on an otherwise smooth lumen of a blood vessel may allow platelets to begin "sticking" there, forming a type of clot called a **thrombus.** A thrombus that forms in the vascular system of the heart can partially or totally block blood flow to a portion of the heart, resulting in a coronary thrombosis, which can cause a heart attack. The degree of blockage along with the heart area affected determines the severity of the attack. If allowed to increase in size as more blood cells attach to it, total blockage of blood flow can happen.

Another scenario is the potential for a portion, or several portions, of the thrombus to break off and flow through the circulatory system like an iceberg at sea. This floating thrombus, called an **embolus,** is not a problem until it travels down too narrow a blood vessel and becomes lodged, partially or totally blocking downstream blood flow. A cerebral embolus would affect blood flow to the brain, causing a stroke; a pulmonary embolus would lodge in the lung region and affect your ability to get oxygen into your blood, as you will see in Chapter 13.

Blood that is not traveling through the vessels at the rate it should can also lead to unwanted clot formation. People who are bedridden, on long plane flights or bus or car rides, or are immobile for extended periods of time are susceptible to thrombus formation. It also appears that women who smoke and use oral contraceptives and individuals on some types of chemotherapy are at a higher risk for clot formation.

Substances that decrease the blood's ability to coagulate, such as aspirin or heparin, help prevent unwanted clotting. Once a clot forms, "clot busters" such as the drug streptokinase, are given to regain proper blood flow.

TEST YOUR KNOWLEDGE 12-3

Choose the best answer:

1. The universal donor blood type is
   a. O-positive
   b. AB-positive
   c. Rh-positive
   d. B-positive
2. The smallest form of arteries are
   a. arterules
   b. capillaries
   c. arterioles
   d. vessicles
3. A type of unwanted blood clot is a
   a. bolus
   b. thrombus
   c. omnibus
   d. skoolbus

Complete the following:

4. List the three layers commonly found in a blood vessel:
   a. _____.
   b. _____.
   c. _____.

COMMON DISORDERS OF THE CARDIOVASCULAR SYSTEM

The following are several types of cardiovascular conditions. This section discusses heart problems, blood vessel problems, and blood disorders.

Pump Problems

So far, we have discussed how a healthy heart works. However, certain events can affect the efficiency of the heart's pumping action. Remember that this is a *two-pump* system. What may damage one pump may not always damage the other pump.

cor pulmonale
(KOR pull moh NAH lee)

Let's look at the right side of the heart first. **Cor pulmonale** is a potentially serious condition in which the right-side pump can't move blood as efficiently as it should. This is a result of the heart muscles working harder than they normally do. As with any muscle that you exercise, heart muscle also becomes larger. In this case, the muscles on the right side of the heart become too large and can no longer efficiently pump blood. Disease conditions such as polycythemia, in which the blood is thicker than normal and is harder to pump, or blood vessels in the lungs that constrict more than normal, making it harder to push blood through them, can cause the heart muscles to work harder. Because these two conditions are related to certain lung diseases, it is no surprise that 85 percent of the patients with chronic obstructive pulmonary disease develop cor pulmonale.

Congestive heart failure is a potentially life-threatening condition that can affect the right or left side of the heart. This is a situation in which the pumping action of the heart cannot overcome an increase of pressure either in the pulmonary vasculature (right pump) or the body systems (left pump). As a result of this increasing vascular pressure, fluid begins to leak out of the vessels and into the tissues of the body.

Let's first look at right-sided congestive heart failure. Remember that the left side is pumping normally, and we are working with a closed system, much like a water pump and cooling system in a car. As the left side pumps blood through your body and back to the right side, the right side cannot take all of the returning blood to pump it to the lungs. As a result, the blood begins to back up. The vessels in the body are flexible and can expand a little to take that extra volume of blood, so extended neck veins can be a sign of cor pulmonale. Certain organs can hold more blood than usual, so an engorged liver and spleen can be a sign of cor pulmonale. Tissues in the periphery can hold extra fluid, so swollen ankles, feet, and/or hands can also be a sign of right-sided heart failure.

Now, let's consider left-sided congestive heart failure. The healthy right pump pushes blood through the vasculature of the lungs on its way to the left-side pump. If the left side can't keep up with the blood being delivered to it, the blood backs up into the lungs, increasing the pressure in those blood vessels. Once that pressure reaches a certain point, fluid leaks out of the vessels and into the lung tissue. Pulmonary edema is the term for fluid that forms in the lungs and causes difficulty breathing. See Figure 12–14 ■.

Sometimes the heart muscle is fine, but there is a problem with one or more of the heart valves that seal off the chambers during contraction. There are two possible types of problems: either the passageway through the valve is too small (stenotic) and restricts sufficient blood flow, or the passageway is too large and blood squirts backward into the chamber on contraction (valvular insufficiency). A problem that can occur in either case is the increased tendency to form clots in the damaged valve area. Such clots can detach, flow through the blood vessels, and cause a pulmonary embolus in the lungs or can travel to the brain and cause a stroke. There are also potential problems with the small, spe-

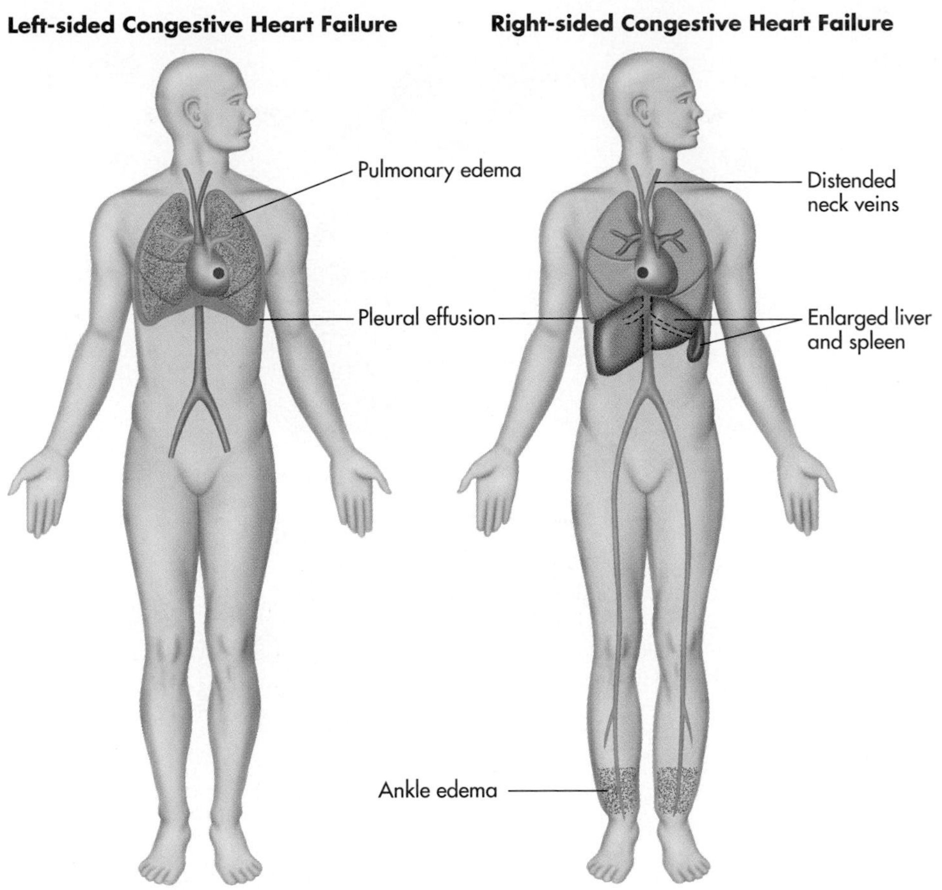

FIGURE ■ 12–14

Left-side and right-side congestive heart failure.

cialized muscles called the papillary muscles that attach to the undersides of the cusps and contract when the ventricles contract so the cusps don't flap back up into the atria. The failure of the papillary muscles to properly contract will allow blood to flow backward into the atrium instead of flowing forward.

Vessel Problems

A common problem with blood vessels occurs to some degree for all of us as we age. **Arteriosclerosis,** also known as *hardening of the arteries*, is a result of the thickening of the intima, which causes the involved vessels to become less flexible or even brittle. Blood vessels in this condition have a tendency to rupture. Since these vessels are less flexible and can't readily accommodate increases in blood volume, the body is more susceptible to high blood pressure.

arteriosclerosis
(ar tee ree oh skleh ROH sis)
sclerosis = *hardening*

Normally, blood vessels have a smooth inner lining, which promotes efficient blood flow by decreasing resistance. **Atherosclerosis** is a potentially life-threatening condition in which fatty deposits, called **plaque,** build up on the inner lining of blood vessels. As a result, blood flow can become greatly restricted or totally blocked. The fatty material that makes up plaque is composed mostly of **cholesterol.** Interestingly, all blood vessels are susceptible to atherosclerosis, but the aorta and coronary arteries seem particularly susceptible to developing this condition. Cerebral arteries can also be affected (see Figure 12–15 ■).

atherosclerosis
(ath er oh skleh ROH siss)
athero *fatty or porridge like*
sclero = *hardness*

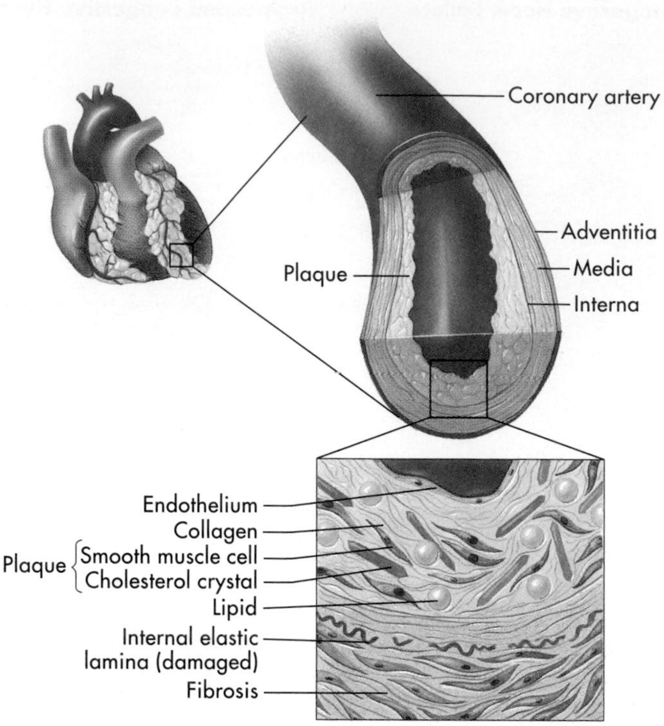

FIGURE ■ 12–15

Atherosclerosis.

infarct *(in FARKT)*

ischemia *(iss KEE mee ah)*

aneurysm *(AN yoo rizm)*

If blood flow is restricted through one or more coronary artery, heart muscle may become oxygen starved and cause tissue death. This would be a myocardial **infarct** (MI), or heart attack. If there is blockage of blood flow to the brain, a cerebral vascular accident (CVA) or stroke can occur. Reduced blood flow to tissues that leads to tissue *injury* but not tissue *death* is called tissue **ischemia.**

Heredity seems to be one factor for atherosclerosis, and atherosclerosis is also a common complication of diabetes. It is interesting that many medical professionals feel that diabetes should be classified as a cardiovascular disease. Diet and lifestyle also seem to predispose some individuals to atherosclerosis.

Arteries are designed to handle the increased pressures generated by a beating heart. In some individuals, those walls may not always be able to maintain their integrity. An **aneurysm** is a localized weakened area of blood vessel wall that may have been caused by a congenital defect, disease, or injury. There also appears to be a familial tendency for abdominal aneurysms, which often present no warning symptoms. The danger is when the aneurysm expands to the point that it ruptures, causing hemorrhaging. If it is a major artery, an individual can bleed out in a matter of minutes. If the aneurysm is detected on an X-ray or ultrasound, surgical intervention can remedy the situation. Early detection is important.

Blood Problems

Secondary polycythemia is a condition in which chronic low levels of oxygen (due to lung disease or living in high altitudes) cause the body to produce more than normal amounts of erythrocytes to transport more efficiently the smaller amounts of available oxygen. Primary polycythemia does the same thing but can be caused by bone marrow cancer.

Anemia is a blood condition in which there is a less than normal number of red blood cells or there is abnormal or deficient hemoglobin. Anemia can be a result of bone marrow dysfunction, low levels of iron or vitamins, or the improper formation of red blood cells. Individuals with anemia share these common symptoms:

anemia *(ah NEE mee ah)*

- pale skin tone (pallor)
- pale mucous membrane and nail beds
- fatigue and muscle weakness
- shortness of breath
- chest pains in some heart patients due to decreased levels of oxygen being supplied to the heart.

Sickle cell anemia is an inherited condition in which red blood cells and hemoglobin molecules do not form properly. The resultant red blood cells are crescent or sickle shaped and have a tendency to rupture. As they are destroyed, the body is stimulated to produce greater numbers of red blood cells to replace them. Unfortunately, at that high production rate, the blood cells cannot mature fast enough. The ruptured cells also clog up smaller blood vessels. Clogged vessels combined with the increased thickening of the blood from excess red blood cells and cell parts lead to increased clotting and an impaired ability to carry oxygen.

There are several blood problems involving white blood cells. **Leukemia,** usually due to bone marrow cancer, is a condition in which a higher than normal number of white blood cells are produced. You might think this would be a good thing; however, the problem is that the white blood cells produced are immature and therefore ineffective in protecting the body from infection. **Leukocytosis** also exhibits as a situation in which there is a higher than normal number of white blood cells. In this case, the cause is often an infection that is being fought. **Leukopenia** is a condition in which the number of white blood cells is lower

Clinical Application

HEART ATTACKS

A true heart attack occurs when there is an insufficient supply of blood from the coronary artery to the tissues of the heart. This could be a result of plaque build-up in the arteries decreasing flow or a piece of that plaque breaking off and occluding the artery. A clot that forms and blocks the artery can be another scenario. If the decreased blood flow is sufficient to kill heart tissue, the condition is called myocardial infarction (MI). You may think that the classic heart attack is when the victim clutches his or her chest in extreme pain and falls over. However, most heart attacks start out slowly with little or no pain (often called a *silent MI*) and may progress over a few hours, days, or even weeks, showing only subtle signs.

Symptoms that can be indicative of an MI are centrally located chest pain, chest heaviness, or vague discomfort; pain in the left shoulder or shoulder blade, neck, and jaw (where it mimics a toothache), radiating down the left arm; nausea, heartburn, weakness, or a clammy, sweaty feeling. Shortness of breath and/or dizziness can also be a warning sign. Women often exhibit "nontraditional" signs and symptoms, such as pain in the shoulder blade or jaw, and such symptoms are missed as indicators of a heart attack, often with tragic results.

Another big problem is that the victim often goes into denial, trying to explain away the symptoms as the result of some other problem, such as indigestion, from eating too much or food that "doesn't agree with me" or feeling that it's gallbladder problem, or a pulled muscle. This can cost the patient valuable time in the treatment for a heart attack. Indeed, the first hour is when much of the heart damage occurs.

Call 911 *immediately* if you even suspect a heart attack. Research shows that an individual who is experiencing a heart attack should also immediately chew and swallow an aspirin tablet, preferably a baby aspirin or a plain, nonenteric coated adult aspirin. The anticoagulating ability of aspirin helps to keep blood flowing through the coronary vasculature, hopefully decreasing the amount of damage to the heart muscle. Most heart attacks are survivable *if* you act quickly and seek treatment immediately. It is better to be safe than sorry!

12-6 To view animations and videos on heart attacks, dysrhythmias, coronary artery disease, angina, coronary heart disease, and shock, please go to your CD-ROM for this chapter.

12-7 To view videos and animations on sickle cell anemia and leukemia, please go to your CD-ROM for this chapter.

than normal. This can be a result of drugs that suppress their production, such as corticosteroids and anti-cancer agents. Chronic infections can also wear the body down to the point that it cannot produce the necessary numbers of white blood cells.

hemophilia *(HEE moh FILL ee ah)*

thrombocytopenia *(THROM boh sigh toh PEE nee ah)*

Sometimes, there is a problem with the ability of blood to clot properly. **Hemophilia** is a general term used to describe inherited blood conditions that prohibit or slow down the blood's ability to clot. **Thrombocytopenia** is a condition in which there are fewer than normal circulating platelets. If the platelet count is low enough, even normal movement can lead to bleeding. This condition can be caused by liver dysfunction, vitamin K–deficiency, radiation exposure, or bone marrow cancer.

THE LYMPHATIC CONNECTION

The lymphatic system, the topic of Chapter 14, has an important relationship with the cardiovascular system (see Figure 12–16 ■). The lymphatic system runs parallel to the cardiovascular system and has three major responsibilities:

1. Help maintain the body's fluid balance by returning interstitial fluid to the venous side of the cardiovascular system.
2. Assist the cardiovascular system in distributing nutrients and hormones that may not easily enter the blood system directly, and assist in the removal of waste products from tissues.
3. Help prevent infection and disease by utilizing lymphocytes.

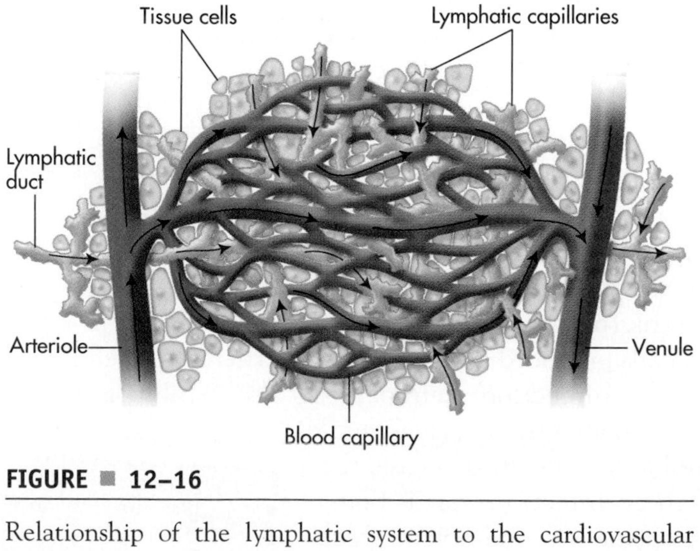

FIGURE ■ 12–16

Relationship of the lymphatic system to the cardiovascular system.

SUMMARY

Snapshots from the Journey

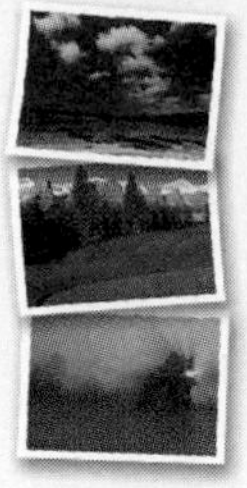

- The cardiovascular system is a closed, pressurized system much like the engine cooling system of a car.
- Like a system of rivers and canals, the cardiovascular system is responsible for transportation of oxygen, hormones, and nutrients to the tissues of the body and for removing the byproducts of metabolism by the cells.
- The cardiovascular system also helps maintain proper fluid balance of the body and assists in the control of body temperature.
- The cardiovascular system is a major player in the body's defense from infection.
- The heart is an organ that is actually two pumps working together to move blood.
- The heart's right pump moves blood collected from the body to the lungs, where oxygen is loaded and carbon dioxide is removed to be exhaled by the lungs.
- The heart's left pump takes the freshly oxygenated blood and pushes it through the body so tissue cells can be kept healthy.
- Arteries carry blood away from the heart.
- Veins carry blood to the heart.
- Capillaries are blood vessels with walls the thickness of only one cell, which readily allows for the transfer of oxygen and nutrients to the tissues in the body.
- This thinness of capillary walls also allows for waste products of the cells' metabolism to be picked up by the blood for removal.
- The major components of blood are plasma, erythrocytes (red blood cells, the main transporter of oxygen), leukocytes (white blood cells, protectors from infection), and platelets (aid in the clotting of blood).

Case Study

A 55-year-old male presents to the emergency department complaining about vague chest pains for the past several days. A quick patient history revealed the following: a two-pack-a-day smoker since the age of 15; height of 67 inches; weight 240; lives alone and doesn't prepare meals, preferring cookies, snack foods, and diet cola; sedentary lifestyle; uses oxygen daily to relieve shortness of breath, and complains of occasional chest pains.

Given these facts, what disease process do you think this individual may be experiencing?

What suggestions would you give to the patient and his doctor?

REVIEW QUESTIONS

Multiple Choice

1. A condition in which one side or the other of the heart cannot pump efficiently enough to overcome vascular resistance, resulting in leakage from the vessels into tissues, is
   a. congestive heart failure
   b. cardiac tamponade
   c. vesiculitis
   d. atherosclerosis

2. Plaque deposits in blood vessels are composed mostly of
   a. platelets
   b. cholesterol
   c. fibrin
   d. heme

3. A localized weakness in the walls of a blood vessel is called a(n)
   a. aneurysm
   b. altruism
   c. embolism
   d. stint

4. Which of the following symptoms would *not* normally be related to anemia?
   a. shortness of breath
   b. fatigue
   c. increased urine output
   d. pallor

5. A general term to describe an inherited blood-clotting disorder is
   a. hemorahgeia
   b. hemophilia
   c. hemoglobin
   d. polycythemia

Fill in The Blanks

1. List the three main responsibilities of the lymphatic system:
   a. ______________________________.
   b. ______________________________.
   c. ______________________________.

2. Decreased blood flow to cardiac muscle that only *injures* the tissue creates a condition known as ______________.

3. The structures composed of smooth muscle that direct the flow through capillary beds are called ______________.

4. ______________ is an important vitamin that is needed for the proper clotting of blood.

5. ______________ is a term used for the dividing wall between the ventricles.

Short Answer

1. Why is the direction of the wave of contraction so important in the heart?

2. Describe the flow of blood beginning at the right atrium and ending at the aorta.

3. Provide one reason the proper amount of iron is so important in your diet.

4. Why can polycythemia potentially cause a heart problem?

Suggested Activities

1. Make arrangements for a tour of a local blood bank to better understand the screening process for donors, how blood is typed, how it is stored, and how it is broken down into useful components.

2. Research and present to the class your findings on all of the useful components of a donated unit of blood.

3. Partner off and take each other's blood pressure and pulse while sitting in a chair, while laying down, and right after walking up a flight of stairs. Compare your results with your classmates'. Discuss any similarities or differences.

12-8

Now that you have completed your journey through this chapter, please go to the CD-ROM for interactive games and puzzles concerning the medical terms and concepts contained in this chapter. By playing the games you will reinforce your learning of medical terminology in a fun way.

Greetings from THE RESPIRATORY System

It's a Gas

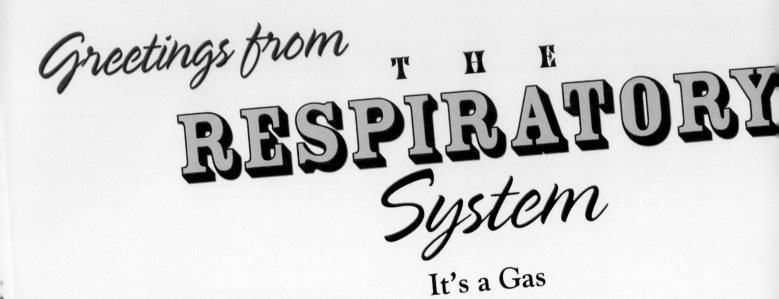

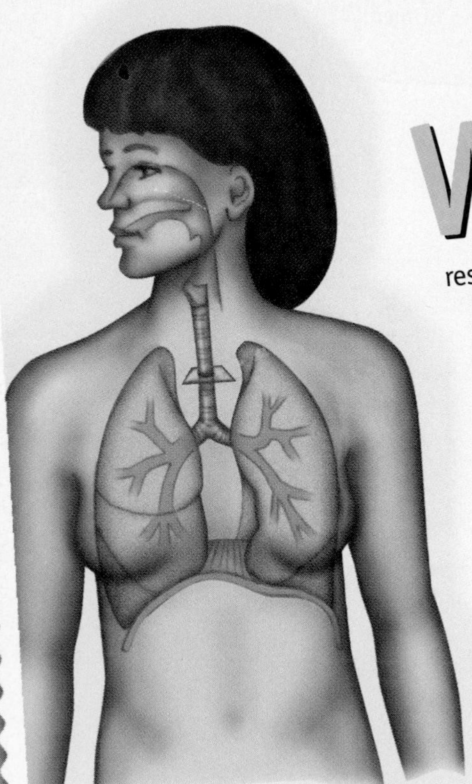

Without fuel, we wouldn't get very far on our trip. Our car won't start without gasoline, our plane would be grounded without jet fuel, and our bodies would die without the fuel necessary for metabolism. The respiratory system's primary function is to transport the vital fuel oxygen from the atmosphere into the bloodstream to be utilized by cells, tissues, and organs for the processes necessary to sustain life. This amazing system is often taken for granted. We don't even consciously realize that the respiratory system is moving 12,000 quarts of air a day in and out of our lungs. On our journey, the fuel for our means of transportation also produces a waste by-product, or exhaust. For example, our car produces waste gases that it eliminates through its exhaust system. The body also produces a waste gas, carbon dioxide, during metabolism that needs to be eliminated via the respiratory system so it does not build up in toxic levels. In this chapter, we explore the journey oxygen molecules must take from the outside atmosphere to our cells and tissues. In addition, we travel with carbon dioxide as it leaves the respiratory system and is placed back into the atmosphere. Hopefully, your journey through the respiratory system will be a "breath-taking" experience.

Chapter 13

LEARNING OBJECTIVES

At the end of the journey through this chapter, you will be able to:

- List and state the basic functions of the components of the respiratory system
- Differentiate between respiration and ventilation
- Explain how the respiratory system warms and humidifies inhaled air
- State the purpose and function of the mucociliary escalator
- Discuss the process of gas exchange at the alveolar level
- Describe the various skeletal structures related to the respiratory system
- Explain the actual process of breathing
- Discuss several common respiratory system diseases

MULTIMEDIA APPLICATIONS

CD-ROM Interactive Exercises

- Animation on gas exchange, 13.1
- 3-D animation of the respiratory system and an interactive drag-and-drop labeling exercise, 13.2
- Videos on various oxygen-delivery devices and respiratory treatments, 13.3
- Interactive drag-and-drop labeling exercise concerning the alveolar area, 13.4
- Interactive exercise on labeling the muscles of ventilation, 13.5
- Animations and videos on COPD, asthma, ARDS, allergic rhinitis, apnea, and tuberculosis, 13.6
- Interactive games and puzzles, 13-7

www.prenhall.com/colbert

- Professional Profiles
  - Respiratory Therapist
  - Perfusionist
- Related Internet Links
- Additional Review Questions

Pronunciation Guide

Correct pronunciation is important in any journey so that you and others are completely understood. Here is a "see and say" Pronunciation Guide for the more difficult terms to pronounce in this chapter.

adenoid (AD eh noid)
alveoli (al VEE oh lye)
atelectasis (at eh LEK tah sis)
bronchi (BRONG kye)
bronchioles (BRONG kee ohlz)
carina (kuh RINE uh)
cilia (SIL ee ah)
conchae (KONG Kay)
diaphragm (DIE ah fram)
emphysema (em fih SEE mah)
empyema (em pye EE mah)
epiglottis (ep ih GLOT is)
erythropoiesis (eh rith roh poy EE sis)
hilum (HIGH lim)
laryngitis (lar in JIGH tis)
laryngopharynx (lah ring goh FAIR inks)
larynx (LAIR inks)
lingula (LING gu lah)
mediastinum (mee dee ah STY num)
nasopharynx (nay zoh FAIR inks)
parietal pleura (pah RYE eh tal PLOO rah)
pharyngitis (far in JIGH tis)
pharynx (FAIR inks)
oropharynx (oh roh FAIR inks)
tuberculosis (too ber kew LOH sis)
trachea (TRAY kee ah)

SYSTEM OVERVIEW

Along your journey, you will undoubtedly have plenty of exercise walking to see the sights. Have you ever wondered why you feel out of breath or why breathing faster and deeper helps you to recover from strenuous exercise? Our body uses energy from the food we eat, but cells can obtain the energy from foodstuffs only with the help of the vital gas oxygen (O_2), which allows for cellular respiration. Luckily, oxygen is found in relative abundance in the atmosphere and therefore in the air we breathe. However, when the cells use the oxygen, they produce the gaseous waste carbon dioxide (CO_2). If allowed to build up in the body, carbon dioxide would become toxic, so the bloodstream carries the carbon dioxide to the lungs to be exhaled and eliminated from the body. The respiratory system's primary role, therefore, is to bring oxygen from the atmosphere into the bloodstream and to remove the gaseous waste by-product carbon dioxide. As you can see from this discussion, the respiratory system is closely interrelated with the heart and circulatory system. Due to their close relationship, these two systems can be grouped together in medicine to form the **cardiopulmonary system.**

Amazing Body Facts

AUTOCONTROL OF CARDIOPULMONARY SYSTEM

The cardiovascular and respiratory or pulmonary systems function without any conscious effort on your part. You probably didn't realize it, but as you read the previous paragraph and these last two sentences, your heart beat approximately 70 times and pumped approximately 5 liters of blood around your body. During that same time, you breathed approximately 12 times, moving over 6,000 milliliters of air.

cardio = *heart*
pulmono = *lungs*

The respiratory system consists of the following major components:

- Two lungs, the vital organs of the respiratory system
- Upper and lower airways that *conduct* or move gas in and out of the system
- Terminal air sacs called alveoli surrounded by a network of capillaries that provide for *gas exchange*

- A thoracic cage that houses, protects, and facilitates function for the system
- Muscles of breathing that include the main muscle, the diaphragm, and accessory muscles

thorac/o = *chest*

Please take a few minutes to look at Figure 13–1 ■. We will explore each of these components as we travel through the respiratory system.

Ventilation Versus Respiration

Before beginning our journey, it is important to pave the way with a solid understanding of some commonly confused concepts. The air we breathe is a mixture of several gases, as can be seen from Table 13–1. The predominant gas is nitrogen (N_2), but this is an *inert* gas, which means it does not combine or interact in the body. Even though nitrogen travels into the respiratory system and comes out virtually unchanged, it is vitally

13-1 To view an animation on gas exchange, please go to the CD-ROM for this chapter.

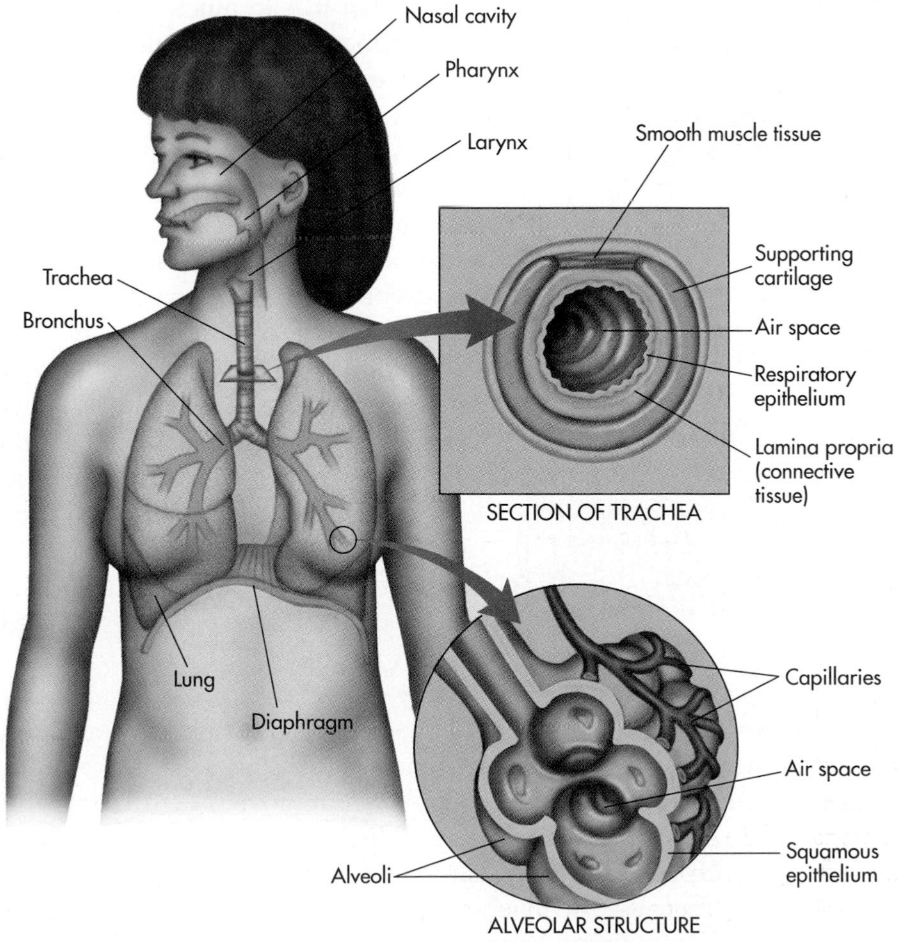

FIGURE ■ 13–1

The components of the respiratory system.

TABLE 13–1 Gases in the Atmosphere

GAS	% OF ATMOSPHERE
nitrogen (N_2)	78.08
oxygen (O_2)	20.95
carbon dioxide (CO_2)	.03
argon	.93

Note: The atmosphere also contains trace gases such as neon and krypton.

Applied Science

GAS EXCHANGE IN PLANTS

Fortunately for the earth's ecosystem, plant physiology of gas exchange is exactly opposite that of humans. Plants take in the CO_2 in the atmosphere and utilize it for energy, then release oxygen into our atmosphere. The earth's largest source of oxygen released is the Amazon rainforest, which is unfortunately being destroyed at a high rate every day. We truly need a green earth to survive, so thank the next plant you see.

The respiratory therapist's main job is to insure proper ventilation of the respiratory system through a variety of treatment modalities. Perfusionists, on the other hand, run a machine that actually performs gas exchange. For example, during a heart or lung transplant, the blood supply is temporarily rerouted through a respirator until the new heart or lung is transplanted. Because this procedure requires a lot of time, the rerouted blood must be oxygenated and carbon dioxide removed via a special mechanical membrane. To learn more about these two related and exciting professions, please visit the companion Web site.

important as a support gas that keeps the lungs open with its constant volume. The next greatest concentrated gas is oxygen, and it is very physiologically active within our bodies. You'll notice that carbon dioxide is in low concentration in the air we inhale, but it is in much higher concentration in the air we exhale.

The respiratory system contains a very intricate set of tubes that move, or conduct, gas from the atmosphere deep into the lungs. This movement of gas is accomplished by what we call breathing. However, a more precise look at the process of breathing shows that it is actually two separate processes. The first is **ventilation,** which is the bulk movement of the air down to the terminal end of the lungs where the actual *gas exchange* takes place with the bloodstream. The process of gas exchange, in which oxygen is added to the blood and carbon dioxide is removed, is termed **respiration.** Since the gas exchange in the lungs occurs between the blood and the air in the external atmosphere, it is more precisely called *external respiration*. The oxygenated blood is transported internally via the cardiovascular system to the cells and tissues where gas exchange is now termed *internal respiration*, and oxygen moves into the cells as carbon dioxide is removed. Ventilation, therefore, is not the same thing as respiration. When you watch a television show that says place the patient on a respirator, it is incorrect and the person should say "a ventilator" because the machine is only moving the gas mixture (ventilating) the patient and not causing gas exchange. See Figure 13–2 ■ which contrasts these important processes.

ventilation *(ven tih LAY shun)*
respiration *(ress pih RAY shun)*
perfusion = *blood flow*

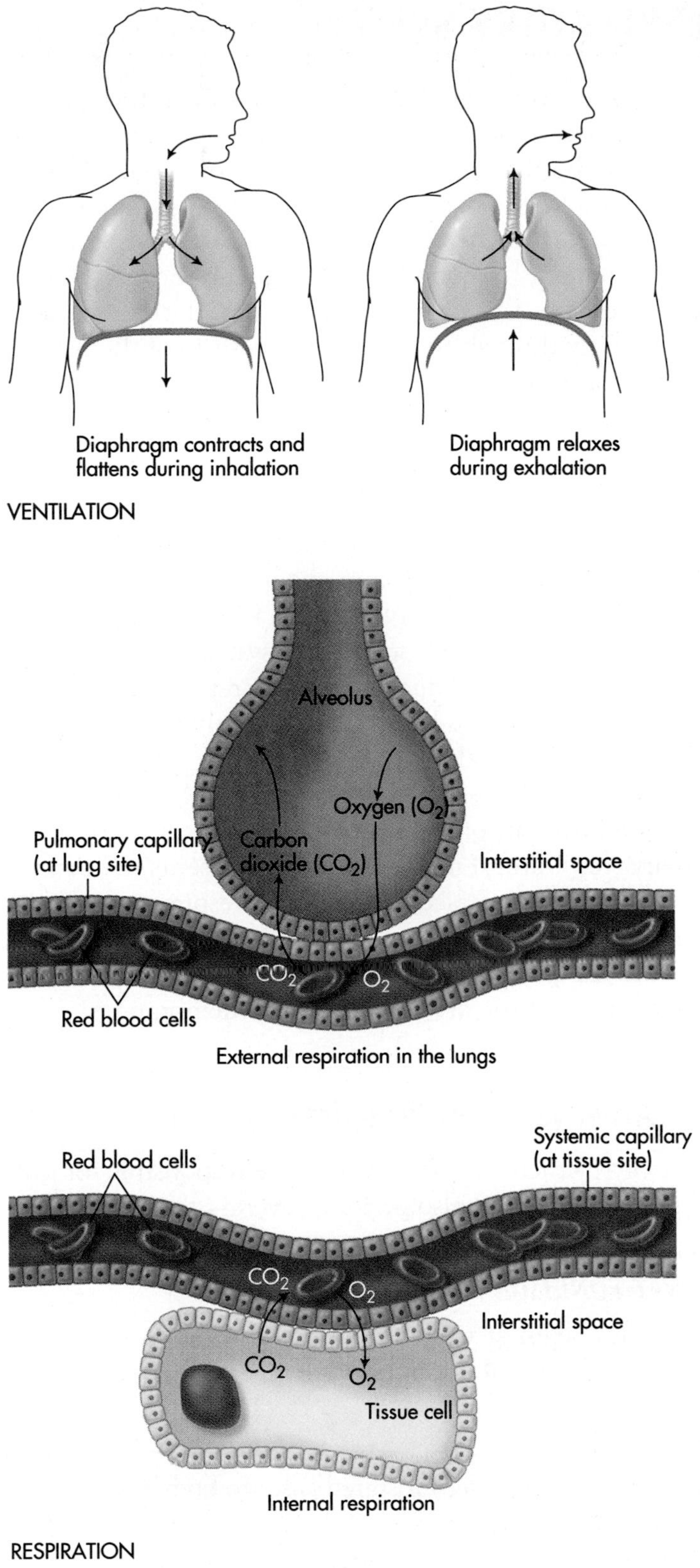

FIGURE ■ 13–2

Contrast of ventilation and external and internal respiration.

THE RESPIRATORY SYSTEM

The respiratory system is responsible for providing all of the body's oxygen needs and removing carbon dioxide. Unlike cars that have large gas tanks for fuel storage, the human body has a very small reserve of oxygen. In fact, its oxygen reserve lasts only about 4 to 6 minutes. If that reserve is used up and additional oxygen is unavailable, then death is the obvious outcome. Therefore, the body must continually replenish its oxygen by bringing in the oxygen molecules from the atmosphere. Again, this process is called ventilation. We now begin our breathtaking journey through the internal structures of the respiratory system by following the path oxygen molecules take.

The Airways and the Lungs

bronchi *(BRONG kye)*
bronchioles *(BRONG kee ohlz)*
alveoli *(al VEE oh lye)*

In a general sense, the respiratory system is a series of branching tubes called **bronchi** and **bronchioles** that transport the atmospheric gas deep within our lungs to the small air sacs called **alveoli,** which represent the terminal end of the respiratory system. To better visualize this system, look at a stalk of broccoli held upside down. The stalk and its branchings represent the airways, and the green bumpy stuff on the end is like the terminal alveoli. See, not only is broccoli good for you, but it can also be a learning tool.

capillaries *(KAP ih lair eez)*

Each alveolus is surrounded by a network of small blood vessels called **capillaries.** This combination of the alveoli and the capillary is called the alveolar–capillary (respiratory) membrane and represents the connection, or for you computer buffs, the interface, between the respiratory and cardiovascular systems. This is where the vital process of gas exchange takes place. Before getting in depth into this process, let's trace the journey that oxygen molecules must take in order to arrive at the alveolar–capillary membrane.

The Upper Airways of the Respiratory Tract

The upper airways, which start at the nose, are responsible for initially conditioning the inhaled air. They also perform several other important functions.

UPPER AIRWAY FUNCTIONS

nares *(NAIR eez)*

The upper airways begin at the two openings of the nose, called **nostrils** or **nares,** and end at the **vocal cords** (see Figure 13–3 ■). The functions of the upper airway include:

- Heating or cooling (inhaled) inspired gases to body temperature (37 degrees Celsius)
- Filtering (inhaled) particles from the inspired gases
- Humidifying inspired gases to a relative humidity of 100 percent
- Providing for the sense of smell, or *olfaction*
- Producing sounds, or *phonation*
- Ventilating, or conducting, the gas down to the lower airways

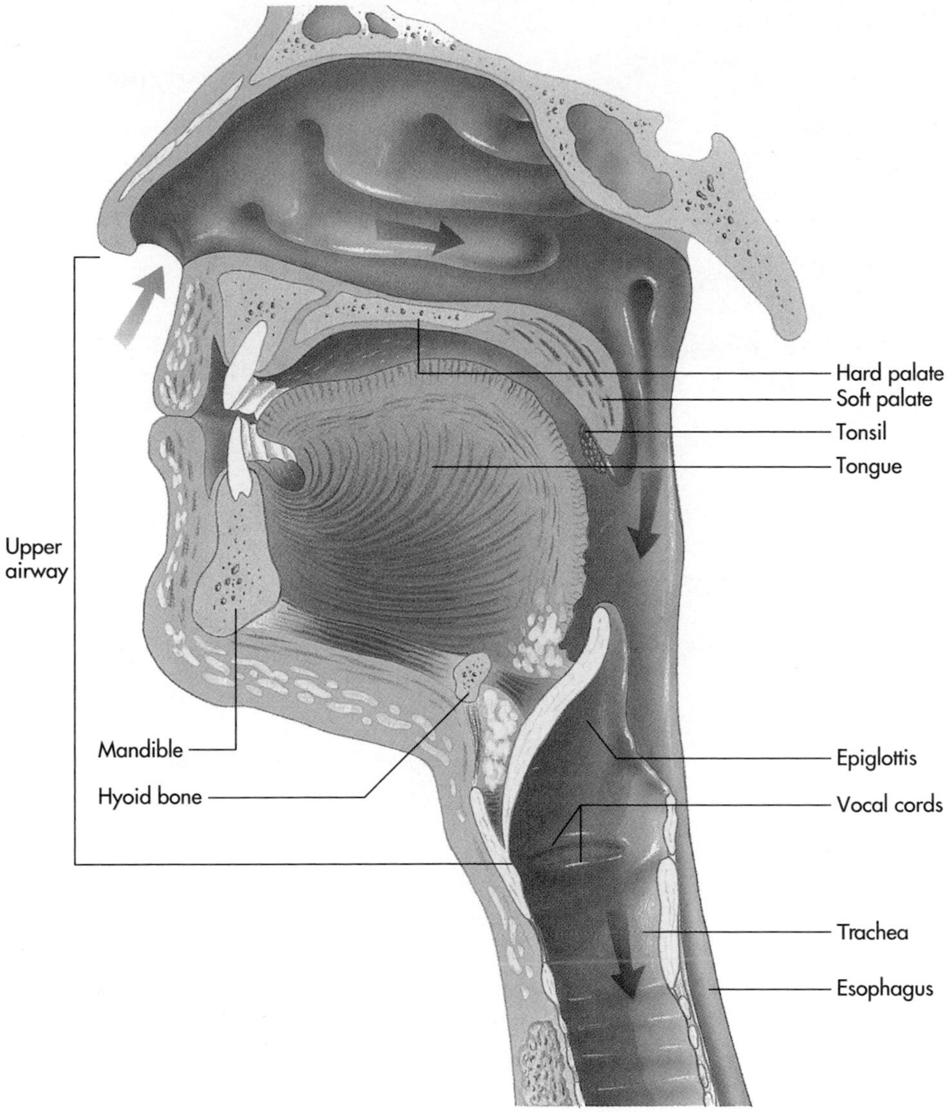

FIGURE ■ 13–3

The upper airway.

THE NOSE

While some people do breathe in through their mouths, under normal circumstances we were meant to breathe in through our nose for reasons that become clear as this discussion progresses. The nose is a rigid structure made of cartilage and bone. There are three main regions contained within the space behind the nose, called the **nasal cavity.** The two nasal cavities are separated by a wall called the *septal cartilage*. The regions contained within each nasal cavity are the vesitubular, olfactory, and respiratory region of the nose. Please see Figure 13–4 ■.

nasal cavity *(NAY zl CAV ih tee)*

The vestibular region is located inside the nostrils and contains the coarse nasal hairs that act as the first line of defense for the respiratory system. These hairs, called *vibrissae*, are covered with sebum, a greasy substance secreted by the sebaceous glands of the nose. Sebum helps to trap large particles and also keeps the nose hairs soft and pliable—those unwanted nose hairs really do have a

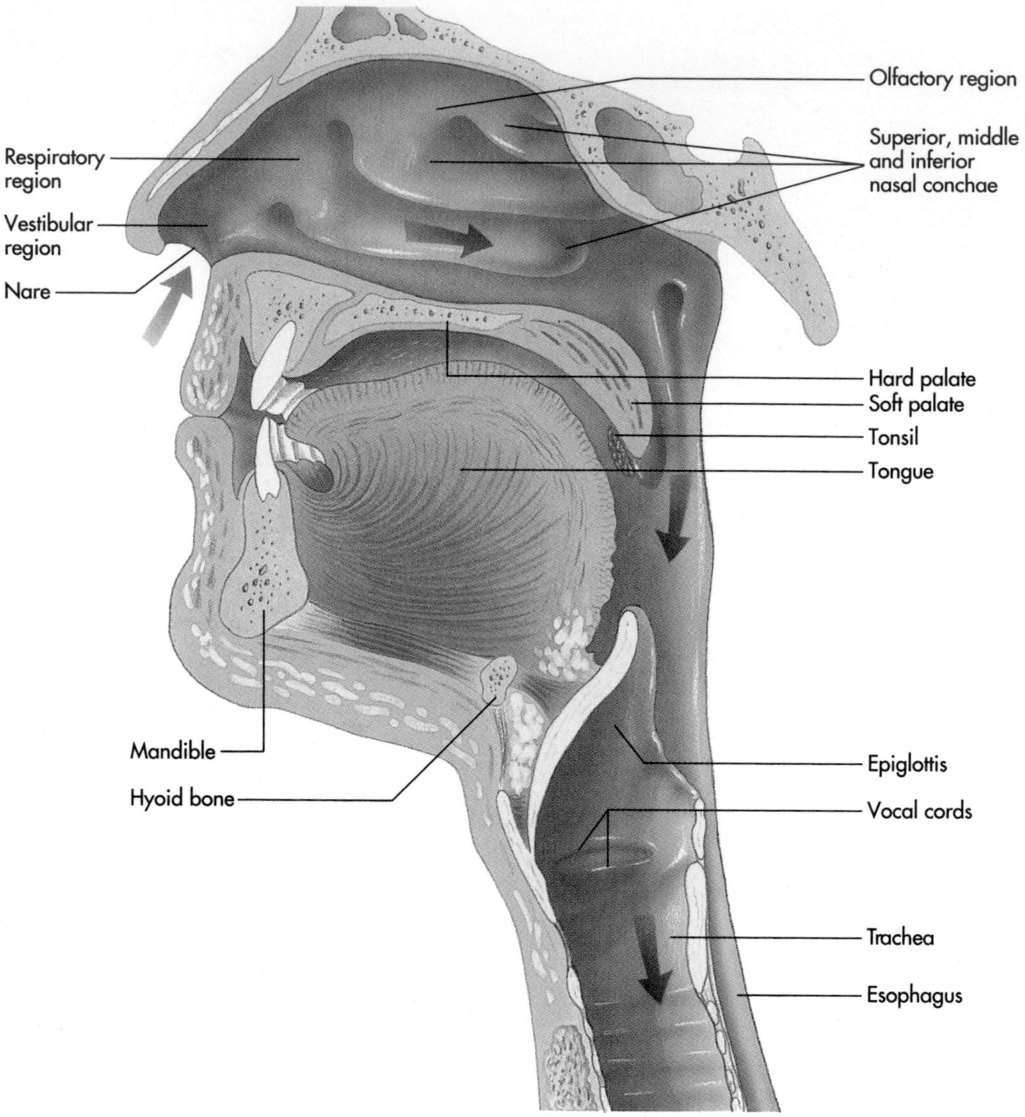

FIGURE 13–4

The nasal regions.

> *Applied Science*
>
> **FALSE ADVERTISING AND OXYGEN**
>
> Oxygen is a colorless, odorless, tasteless gas. However, a recent trend began in 2000: so-called oxygen bars where you can treat yourself to supplemental oxygen. Interestingly, they offer oxygen in different flavors, like raspberry and chocolate. You now know this is impossible. The tasteless, odorless oxygen remains tasteless and odorless, but the plastic tubing that delivers the oxygen is scented in assorted "flavors." So much for truth in advertising.

role as a gross particle filter. "Gross" in this case means large. The vestibular region helps to filter out large particles so they do not enter the lungs, where they could irritate and clog the airways.

The olfactory region is strategically placed on the roof of the nasal cavity. The advantage to this is that sniffing inspired gas into this region keeps it there and does not allow the gas to reach deeper into your lungs. This is a safe way to sample a potentially noxious or dangerous gas without taking a deep breath into the lungs, where it could cause severe damage. It is interesting to note that your ability to taste is related to your sense of smell. If you ever had a nasty head cold and could not taste your food, you now know why.

The air from the atmosphere must be warmed to body temperature and must also be moistened so the airways and the lungs do not dry out. This is a job for the respiratory region. Keep in mind that the respiratory region resides in the nasal cavity, which is lined with mucous membranes that are richly supplied with blood. The respiratory region possesses three scroll-like bones known as **turbinates,** or **conchae** (again see Figure 13–4). These split up the gas into three channels, thereby providing more surface area for incoming air to make contact with the nasal mucosa. While the respiratory region has a small volume of 20 milliliters, if you could unfold the turbinates, you would have a surface area of 106 *square centimeters!*

conchae *(KONG Kay)*

In addition, because the nasal cavity is no longer a straight passageway, the air current becomes turbulent so more air makes contact with these richly vascularized mucous membranes that transmit heat and moisture to the inspired gas. Incredibly, these moist mucous membranes add 650 to 1000 milliliters of water each day to moisten inspired air to 80 percent relative humidity within the respiratory region of the nose. In such a short distance, this is a pretty impressive humidification process. When the furnace in your house turns on in cold weather, this may dry the inspired air significantly and make it harder for your respiratory region to work. Therefore, humidifying this dry gas with water, such as from a room humidifier, may keep added stress off of your body's natural humidification system.

Amazing Body Facts

WHY DO WE BREATHE THROUGH OUR MOUTH?

You may have seen your favorite football player wearing an odd-looking strip of plastic across the nose. This is to help make breathing easier by increasing the diameter of the nostrils. The nose is responsible for one half to two thirds of the total airway resistance in breathing. Airway resistance represents the work required to move the gas down the tube. The larger the tube, the less resistance and therefore less work involved in breathing. Therefore, mouth breathing predominates during stress and exercise because it is easier for the gas (less resistant) to travel through the larger oral opening. Of course, when you get a head cold and your nasal passages become blocked by secretions, it becomes necessary to breathe through the easier or open route of the mouth. On your journey, you must always be ready for detours.

TEST YOUR KNOWLEDGE 13-1

Choose the best answer:

1. Which gas is found in the atmosphere?
   a. oxygen
   b. nitrogen
   c. carbon dioxide
   d. all the above

2. The process of moving gas into and out of the respiratory system is
   a. ventilation
   b. external respiration
   c. internal respiration
   d. diffusion

3. The process of gas exchange at the tissue sites is called
   a. ventilation
   b. external respiration
   c. internal respiration
   d. osmosis

4. Gas exchange takes place across the
   a. bronchi
   b. bronchioles
   c. alveolar–capillary membrane
   d. heart

5. The bones in the respiratory region of the nose are called
   a. sinuses
   b. turbinates
   c. tetonic plates
   d. bronchioles

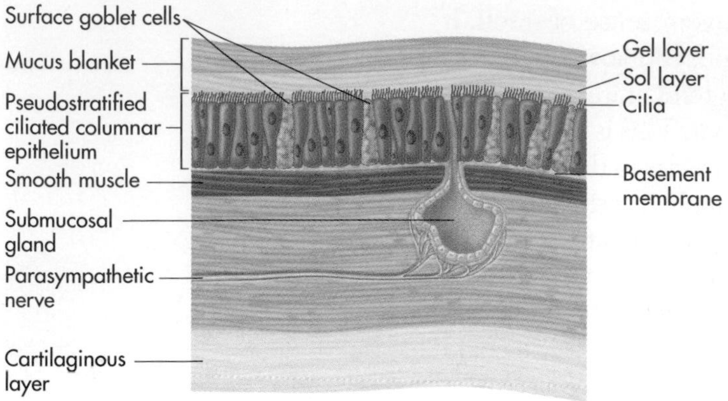

FIGURE ■ 13–5

The mucociliary escalator.

GOING TO RIDE THE MUCOCILIARY ESCALATOR

The epithelial lining of the respiratory region of the nose plays a very important role in keeping this region of the nose clean and free of debris build-up. Cells in the epithelial layer (or respiratory mucosa) are called *psuedostratified ciliated columnar cells* and are found not only in the respiratory region of the nose but throughout most of the airways. See Figure 13–5 ■. The epithelium is a single layer of tall, column-like cells with nuclei located at different heights, giving the false appearance of two layers of cells when in fact there is only one—hence the term *pseudostratified columnar*. Now all we need to add is the cilia. Each columnar cell has 200 to 250 cilia on its surface. **Cilia** are hairlike projections that can beat at a fantastic rate. Think of them as super-duper rowers in a boat.

pseudo = *false*
stratified = *layers*

Goblet cells and submucosal glands are interspersed in the respiratory mucosa and produce about 100 milliliters of mucus per day. The mucus actually resides as two layers. The cilia reside in the sol layer, which contains thin, watery fluid that allows them to beat freely. The gel layer is on top of the sol layer; as its name suggests, it is more viscous or gelatinous in nature. This sticky gel layer traps small particles, such as dust or pathogens, on the mucus blanket, much like flypaper. Once the debris are trapped on the mucus blanket, it must be removed from the lung.

cilia *(SIL ee ah)*

So how does this mucous layer actually work? The microscopic, hairlike cilia act as tiny "oars," and in Figure 13–5, you can see that these oars rest in the watery sol layer. They beat at an incredible rate of 1,000 to 1,500 times per minute and propel the gel layer and its trapped debris onward and upward about 1 inch per minute to be expelled from the body. When this process occurs in the nose, the debris-laden secretions are pushed toward the front of the nasal cavity to be expelled through the nose. The psuedostratified ciliated columnar epithelium, located in the airways of the lungs, propels the gel layer toward the oral cavity to be either expectorated with a cough or swallowed into the stomach. Some texts refer to this epithelial layer as the *mucociliary escalator,* which gives a better picture of what it does. This escalator works 24/7, that is unless something paralyzes it, such as smoking.

para = *around*
nasal = *referring to nose*
sinuses =

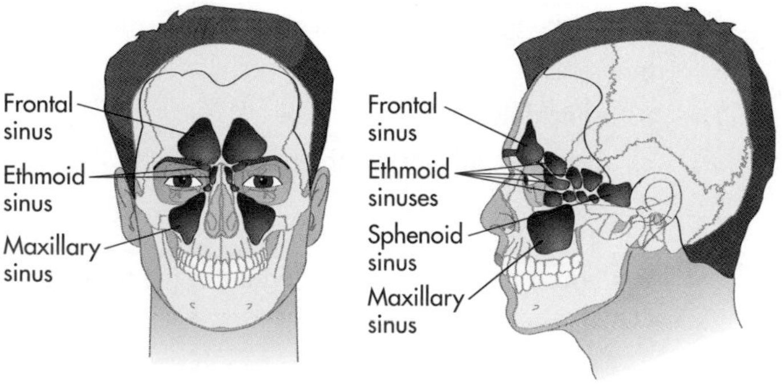

FIGURE ■ 13–6

The paranasal sinuses.

The Sinuses

Have you ever heard of someone being called an airhead? Technically, we are all airheads because the skull contains air-filled cavities (commonly called **sinuses**) that connect with the nasal cavity via small passageways. Because these are located around the nose, they are called paranasal sinuses. They are lined with respiratory mucosa that continually drain their secretions into the nose. The sinuses are named for the specific facial bones in which they are located (see Figure 13–6 ■).

These cavities of air in the bones of the cranium are believed to help in the prolongation and intensification of sound produced by the voice. If you ever shouted inside a cave, you noticed a more resonant quality to the sound. In addition, it is theorized the air-filled sinuses help to lighten the heavy head that sits atop the neck.

Sinuses do not exist at birth but develop as you grow and influence facial changes as you mature. Sinuses also provide further warming and moisturizing of inhaled air.

The Pharynx

The pharynx is a hollow, muscular structure lined with epithelial tissues. The throat (called **pharynx** by trained professionals) begins behind the nasal cavities and is divided into the following three sections, as shown in Figure 13–7 ■.

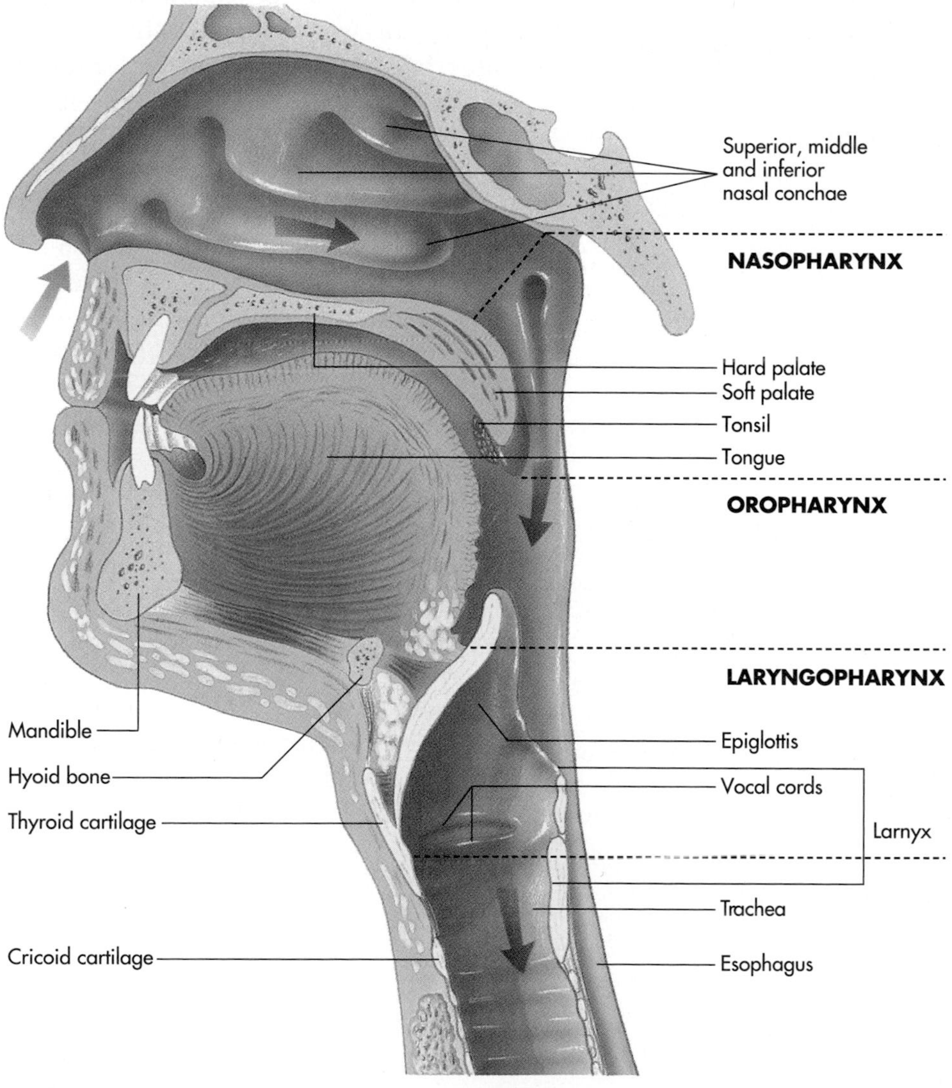

FIGURE ■ 13–7

The nasopharynx, oropharynx, and laryngopharynx.

- nasopharynx
- oropharynx
- laryngopharynx

hypo = *below*
adenoid *(AD eh noid)*
eustachian tubes *(yoo STAY she ehn)*
palatine tonsils *(PAL ah tighn TAHN sill)*

The **nasopharynx** is the uppermost section of the pharynx and begins right behind the two nasal cavities. Air that is breathed through the nose passes through the nasopharynx. This section also contains lymphatic tissue of the immune system, called the **adenoids,** and passageways to the middle ear called **eustachian tubes.** You can understand how an infection located in the nasal cavities can lead to an ear infection, and vice versa.

The **oropharynx** is the next structure and is located right behind the oral or buccal cavity. Air that is breathed through the mouth as well as air that is breathed through the nose passes through here. It is important to note that anything that is swallowed also passes through this section. Therefore, the oropharnyx conducts not only atmospheric gas but also food and liquid.

The oral entrance is a strategic area to place "guardians" for the immune system because this is where pathogens can easily enter the body. Lymphoid tissue, or tonsils, such as the **palatine tonsils,** are located in this area. Another set of tonsils, the lingual tonsils, are found at the back of the tongue. During the process of swallowing, the uvula and soft palate move in a posterior and superior position to protect the nasopharynx and nasal cavity from allowing food or liquid to enter. Actually swallow and feel this happening within your oral cavity. This protection can be overcome by forceful laughter, and that is why when you laugh with liquid or food in your mouth, the food or liquid can sometimes come up through your nose.

Clinical Application

KEEPING THE VITAL AIRWAY OPEN

Just like any vital highway, the airway needs to remain open to a flow of traffic, or the oxygen molecules will cease to flow into the alveoli and therefore not get into the bloodstream to supply the tissues. While a traffic jam can last for hours, oxygen flow can be disrupted for only a few minutes without tragic results. For example, if the upper airway swells shut from a severe allergic reaction to a bee sting, an emergency airway must be established. Referring back to Figure 13–7, you see space between the thyroid and cricoid cartilages and this is where an emergency cricoidthyroidotomy is performed. This space has few blood vessels or nerves, which makes it ideal in an emergency situation to place a temporary breathing tube.

Sometimes a longer-term breathing tube must be inserted into the lungs via a technique called intubation. This tube passes through the vocal cords and sits above the juncture (carina) between the right and left lung. A machine called a ventilator can move air into and out of the damaged lungs at this juncture. The tube has an inflatable cuff to seal the airway once it is in place. Knowledge that the vocal cords open and close during breathing becomes clinically significant. Adduction seals the vocal cords and occurs during expiration, while abduction opens the cords, increasing the size of the glottic opening during inspiration. If the patient is breathing, it is better to pass the tube with the deflated cuff through the narrow opening of the vocal cords during a breath in when the cords are open. Conversely, when removing the tube (extubation), the health care professional must always remember to deflate the cuff so it doesn't damage the cords as the tube is pulled back through them. It should go without saying (no pun intended) that a patient cannot talk when intubated because the vocal cords cannot function properly. If you ever see a TV soap opera or movie where someone is talking with a tube going down his or her mouth into the lungs, you will know it is impossible. More permanent airways, called tracheostomy tubes, can be placed in the neck and are made so the patient can talk.

The Larynx

The larynx houses the important structure needed for speech. The **laryngopharynx** is the lowermost portion of the pharynx; an older term for it was the *hypopharynx* because of its position. Commonly known as the voice box, the larynx is a semi-rigid structure composed of several types of cartilage connected by muscles and ligaments that provide for movement of the vocal cords to control speech. The "Adam's Apple" is the largest of the cartilages found in the larynx. This cartilage is also anatomically known as the thyroid cartilage, beneath which is the cricoid cartilage. Both cartilages in the exposed areas of airways found in the neck are necessary to provide structure and support for airways so they do not collapse and block the flow of air in and out of the lungs.

Air that is breathed and anything that is swallowed passes through the laryngopharynx. Swallowed materials *should* pass through the **esophagus** to get to the stomach, and air *should* travel through the larynx and then the trachea on its way to the lungs. What directs the flow of "traffic" (air to the lungs and food and liquid to the stomach)? Is it a tiny highway worker directing traffic? No, it is directed by a mechanism termed the *glottic mechanism* (swallowing reflex). The space between the vocal cords is called the *rima glottis*, or simply the glottis. The **glottis** is the opening that leads into the larynx and eventually the lungs. Fortunately, there is a leaf-shaped, fibrocartilage, flaplike structure located above the opening, or glottis, called the **epiglottis.** The epiglottis closes over the opening to the larynx when you swallow and opens up when you breathe. This selective closure is called the glottic or sphinchter mechanism and facilitates the closing of the epiglottis over the glottic opening, thus sealing it so food does not enter the lungs.

esophagus *(eh SOFF ah guss)*

glottis *(GLOT is)*

epiglottis *(ep ih GLOT is)*
epi = *above*

Therefore, the lungs are closed to traffic when swallowing and the food and liquid travels down the only open tube or route, which is now the esophagus, leading into the stomach. When we breathe in, the gas preferentially travels into the lungs through a process that actually draws it into the lungs because of pressure differences. More on this soon.

The vocal cords are the area of division between the upper and lower airways, representing the point of transition to the lower airways. The lower airways start below the vocal cords, and we soon continue our journey down the lower airways all the way down to the end point, or alveoli.

otomy = *cutting into*

TEST YOUR KNOWLEDGE 13-2

Choose the best answer:

1. The hairlike structures that propel mucus in the airways are
   a. sol layer
   b. gel layer
   c. pathogens
   d. cilia

2. Which of the following is *not* true about the sinuses?
   a. air-filled cavities
   b. located in the skull and around the nose
   c. help to lighten the head
   d. gas exchange occurs there

3. Food is prevented from entering the _____ when eating by the closure of the _____.
   a. esophagus, glottis
   b. esophagus, epiglottis
   c. trachea, epiglottis
   d. epiglottis, glottis

4. The vocal cords are found in the
   a. laryngopharynx
   b. nasopharynx
   c. oropharynx
   d. alveoli

THE LOWER RESPIRATORY TRACT

trachea *(TRAY kee ah)*

The airway that leads to the lungs and then branches out into the various lung segments resembles an upside down tree and is sometimes called the tracheobronchial tree. See Figure 13–8 ■. Upon leaving the vocal cords in the larynx, the inspired air enters the **trachea,** the lay term for which is windpipe. The trachea extends from the cricoid cartilage of the larynx to the sixth cervical vertebrae (approximately to the midpoint of the chest). The cartilage found in the trachea is in the form of C-shaped structures in the anterior portion of the trachea to provide rigidity and protection for the exposed airway in the neck. This C shape also serves another important purpose: the esophagus lies in the area where the C opens up posteriorly. Without the cartilage, there is some "give" in the posterior aspect of the larynx and trachea, so the esophagus can expand when you swallow larger chunks of food and they won't get stuck against the rigid cartilage of the trachea.

The trachea is the largest bronchus and can be thought of as the trunk of the tracheobronchial tree. Often it is represented as generation 0 (zero) because it is the trunk or start of the tree that has not yet begun to branch. Once the trachea reaches the center of the chest, it begins its first branching, or bifurcates, into two bronchi (bronchus is the singular form), the right mainstem and the

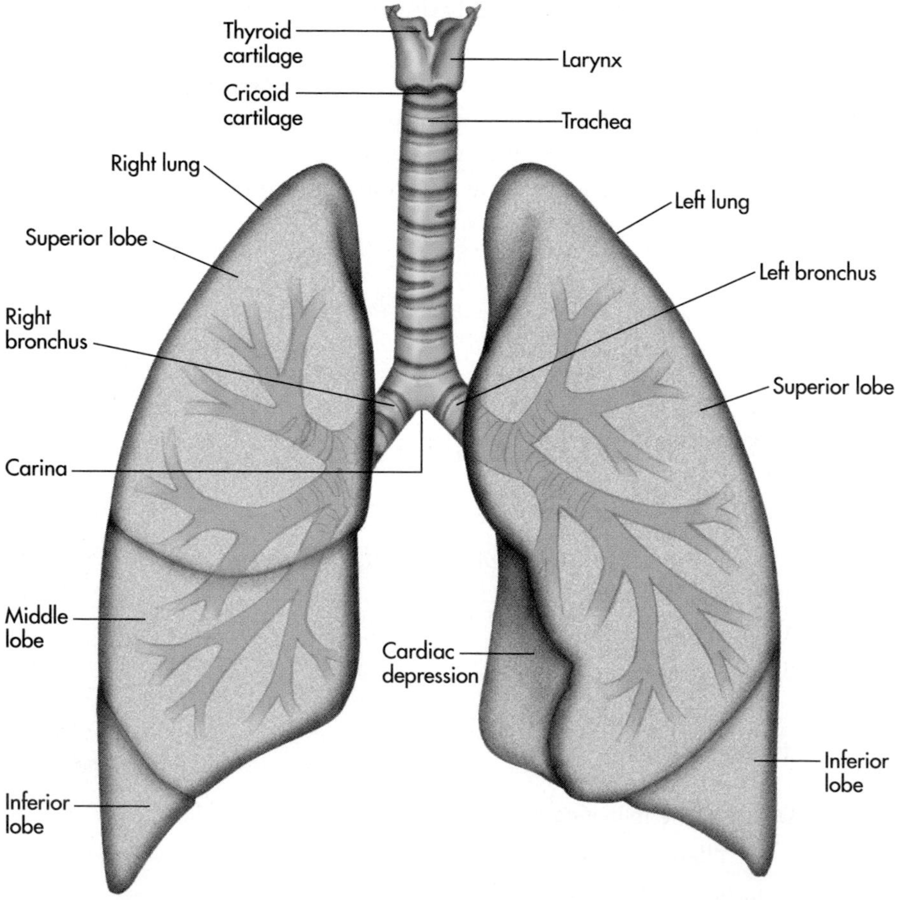

FIGURE ■ 13–8

The tracheobronchial tree.

left mainstem, which can be termed generation 1 because they represent the first branching of the tree. Each new branching is considered another generation. The site of bifurcation is called the **carina** (again, see Figure 13–8). One bronchus goes to the right lung and the other bronchus goes to the left lung. The mainstem bronchi are sometimes also referred to as the primary bronchi. Now the bronchi must branch into the five lobar bronchi (generation 2) that correspond to the five lobes of the lungs.

Each lung lobe is further divided into specific segments, and the next branching of bronchi are called the segmental bronchi (generation 3). At the point from the trachea down to the segmental bronchi, the tissue layers of the bronchi are all the same, only smaller, as they branch downward. The layers are the epithelial layer, which is the mucociliary escalator—or pseudostratified ciliated columnar cells—that keeps the area clean of debris. A middle lamina propria layer contains smooth muscle, lymph, and nerve tracts. The third layer is the protective and supportive cartilaginous layer (see Figure 13–9 ■).

> **Clinical Application**
>
> **THE ANGLE MAKES A DIFFERENCE**
>
> The angle of branching is not the same for both sides of the tracheobronchial tree. The right mainstem branches off at a 20 to 30 degree angle from the midline of the chest. The left mainstem branches off at a more pronounced 40 to 60 degree angle. This is important because the lesser angle of the right mainstem branching allows foreign bodies that are accidentally breathed in to more often lodge in the right lung. This is nice to know if a child has aspirated (taken into the lung) an object and the physician must enter the lung with a bronchocope to remove the object. Time may be critical, and it may make a difference if the search is begun immediately in the right lung because its anatomic structure makes it a high probability that the object has lodged there. In addition, a breathing tube or endotracheal tube may be placed too far into the lung and instead of sitting above the carina so both lungs are ventilated most likely will pass into and ventilate only the right lung. This is why an X-ray for proper tube placement is so important.

> **13-2** To view a 3-D representation of the respiratory system and to perform an interactive drag-and-drop labeling exercise on the lungs, please go to your CD-ROM for this chapter.

The branching becomes more numerous with tiny subsegmental bronchi (generations 4 to 9) branching deep within each lung segment. The diameter of subsegmental bronchi ranges from 1 to 6 millimeters. Cartilaginous rings are now irregular pieces of cartilage and will soon fade away completely. Notice as we move toward the gas exchange regions that the airways simplify to make it easier for gas molecules to pass through. Now we reach the very tiny airways called bronchioles (generations 10 to 15) that average only 1 millimeter in diameter. They have no cartilage layer, and the epithelial lining becomes ciliated cuboidal (short squat cells as opposed to large columns). The cilia, goblet cells, and submucosal gland are almost all gone by generation 15. There is no gas exchange yet, just simple conduction of the gas mixture containing the oxygen molecules down the tree. Now we reach the terminal bronchioles (generation 16), which have an average diameter of .5 millimeters, no goblet cells, no cartilage, no cilia, and no submucosal glands. This marks the end of the conducting areas, and we now journey into the gas exchange or respiratory zone of the lung.

The next airway beyond the terminal bronchiole is called the respiratory bronchiole (generations 17 to 19) because a small portion of gas exchange takes place here. The epithelial lining is simple cuboidal cells interspersed with actual alveoli-type cells, which are flat, pancake-like cells called *simple squamous*

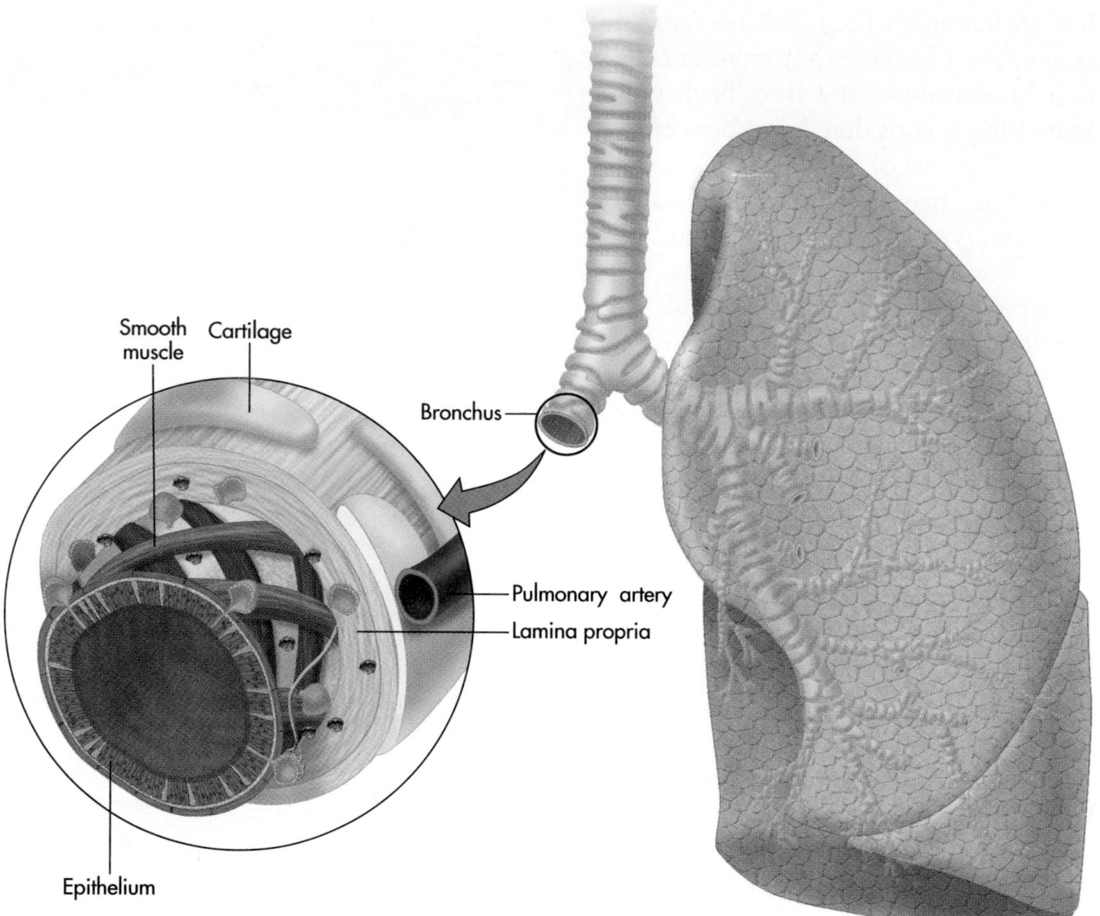

FIGURE ■ 13–9

Tissue layers in the bronchi.

Clinical Application

THERAPEUTIC OXYGEN

Often, a distressed respiratory system and sometimes the cardiac system needs supplemental oxygen to assist its function and meet its needs. There are many ways to deliver an enriched oxygen supply to the lungs, including an oxygen mask, nasal cannula (tube), and specialized devices to deliver both oxygen and extra humidity to the lungs to assist their function.

13-3 To view videos of various oxygen-delivery devices and respiratory treatments, please go to your CD-ROM for this chapter

pneumocytes. Alveolar ducts (generations 20 to 22) originate from the respiratory bronchioles wherein the walls of the alveolar ducts are completely made up of simple squamous cells arranged in a tubular configuration. The alveolar ducts give way to the grape bunch–like structures of several connected alveoli, better known as the alveolar sacs (generation 23). See Figure 13–10 ■.

The Alveolar Capillary Membrane: Where the Action Is

The alveoli are the terminal air sacs that are surrounded by numerous pulmonary capillaries and together make up the functional unit of the lung known as the

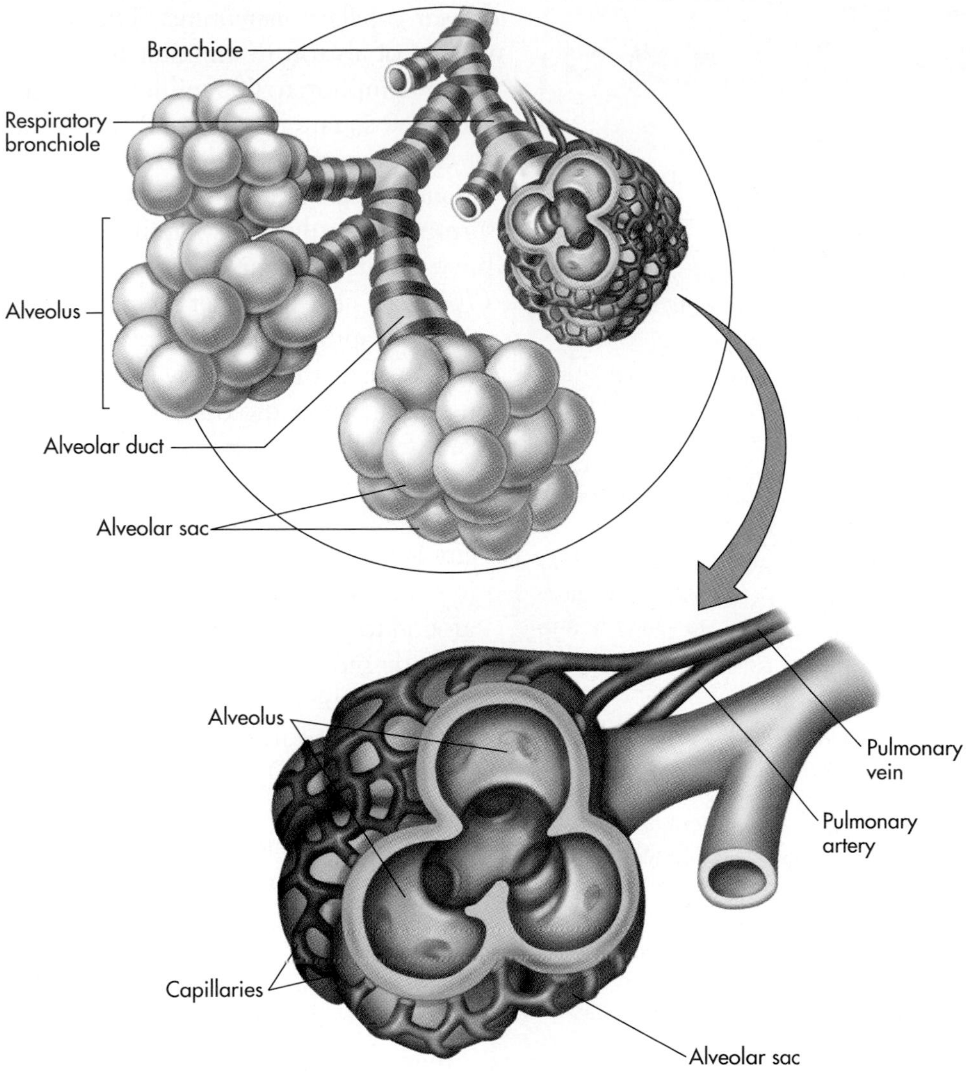

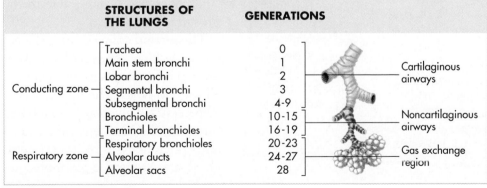

	STRUCTURES OF THE LUNGS	GENERATIONS	
Conducting zone	Trachea	0	Cartilaginous airways
	Main stem bronchi	1	
	Lobar bronchi	2	
	Segmental bronchi	3	
	Subsegmental bronchi	4-9	
	Bronchioles	10-15	Noncartilaginous airways
	Terminal bronchioles	16-19	
Respiratory zone	Respiratory bronchioles	20-23	Gas exchange region
	Alveolar ducts	24-27	
	Alveolar sacs	28	

FIGURE ■ 13–10

Conduction and gas exchange structures and functions.

> **13-4** To perform an interactive drag-and-drop labeling exercise concerning the alveolar area, please go to your CD-ROM for this chapter.

Clinical Application

WHAT CAN GO WRONG WITH GAS EXCHANGE?

The membrane between the alveoli and the capillaries is quite thin. In fact, it is only 0.004 millimeters thick! The thinness of this membrane aids in the diffusion of the gases between the lungs and the blood. Anything that would act as a barrier to oxygen molecules getting to or through this barrier would decrease the amount of oxygen that gets into the blood. For example, excessive secretions and fluid such as in pneumonia act as a barrier and reduce the oxygen levels in the blood, which can be measured by sampling arterial blood and analyzing the amount of each gas dissolved in it. This is called an arterial blood gas, or ABG. In the case of severe pneumonia, the level of oxygen known as the PaO_2 goes down because less oxygen can get into the blood, and the $PaCO_2$ in the arterial blood goes up because less CO_2 crosses into the lungs to be exhaled.

The blood cells can also be affected. Red blood cells, or **erythrocytes,** are responsible for the bulk of the transportation of oxygen and carbon dioxide in the blood via a protein-and iron-containing molecule called **hemoglobin,** which performs the actual transportation. It is estimated that there are about *280 million* hemoglobin molecules found in *each* erythrocyte!

In general, if the hemoglobin is carrying large amounts of oxygen, the blood will be bright red. If there is less oxygen and more carbon dioxide being carried, then the blood will be darker in color or may have a bluish tint. An obvious example of this can be seen when you look at the veins in your arm. Venous blood has lower levels of oxygen and higher levels of carbon dioxide. As a result, venous blood has a dark red tint. Low levels of red blood cells or anemia would limit the number of hemoglobin molecules that could transport oxygen and thus greatly reduce the amount in the blood available for the tissues. Therefore, the number of red blood cells and the amount of hemoglobin in your blood (both of which can be measured) is important in oxygen delivery to your tissues.

Your body can attempt to respond to low hemoglobin levels by producing more red blood cells by a process called **erythropoiesis.** This process begins once the kidneys detect low levels of oxygen coming to them from the blood. The kidneys release into the bloodstream a hormone called **erythropoietin.** This substance travels through the blood and eventually reaches specialized cells found in the red bone marrow. Once stimulated, these specialized cells begin to increase their production of erythrocytes until demand is met. Having too little iron in the body can also affect oxygen delivery because the iron in the hemoglobin is what holds onto the oxygen molecules. The terms *iron-poor* blood and *tired* blood come from the fact that a patient with low levels of iron tires easily due to low oxygen levels.

alveolar capillary membrane. The average number of alveoli in an adult lung ranges from 300 million to 600 million. This gives a total 80 square meters (m^2) surface area for the oxygen molecule to diffuse across (about the size of a tennis court) into the surrounding pulmonary capillaries, which have about the same cross-sectional area (70 m^2). The blood entering the pulmonary capillaries comes from the right side of the heart and is low in oxygen and high in carbon dioxide because it just came from the body tissues. Gas exchange or external respiration takes place, and the blood leaving the pulmonary capillary is high in oxygen and travels to the left side of the heart to be pumped around to the tissues. Conversely, carbon dioxide molecules are in high concentration in the pulmonary capillary blood and very low in the lung (remember, there is little CO_2 in the atmosphere), so CO_2 leaves the blood and enters the lung to be exhaled.

Upon closer inspection of the alveolar capillary membrane, you will see four distinct components. The first layer is the liquid **surfactant** layer that lines the alveoli. This phospholipid helps lower the surface tension in these very tiny spheres (alveoli) that would otherwise collapse due to the high surface tension.

The second component is the actual tissue layer, or alveolar epithelium, comprised of simple squamous cells of two types. The majority type (95 percent) of alveolar surface is flat, thin, pancake-like cells called squamous pneumocytes or Type I cells. These are where the gas molecules can easily pass through in the process of gas exchange. The alveoli also need to produce the valuable surfactant, and this is where the plump Type II, or granular pnuemocytes, come in. These highly metabolic cells not only produce surfactant but aid in cellular repair responsibilities. Finally, this area needs to be free of debris that would act as barriers to the vital process of gas exchange. This is where the "clean-up" cells called Type III cells or wandering macrophages ingest foreign particles as the macrophages wander throughout the alveoli. There are even small holes between the alve-

erythr/o = *red*
poiesis = *to make*
erythrocytes *(eh RITH roh sights)*
hemoglobin *(HEE moh GLOH binn)*
erythropoiesis *(eh RITH roh poy EE suss)*
erythropoietin *(eh RITH roh poy EH tin)*
surfactant *(sir FAC tent)*

oli called *pores of Kohn* that allow the macrophages to move from one alveolus to another.

pneumo = *air or lung*
cyte = *cell*

The third component of the alveolar capillary membrane is the *interstitial space*. This is the area that separates the basement membrane of alveolar epithelium from the basement membrane of the capillary endothelium and contains interstitial fluid. This space is so small that the membranes of the alveoli and capillary appear fused. However, if too much fluid gets into this space (interstitial edema), the membranes separate, which makes it harder for gas exchange to occur because the gas has to travel a greater distance and through a congested, fluid-filled space.

The fourth component is the *capillary endothelium* that forms the wall of the capillary. The capillary contains the blood with the red blood cells that carry the precious gas cargo to its destination.

Applied Science

THE AMAZING SURFACTANT

Not only does surfactant lower the surface tension when the alveoli are small (end-expiration), thereby preventing alveoli collapse, but when you take a deep breath (end-inspiration), your alveoli get larger and the surfactant layer thins and becomes less effective, its surface tension increasing because of its thinning. This prevents overexpansion or rupture of the alveoli. Lack of surfactant can cause stiff lungs that resist expansion. Surfactant develops late in fetal development, and premature babies therefore may not have sufficient levels. Without immediate intervention, their tiny lungs would collapse (*atelectasis*) and thus prevent vital gas exchange. If they are given too much volume to re-expand their stiff lungs, the alveoli may rupture, again because surfactant is not there to prevent overexpansion. Surfactant also has an antibacterial property that helps to fight harmful pathogens. Fortunately, medical science has developed surfactant replacement therapy that can instill surfactant into the lungs to maintain their function until babies have matured and can produce it on their own.

TEST YOUR KNOWLEDGE 13-3

Choose the best answer:

1. The largest bronchus or trunk of the tracheobronchial tree is the
   a. right mainstem bronchus
   b. left mainstem bronchus
   c. bronchiole
   d. trachea

2. The site of bifurcation of the right and left lungs is called the
   a. alveoli
   b. carina
   c. trachea
   d. capillary

3. If an object is aspirated into the airways, it is most likely to go to
   a. the right lung
   b. the left lung
   c. the stomach
   d. the oropharynx

4. The first portion of the airway where gas exchange begins is the
   a. terminal bronchiole
   b. trachea
   c. mainstem bronchus
   d. respiratory bronchiole

5. The alveolar layer that lowers surface tension to keep the alveoli expanded is the
   a. surfactant layer
   b. capillary layer
   c. epithelium layer
   d. macrophage layer

6. The alveolar cell that allows for gas exchange is the
   a. squamous cell
   b. granular cell
   c. macrophage cell
   d. Kohn cell

The Housing of the Lungs and Related Structures

mediastinum *(mee dee ah STY num)*

The lungs reside in the thoracic cavity and are separated by a region called the **mediastinum,** which contains the esophagus, heart, great vessels (superior and inferior vena cava and aorta), and trachea (see Figure 13–11 ■).

Breathing in and out causes the lungs to move within the thoracic cavity. Over time, an irritation could occur as the lungs rub the inside of the thoracic cage. To prevent such damage, each lung is wrapped in a sac, or serous membrane, called the **visceral pleura.** The thoracic cavity and the upper side of the diaphragm are lined with a continuation of this membrane called the **parietal pleura.** Between these two pleural layers is an intrapleural space (pleural cavity) that contains a slippery liquid called *pleural fluid.* This fluid greatly reduces the friction as an individual breathes.

visceral pleura *(VISS er al PLOO rah)*

parietal pleura *(pah RYE eh tal PLOO rah)*

The Actual Lungs

The right and left lungs are conical-shaped organs; the rounded peak is called the apex of the lung. The apices of the lung extend 1 to 2 inches above the clavicle. The bases of the lungs rest on the right and left hemidiaphragm. The right lung base is a little higher than the left to accommodate the large liver lying underneath. The medial surface of the lung has a deep, concave cavity that contains the heart and therefore is called the cardiac impression and is deeper on the left side. The **hilum** is the area where the root of each lung is attached. Each root contains the mainstem bronchus, pulmonary artery and vein, nerve tracts, and lymph vessels.

hilum *(HIGH lim)*

lingula *(LING gu lah)*

The right lung has three lobes—the upper, middle, and lower lobes—that are divided by the horizontal and oblique fissures. The left lung has only one fissure, the oblique fissure, and therefore only two lobes, called the left upper and left lower lobes. You may hear the term **lingula.** This is an area of the left lung that corresponds with the right middle lobe. Why only two lobes in the left, you may ask? Remember that the heart is located in a space (cardiac impression) in the left anterior area of the chest and therefore takes up some space of the left lung. In fact, the right lung is larger and about 60 percent of gas exchange occurs there. The lobes are even further divided into specific segments related to their anatomical position. For example, the apical segment of the right upper lobe is the top portion or tip of the right upper lobe.

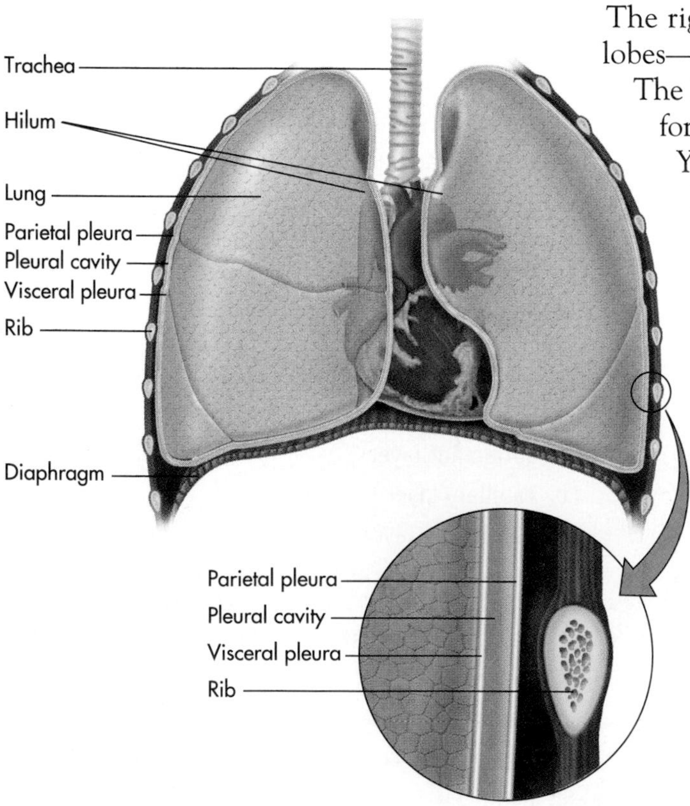

FIGURE ■ 13–11

Structures of the thoracic cavity.

The Protective Bony Thorax

The lungs, heart, and great vessels are all protected by the *bony thorax*. This bony and cartilaginous frame provides protection and also movement of the thoracic cage to accommodate breathing. The bony thorax includes the rib cage, the sternum or breastbone, and the corresponding thoracic vertebrae to which the ribs attach (see Figure 13–12 ■).

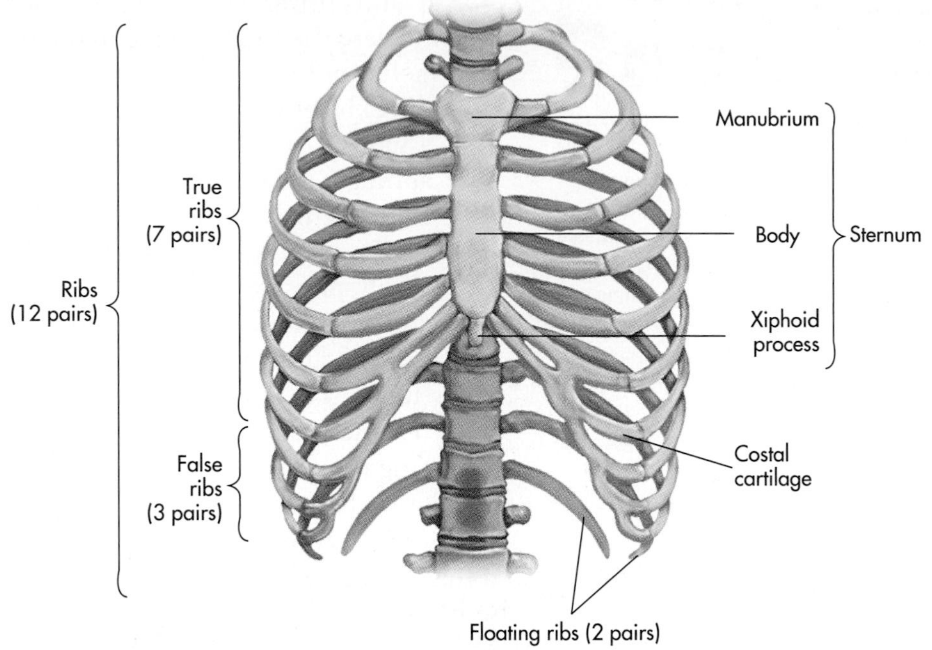

FIGURE ■ 13–12

The thoracic cage.

The **sternum,** or breastbone, is centrally located on the anterior portion of the thoracic cage and is comprised of the manubrium, body, and xiphoid process. This anatomical landmark is very important for proper hand placement in CPR. The hand is placed over the body of the sternum where compressions squeeze the heart between the body of the sternum and the thoracic vertebrae. If the hand placement is too low on the xiphoid process, it can break off and lacerate the internal organs.

sternum *(STER num)*

The **thoracic cage** consists of 12 pairs of elastic arches of bone called ribs. The ribs are attached by cartilage to allow for their movement while breathing. The true ribs are pairs 1 through 7 and are called *vertebrosternal* because they connect anteriorly to the sternum and posteriorly to the thoracic vertebrae of the spinal column. Pairs 8, 9, and 10 are called the false ribs, or *vertebrocostal*, because they connect to the costal cartilage of the superior rib and again posterior to the thoracic vertebrae. Rib pairs 11 and 12 are called the floating ribs because they have no anterior attachment.

thoracic cage *(tho RASS ik)*

How We Breathe

The control center that tells us to breathe is located in the brain in an area known as the **medulla oblongata.** Inspiration is an active process of ventilation in which the main breathing muscle, the **diaphragm** (a dome-shaped muscle when at rest), is sent a signal via the phrenic nerve and contracts and flattens, thereby increasing the space in the thoracic cavity (see Figure 13–13 ■). The increase in volume in the thoracic cavity causes a decrease in pressure because volume and pressure are indirectly related. This creates a lower than atmospheric pressure in the thoracic cavity, allowing air to rush into the lungs. The external intercostal muscles also assist by moving the ribs

medulla oblongata *(meh DULL lah ob lon GOT ah)*

diaphragm *(DIE ah fram)*

Amazing Body Facts

EXHALED CO_2 AND MOSQUITOES

Since mosquitoes are too small to carry flashlights, how do they find you in the dark? They do it by using carbon dioxide sensors to locate increased concentrations of CO_2 emitted by, you guessed it, your exhaled breath. Once they detect your exhaled CO_2, they use their heat sensors to find an area of skin on which to begin their banquet!

Another amazing carbon dioxide fact is that many people believe swimmers hyperventilate to get more oxygen in their systems before a sustained underwater dive. In reality, they are "blowing off" CO_2 to get their levels low. Since higher levels of CO_2 cause us to want to breathe, the body is fooled into believing it doesn't need to for a while longer, so swimmers can remain underwater longer. Unfortunately, the body still uses up its oxygen at a regular rate and sometimes uses enough of the reserve that swimmers risk losing consciousness.

up and outward during inspiration to increase the total volume in the thoracic cavity.

Exhalation, on the other hand, is usually a passive act. As the diaphragm relaxes, it forms a dome shape, which decreases the amount of space in the thoracic cavity. As a result, pressure in the lungs becomes greater than the atmospheric pressure and the air is pushed out of the lungs. The fact that the lungs are elastic tissue that is stretched during inspiration also aides in expiration because this elastic tissue now wants to return to rest, much as a stretched rubber band that is released.

What makes the brain tell the lungs how fast or how slowly to breathe? Although we can consciously speed up or slow down our breathing, **OUR BREATHING RATE IS NORMALLY CONTROLLED BY THE LEVEL OF CARBON DIOXIDE IN OUR BLOOD.** If carbon dioxide levels rise, it means that not enough CO_2 is being ventilated, so the medulla sends signals to the respiratory muscles to increase the rate and depth of breathing.

Sometimes the body needs help to breathe beyond resting or normal breathing. For example, during increased physical activity or in disease states in which more oxygen is required, **accessory muscles** are used to help pull up your rib cage to make an even larger space in the thoracic cavity. The accessory muscles used are the scalene muscles in the neck, the sternocleidomastoid, and pectoralis major and pectoralis minor muscles of the chest.

Although exhalation is a passive process, there are times, especially with certain disease states, when exhalation may need to be assisted. Again, the body has accessory muscles of exhalation that assist in a more forceful and active exhalation by increasing abdominal pressure. The main accessory muscles of exhalation are the various abdominal muscles that push up the diaphragm or the back muscles that pull down and thus compress the thoracic cage. See Figure 13–14 ■ for the specific accessory muscles of exhalation.

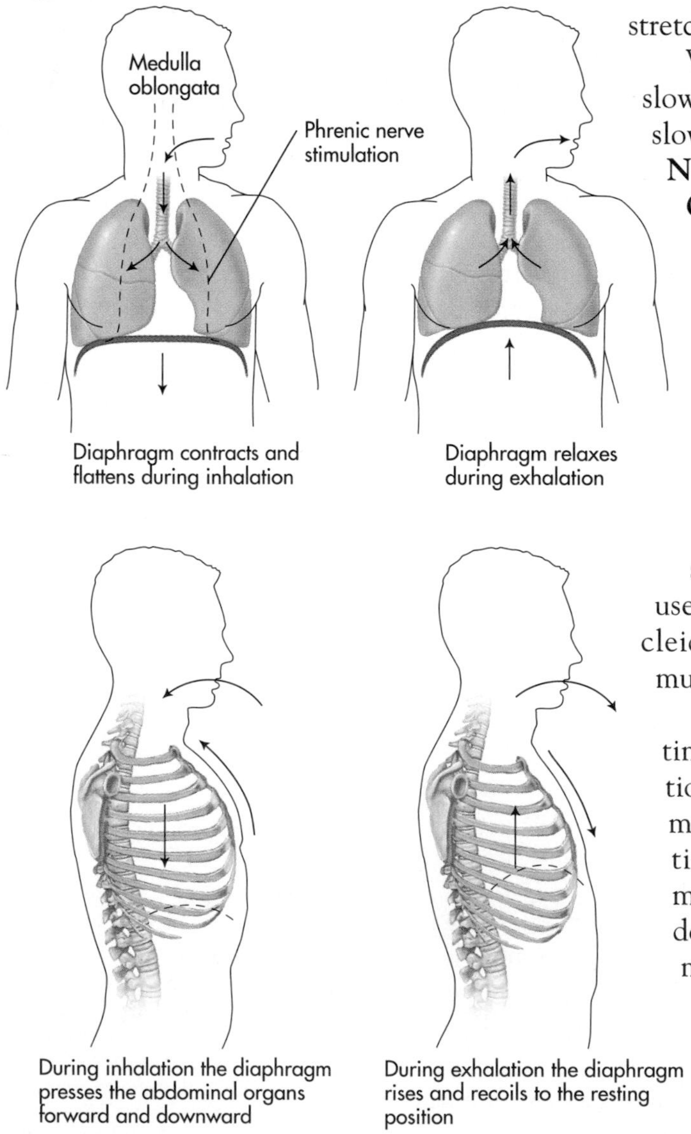
Medulla oblongata
Phrenic nerve stimulation
Diaphragm contracts and flattens during inhalation
Diaphragm relaxes during exhalation
During inhalation the diaphragm presses the abdominal organs forward and downward
During exhalation the diaphragm rises and recoils to the resting position

FIGURE ■ 13–13

How we breathe.

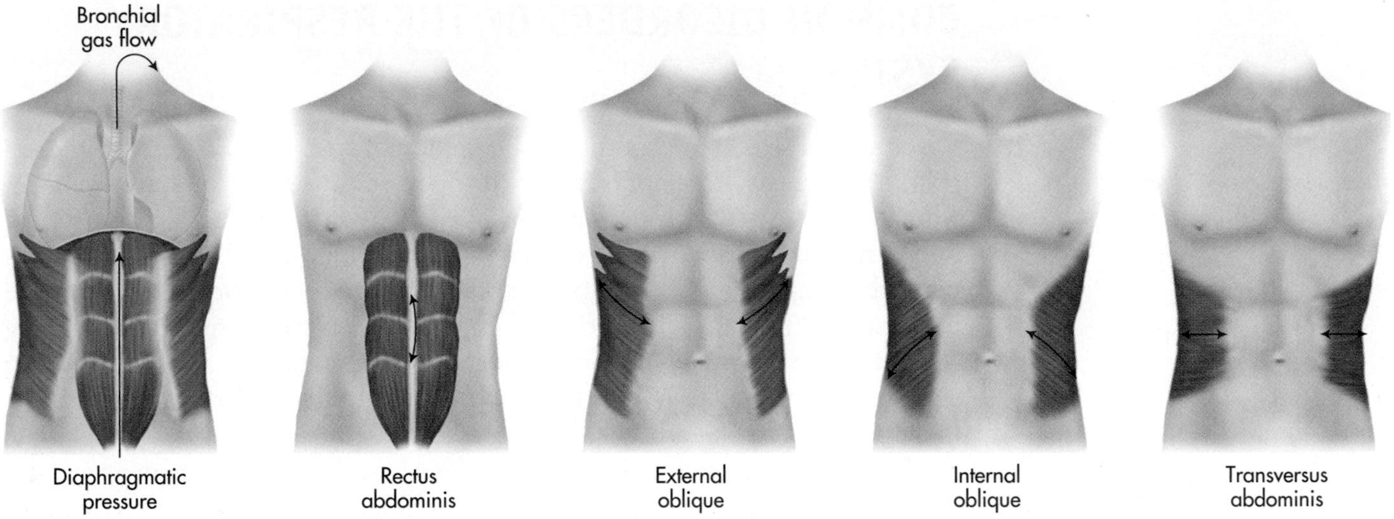

FIGURE ■ 13–14

The accessory muscles of exhalation.

13-5 For an interactive exercise on labeling the muscles of ventilation, please view the CD-ROM for this chapter.

TEST YOUR KNOWLEDGE 13-4

Choose the best answer:

1. The _____ pleural lines the thoracic cavity.
   a. visceral
   b. parietal
   c. mediastinum
   d. chest

2. The portion of the sternum where CPR is performed is the
   a. xiphoid process
   b. ribs
   c. manubrium
   d. body

3. The _____ nerve innervates the main breathing muscle, called the _____.
   a. thoracic; internal intercostals
   b. thoracic; diaphragm
   c. phrenic; external intercostals
   d. phrenic; diaphragm

4. Rib pairs 1 to 7 are attached to
   a. the vertebral column only
   b. the vertebral column and the sternum
   c. the sternum only
   d. are free floating

COMMON DISORDERS OF THE RESPIRATORY SYSTEM

atelectasis *(at eh LEK tah sis)*

Respiratory disease is one of the most common diseases seen in health care settings. **Atelectasis,** commonly found in the hospital setting, is a condition in which the air sacs of the lungs are either partially or totally collapsed. Atelectasis can occur in patients who cannot or will not take deep breaths to fully expand the lungs and keep the passageways open. Surgery or an injury of the thoracic cage (such as broken ribs) often makes deep breathing painful. Taking periodic deep breaths is important not only to expand the lungs but also to stimulate the production of surfactant, which helps to keep the small alveolar sacs open between breaths.

Patients with large amounts of secretions who cannot cough them up are also at risk for atelectasis because the secretions block airways and lead to areas of collapse. Quite often, if atelectasis is not corrected and secretions are retained, **pneumonia** can develop within 72 hours. Pneumonia is a lung infection that can be caused by either a virus, fungus, or bacterium. Inflammation occurs in the infected areas, with an accumulation of cell debris and fluid. In certain pneumonias, lung tissue is destroyed. Pneumonias, if severe enough, can lead to death.

COPD, or chronic obstructive pulmonary disease, is group of diseases in which patients have difficulty getting all the air out of their lungs and often large amounts of secretions and lung damage is involved. COPD refers to one of or a combination of **asthma, emphysema,** and **chronic bronchitis.**

asthma *(AZ mah)*
emphysema *(em fih SEE mah)*
chronic bronchitis *(brong KYE tiss)*

Asthma is a potentially life-threatening lung condition in which the body reacts to an allergy by causing constriction of the airways of the lungs, known as *bronchospasm* (see Figure 13–15 ■). It is difficult to get air in and even more difficult to get air out of the lungs. The inability to get air out of the lungs is known as *gas trapping*. As a result of gas trapping, fresh air cannot get into the lungs, so the victim breathes the same air over and over. This lowers the amount of oxygen in the blood and increases the blood levels of carbon dioxide. Because this is an inflammatory process of the airways, there is also an increase in the amount of mucus secretions that the airways produce. These increased secretions can block the airways (a phenomena known as *mucus plugging*) and further reduce the flow of fresh air to the lungs. Although asthma can be a life-threatening disease, it can be controlled with the use of medication.

Emphysema is a nonreversible lung condition in which the alveolar air sacs are destroyed and the lung itself becomes "floppy" (see Figure 13–15 ■), much like a worn area or bubble in a tire. As the alveoli are destroyed, it becomes more difficult for gases to diffuse between the lungs and the blood. The lung tissue becomes fragile and can easily rupture (again, much like a worn tire), causing air to escape into the thoracic cavity and further inhibit gas exchange. This causes a pneumothorax which is explained shortly.

Chronic bronchitis is a potentially reversible lung disease in which there are inflamed airways and large amounts of sputum being produced. As inflammation occurs, the airways swell and the inner diameter of the airways get smaller. As they get smaller, it becomes difficult to move air in and out, which increases the work of breathing. Because of this increased work level, more oxygen is used and more carbon dioxide is produced.

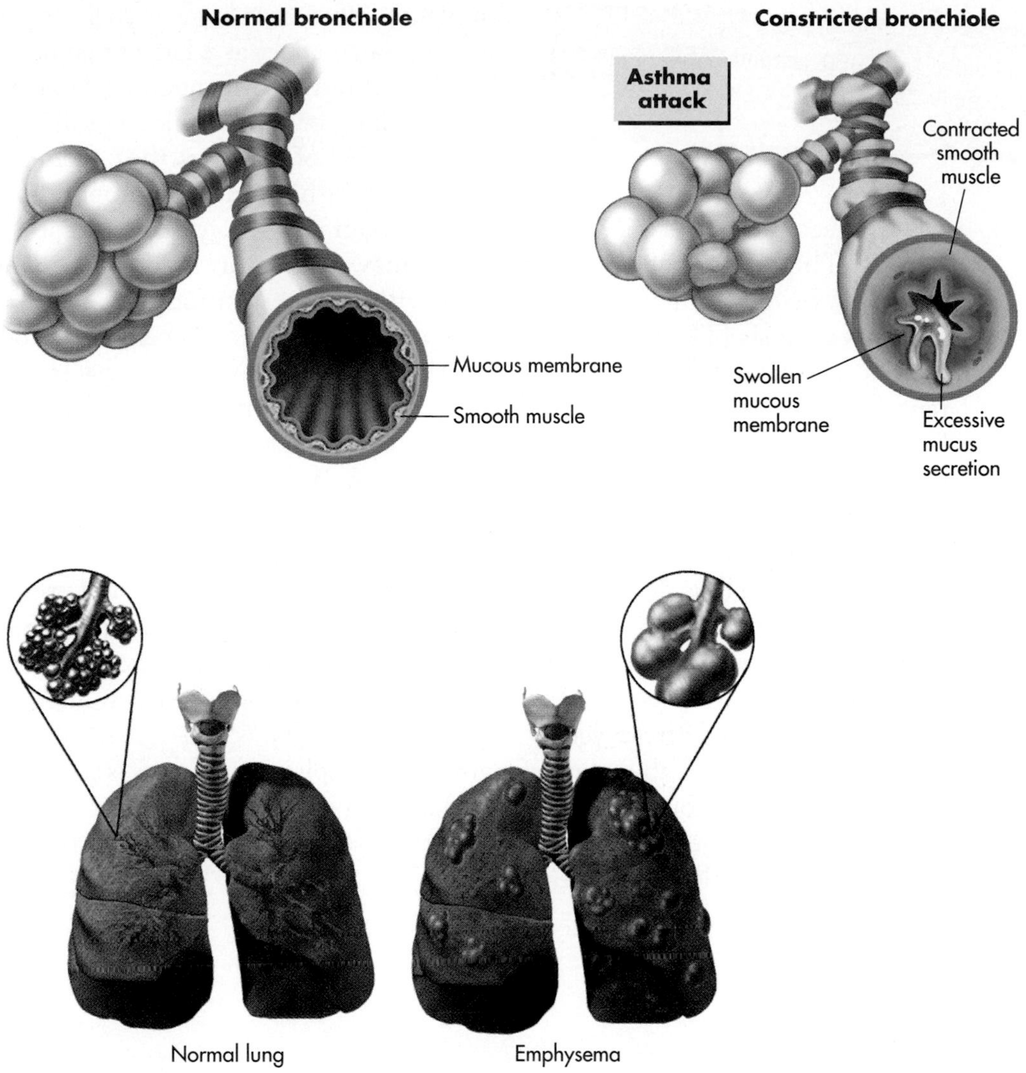

FIGURE ■ 13–15

Asthma and emphysema.

A **pneumothorax** is a condition in which there is air inside the thoracic cavity and outside of the lungs. Air can enter the thoracic cavity from two directions. A stab wound or gunshot wound to the chest would allow air to rush into the thoracic cavity from the outside. The lung might develop a leak as a result of either a structural deformity or a disease process (such as in emphysema). In this situation, air would enter the thoracic cavity from the lung as air is breathed in. In either case, if the gas cannot escape, it will continue to fill a space in the thoracic cavity and provide less space for the lung or lungs to expand when breathing. If the lungs are too greatly restricted to expand, a life-threatening situation may occur.

pneumothorax *(NOO moh THOH raks)*

A **pleural effusion** is a condition in which there is an excessive build-up of fluid in the pleural space between the parietal and the visceral pleura. This fluid may be pus (in which case it is known as **empyema**), serum from the blood (called a **hydrothorax**), or blood (called a **hemothorax**). Because fluids are affected by gravity, pleural effusions tend to move to the lowest point in the pleural space.

pleural effusion *(PLOO ral eh FYOO zhun)*

empyema *(em pye EE mah)*

hydrothorax *(HIGH dro THOH raks)*

hemothorax *(HEEM oh THOH raks)*

13-6 To view animations and videos on COPD, asthma, ARDS, apnea, allergic rhinitis, and tuberculosis, please go to your CD-ROM for this chapter.

If a pleural effusion is large enough, it can have the same effect as a large pneumothorax. It can restrict the amount of expansion of a lung or lungs. Since less air can flow in and out of the lungs, the patient has to work harder by breathing in and out more rapidly to meet the body's demands for more oxygen and the removal of carbon dioxide. This additional work of breathing may exhaust an individual to the point that he or she can no longer breathe without intervention.

tuberculosis *(too ber kyoo LOH siss)*

Tuberculosis (TB) is an infectious disease that has seen a recent rise in occurrence. Tuberculosis thrives in areas of the body that have high oxygen content such as is the lung. Tuberculosis can lay dormant in the body for years before beginning to multiply. If it continues unchecked, vast lung damage can occur. There has been recent concern about a multidrug-resistant form of tuberculosis that is very resistant to the drugs we normally use to treat TB, and has a high mortality rate.

Patients with lung disease may exhibit signs and symptoms such as dyspnea, tachypnea, cyanosis due to low oxygen levels, and use of accessory muscles of ventilation to assist normal breathing. In addition, the cardiac system may exhibit tachycardia to speed up oxygen delivery and may increase the number of red blood cells that carry oxygen.

The major preventable cause of many of the respiratory diseases is smoking. The annual number of smoking-related deaths in the United States is equivalent to one jumbo jet filled with passengers crashing every day with no survivors, or 450,000 deaths per year.

SUMMARY

Snapshots from the Journey

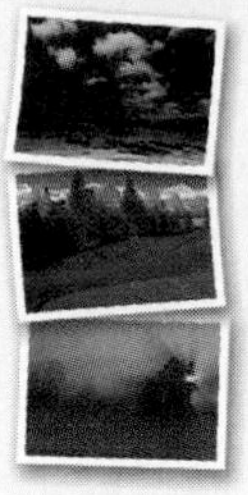

- Moving approximately 12,000 quarts of air each day, the respiratory system is responsible for providing oxygen for the blood to take to the body's tissues and removing carbon dioxide, one of the waste products of cellular metabolism.
- Ventilation is the movement of gases in and out of the lungs; during respiration oxygen is added to the blood and carbon dioxide is removed.
- The lungs contain continually branching airways called bronchi and bronchioles.
- At the end of bronchioles are alveolar sacs.
- Each alveolar sac is surrounded by a capillary network where gas exchange occurs with the blood.
- The purpose of the upper airways is to filter, warm, and moisten inhaled air for its journey to the lungs.
- In addition, the upper airways provides for *olfaction* (sense of smell) and *phonation* (speech).
- The mucociliary escalator captures foreign particles, and the hairlike cilia constantly move a layer of mucus up to the upper airways to be swallowed or expelled.
- Adenoids and tonsils aid in preventing pathogens from entering the body.
- Since activities of breathing and swallowing share a common pathway, the epiglottis protects the airway to the lungs from accidental aspiration of food and liquids.
- Vocal cords are the gateway between the upper and lower airways.
- The tracheobronchial tree is like an upside down tree with ever-branching airways, where the trunk of the tree is represented by the trachea and the leaves by the alveoli.
- The alveolar capillary membrane is where external respiration or gas exchange occurs.
- The bony thorax provides support and protection for the respiratory system.
- The main muscle of breathing is the diaphragm, and accessory muscles assist in times of need such as exercise and disease.
- The medulla oblongata in the brain is the control center for breathing and sends impulses via the phrenic nerve to the diaphragm.

Case Study

A patient comes to the emergency department with wheezing and thick secretions. His heart rate, breathing rate, and blood pressure are all increased. He is using accessory muscles of ventilation to breathe and has peripheral cyanosis. He has a history of asthma and has had a "bad cold" for several days.

What are two possible respiratory conditions he may have?

Can you think of some recommended treatments for this patient?

What would be some positive indicators that your treatment is working? For example, after the treatment, you notice less accessory muscle use. Can you think of at least two more?

REVIEW QUESTIONS

Multiple Choice

1. The process of gas exchange between the alveolar area and capillary is
   a. external ventilation
   b. internal ventilation
   c. internal respiration
   d. external respiration

2. The bulk movement of gas within the lung is called
   a. internal respiration
   b. ventilation
   c. diffusion
   d. gas exchange

3. Which of the following is *not* a function of the upper airway?
   a. humidification
   b. gas exchange
   c. filtration
   d. heating or cooling gases

4. The largest cartilage in the upper airway is the
   a. cricoid
   b. eustachian
   c. mega cartilage
   d. thyroid

5. Which structure controls the opening to the trachea?
   a. esophagus
   b. hypoglottis
   c. epiglottis
   d. hyperglottis

Fill in the Blank

1. Small bronchi are called ______________.

2. The sense of smell is termed ______________, and the act of speech is called ______________.

3. The hairlike projections called ______________ beat within the ______________ layer and propel the ______________ layer toward the oral cavity to be expectorated.

4. The ______________ are thought to lighten the head and provide resonance for the voice.

5. The ______________ and the ______________ are part of the immune system and are found in the nasopharynx and oral pharynx.

Short Answer

1. Describe the tissue layers in the bronchi.

2. Explain how gas exchange takes place in the lungs.

3. Discuss the importance of surfactant.

4. Describe the process of normal breathing beginning with the brain.

Suggested Activities

1. Research the effects of second-hand smoking and smokeless tobacco, and share results with the class or develop posters on these subjects.

2. Working as a group, research occupational causes of lung diseases and see how long a list you can develop.

13-7

Now that you have completed your journey through this chapter, please go to the CD-ROM for interactive games and puzzles concerning the medical terms and concepts contained in this chapter. By playing the games you will reinforce your learning of medical terminology in a fun way.

Greetings from THE LYMPHATIC AND IMMUNE Systems

Your Defense Systems

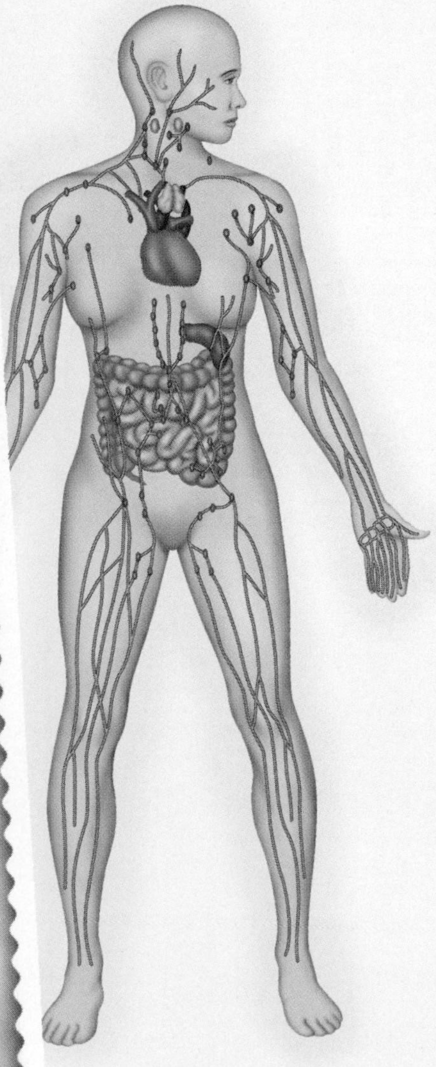

So far in our travels, we have visited control systems, transport systems, and infrastructure, to name just a few. We have seen how each separate system works together to allow the body to function as an integrated unit. However, like all cities, the body must be protected. Cities have police and fire departments. On a larger scale, countries have armies and bases. Similarly, your body has the immune and lymphatic systems with a variety of protective mechanisms and cells each performing specific duties. These systems help to protect the body from pathogens that can produce disease. Without your immune and lymphatic systems, your journey would be a very short one—the first exposure to a potential pathogenic organism would wreak havoc in your body and literally stop the journey before it began.

Chapter 14

LEARNING OBJECTIVES

Upon completion of your journey through this chapter, you will be able to:

- List and describe the major components of the immune system and their function(s).
- Explain the antigen–antibody relationship.
- Name and describe the functions of the blood cells responsible for protecting the body from invasion.
- Discuss how inflammatory responses and fevers relate to infection.
- Compare innate immunity to adaptive immunity.
- Describe the function of lymphocytes and helper cells in the immune response.
- List and describe several common diseases of the immune system.

MULTIMEDIA APPLICATIONS

CD-ROM Interactive Exercises

- Video on lymphatic drainage massage therapy, 14.1
- 3-D illustration of the lymphatic system, 14.2
- Drag-and-drop exercise of the lymphatic system, 14.3
- Pathology spotlight on skin cancer, 14.4
- Video on proper hand-washing technique, 14.5
- Animation of T cell destruction by HIV, 14.6
- Pathology spotlight on leukemia, 14.7
- Animation of the treatment of severe allergic reactions with an EpiPen and video on allergic rhinitis, 14.8
- Interactive puzzles and games, 14.9

www.prenhall.com/colbert

- Professional Profiles
  - Nuclear Medicine
  - Pharmacy
- Related Internet Links
- Additional Review Questions

Pronunciation Guide

Correct pronunciation is important in any journey so that you and others are completely understood. Here is a "see and say" Pronunciation Guide for the more difficult terms to pronounce in this chapter.

basophils (BAY soh fills)
cytokines (SIGH tow kines)
cytotoxic T cells (sigh tow TOX ick)
dendritic cells (DEN dri tick)
eosinophils (ee oh SIN oh fillz)
histamine (HISS tah meen)
interferon (in ter FIR on)
interleukins (in ter LOO kins)
leukocytes (LOO koh sights)
lymph nodes (LIMF nohdz)
macrophages (MAC reh fage ez)
neutrophils (NOO troh fill)
T lymphocytes (T LIMF oh sights)
thoracic duct (thoh RASS ik)
thymus (THIGH muss)
tumor necrosis factor (neh KROH siss)

THE DEFENSE ZONE

Although war is a severe analogy to use, it is the reality of what happens when a potentially dangerous threat invades the body. Suppose that a nasty army of pathogens attempts to invade your body. First, it must get past your barriers. Many invaders will be repelled simply by your intact skin or the secretions of your mucous membranes. If the invader does get inside your body, it is recognized as *not* belonging in your body. This recognition stimulates a series of responses to neutralize the foreign invader. Weapons in the form of specialized cells are engaged by the immune and lymphatic systems to fend off the pathogens. In addition, the immune and lymphatic systems release powerful chemicals to help to fight off the invaders.

These chemicals also stimulate the inflammatory response and leave a chemical mess to clean up. The "war" also leaves behind an area of neutralized pathogens and excessive debris and fluid that has collected around the battlefield and must be cleaned up. This again is accomplished by the combined and integrated efforts of the immune and lymphatic systems until the danger is over and your body can return to normal functioning. Let's begin the discussion with the lymphatic system, then bring in the immune system, and finally show how the two work in concert to keep your body healthy.

THE LYMPHATIC SYSTEM

lymphatic *(lim FAT ik)*

The **lymphatic** system is both the transport system and barracks of your immune system. It is a second circulatory system parallel to the cardiovascular system. As you will soon see, it works closely with the cardiovascular system, and their close proximity is needed for mutual benefit. The lymphatic system has the following four functions:

pathogen *(PATH oh jenn)*
path = *disease*
gen = *to create*

- recycling fluids lost from the cardiovascular system
- transporting **pathogens** to the lymph nodes where they can be destroyed

- storage and maturation of some types of white blood cells.
- absorption of glycerol and fatty acids from food (see digestive system for details)

> **14-1** The lymph system is a very low-pressure system and sometimes the nodes or filters can become clogged and circulation impaired. Lymphatic drainage massage is a technique to optimize lymphatic circulation, and you can go to your CD-Rom to view a short video on this important therapy.

Given that the lymphatic system is intimately connected to the function of the cardiovascular system, it should come as no surprise that the smallest pipes of the lymphatic system, called **lymph capillaries,** run parallel to blood capillaries. Lymph capillaries, tubes that form a network between the cells of connective tissues, are so named because they are structurally similar to blood capillaries, but unlike blood capillaries, lymph capillaries are open ended. The lymphatic system is not a closed system like the cardiovascular system. The fluid filling the lymph capillaries is known as **lymphatic fluid,** or simply **lymph.** (For a map of the lymphatic system, see Figure 14–1 ■)

lymph capillaries *(LIMF KAP ih lair eez)*

lymphatic fluid *(lim FAT ik FLOO id)*
lymph *(LIMF)*

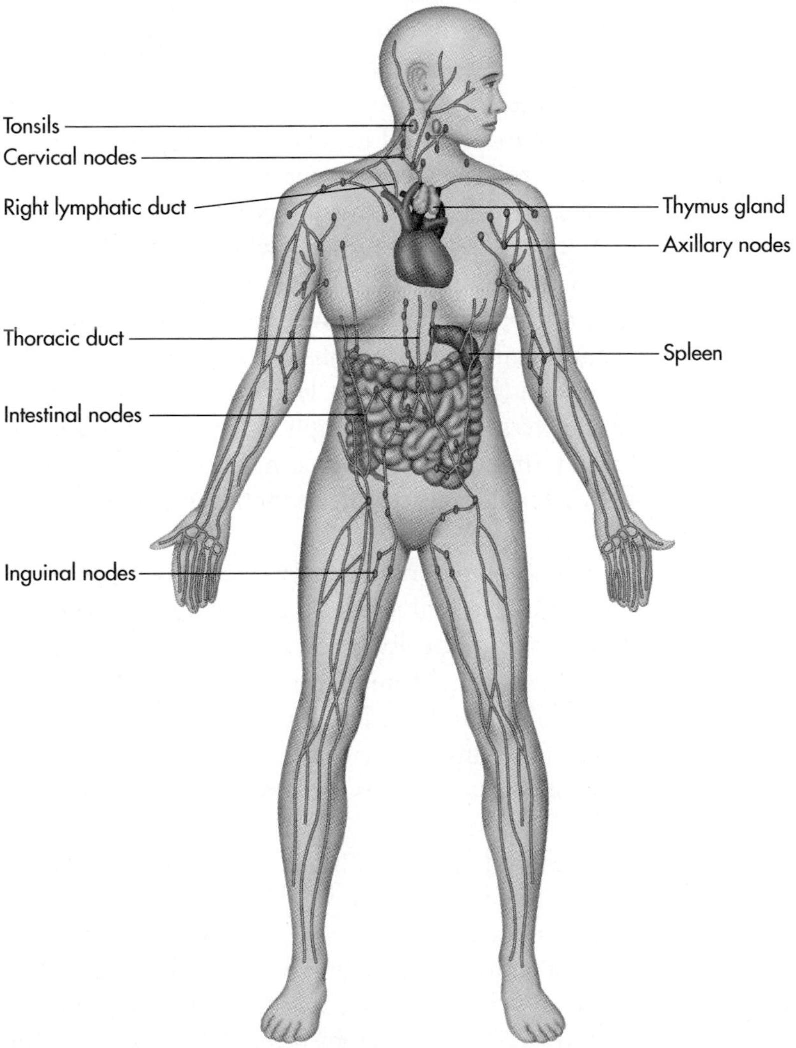

FIGURE ■ 14–1

The lymphatic system.

lymphatic vessels *(lim FAT ik)*
lymph nodes *(LIMF nohdz)*

Several lymph capillary networks empty into **lymphatic vessels,** which are structurally similar to veins, including having valves. Body movement and contraction of smooth muscle in the vessel walls propel lymph through the system. Small lymphatic vessels empty into larger lymphatic vessels. Larger lymphatic vessels empty into **lymph nodes.** Ranging in size from a pin head to an olive, the lymph nodes can be thought of as filters strategically placed all along the pathways or vessels of the lymphatic system. Think about a water filtration system for a city where a system of pipes (vessels) bring the dirty water into a plant with a filtration system (node) that then recycles clean water back into the system.

14-2 Go to your CD-Rom for this chapter for a 3-D illustration of the lymphatic system.

lymphatic trunks *(lim FAT ik)*
thoracic duct *(thoh RASS ik)*
right lymphatic duct *(lim FAT ik duct)*

Lymph nodes are small, encapsulated bodies divided into sections (see Figure 14–2 ■). Inside the nodes are sections of lymphatic tissue containing white blood cells known as lymphocytes. The lymphatic tissue is surrounded by lymphatic sinuses filled with lymph fluid. A number of lymphatic vessels enter or exit each lymph node. This in essence ensures that all lymph fluid must pass through a lymph node for filtration and destruction of pathogens by the white blood cells and also ensures that flow slows enough to allow the lymphocytes and macrophages to destroy pathogens.

Lymph nodes are concentrated in several areas around the body and are identified by their regional location: cervical, axillary, inguinal, pelvic, abdominal, thoracic, and supratrochlear. (Notice that the lymph nodes are concentrated to catch pathogens where they are most likely to enter the body, such as in the lungs, digestive system, and reproductive system.) Lymphatic tissue is also found in the pharynx, in patches commonly known as tonsils and adenoids, and in the thymus and spleen (more on these lymphatic structures later).

Lymphatic vessels exiting lymph nodes empty into one of several **lymphatic trunks.** These trunks, named for their location, are the lumbar, intestinal, intercostal, bronchomediastinal, subclavian, and jugular.

Lymphatic trunks empty into one of two collecting ducts. The lumbar, intestinal, and intercostal trunk all empty into the **thoracic duct,** a large duct that runs from the abdomen up through the diaphragm and into the left subclavian vein. More than two thirds of the lymphatic system drains into the thoracic duct. The bronchomediastinal, subclavian, and jugular trunks empty into the **right lymphatic duct,** a smaller duct within the right thorax that empties into the right subclavian vein (see Figure 14–3 ■).

So what we have is a major recycling plant within the body. The circulation of lymphatic fluid, then, follows this pattern: blood to tissue to lymphatic capillaries to lymphatic vessels to lymph nodes to lymphatic vessels to collecting ducts to lymphatic trunks to subclavian veins and then back to the blood. The fluid that moves from blood capillaries into tissues is thereby filtered through the white blood

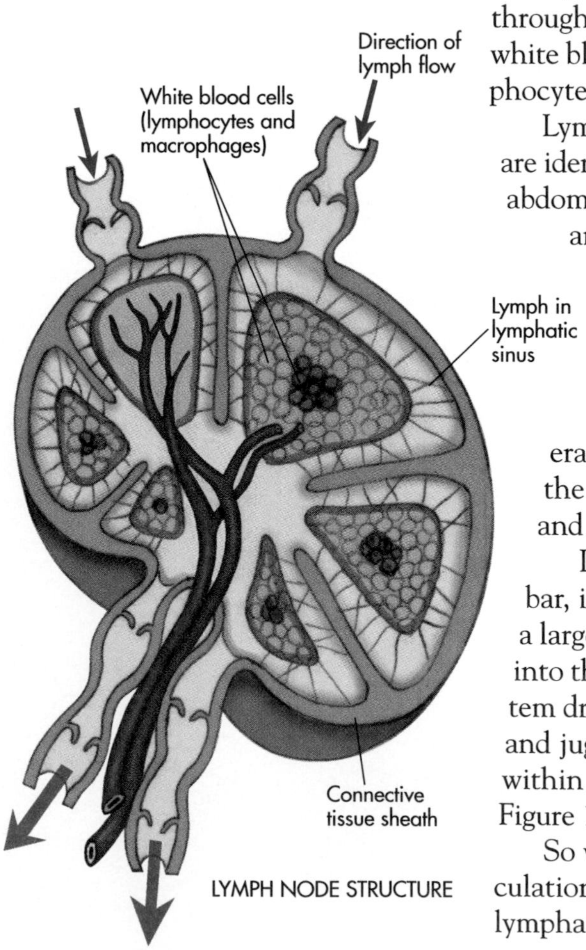

FIGURE ■ 14–2

The lymph node structure.

cells in the lymph nodes where pathogens are removed and destroyed and recycled back to the cardiovascular system.

As previously mentioned, there are two larger collections of lymphatic tissue, known as lymph organs. These lymph organs are the thymus and the spleen. While they are not strictly lymph nodes and are not part of lymph circulation, they are so similar to lymph nodes that they are classified as part of the lymph system.

The **spleen** (see Figure 14–3) is a spongy organ in the upper left quadrant of the abdomen. It is structurally similar to lymph nodes but instead of having lymphatic sinuses, the spleen has blood sinuses. Surrounded by the blood sinuses are islands of white pulp containing lymphocytes and islands of red pulp containing both red blood cells and white blood cells. One of the functions of the spleen is to remove and destroy old, damaged, or fragile red blood cells. Can you guess the second function of the spleen, given its anatomy? Since it is similar to a lymph node, the spleen also filters pathogens from the blood stream and destroys them in the same way that lymph nodes filter pathogens from lymph.

While the spleen is a very important organ, it is not one of the vital organs and in some cases, such as trauma, may need to be surgically removed. While its removal in children can severely compromise their ability to ward off disease, the spleen's removal in an adult has much less effect. You'll soon see one reason for this is that as we age, the body becomes better at fighting off infections that it has seen in the past, but new invaders present more of a challenge when we are first exposed to them as children. Because of the spleen's rich supply of blood vessels, injury to the spleen can often cause internal bleeding.

The **thymus** is a soft organ located between the aortic arch and sternum (again, see Figure 14–3). The thymus is very large in children because of all the new infections it must be ready to fend off. It gets smaller or even disappears in adults as the immune system fully matures in its ability to fight infection. The thymus is packed with lymphocytes, which mature into a type of white blood cell called a T lymphocyte. The thymus also secretes a hormone that stimulates the maturation of T lymphocytes in lymph nodes.

thymus *(THIGH muss)*

14-3 Go to your CD-ROM for this chapter for a drag-and-drop exercise on the lymphatic system.

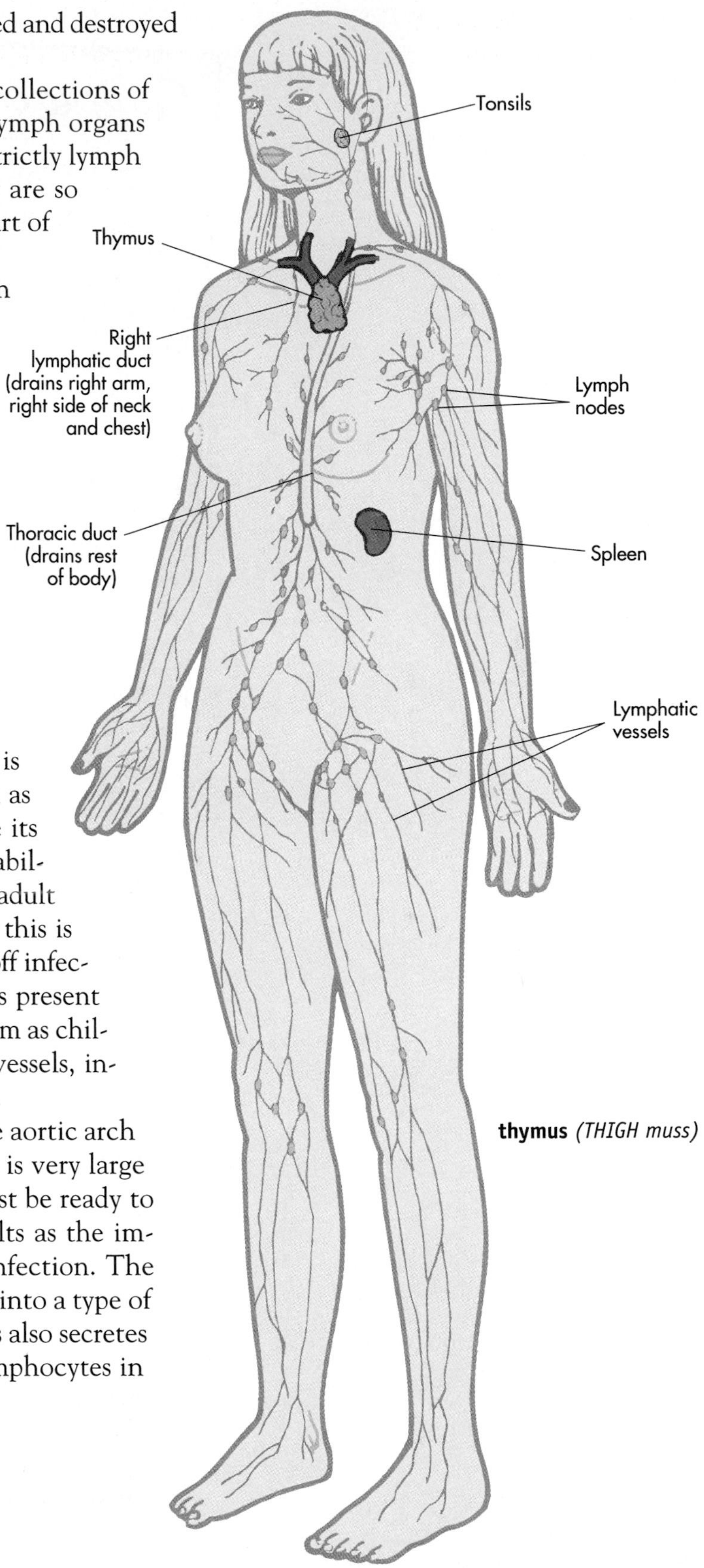

FIGURE ■ 14–3

The spleen and thymus.

Clinical Application

CANCER STAGES

When patients are diagnosed with cancer, they are often told they have a certain "stage" of cancer. Cancer is staged and prognosis is determined by the amount of metastasis (spread). The lymphatic system is amazingly efficient at capturing and transporting pathogens from connective tissue to lymph nodes for destruction. Unfortunately, this ability can also be a liability when cancerous cells develop in one part of the body and use the lymphatic system to hitch a ride to distant areas of the body. Once the cancerous cells make their way from their point of origin into lymphatic capillaries, and if the lymphocytes in the lymph nodes do not overpower the tumor cells, cancer cells can easily move around the body, invading many different areas simultaneously.

Cancers that are diagnosed after they have already spread are much more likely to be fatal than cancer that is treated before cells have a chance to spread. This is why screening for certain types of cancer is so important and often why lymph nodes are removed for study around surgical sites of cancer. The earlier a patient is diagnosed, the better his or her chances of beating the disease. Though most types of cancer have specific staging criteria, cancer stages generally follow this pattern:

- Stage 1, no spread from origin
- Stage 2, spread to nearby tissues
- Stage 3, spread to nearby lymph nodes
- Stage 4, spread to distant tissues and organs

Stage 4 cancers are often terminal.

14-4 Go to your CD-ROM for a pathology spotlight video on skin cancer that has the potential to be spread via the lymphatic system.

Nuclear medicine deals with the treatment of various types of cancer and attempts to prevent the spread of the cancer through the lymphatic system. Please go to the companion Web site to learn more about nuclear medicine and the related professional profiles of opportunities that exist in this field.

TEST YOUR KNOWLEDGE 14-1

Choose the best answer:

1. Any organism that invades your body and causes disease is known as a
   a. bacteria
   b. fungus
   c. virus
   d. pathogen

2. Which of the following areas do *not* have large number of lymph nodes?
   a. cervical
   b. axillary
   c. abdominal
   d. adrenal

3. Cancer that has entered the lymph nodes is in this stage:
   a. first
   b. second
   c. third
   d. center

4. Which cells are housed in lymph nodes?
   a. red blood cells
   b. white blood cells
   c. platelets
   d. lymph nodules

5. The thoracic duct of the lymphatic system empties into this blood vessel.
   a. right subclavian vein
   b. left subclavian vein
   c. aorta
   d. hepatic portal vein

6. The function of the thymus is to
   a. remove pathogens from blood
   b. destroy damaged red blood cells
   c. both a & b
   d. none of the above

THE IMMUNE SYSTEM

If the lymphatic system can be considered a transport and storage system for the body's defense systems, then the components of the immune system are the weapons and the actual troops, much like the National Guard, can be called in to protect a city in times of extreme need. The immune system is a series of cells, chemicals, and barriers that protect the body from invasion by pathogens. Some of the weapons are active, some are passive, some are inborn, others change with experience. Together they form a system that is remarkably good at keeping the body free of infection.

Antigens and Antibodies

As you should remember from our discussion of blood types in Chapter 12, cells have molecules on the outer surface of their membranes to distinguish whether they are friend or foe. These molecules are called **antigens.** Each human being has his or her own unique cell surface antigens, as do all other living things, including bacteria, viruses, animals, and plants. The presence of these unique fingerprints or antigens allows the immune system to distinguish between cells that are naturally yours and cells that are not. This ability, called **self-recognition** and **nonself-recognition,** is at the heart of immune system function.

antigen *(AN tih jenn)*

Antigens are like the identity codes sent out by airplanes. Air traffic controllers and fighter jets on patrol over a no-fly zone depend on the identity codes to tell which aircraft are friendly. Antigens do the same for your immune system. A well-functioning immune system ignores your antigens (self) and attacks other antigens (nonself). We discuss this in more depth later in this chapter.

As part of its defense system, the body can make proteins that bind to antigens, eventually leading to their destruction. Can you remember these proteins from the discussion of blood types? You got it! They are **antibodies,** one of the most potent weapons in the body's defensive arsenal. Therefore, antibodies are called into action when a foreign antigen invades the body.

Innate Versus Adaptive Immunity

The immune system defends the body on two fronts, by **innate immunity** and **adaptive immunity.** Innate immunity is the first line of defense against invasion. Innate immunity, as the name suggests, is the body's inborn ability to fight infection. Innate immunity prevents invasion, or if pathogens do get inside, innate immunity recognizes the invasion and takes steps to stop the infection from spreading. However, innate immunity can only recognize that something is not you, it can't identify the invaders. Innate immunity *cannot* improve with experience, and because it does not recognize specific pathogens, it cannot "remember" an infection the body has encountered before.

Innate immunity consists of a collection of relatively crude mechanisms for defending the body from infection, sort of like building a wall around a city or having metal detectors at the airport. Walls can keep out some invaders and metal detectors can tell if someone might be carrying a metallic weapon, but neither can respond to specific threats. (There is a world of difference between car keys and pocket knives, but metal detectors cannot tell them apart. That's why you have to take your change out of your pocket when you go through a metal detector!) Other parts of innate immunity are like weapons of mass destruction, indiscriminately killing pathogens and healthy tissue alike.

Innate immunity is backed up by a platoon of mechanisms that specifically target invaders, can remember invaders from previous encounters and therefore prepare for future invasions, and can improve their responses with experience. These mechanisms are known as *adaptive immunity* because the mechanisms "learn" and change each time they are engaged. The components of adaptive immunity can be trained as an elite fighting force for particular pathogens. Their goals are "surgical strikes" targeting particular invaders and sparing as much of the healthy body tissue as possible.

It is tempting to think of these two parts of immunity as separate entities. However, the two work closely together. Innate immunity prepares the way for adaptive immunity, weakening some pathogens and stimulating components of adaptive immunity. Adaptive immunity in turn further stimulates innate immunity. It is through the mutual cooperation of both innate and adaptive immunity attacking the pathogen on two fronts that invaders can be removed from the body.

TEST YOUR KNOWLEDGE 14-2

Choose the best answer:

1. Cell surface molecules that can be used to identify cells are called
   a. antibodies
   b. antigens
   c. antihistamines
   d. antibiotics

2. Proteins that bind to antigens are called
   a. binding proteins
   b. receptors
   c. hormones
   d. antibodies

3. This type of immunity has no memory and is not specific:
   a. adaptive
   b. acquired
   c. innate
   d. nonspecific

Components of the Immune system

We often think the immune system begins in the blood with the white blood cells. However, physical barriers exist to act as a first line of defense to attempt to stop the infective agents from getting into the body in the first place. This is much like concrete traffic barriers you see in front of public buildings.

BARRIERS

Anything that prevents invaders from getting inside your body prevents infection. Therefore, your body has many barriers located in the places where invaders are most likely to gain entrance. Physical barriers include skin and the mucous membranes of the eyes, digestive system, respiratory system, and reproductive system. Not only are these surfaces difficult to penetrate, they are packed with white blood cells and lymph capillaries to trap any invaders that might get through. The fluids associated with these physical barriers contain chemicals that act as chemical barriers. These chemicals are contained in tears, saliva, urine, mucous secretions, and sweat. One example is the oil secreted by the sebaceous glands of your integumentary system, which can be antibacterial. These barriers, both chemical and physical, prevent some invaders from ever getting inside the body. They are the "fortress" of the body, part of your innate immunity. After reading this information, can you see why wounds are frequent sources of infection?

CELLS

If an invader has an opportunity to enter the body, white blood cells (**leukocytes**) are responsible for defending the body against invaders. You learned about red blood cells and platelets in Chapter 12. Red blood cells are responsible for carrying oxygen throughout the body, and platelets are responsible for blood's ability to clot. White blood cells, on the other hand, are the mobile units of the immune system. White blood cells, which form in the bone marrow like red blood cells and platelets, move to other parts of the body to grow and mature until they are needed during an invasion. They are generally not released into the bloodstream in large numbers unless an infection is present.

leukocytes *(LOO koh sights)*
leuko = *white*
cyte = *cells*

> 14-5 Proper hand-washing technique is the number one way of preventing the spread of disease in a hospital and also helps to protect your immune system from invasion. To view a video on proper hand-washing technique, please go to the CD-ROM for this chapter.

Leukocytes can be divided into two groups. Polymorphonuclear granulocytes are cells with granules or spots in their cytoplasm. Agranulocytes or mononuclear cells have no granules in their cytoplasm. These two groups contain several different types of cells that play a role in the body's defense against infection. Figure 14–4 ■ shows the major white blood cells found in the plasma.

TYPES OF WHITE BLOOD CELLS

In a police department of a large city, several types of jobs are needed for the entire department to function: traffic control officers, homicide detectives, forensic crime scene technicians, evidence control officers, internal affairs investigators, and more. Each has a specific duty and is called upon as needed, but in essence they all have the same goal—fighting crime. Similarly, the body has various types of white blood cells that are required to protect the body in varying circumstances. The following represents a description of the major white blood cells in the plasma and the additional specialized white blood cells of the lymphatic system.

neutrophil *(NOO troh fill)*

Neutrophils **Neutrophils** are granulocytes whose function is phagocytosis. (Remember phagocytosis from Chapter 3?) Phagocytic cells ingest pathogens and cellular debris. (Think PacMan.) Neutrophils originate in the bone marrow and are the most common leukocyte in the bloodstream. Neutrophils are the first cells to arrive at the site of damage. They immediately begin to clean up the area by ingesting pathogens, and they release chemicals that increase tissue damage and inflammation, stimulating immune response. Neutrophils are part of innate immunity.

macrophages *(MAC reh fage ez)*

Macrophages **Macrophages** are modified monocytes, a type of agranulocyte, which leave the bloodstream and enter tissues. They are also phagocytic cells, which are active in the later stages of an infection. In addition to phagocyto-

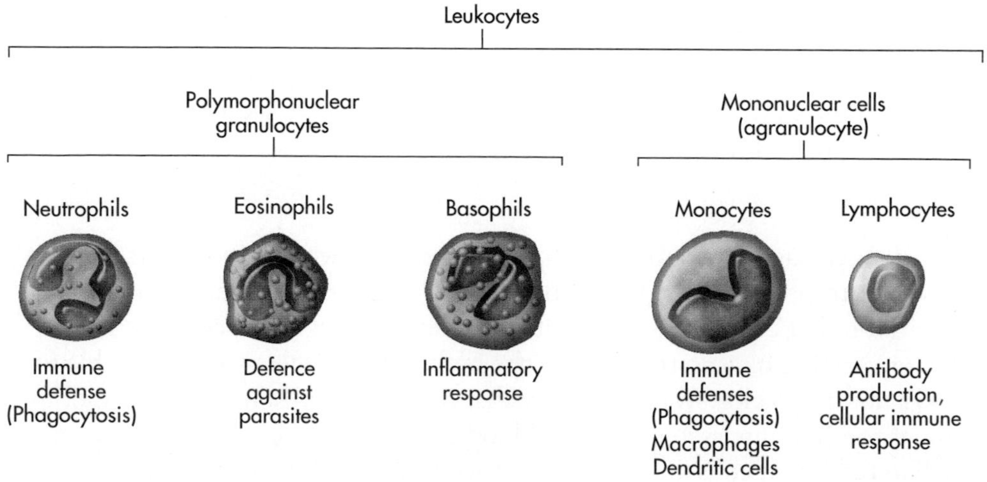

FIGURE ■ 14–4

Major Leukocytes.

sis, these cells release chemicals to stimulate the immune system. Macrophages are also part of innate immunity.

Basophils and Mast Cells **Basophils** and **mast cells** release chemicals to promote inflammation. Basophils are granulocytes, which are mobile, entering infected tissues from the bloodstream. Basophil numbers are very low unless an active infection is present. Mast cells are not mobile and are found stationed throughout the body. They are always found in connective tissue. For example, when the mast cells in the connective tissue of the nose are stimulated, chemicals are released that lead to rhinitis, more commonly called "runny nose." Mast cell stimulation in the lungs can trigger an asthmatic attack. Both basophils and mast cells are part of innate immunity.

basophil *(BAY soh fill)*

Eosinophils **Eosinophils** are granulocytes that counteract the activities of basophils and mast cells. The function of eosinophils is to break down the chemicals released by basophils and mast cells, thereby slowing or stopping inflammatory response so it doesn't go too far. Eosinophil numbers are generally low in the bloodstream unless active infection or allergies are present. Eosinophils also have a role in fighting invasion by parasitic worms and are part of innate immunity.

eosinophil *(ee oh SIN oh fill)*

Dendritic cells **Dendritic** cells are another member of a group of cells that are modified monocytes. All of these cells are weakly phagocytic. However, their most important job is as **antigen displaying cells,** or ADC's. These cells are able to ingest a foreign cell and place the foreign antigens into their own cell membrane. Then the dendritic cell cruises the lymph nodes, displaying the foreign antigens and looking for the lymphocytes that match the antigen. This is an important trigger of adaptive immunity. ADCs are the red flags or "all points bulletins" that alert your adaptive immune system to respond. They are an important bridge between innate and adaptive immunity.

dendritic cells *(den DRID ick)*

Natural Killer Cells **Natural killer cells** (NK cells) are a type of a lymphocyte. These lymphocytes are part of innate immunity. NK cells are crude weapons, releasing chemicals to kill any cells displaying foreign antigens, whether they are pathogens or the body's own infected cells. NK cells take out the neighborhood. These cells patrol the body, wiping out any infected cell they encounter. Some early symptoms of a cold or flu are actually due to the action of the NK cells damaging tissues, not from the infection.

T Lymphocytes **T lymphocytes** (T cells) are lymphocytes responsible for a portion of adaptive immunity known as cell-mediated immunity. There are several different types of T cells, including **cytotoxic T cells** (literally "cell poison"), which kill infected cells and release immune stimulating chemicals; **helper T cells,** which help activate other parts of adaptive immunity; **regulatory T cells,** which regulate immune response; and **memory T cells,** which remember pathogens after exposure.

T lymphocytes *(T LIMF oh sights)*

B Lymphocytes **B lymphocytes** (B cells) are lymphocytes responsible for the part of adaptive immunity known as antibody-mediated immunity. There are two types of B cells: **plasma cells,** which produce antibodies to nonself-antigens, and **memory B cells,** which remember pathogens.

B lymphocytes *(B LIMF oh sights)*

plasma cells *(PLAZ mah)*

CHEMICALS

cytokines *(SIGH tow kines)*

Not only do blood cells fight invaders, but chemicals found in the body can also assist in neutralizing and destroying invaders. **Cytokines** are proteins produced by damaged tissues and white blood cells that stimulate immune response in a variety of ways, including increasing inflammation, stimulating lymphocytes, and enhancing phagocytosis. Cytokines are involved in both innate and adaptive immunity.

interferon *(in ter FIR on)*

Interferon is a cytokine produced by cells that have been infected by a virus. Interferon binds to neighboring, uninfected cells and stimulates them to produce chemicals that may protect these cells from viruses. Interferon has also had some success as an anticancer drug, but it is still considered experimental.

tumor necrosis factor *(neh KROH siss)*

interleukins *(in ter LOO kins)*

Tumor necrosis factor, or TNF, is a cytokine produced by white blood cells. It stimulates macrophages and also causes cell death in cancer cells. A new class of drugs that inhibit TNF have been very successful in treating rheumatoid arthritis. Many cytokines are types of molecules called **interleukins.** There are at least 10 different interleukins. They are involved in nearly every aspect of innate and adaptive immunity. Interleukins also have been used with moderate success in treating some forms of cancer.

lysis = *to breakdown or destroy*
lysis *(LYE siss)*

Complement cascade is a complex series of reactions that activate 20 proteins that are usually inactive in the blood unless activated by a pathogen invasion. When these proteins are activated, they have a variety of effects, including **lysis** of bacterial cell membranes, stimulation of phagocytosis, attraction of white blood cells to the site of infection, clumping of cells with foreign antigens, and alteration of the structure of viruses. Complement cascade is part of both innate and adaptive immunity.

INFLAMMATION

Inflammation, or the inflammatory response, is one of the most familiar weapons in the body's arsenal. You have all experienced the swelling, pain, heat, and redness associated with inflammation at one time or another. Think back several chapters ago to our example of hitting your thumb with a hammer. What would happen to your thumb within a few minutes of injury? It would swell, turn red, get hot to the touch, and hurt for some time after the injury. What about an infected cut? Or a sore throat when you have a cold or the flu? Again, the symptoms are the same: redness, heat, swelling, and pain. This reaction is a deliberate action of your body in response to tissue damage, whether a mechanical injury, like hitting your thumb with a hammer, or damage due to the invasion of a pathogen, as in a wound infection or a strep throat. Part of this response helps to wall off the infected area to prevent further spread and allow the battle to focus at this site. This process is called *margination* and is an attempt to isolate the problem.

histamine *(HISS tah meen)*

When tissue is damaged, the cells send out chemicals such as **histamine,** a cytokine, which have several effects. These chemicals attract white blood cells to the site of injury, increase the permeability of capillaries, and cause local vasodilation. Extra fluid moves from the capillaries into the damaged tissue, causing swelling. More blood comes to the site, increasing the temperature of the tissue. White blood cells enter the area, destroying pathogens and clearing away dead and dying cells. The increase in fluid and cells coming to the area

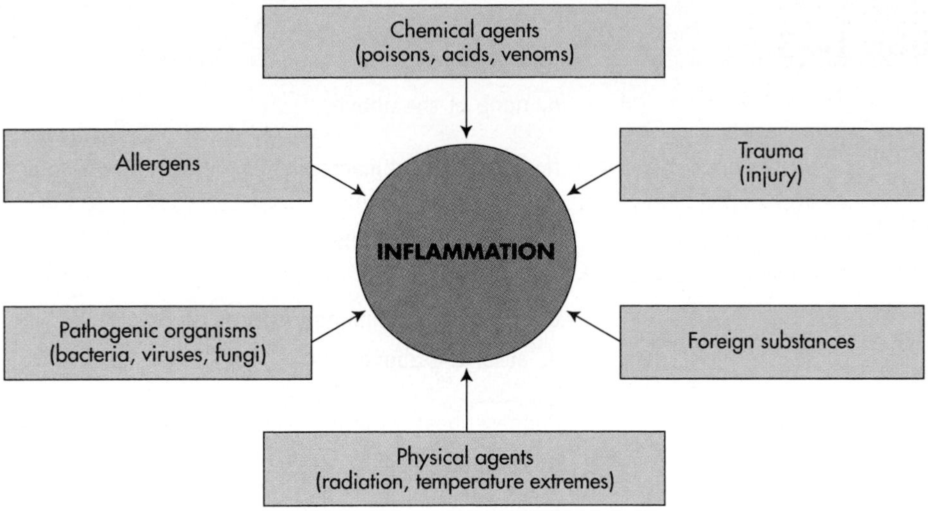

FIGURE ■ 14–5

Causes of the inflammatory response.

increases the pressure and is part of the reason the area remains painful even as the damage is being repaired. Inflammation is an innate immune mechanism, but it is also an important player in adaptive immunity. There are several causes of an inflammatory response. Please see Figure 14–5 ■.

FEVER

During an infection, tissues and components of the immune system release a number of cytokines, which promote inflammation and immune responses. These cytokines circulate through the bloodstream and often reach distant targets, including the brain. One of the cytokine targets in the brain is the hypothalamus, which is responsible for setting and maintaining body temperature. Under the stimulation of cytokines, the hypothalamus raises the body's temperature setpoint. You feel cold and begin to put on more clothes, to huddle under more blankets and even to shiver. Eventually, body temperature rises to the new setpoint and a fever results. While unpleasant to experience, this rise in body temperature is a deliberate attempt by the immune system to destroy the pathogens that have invaded the body. Like the rest of the innate response system, fever is a crude weapon against invaders. It might help fight off the infection, but it also causes overall discomfort.

Clinical Application

INFLAMMATION: A DOUBLE-EDGED SWORD

Inflammation, like many of the body's weapons, has a positive feedback loop. Once inflammation starts, it continues until turned off. This kind of runaway positive feedback can cause problems if localized swelling increases pressure, causing more tissue damage. One of the reasons you "ice" a sprained ankle is to decrease inflammation to prevent further damage. Inflammation is a particular problem in enclosed or small spaces like the brain, spinal cord, respiratory system, and extremities where a small buildup of pressure can cause serious damage. Even more dangerous is inflammation that becomes systemic, spreading throughout the whole body. This type of inflammation, called anaphylaxis, often causes blood pressure to plummet due to widespread vasodilation. Some people who are allergic to insect stings may experience this kind of inflammation. Anaphylaxis can be fatal unless treated by a medical professional immediately.

TEST YOUR KNOWLEDGE 14-3

Choose the best answer:

1. Which of the following is *not* a function of complement cascade?
   a. lysis of bacterial cell membrane
   b. stimulation of macrophages
   c. chemotaxis
   d. swelling

2. These chemicals may protect the body against viruses and some cancers:
   a. complement
   b. cytokines
   c. interferons
   d. immunoglobulins

3. B lymphocytes are directly responsible for
   a. cell-mediated immunity
   b. inflammation
   c. complement cascade
   d. none of the above

4. Neutrophils and macrophages aid the innate immune system by doing this:
   a. secreting cytokines
   b. phagocytosis
   c. stimulating immune response
   d. all of the above

5. Redness, heat, swelling, and pain are all symptoms of
   a. complement
   b. fever
   c. inflammation
   d. infection

HOW THE IMMUNE SYSTEM WORKS

Think back to when you were in grade school and all the colds and sore throats you and your friends suffered through, not to mention chicken pox and measles for you older students. Compare that to the frequency of colds and sore throats you get as an adult. Chances are the number is much lower. What has happened?

Innate Immunity

As we have seen, for a pathogen to successfully invade your body, it must first get past your physical and chemical barriers. (Think of your body as a castle and the barriers of innate immunity as the alligator-filled moat protecting the castle from the marauding hoards.) Most of the millions of pathogens you encounter each day are kept out by these barriers. However, some pathogens—influenza or the cold virus, for example—are very good at getting past barriers.

When a pathogen does get past the barriers, the more active portions of innate immunity are activated. The presence of a foreign antigen is detected by neutrophils. Neutrophils ingest the foreign antigen, destroying it, and release chemicals (cytokines, for example) that attract other white blood cells to the site of infection and stimulate inflammation. (Continuing our castle analogy, the neutrophils are the guards who greet any marauders who manage to survive the alligators.)

The release of cytokines and stimulation of inflammation attract macrophages and NK cells to the infection site. Macrophages destroy more infected cells by phagocytosis. NK cells use chemicals to destroy infected cells.

Both cells release chemicals that further stimulate inflammation, activate more immune cells, and trigger the complement cascade. (The castle guards sound the alarm that the castle has been breached, summoning more troops to fight the invaders.)

At this point, the infected cells, or the pathogens themselves, are under attack on several fronts: phagocytosis, noxious chemicals, membrane rupture, clumping, and even alteration of their molecular structure. Chemicals have signaled your hypothalamus to raise your body temperature, and you run a fever. You feel like . . . , well you know how you feel. There is no question in your mind that you are ill. (Even though the guards are protecting the castle, the castle will be damaged.)

You would think this would be enough to fight off most pathogens. But keep in mind that this is crude warfare. Innate immunity simply destroys anything nonself. It does not use surgical strikes or specific weapons. Innate immunity lays waste to the infected area with almost indiscriminate attacks. Defending the castle is warfare in the crudest sense—no specialized weapons, just desperate attempts to defeat the invaders. Uninfected cells can be destroyed in the process.

In some cases, these mechanisms are enough, but often the innate immune system is buying time for adaptive immunity to ready the "big guns," the B and T cells of adaptive immunity. Indeed, the activities of innate immunity stimulate adaptive immunity. Chemicals released by NK cells, neutrophils, and other cells help activate adaptive immunity. When phagocytic cells ingest pathogens, they display the foreign antigen on their cell membranes. *This ability to display foreign antigens without being infected is absolutely necessary for activation of B and T cells.*

Adaptive Immunity

Fighting specific pathogens is the job of adaptive immunity. This part of the immune system has memory, "learns" with experience, and recognizes specific pathogens. It is because of adaptive immunity that people get the chicken pox only once. (Thank goodness for that!) The cells responsible for the adaptive immune system, B and T lymphocytes, remember pathogens and mount specific responses to those pathogens if they meet again. It is because of adaptive immunity that immunizations are able to prevent illness. When was the last time you heard of somebody in the United States getting polio? Just 60 years ago, polio was an epidemic in the U.S. Keep in mind that innate and adaptive immunity work hand in hand. One cannot do its job without the other.

LYMPHOCYTE SELECTION

In order to function, lymphocytes must be able to recognize pathogens and to ignore the body's own tissues. Think of these cells as members of the local fire company. They have a very specific job—putting out fires. Like any professional firefighter, lymphocytes must be **selected.** During **positive selection,** lymphocytes that actually recognize and bind to antigens are allowed to survive. Lymphocytes that fail to do their job do not survive, much like a firefighter who cannot carry a hose or climb a ladder will not become part of the company. Unfortunately, some of these selected lymphocytes actually recognize and bind to your antigens.

If not destroyed, they will attack and destroy your own tissues. By the same token, fire companies take care not to select arsonists to work for the fire department! The destruction of self-recognizing lymphocytes is known as **negative selection.** Both positive and negative selection must work in order for your immune system to function appropriately. You must have lymphocytes that attack invaders but don't attack you!

LYMPHOCYTE ACTIVATION

Lymphocytes develop and mature when you are a baby or a very young child. Just like you, they begin as an undifferentiated cell, meaning they have the potential to become anything. They must then undergo a maturation process to become **differentiated** or, in other words, to grow up to be a specialized cell with a specialized function. While undifferentiated lymphocytes are produced in the bone marrow, some migrate to the thymus and are destined to become T cells. Others stay, develop, and mature in the bone marrow to become B cells.

After they are specialized, the lymphocytes hang out in the lymph nodes waiting for a pathogen to come along that they recognize. The lymphocytes can go into suspended animation for all that time. In order for the lymphocytes to fight off the pathogen, they must have a wake-up call. Picture the fire company sleeping in the middle of the night and the alarm going off. This wake-up call is called **lymphocyte activation.** It causes lymphocytes to circulate continuously in the bloodstream and lymph system to combat the pathogen. See Figure 14–6 ■ to see how the immune system activates and differentiates lymphocytes.

Let's go back to innate immune response for a minute. When a pathogen invades your tissues, your innate immunity mounts a response to the pathogen. One part of innate immunity is phagocytosis of infected cells or bits of pathogen. When these cells, macrophages, dendritic cells, and others, eat the pathogen, the pathogen's antigens are displayed on the outside of the phagocytic cells, kind of like little wanted posters. These cells then prowl the lymph nodes, displaying these tiny bits of pathogen, searching for the lymphocytes that can recognize the pathogen bits. When the right lymphocytes meet the right antigen display, the lymphocytes are activated (their wake-up call for battle). This activation is the beginning of adaptive immunity. Remember, water doesn't come out of a fire hose until the hose is turned on.

LYMPHOCYTE PROLIFERATION

The body has only a few lymphocytes that recognize each invader to which it has been exposed. But in order to fight off an infection, hundreds of thousands of lymphocytes are needed to attack the infection. Simple activation of lymphocytes is not enough. The activated lymphocytes must make thousands of copies of themselves in order to fight off the thousands of pathogens reproducing in the body. This reproduction of lymphocytes is called **lymphocyte proliferation** (see Figure 14–7 ■). Just like one platoon would not be enough to repel a full-scale invasion of a country, or one fire company enough to save a city block from burning down, a few lymphocytes are not enough to defend the entire body.

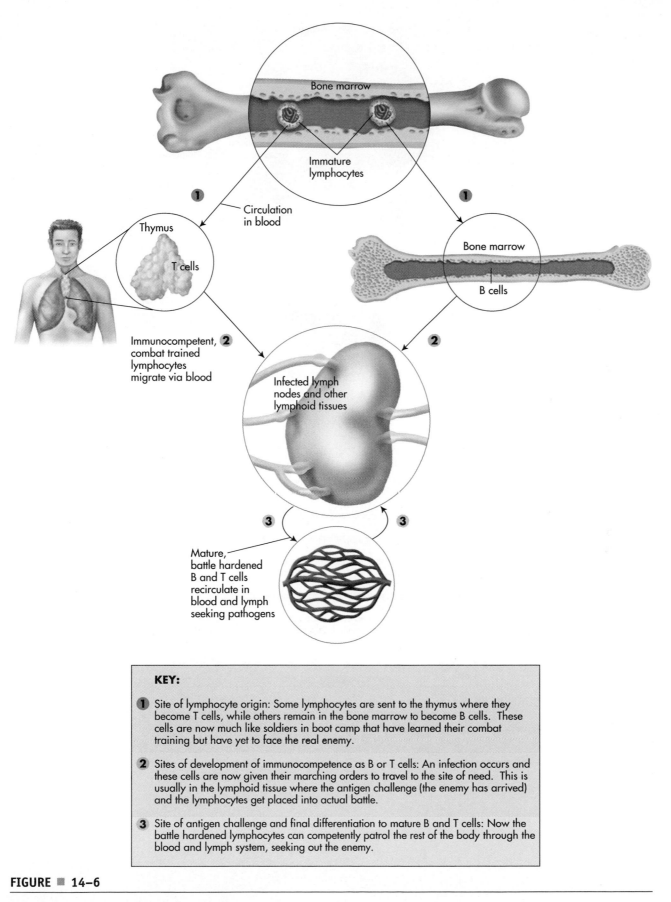

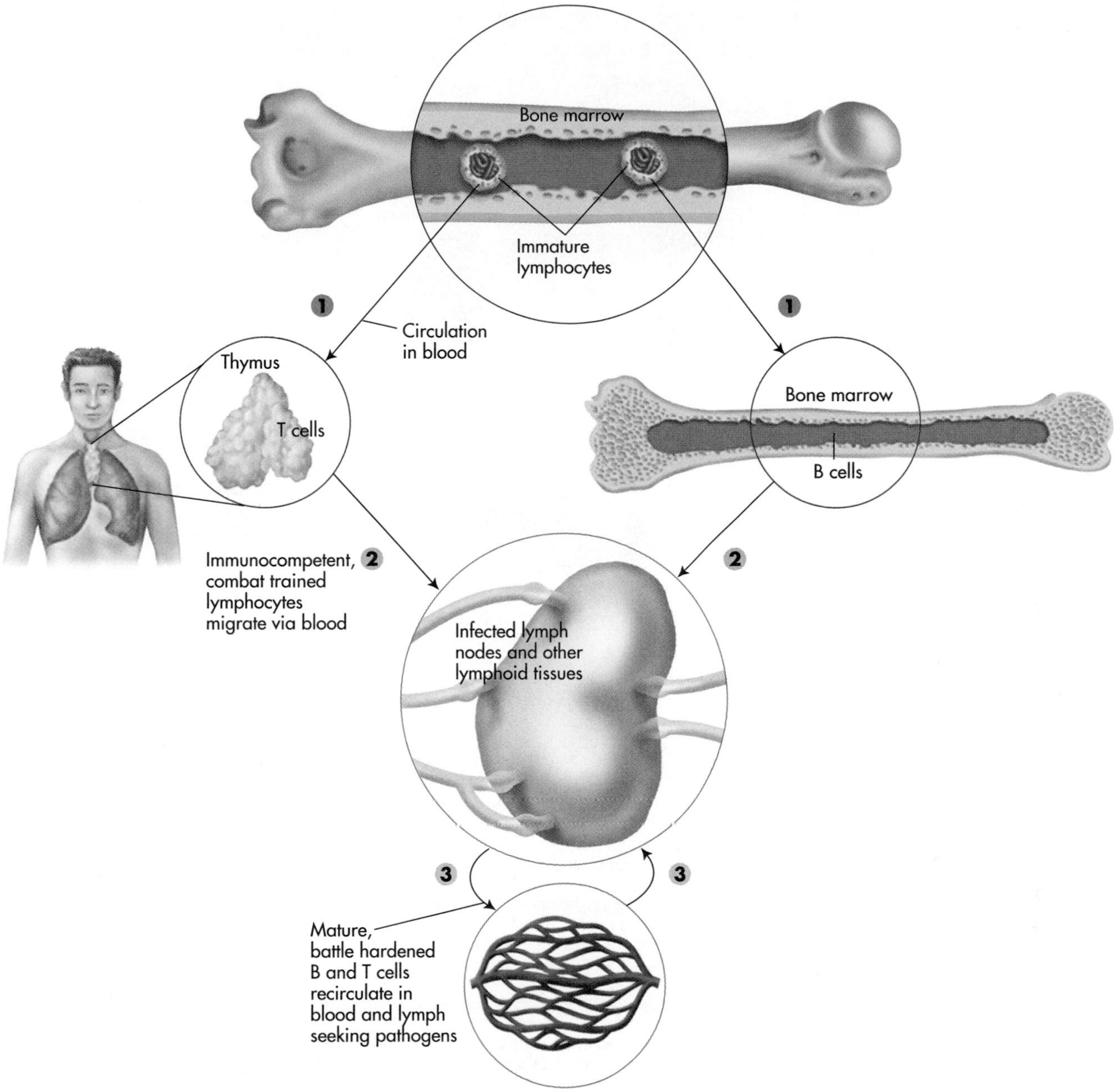

KEY:

1. Site of lymphocyte origin: Some lymphocytes are sent to the thymus where they become T cells, while others remain in the bone marrow to become B cells. These cells are now much like soldiers in boot camp that have learned their combat training but have yet to face the real enemy.

2. Sites of development of immunocompetence as B or T cells: An infection occurs and these cells are now given their marching orders to travel to the site of need. This is usually in the lymphoid tissue where the antigen challenge (the enemy has arrived) and the lymphocytes get placed into actual battle.

3. Site of antigen challenge and final differentiation to mature B and T cells: Now the battle hardened lymphocytes can competently patrol the rest of the body through the blood and lymph system, seeking out the enemy.

FIGURE ■ 14–6

Lymphocyte differentiation and activation.

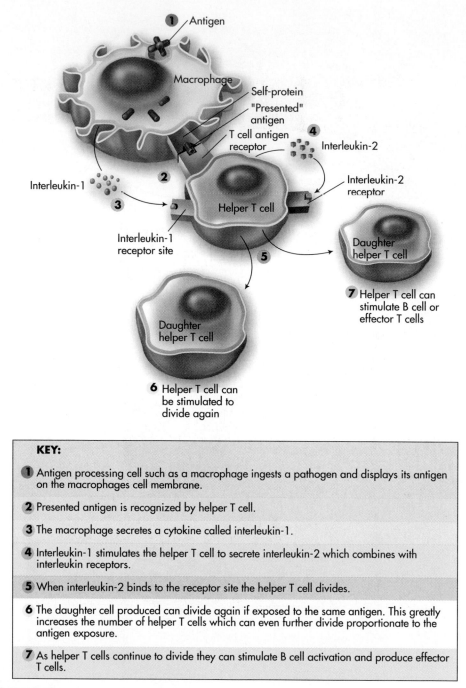

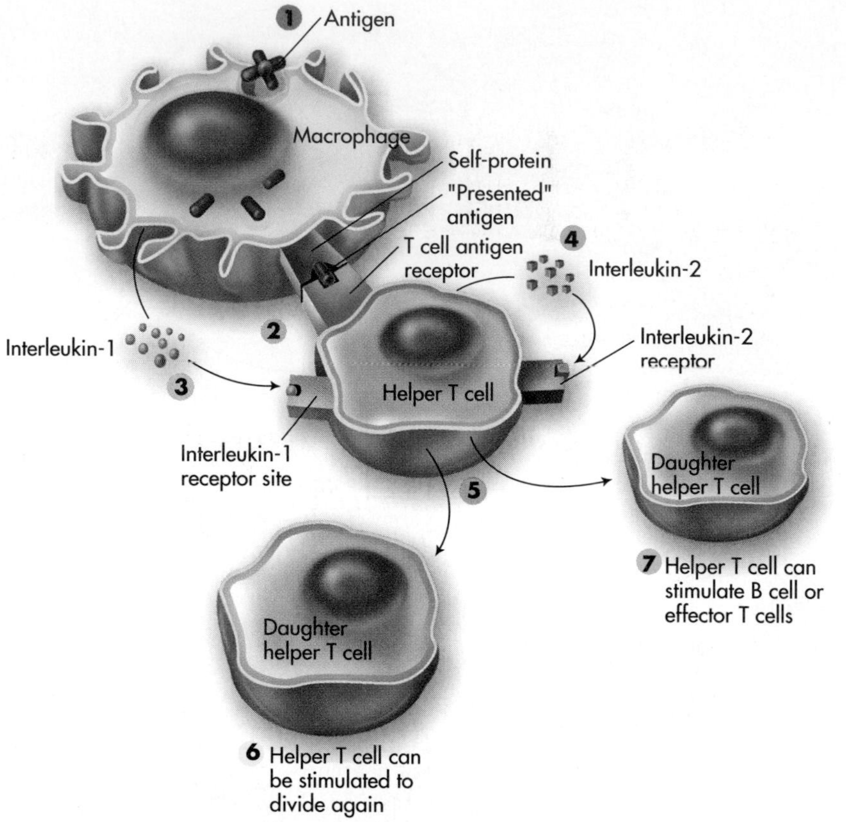

KEY:
1 Antigen processing cell such as a macrophage ingests a pathogen and displays its antigen on the macrophages cell membrane.
2 Presented antigen is recognized by helper T cell.
3 The macrophage secretes a cytokine called interleukin-1.
4 Interleukin-1 stimulates the helper T cell to secrete interleukin-2 which combines with interleukin receptors.
5 When interleukin-2 binds to the receptor site the helper T cell divides.
6 The daughter cell produced can divide again if exposed to the same antigen. This greatly increases the number of helper T cells which can even further divide proportionate to the antigen exposure.
7 As helper T cells continue to divide they can stimulate B cell activation and produce effector T cells.

FIGURE ■ 14–7

Activation and proliferation of helper T cells.

When you first met lymphocytes, earlier in our tour of the troops, you discovered that B cells and T cells have very different roles in the defense of the body. While activation and selection is, for our purposes, the same for both B and T cells, proliferation is different depending on the type of lymphocyte that is being reproduced.

There are two types of proliferation: proliferation of helper T cells and proliferation of all other types of lymphocytes. Remember, the job of helper T cells is to help other lymphocytes. There must be lots of helper T cells before any other lymphocytes can be activated. Helper T cells are stimulated to divide by binding to antigen-displaying cells (from innate immunity) and by stimulation by cytokines (some secreted by cells from the innate immune response and inflammation). The helper T cells continue to divide, producing more helper T cells, and then help (hence their name) in the proliferation of B cells and other types of T cells (again, see Figure 14–7).

Helper T cells are absolutely necessary for the reproduction of B cells and other types of T cells. This is why HIV, the virus that causes AIDS, is so devastating to the immune system. HIV targets helper T cells specifically. To understand the role of the helper T cells, imagine a huge game of tag in which no lymphocytes can be activated or reproduced until they have been tagged by a helper T cell.

Clinical Application

AIDS

AIDS, acquired immune deficiency syndrome, is caused by infection with the human immunodeficiency virus (HIV), a virus that specifically targets and destroys a type of helper T cell called CD-4. CD-4 cells are necessary for the proliferation of B cells and cytotoxic T cells. As helper T cells are infected with HIV and begin to die, their numbers decrease dramatically, so B cell and T cell proliferation is too slow to respond to an infection. Patients with full-blown AIDS often die from massive infections that they would otherwise be able to fight easily. These same infections are also found in patients with other types of immune deficiency diseases or who are taking immunosuppressant drugs to prevent post transplant organ rejection or to treat autoimmune diseases.

14-6 Go to your CD-ROM to view an animation of T cell destruction by HIV.

TEST YOUR KNOWLEDGE 14-4

Choose the best answer:

1. In order to be activated, B and T cells must bind with
   a. an antigen displaying cell
   b. a pathogen
   c. a damaged cell
   d. all of the above

2. Selection for immune-competent cells is called
   a. negative selection
   b. positive selection
   c. immune selection
   d. make a selection

3. After a lymphocyte is activated, what must it do before it can fight off a pathogen?
   a. die
   b. agglutinate
   c. proliferate
   d. congregate

4. The primary function of these cells is the activation of other lymphocytes:
   a. cytotoxic T cells
   b. helper T cells
   c. memory T cells
   d. regulatory T cells

B and T Cell Action

So, let's get back to the body's response to invasion. The innate immune system has been attacking the pathogen or cells infected with the pathogen on a number of fronts, using phagocytic cells, NK cells, fever, and a variety of noxious chemicals. A number of the body's own cells have been destroyed in the process, but the pathogen has not been defeated. However, while innate immunity has been holding down the fort Antigen Displaying Cells (ADCs) have sent out a signal calling on the weapons of adaptive immunity, B cells and T cells.

B CELLS

B cells are responsible for a type of adaptive immunity known as **antibody-mediated immunity.** B cells fight pathogens by making and releasing antibodies to attack a specific pathogen. As we saw previously, B cells develop into **plasma cells** and **memory B cells.** Antibodies are made by plasma cells and released into the bloodstream. Antibodies bind to the antigens of infected cells or the antigens on the surface of freely floating pathogens. They are missiles programmed to home in on a specific target. Antibodies destroy pathogens using several methods, including inactivating the antigen, causing antigens to clump together, activating complement cascade, causing the release of chemicals to stimulate the immune system, and enhancing phagocytosis. This response to the pathogen is called **primary response.**

All of these antibody-mediated mechanisms not only destroy pathogens specifically, they also further stimulate both adaptive and innate immune response, continually increasing response to the pathogen. Remember that immune response is a positive feedback loop that must be deliberately turned off. It will not stop on its own. This makes sense if you think in terms of protection. Your protective systems should not give up until the danger is past. Smoke alarms keep wailing until there is no more smoke.

Other B cells, memory B cells, are stored in lymph nodes until they are needed at some future date. If the body is exposed to the same pathogen in the future, memory cells allow it to mount a much faster response to the invasion. This response is known as **secondary response** and is responsible for the ability of adaptive immunity to improve with experience (see Figure 14–8 ■).

T CELLS

As previously explained, there are at least four types of T cells: helper T cells, cytotoxic T cells, regulatory T cells (formerly known as suppressor T cells), and memory T cells. We have already seen the action of helper T cells. Helper T cells are responsible for activation of B and T lymphocytes.

cytotoxic = *cell death*
cytotoxic T cells *(sigh tow TOX ick)*
perforin = *causes the cell to become perforated and die*

Cytotoxic T cells are responsible for a part of adaptive immune response known as **cell-mediated immunity,** so called because the cytotoxic T cells are directly responsible for the death of pathogens or pathogen-infected cells. Cytotoxic T cells release a cytokine called **perforin,** which causes infected cells to develop holes in their membranes and die. Cytotoxic T cells also release other cytokines that stimulate both innate and adaptive immunity, especially attracting macrophages to the site of infection to dispose of cellular

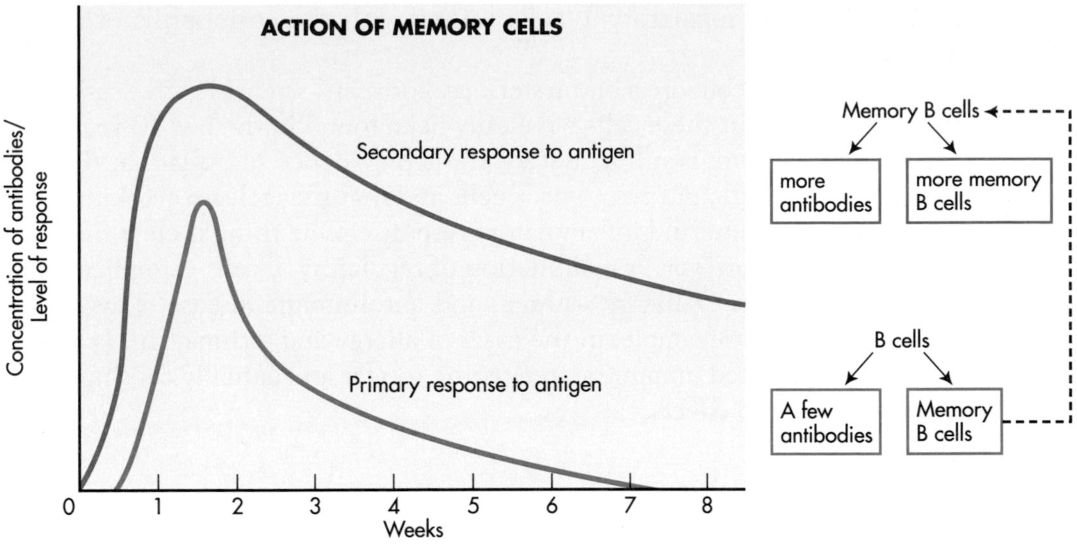

FIGURE ■ 14–8

The primary response causes B cells to produce *memory* B cells and a few antibodies. The second exposure causes the secondary response to produce more memory B cells and even more antibodies to fight the invaders. Now that the body has antibodies and more memory B cells, the secondary response begins more rapidly after exposure, produces more antibodies, and lasts a longer time.

debris. The response of cytotoxic T cells is the primary response of cell-mediated immunity. Some T cells, rather than becoming cytotoxic T cells, give rise to memory T cells. Like memory B cells, memory T cells are responsible for secondary response, storing the recognition of the pathogen until the next encounter (see Figure 14–9 ■). This memory of the pathogen is responsible for the secondary response.

Regulatory T cells are the off-switch for the immune system. Immunity is controlled largely by positive feedback. Tissue damage causes the release of stimulatory chemicals that cause inflammation and increased immune response. Increased immune response results in the release of more chemicals, which causes more stimulation, which causes more chemicals to be released, and so on. Something must actively work to turn off the response when the threat is over or the immune response could become rampant and out of control and thus cause damage. This

Clinical Application

HOW YOU ACQUIRE IMMUNITY TO PATHOGENS

Your adaptive immune system is able to acquire immunity to new pathogens by creating memory cells each time you meet a pathogen. This process, called immunization, whether natural or done by medical procedures, trains your immune system by creating memory cells for a pathogen. When you are exposed to the pathogen a second time, you do not get ill. Your immune system fights off the pathogen very quickly. In active acquired immunity, *you make* antibodies to fight the pathogens. In passive acquired immunity, antibodies *are introduced* to your body and therefore you don't make your own.

You can acquire immunity in several different ways. **Natural active immunity** is acquired in the course of daily life. When you catch a virus or a bacterium, your immune system fights it off, and memory cells are created for the next meeting. Anybody old enough to have had the chicken pox as a child (before the vaccine became available) is usually protected from a second round of chicken pox.

Artificial active immunity is acquired during vaccinations. Getting a measles shot exposes you to small amounts of weakened virus, not enough to make you sick, but enough for your immune system to create memory cells. If you meet the virus later in life, you will be able to fight it off. Babies acquire **natural passive immunity** to many pathogens via antibodies passed across the placenta or during breast feeding. These antibodies, which babies can't yet make, protect them from infection for several months after birth. **Artificial passive immunity** is acquired when antibodies from one person are injected into another to help fight infection. See Figure 14–10 ■.

is the job of the regulatory T cells (along with the eosinophils of innate immunity).

Regulatory T cells are a bit mysterious. For years, scientists have suspected their existence, but these cells have only been found in the last 10 years. Exactly how they work is still a mystery, though evidence suggests that they directly inhibit B cells and cytotoxic T cells and that they release cytokines that decrease immune and inflammatory response. One thing is clear from the research, however. A malfunction of regulatory T cells is implicated in some types of allergy, asthma, and autoimmune disease. This makes sense, for example, in the cases of allergy and asthma, this is an unregulated immune system going too far and actually causing widespread effects.

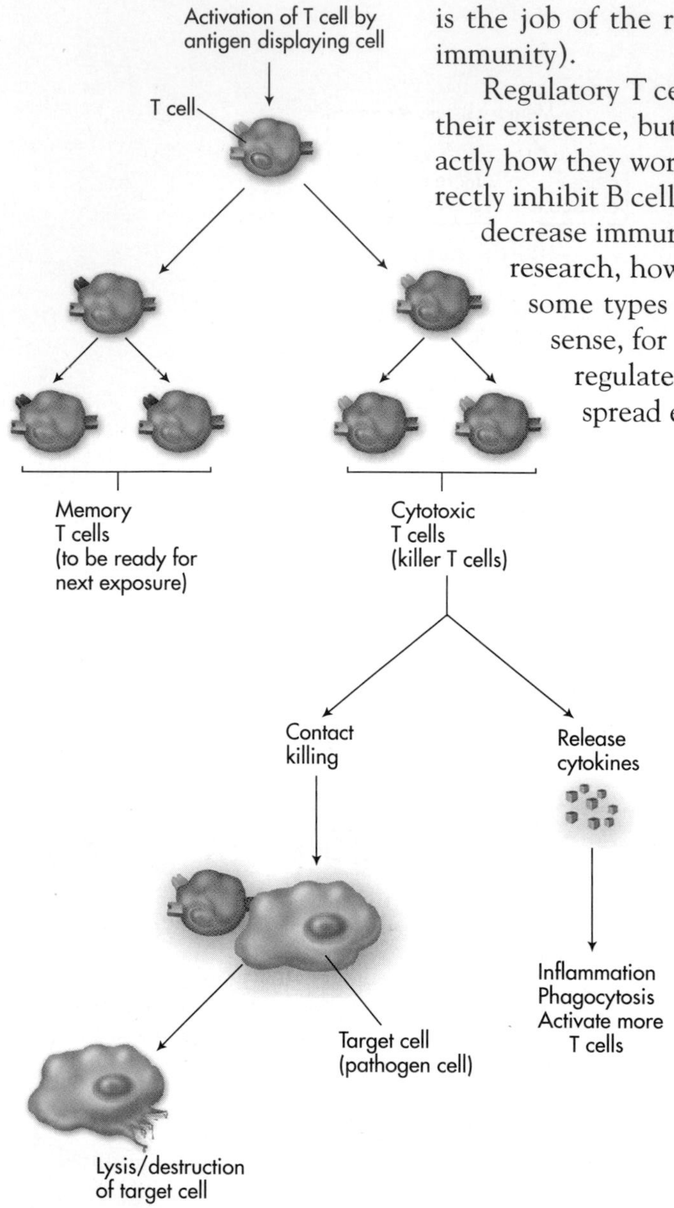

FIGURE ■ 14–9

Cell-mediate immunity, primary and secondary response.

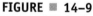

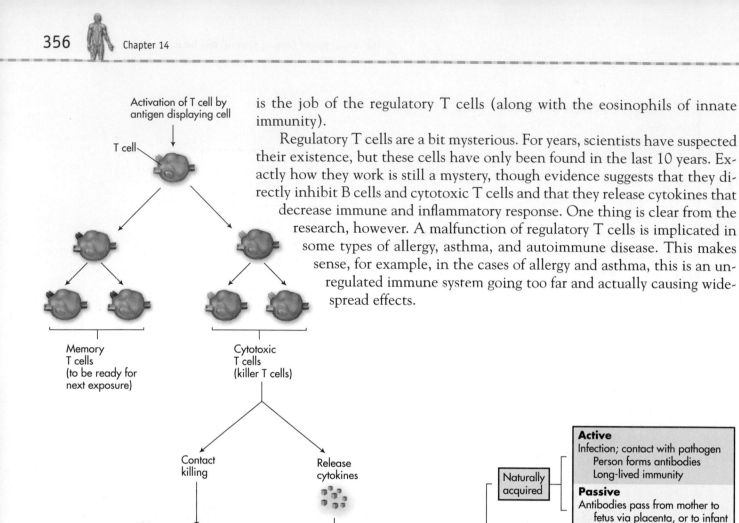

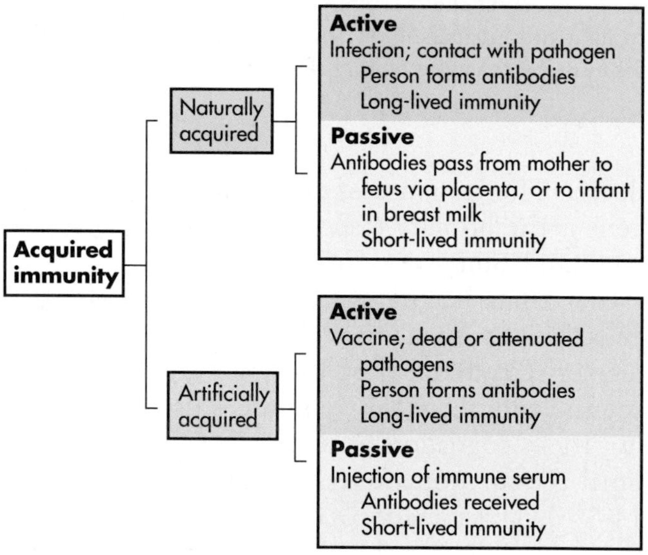

FIGURE ■ 14–10

Types of immunities.

TEST YOUR KNOWLEDGE 14-5

Choose the best answer:

1. B cells, once activated, can become two different kinds of cells: memory B cells and
   a. cytotoxic T cells
   b. natural killers
   c. plasma cells
   d. macrophages

2. Secondary response is mediated by
   a. cytotoxic T cells
   b. macrophages
   c. memory cells
   d. all of the above

3. _____ cells are responsible for antibody mediated immunity while cell mediated immunity is performed by _____ cells.
   a. B cells, cytotoxic T cells
   b. B cells, cytotoxic T cells
   c. B cells, plasma cells
   d. plasma cells, memory cells

4. These cells, which were only discovered recently, are part of the "off-switch" for the immune system.
   a. cytotoxic T cells
   b. memory T cells
   c. regulatory T Cells
   d. helper T cells

THE BIG PICTURE

At this point we have talked about the lymphatic system, innate immunity, and adaptive immunity as separate means to the same end: ridding the body of invading pathogens. We have mentioned repeatedly that the divisions are *not* separate but are intimately connected. Now that we have inspected them separately, it is time to put the entire defense system back together as a single, integrated fighting force (see Figure 14–11 ■).

A nasty army of pathogens attempts to invade your body. First, they must get past your barriers. Many invaders will be repelled simply by your intact skin or the secretions of your mucous membranes. If the invader gets inside your body, a series of weapons are stimulated by the introduction of a nonself-antigen. Cells (neutrophils, macrophages, basophils, etc.) are stimulated. Chemicals (cytokines) are released, which stimulate inflammation and phagocytosis.

Macrophages and other cells, which have ingested some of the invaders and are now wearing the foreign antigens, move to the lymphatic system and search the lymph nodes, looking for the T and B cells that will recognize the intruder. Helper T cells are activated. Helper T cells activate and cause the proliferation of B cells and cytotoxic T cells as well as release chemicals that further stimulate the phagocytic cells and inflammation. B cells produce antibodies that destroy the invaders and further stimulate immune response. Cytotoxic T cells destroy invaders directly and release chemicals that further stimulate immune response.

Immune response, both innate and adaptive, will continue to be stimulated until the feedback loop is stopped, at least in part by regulatory T cells. Memory B cells and T cells will be stored in the lymph nodes for later use if another army of those same type of pathogens attempt another invasion. Macrophages and other phagocytic cells will clean up the debris left by the warfare waged by your immune system. Once the danger is passed, your body will return to normal.

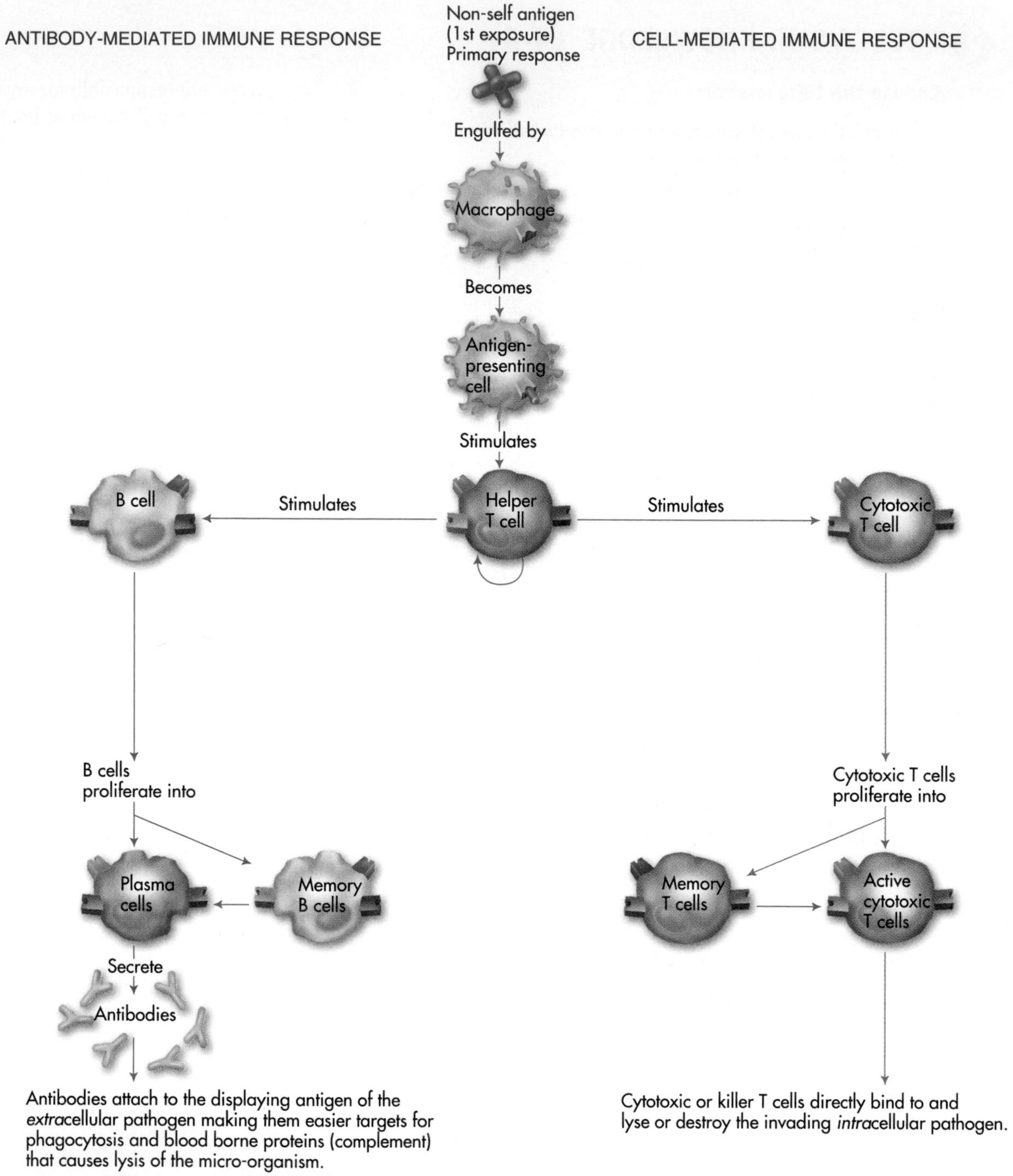

FIGURE ■ 14–11

The battle plan of the body's defenses.

COMMON DISORDERS OF THE IMMUNE SYSTEM

Immune disorders can be life-threatening because of a weakened or immunocompromised body defense system. The system can become compromised by factors outside of the body, such as invading viruses, or by a situation in which the body attacks itself.

Immunodeficiency Disorders

Patients with any of several types of immunodeficiency disorders have immune systems that are underactive. Their immune systems do not respond adequately to the invasion of pathogens and therefore do not protect them from infection. Patients who are immune deficient get sick very easily and do not recover quickly. Minor infections can be fatal. Some immune-deficient patients become infected by pathogens that usually cannot infect humans. Immune deficiency can be caused by viruses, genetics, chemical or radiation exposure, or even medication.

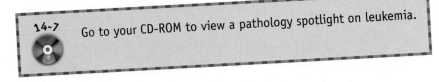

14-7 Go to your CD-ROM to view a pathology spotlight on leukemia.

Immune-compromised patients include those with AIDS, SCID (severe combined immune deficiency, a genetic disorder), leukemia (cancer of the white blood cells), some forms of anemia, and patients undergoing chemotherapy or taking immunosuppressant drugs after organ transplant.

Autoimmune Disorders

Autoimmune disorders are the opposite of immunodeficiency disorders, exactly what you would expect, given their name. Autoimmune disorders occur when the immune system attacks some part of the body. For some reason, the body fails to recognize "self" and destroys its own tissue as if it were an invader. There are literally hundreds of autoimmune disorders. Any part of the body can come under attack by mistake. Some of the more common disorders (and what they attack) are as follows:

- rheumatoid arthritis (joint linings)
- multiple sclerosis (myelin sheath in central nervous system)
- lupus erythematosis (every tissue, perhaps DNA)
- Type 1 diabetes (beta cells in pancreas)
- myesthenia gravis (acetylcholine receptors in skeletal muscle)
- Graves' disease (thyroid gland)
- Addison's disease (adrenal gland)

Just this short list illustrates how devastating an autoimmune disorder can be. Imagine the full power of your immune system turning against your thyroid gland or myelin sheath. The effects are devastating. Most autoimmune disorders can be treated with immunosuppressant drugs, but treatment may not be spectacularly successful and side effects are often severe.

Hypersensitivity Reactions

During a hypersensitivity reaction, more commonly known as an allergy, the immune system mounts a hyperactive response to a foreign antigen, often treating a harmless antigen, like grass or mold or insect bite, as an invading pathogen.

14-8 Go to your CD-ROM to see an animation of the treatment with an EpiPen (device to deliver epinephrine) of severe allergic reactions leading to anaphylactic shock. In addition, you can view a video on a nonfatal but fairly common hypersensitivity reaction called allergic rhinitis or, in simple lay terms, the runny nose.

There are several types of drugs dispensed by a pharmacy to treat autoimmune and allergic disorders. To learn more about the professional opportunities within a pharmacy, please visit the companion website.

Local hypersensitivity reactions, like hay fever, hives, skin rashes, and asthma, are generally mild and not life threatening (asthma is an obvious exception). Systemic hypersensitivity reactions, known as anaphylaxis, are life threatening. During anaphylaxis, mast cells and basophils release immune-stimulating chemicals throughout the body. The chemicals cause widespread vasodilation, which leads to dangerously low blood pressure and heart failure. Hives and asthma may also accompany an anaphylactic reaction. See Figure 14–12 ■, which shows stimulation of the mast cells within the nose due to an allergen, which causes allergic rhinitis (runny nose). Note that mast cells are found throughout the body. If overstimulated in the eyes, mast cells cause red and runny eyes; if overstimulated in the lungs, they cause allergic asthma.

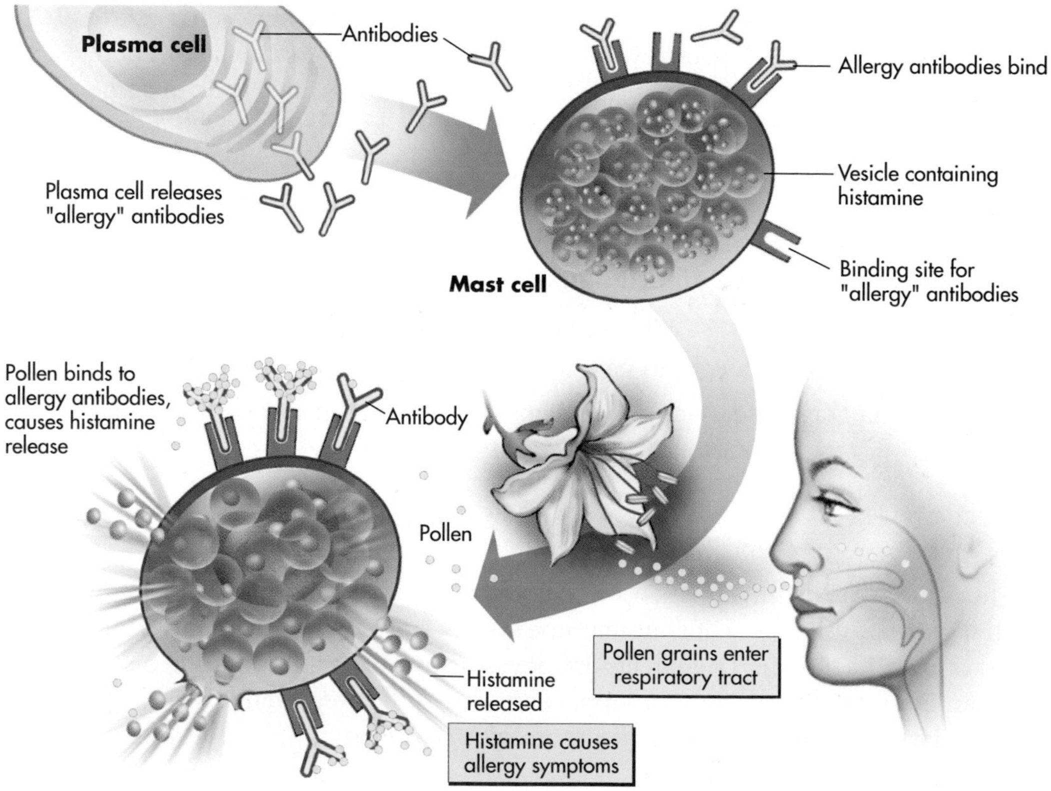

FIGURE ■ 14–12

Allergic rhinitis.

SUMMARY

Snapshots from the Journey

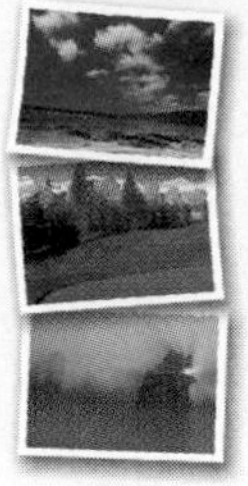

- The lymphatic system is the transport system for the immune system and houses the lymphocytes. It consists of lymph capillaries, vessels, trunks, and ducts containing lymphatic fluid and lymph nodes, which house white blood cells.
- Lymph nodes are concentrated in several regions of the body: cervical, axillary, inguinal, pelvic, abdominal, thoracic, and supratrochlear. These patches are in areas where pathogens are most likely to enter. Tonsils, adenoids, spleen, and thymus all contain lymphatic tissue.
- Fluid leaking from blood capillaries enters tissue fluid and flows into lymph capillaries. The fluid is carried through lymph capillaries to lymph vessels to lymph nodes. In the nodes, any pathogens are destroyed by white blood cells. Fluid then flows from nodes to vessels to lymphatic trunks to collecting ducts and into either the right or left subclavian vein, returning the fluid to the bloodstream.
- The thymus and spleen are lymphatic organs. The spleen contains blood sinuses and removes dead and dying red blood cells as well as pathogens. The thymus is the birthplace of T lymphocytes.
- Immune system function is based on its ability to recognize cell surface molecules called antigens. The immune system must ignore self-antigens (the body's antigens) and respond to nonself-antigens (foreign cells).
- The immune system is divided into two separate but extremely interdependent parts, innate immunity and adaptive immunity. Innate immunity is nonspecific, has no memory, and cannot improve performance with experience. Adaptive immunity is specific, has memory, and can improve performance with experience.
- Barriers prevent pathogens from getting into the body. Barriers can be either physical or chemical. Skin and tears are examples of barriers.
- The immune system uses a dozen or more different types of cells to combat pathogens. All of these cells are leukocytes or modified leukocytes. Some are part of innate immunity and some are part of adaptive immunity. Their functions range from phagocytosis, chemical stimulation of other cells, and antigen display to antibody secretion and direct destruction of pathogens.
- Immune response is stimulated by a variety of chemicals, including the cytokines, histamine, and complement.
- Inflammation, the familiar redness, heat, swelling, and pain associated with infection, is a powerful tool in the immune system's arsenal. During inflammation, white blood cells are stimulated and attracted to the site of infection to destroy pathogens and clean up cellular debris. Inflammation is, like much of immune response, a two-edged sword. Too much inflammation may be more damaging than the infection itself.
- Fever, like inflammation, is a deliberate attempt by the body to destroy a pathogen. Chemicals trick the hypothalamus into raising the temperature setpoint in an attempt to make body temperature too hot for pathogens.
- Innate immune mechanisms are triggered by the presence of foreign antigens in the body. These mechanisms hold off the infection and stimulate adaptive immune mechanisms.

- Adaptive immunity uses T and B lymphocytes to fight specific pathogens. Lymphocytes must be selected during development to recognize foreign antigens but to ignore the body's own antigens. In order to fight a pathogen, lymphocytes must be activated by binding with antigen displaying cells. Once activated, lymphocytes must proliferate, making thousands of copies of themselves. Helper T cells are required for activation of most types of lymphocytes.
- B cells are mediators of antibody-mediated immunity. B cells are activated by binding to antigen-presenting cells and helper T cells. Once B cells begin to proliferate, they become either plasma cells or memory B cells. Plasma cells secrete antibodies during primary response. Antibodies help destroy pathogens by binding to antigens on infected cells. Memory B cells are stored for the next time the pathogen is encountered. They mediate secondary response.
- Cytotoxic T cells mediate cell-mediated immunity by directly killing infected cells. This is the primary T cell response. Like B cells, cytotoxic T cells are activated by helper T cells. Some T cells become memory T cells and mediate secondary response if the pathogen is encountered again.
- Regulatory T cells are one of the off-switches for the immune system. We don't know very much about how these cells work because they were only discovered in the last 10 years.
- Keep in mind that innate and adaptive immunity do not work separately. They work together. One stimulates the other in a huge positive feedback loop. If either innate or adaptive immunity stops working, the whole system breaks down.

Case Study

John has made big changes in his life. An IV drug user for more than 5 yeas, he recently completed an inpatient rehabilitation program and got serious about staying off drugs. His cousin, Bill, suggested that John move west to a quiet rural area and work on Bill's farm. John takes Bill up on his offer, figuring it will be a true fresh start.

John, who had lived in the city for his whole life, had never even seen a farm. He loved the peace and quiet and adjusted to the physical labor. Things went well for a few weeks, and then John fell ill. His head was stuffy, his nose ran, he had a cough, ran a low-grade fever, and his glands (really his cervical lymph nodes) swelled. No matter how much John slept, it was never enough. The mystery illness would hang around for a few days and then seem to go away, only to come back in a few days. Frustrated and a little scared, John finally went to see Bill's doctor.

Given John's history and symptoms, what might the doctor suspect?

The doctor runs some blood tests, including a differential white cell count, and to his delight, John's T cell count is normal and there are no signs of HIV antibodies. However, John's eosinophil, basophil, and neutrophil counts are elevated.

What do the symptoms suggest now that AIDS has been ruled out?

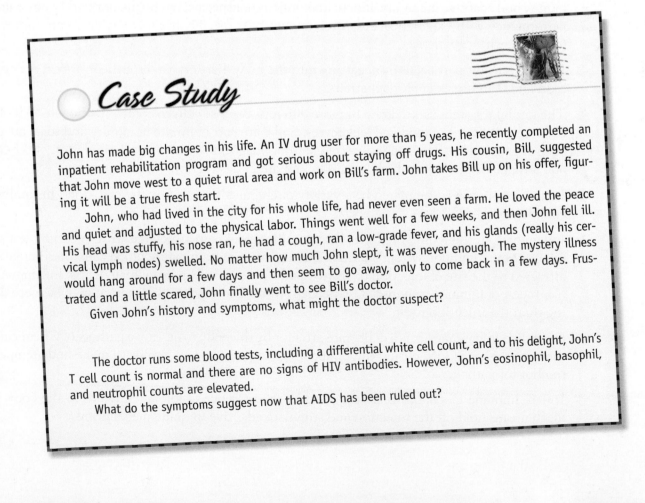

REVIEW QUESTIONS

Multiple Choice

1. Lymphocytes are selected for their ability to
   a. recognize antigens
   b. ignore self antigens
   c. a only
   d. both a and b

2. Mounting an excessive immune response to a harmless antigen is called a(n)
   a. autoimmune disorder
   b. allergy
   c. immunodeficiency
   d. AIDS infection

3. Which of the following is an innate immune cell?
   a. neutrophil
   b. memory cell
   c. helper T cell
   d. plasma cell

4. Lymphocytes are activated by binding with antigens on
   a. bacteria
   b. antigen displaying cells
   c. viruses
   d. lymph nodes

5. Innate immunity is not stimulated by foreign antigens.
   a. true
   b. false
   c. it depends
   d. all of the above

6. Fever and inflammation are both part of what kind of immunity?
   a. auto
   b. adaptive
   c. acquired
   d. innate

Short Answer

1. List the regions of the body containing many lymph nodes.

____

____

____

____

2. Trace the circulation of lymph from the cardiovascular system through the lymphatic system and back to the cardiovascular system.

3. List four types of cells and their functions in immunity.

4. Explain the differences between innate and adaptive immunity.

Suggested Activities

1. Draw a flow chart of innate and adaptive immunity and their interactions.

2. Form a group of students and role-play parts of the immune system. Assign some to be macrophages, others to be NK cells, and others to be B and T lymphocytes. Describe the process of fighting off a pathogen as per your role.

3. Using the Internet, do a quick search of autoimmune disorders. How many can you find? What tissues can be attacked by your immune system?

14-9 Now that you have completed your journey through this chapter, please go to the CD-ROM for interactive games and puzzles concerning the medical terms and concepts contained in this chapter. By playing the games you will reinforce your learning of medical terminology in a fun way.

Greetings from THE GASTROINTESTINAL System

Fuel for the Trip

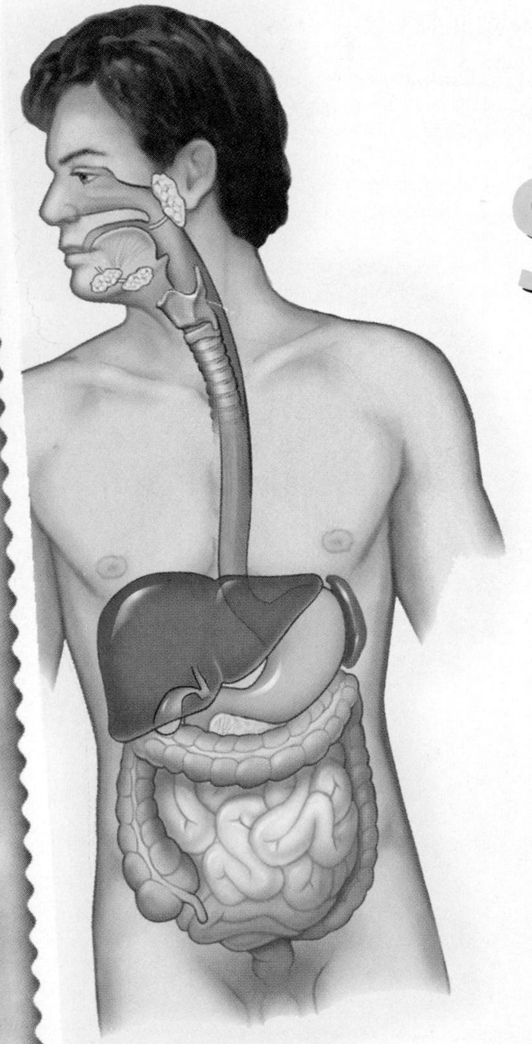

So far, we have discussed a variety of body systems and learned how they are put together and how they function. All of these systems need to function together to create a smooth-running machine. But just like a Ferrari, no matter how well it is designed nor how precisely it is put together, the body cannot function without fuel! This chapter focuses on the **gastrointestinal** (GI) system and how it

- *takes in (ingests)* raw materials,
- *breaks them down (digests)* both physically and chemically to usable elements,
- *absorbs* those elements, and
- *eliminates* what isn't usable.

These processes are accomplished through an amazing array of main and accessory organs and substances. Here is a concept to ponder as we journey through the digestive system: the food that enters your mouth, travels through your digestive system, and is eventually eliminated is never once *inside* your body but basically remains in a tubelike "highway" with materials contained within the food exiting the highway ramps in specific areas!

Chapter 15

LEARNING OBJECTIVES

Upon completion of your journey through this chapter, you will be able to:

- Locate and describe the functions of the main organs of the digestive system
- Locate and describe the function of the accessory organs for digestion
- Differentiate between ingestion and digestion and between chemical and mechanical processing of food
- Trace the journey of a bolus of food from the mouth to the anus
- Discuss the structure of the tooth
- Describe the various enzymes and chemicals needed for digestion
- Describe common disorders of the gastrointestinal system

MULTIMEDIA APPLICATIONS

CD-ROM Interactive Exercises

- 3-D animation of the digestive system, 15.1
- Animation of GERD, 15.2
- Interactive drag-and-drop exercise of the digestive system, 15.3
- Interactive drag-and-drop labeling of the intestinal wall, 15.4
- Videos on anorexia and bulimia, eating disorders, and diabetes, 15.5
- Interactive games and puzzles, 15.6

www.prenhall.com/colbert

- Professional Profile
  - Dental Assistants and Hygienists
  - Medical Profession: Dietician
- Related Internet Links
- Additional Review Questions

Pronunciation Guide

Correct pronunciation is important in any journey so that you and others are completely understood. Here is a "see and say" Pronunciation Guide for the more difficult terms to pronounce in this chapter.

adventitia (add ven TISH ah)
alimentary tract (al ah MEN tar ee)
appendicitis (ah pen dih SIGH tiss)
appendix (ah PEN dicks)
cecum (SEE kum)
cementum (si MEN tum)
cholecystitis (koh lee siss TYE tiss)
cholelithiasis (KOH lee lith EYE ah siss)
chyle (KILE)
chime (KIME)
defecation (deh fih CAY shun)
duodenum (doo ODD eh num)
emulsification (ee mull sih fih KAY shun)
epiglottis (ep ih GLAH tiss)
esophagus (eh SOFF ah guss)
frenulum (FREN you lum)
fundus (FUN duss)
gingivae (JIN jih vay)
hepatic duct (hep PA tic duct)
ilium (ILL ee um)
jejunum (jee JOO num)
labia (LAY bee ah)
mastication (MASS tih CAY shun)
mesentery (MEZ in tare ee)
pancreatitis (PAN kree ah TYE tiss)
peristalsis (pair ih STALL siss)
pharynx (FAIR inks)
plicae circulares (PLY Kay sir cue LAIR es)
pyloric sphincter (pye LOR ik SFINK ter)
pylorus (pye LOR uss)
rugae (ROO gay)
serosa (seh ROSE ah)
villi (VILL eye)

SYSTEM OVERVIEW

alimentary tract *(al ah MEN tar ee)*

anus *(AY nuss)*

The digestive tract (often called the **alimentary tract** or **alimentary canal**), is a muscular tube or tunnel-like structure that contains the organs of the digestive system. This tube begins at the mouth and ends at the **anus.** Between these two points are the pharynx, esophagus, stomach, and small and large intestines. In addition, *accessory organs* (such as teeth, salivary glands, liver, pancreas, and gallbladder) are necessary for processing materials into usable substances. Refer to Figure 15–1 ■ as we journey through the digestive system.

The components of the digestive system work together to perform the following general steps:

1. ingestion
2. mastication
3. digestion
4. secretion
5. absorption
6. excretion (defecation)

mastication *(MASS tih CAY shun)*

Food first enters the mouth, an activity called **ingestion.** Once food is ingested, the tongue and teeth work together to *mechanically process* the food by *physically* breaking it down. The chewing action is called **mastication.** This mechanical mixing process also continues in the muscular motions of the digestive tract, as you will soon see. **Digestion** is the *chemical process*

15-1 To view a 3-D animation of the digestive system, please go to your CD-ROM for this chapter.

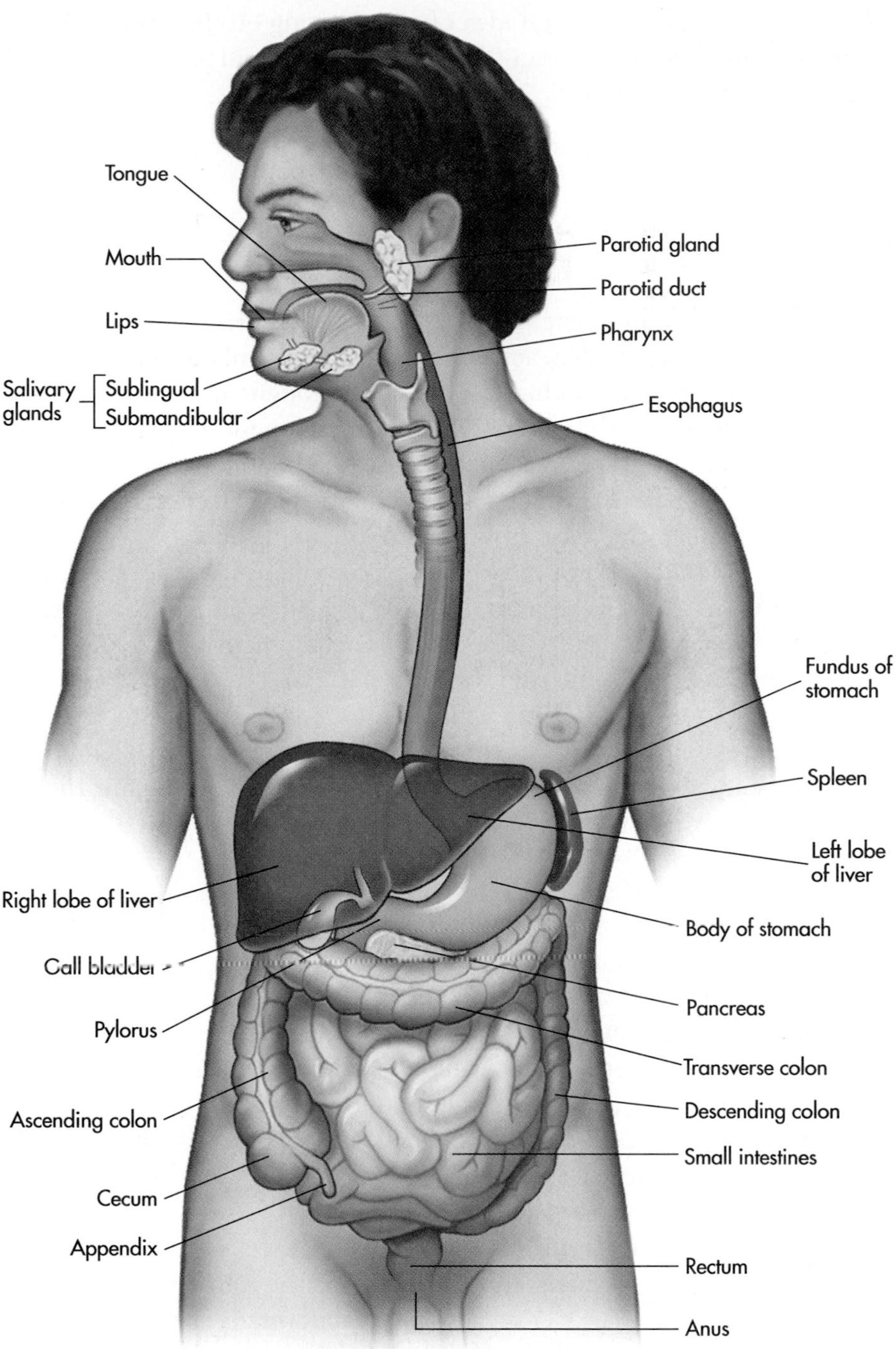

FIGURE ■ 15–1

The digestive system.

of breaking down food into small molecules. This is necessary so nutrients can be absorbed by the lining of the digestive tract.

The **secretion** of acids, buffers, enzymes, and water aid in the breakdown of food. Once the food is broken down both physically and chemically, it is ready for **absorption** through the lining of the digestive tract for use by the body. Finally, waste products and unusable materials are prepared for **excretion** and are eliminated by the body through **defecation.**

Now that you have a general idea of what's going on, let's begin the journey through the digestive system from beginning to end as a slice of double cheese, pepperoni pizza would!

THE MOUTH AND ORAL CAVITY

labia *(LAY bee ah)*
palates *(PAL ahts)*
uvula = *little grape*

pharynx *(FAIR inks)*

Your mouth is the opening that leads to the oral cavity, which is also called the *buccal cavity*. Your lips, or **labia,** act as a door to this chamber. The *hard* and *soft* **palates** create the roof of the chamber, while the **tongue** acts as the floor. The tongue's base (area of attachment) and the *uvula,* that punching bag–shaped object dangling down from the soft palate, act as the boundary between the oral cavity and the next part of the digestive system, the **pharynx.** As we discovered in our travels through the respiratory system, the uvula aids in swallowing because it helps direct food toward the pharynx and helps block food from coming out your nose! There is a pair of lingual tonsils back there too. Although they aren't important for digestion, the tonsils help in fighting infection as part of the lymphatic system. The sides of the cavity are created by your cheeks. Your mouth and oral cavity region receives, or *ingests,* food. The food is tasted, *mechanically* broken down into smaller pieces, and *chemically* broken down to some degree. Liquid is added to make it easier to swallow. See Figure 15–2 ■ to view the oral cavity.

Tongue

bolus *(BOW luss)*

frenulum *(FREN you lum)*
sub = *under*
lingual = *pertaining to tongue*

Your tongue is a muscle that performs many duties. It provides taste stimuli to your brain, senses temperature and texture (as does the rest of your mouth), manipulates food while chewing, and aids in swallowing. As the tongue moves the food around in the oral cavity, saliva is added to moisten and soften the food, while teeth continue to crush the food until it reaches the right consistency. The tongue pushes the food into a ball-like mass called a **bolus** so it can be passed on to the pharynx. If you can push that bolus into the pharynx with your tongue, why don't you swallow your tongue too? A membrane under your tongue, called the lingual **frenulum,** which you can see when you lift up your tongue, prevents this from happening. Not only is the frenulum important for swallowing, it also aids in proper speaking. An abnormally short frenulum prevents clear speech, hence the term "tongue-tied"!

Salivary Glands

parotid salivary gland *(pah RAH tid SAL ih vair ee glands)*

sublingual salivary glands *(sub LIN gwill SAL ih vair ee glands)*
submandibular salivary glands *(sub MAN dih bue lar SAL ih vair ee glands)*

As you can see in Figure 15–3 ■, there are three pairs of salivary glands, which are controlled by the autonomic nervous system. A large **parotid salivary gland** is found slightly inferior and anterior to each ear. These are the ones that swell up and make you look like a chipmunk when you get the mumps. The ducts from these glands empty into the upper portion of the oral cavity. The smallest of the salivary glands, the **sublingual salivary glands,** are located under the tongue. The **submandibular salivary glands** are located on both sides along the inner surfaces of the mandible, or lower jaw.

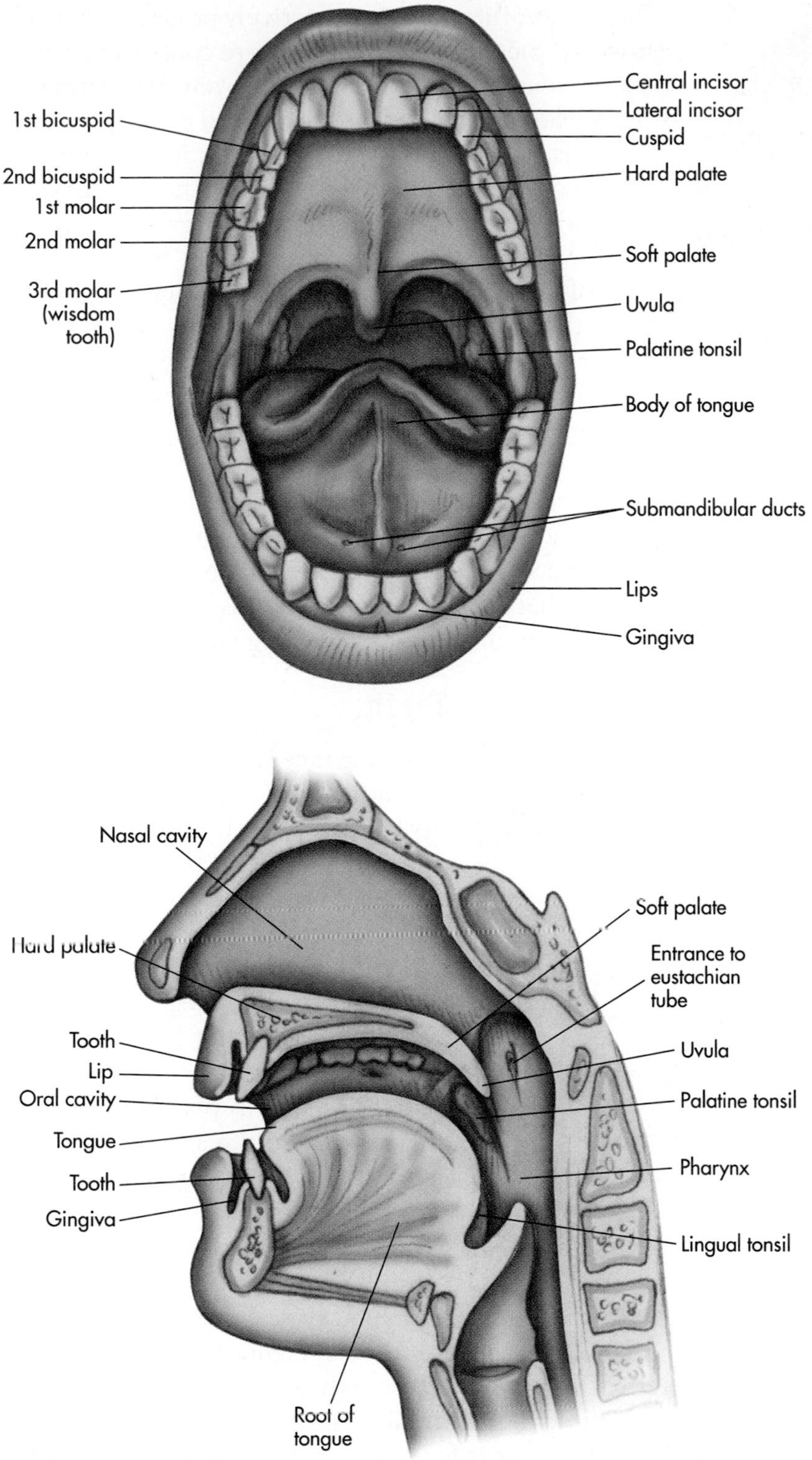
Central incisor
Lateral incisor
Cuspid
Hard palate
Soft palate
Uvula
Palatine tonsil
Body of tongue
Submandibular ducts
Lips
Gingiva
1st bicuspid
2nd bicuspid
1st molar
2nd molar
3rd molar (wisdom tooth)
Nasal cavity
Hard palate
Tooth
Lip
Oral cavity
Tongue
Tooth
Gingiva
Root of tongue
Soft palate
Entrance to eustachian tube
Uvula
Palatine tonsil
Pharynx
Lingual tonsil

FIGURE ■ 15–2

The mouth and oral cavity.

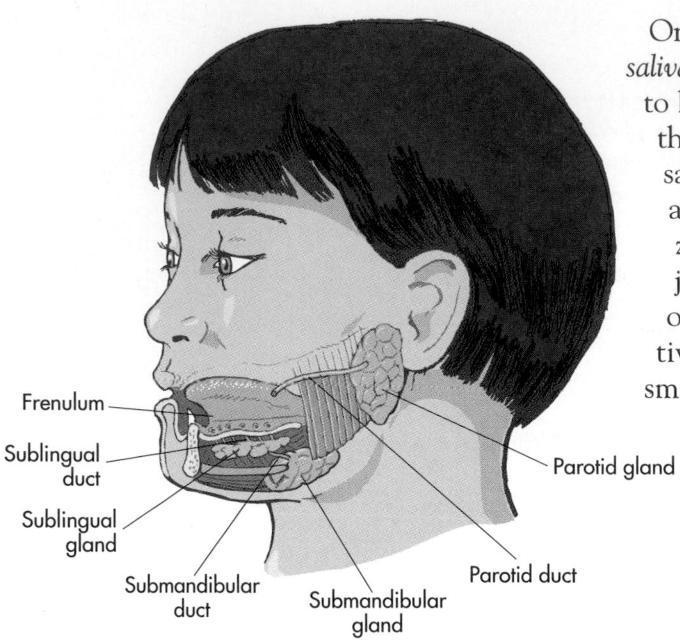

FIGURE ■ 15–3

The salivary glands.

On average, these glands collectively produce *1 to 1.5 liters of saliva daily!* Small amounts of saliva are continuously produced to keep your mouth moist, but once you start eating or even think about eating, look out! The flood gates open! Although saliva is almost totally water (99.4%), it also contains some antibodies, buffers, ions, waste products, and **enzymes.** Enzymes are formed by cells. They are organic catalysts whose job is to speed up chemical reactions. Salivary amylase is one of the digestive enzymes that speed up the chemical activity that breaks down carbohydrates, such as starches, into smaller molecules, such as glucose, that are more easily absorbed by the digestive tract once they get there. So, before you even swallow a bite of pizza, amylase is breaking down the starch in the crust for digestion. Saliva plays an important role even *after* you eat. As the saliva is continuously secreted in small amounts, it cleans the oral surfaces and also aids in reducing the amount of bacteria that grows in your mouth. Just remember, that action is *not* a substitute for brushing your teeth!

> *Clinical Application*
>
> **SUBLINGUAL MEDICATION**
>
> Go to a mirror and open your mouth. Lift your tongue and you will notice that there are blood vessels everywhere just barely underneath the surface of the skin. This sublingual blood vessel network can readily absorb substances such as certain drugs. Rapid absorption into the blood system is vital in some cases, such as for those who need the drug nitroglycerin to treat angina quickly. Angina is caused by insufficient blood flow to the heart and consequently not enough oxygen to coronary tissues. Nitroglycerin improves coronary blood flow and in most cases relieves angina.

Teeth

The final important components of the mechanical aspect of digestion in the oral cavity are the teeth. It is unfortunate that we get only two sets of them in a lifetime.

The first set of teeth are called *baby teeth*, or more properly, **deciduous teeth.** Like the leaves on a deciduous tree, they fall away in time. Beginning at around 6 months of age, they begin to appear, the first being the lower central incisors, with all 20 usually in place by 2 1/2 years of age. Between the ages of 6 and 12 years the Tooth Fairy is kept busy as these teeth are pushed out and replaced by the 32 larger *permanent teeth*. The exception to this are the *wisdom teeth*, which may not appear until an individual is as old as 21 years.

deciduous *(deh SIH jew uss)*

Now, not all teeth are the same, as you can see by their shapes and locations. Each has special responsibilities. Look at Figure 15–4 ■ as we discuss the various types of teeth. The first tooth type is the **incisor** which is located at the front of your mouth, unless you are an aggressive hockey player. Incisors are blade-shaped teeth used to cut food. **Canine teeth** are for holding, tearing, or slashing food. Canine teeth are also known as eyeteeth, or **cuspids,** and are located next to the incisors. Next in line are the **bicuspids,** or premolars, which are transitional teeth. **Molars** are the final type of teeth and have flattened tops. Both the bicuspids and molars are responsible for crushing and grinding.

Regardless of its type, the structure of each tooth is pretty much the same. As you can see in Figure 15–4, each tooth has a **crown, neck,** and **root.** The

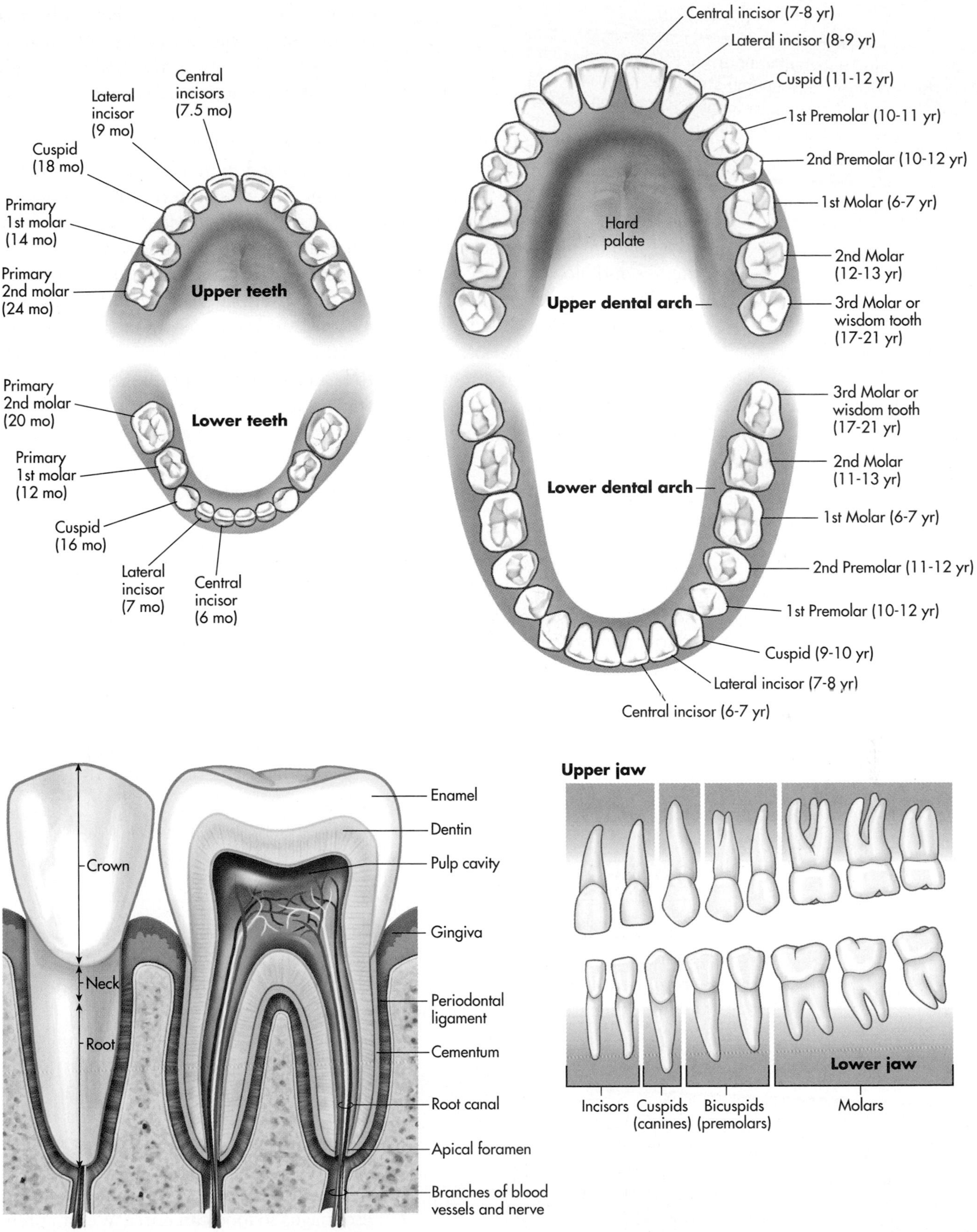
Central incisors (7.5 mo)
Lateral incisor (9 mo)
Cuspid (18 mo)
Primary 1st molar (14 mo)
Primary 2nd molar (24 mo)
Upper teeth
Lower teeth
Primary 2nd molar (20 mo)
Primary 1st molar (12 mo)
Cuspid (16 mo)
Lateral incisor (7 mo)
Central incisor (6 mo)
Central incisor (7-8 yr)
Lateral incisor (8-9 yr)
Cuspid (11-12 yr)
1st Premolar (10-11 yr)
2nd Premolar (10-12 yr)
1st Molar (6-7 yr)
Hard palate
2nd Molar (12-13 yr)
Upper dental arch
3rd Molar or wisdom tooth (17-21 yr)
3rd Molar or wisdom tooth (17-21 yr)
2nd Molar (11-13 yr)
Lower dental arch
1st Molar (6-7 yr)
2nd Premolar (11-12 yr)
1st Premolar (10-12 yr)
Cuspid (9-10 yr)
Lateral incisor (7-8 yr)
Central incisor (6-7 yr)
Crown
Neck
Root
Enamel
Dentin
Pulp cavity
Gingiva
Periodontal ligament
Cementum
Root canal
Apical foramen
Branches of blood vessels and nerve
Upper jaw
Lower jaw
Incisors
Cuspids (canines)
Bicuspids (premolars)
Molars

FIGURE ■ 15–4

Types, location and, structures of teeth.

Dental assistants and hygienists are dedicated to keeping the teeth and surrounding structures clean and free of disease. In addition, they assist in taking X-rays and making impressions for dental cosmetics. To learn more about the professions of dental assistance and hygienist, please go to the companion website.

crown is the visible part of the tooth. It is covered by the hardest biologically manufactured substance in the body, **enamel.** The *neck* is a transitional section that leads to the *root*.

Internally, most teeth are made up of a mineralized, bonelike substance called **dentin.** The next internal layer is a connective tissue called **pulp,** which is located in the *pulp cavity*. The pulp cavity also contains blood vessels and nerves that provide nutrients and sensations. The nerves and blood vessels get to the pulp cavity via the infamous root canal.

cementum *(si MEN tum)*
periodontal *(perr ee oh DON til)*
gingiva *(jin jih VA)*

The root is nestled in a bony socket and is held in place by fibers of the periodontal ligament. In addition, **cementum** covers the dentin of the root, aiding in securing the **periodontal ligament.** Cementun is a soft version of bone. Healthy gums, or **gingiva,** also help to hold the teeth in place. Epithelial cells form a tight seal around the tooth to prevent bacteria from coming into contact with the tooth's cementum.

PHARYNX

epiglottis *(ep ih GLAH tiss)*

The pharynx brings us to the next part of the journey. It is a common passageway not only for food but also for water and air. It has three parts: the *nasopharynx*, the *oropharynx*, and the *laryngopharynx*. The nasopharynx is primarily part of the respiratory system. The oropharynx and the laryngopharynx serve double duty as a passageway for food and water and for air. During swallowing, passageways to the nasal and respiratory regions are protected from the accidental introduction of food and liquids. The nasopharynx is blocked by the soft palate, and a flap of tissue, called the **epiglottis,** covers the airway to the lungs as the trachea rises during swallowing. These actions force the food to enter the only possible route, the esophagus.

ESOPHAGUS

The **esophagus** is approximately 10 inches (25 centimeters) long and is responsible for transporting food from the pharynx to the stomach. It extends from the pharynx, through the thoracic cavity and diaphragm, to the stomach, which is located in the peritoneal cavity (see Figure 15–5 ■).

15-2 Gastroesophageal reflux disease (GERD) is a fairly common disorder in which the lower esophageal sphincter does not properly reseal off and allows the acidic stomach contents to back up (reflux) into the esophagus, causing a burning sensation. If left untreated, it can cause serious damage to the esophagus. To see an animation of GERD, please go to your CD-ROM.

The esophagus is normally a collapsed tube, much like a deflated balloon, until a bolus of food is swallowed. As this bolus moves to the esophagus, a muscular ring at the beginning of this structure, known as the **pharyngoesophageal sphincter,** relaxes. This is like opening the door to the esophagus so food can enter. We can't rely on gravity to move food through the esophagus, so the muscles of the esophagus begin rhythmic contractions that work the food down to the stomach. This rhythmic muscular contraction is known as **peristalsis.** Once the bolus reaches the end of the esophagus, a second door must be opened to allow entry to the stomach. This is the **lower esophageal sphincter,** or **LES,** also known as the *cardiac sphincter,* that relaxes to let food into the stomach and then closes to prevent acidic gastric juices from squirting up into the esophagus. Heartburn (pyrosis) is what happens if that door inadvertently opens.

The esophagus also helps move the bolus by excreting mucus so its walls are slippery. The esophageal walls are lined with stratified squamous epithelium, which makes the esophagus resistant to abrasion, temperature extremes, and irritation by chemicals.

The whole process of swallowing food takes about 9 seconds on average. Dry or "sticky" food may take longer with repeated attempts to work it down (ever try to swallow too large a bite of a peanut butter sandwich and have it stick, pounding on the LES door?). Fluids take only seconds to get to the stomach.

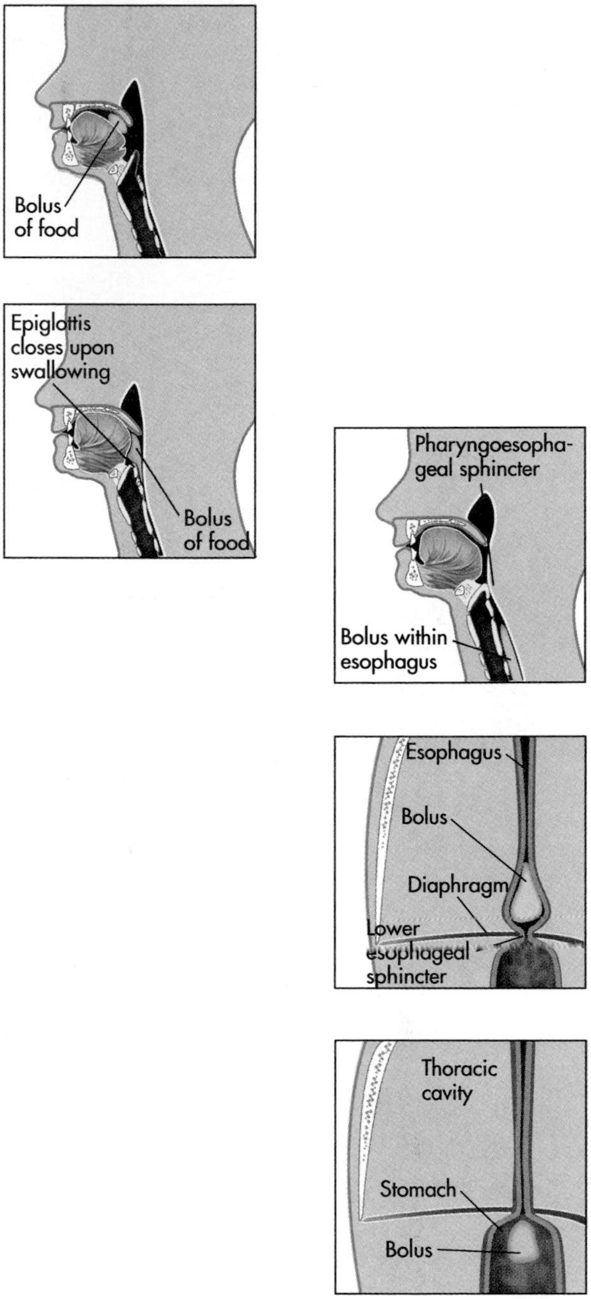

FIGURE ■ 15–5

The movement of a bolus of food from the mouth to the stomach via the esophagus.

THE WALLS OF THE ALIMENTARY CANAL

It is interesting to note that the same four basic tissue types form the wall of the entire alimentary canal from the esophagus onward (see Figure 15–6 ■). The innermost layer that lines the lumen of the canal is the **mucosa.** This layer is composed mostly of surface epithelium with some connective tissue and a thin smooth muscle layer surrounding it. The mucosa also possesses cells that secrete *digestive enzymes* to break down foodstuffs and *goblet cells* that secrete *mucus* for lubrication.

The **submucosa** is the next layer and is composed of soft connective tissue. This layer contains blood and lymph vessels, lymph nodes (called Peyer patches which are similar to your tonsils), and nerve endings. The next layer is the **muscularis externa** and is composed of two layers of smooth muscle. The innermost layer encircles the canal, while the outer layer is longitudinal in nature so it lies in the direction of the canal. There is an additional third layer of oblique smooth muscle, but it is only found surrounding the stomach.

The outermost layer is the **serosa,** composed of a single thin layer of flat, serous, fluid-producing cells supported by connective tissue. For most of the canal, the serosa is the *visceral peritoneum*. The peritoneum is a serous membrane in the abdominopelvic cavity. Like all serous membranes it has two layers. The visceral peritoneum covers the organs and the parietal peritoneum lines the wall of the abdominopelvic cavity. Between the layers is a fluid filled potential space called the peritoneal cavity. This fluid is important for both keeping the outer surface of the intestines moist and allowing friction-free movement of the digestive organs against the abdomenopelvic cavity. Some abdominal organs such as the urinary bladder and the duodenum are not surrounded by peritoneum and are called retroperitoneal organs. The esophagus differs in that it possesses only a loose layer of connective tissue called the **adventitia.**

esophagus *(eh SOFF ah guss)*
pharyngoesophageal sphincter *(fair IN goee SOFF uh geel)*
peristalsis *(pair ih STALL siss)*

retro *(behind)*
adventitia *(add ven TISH ah)*

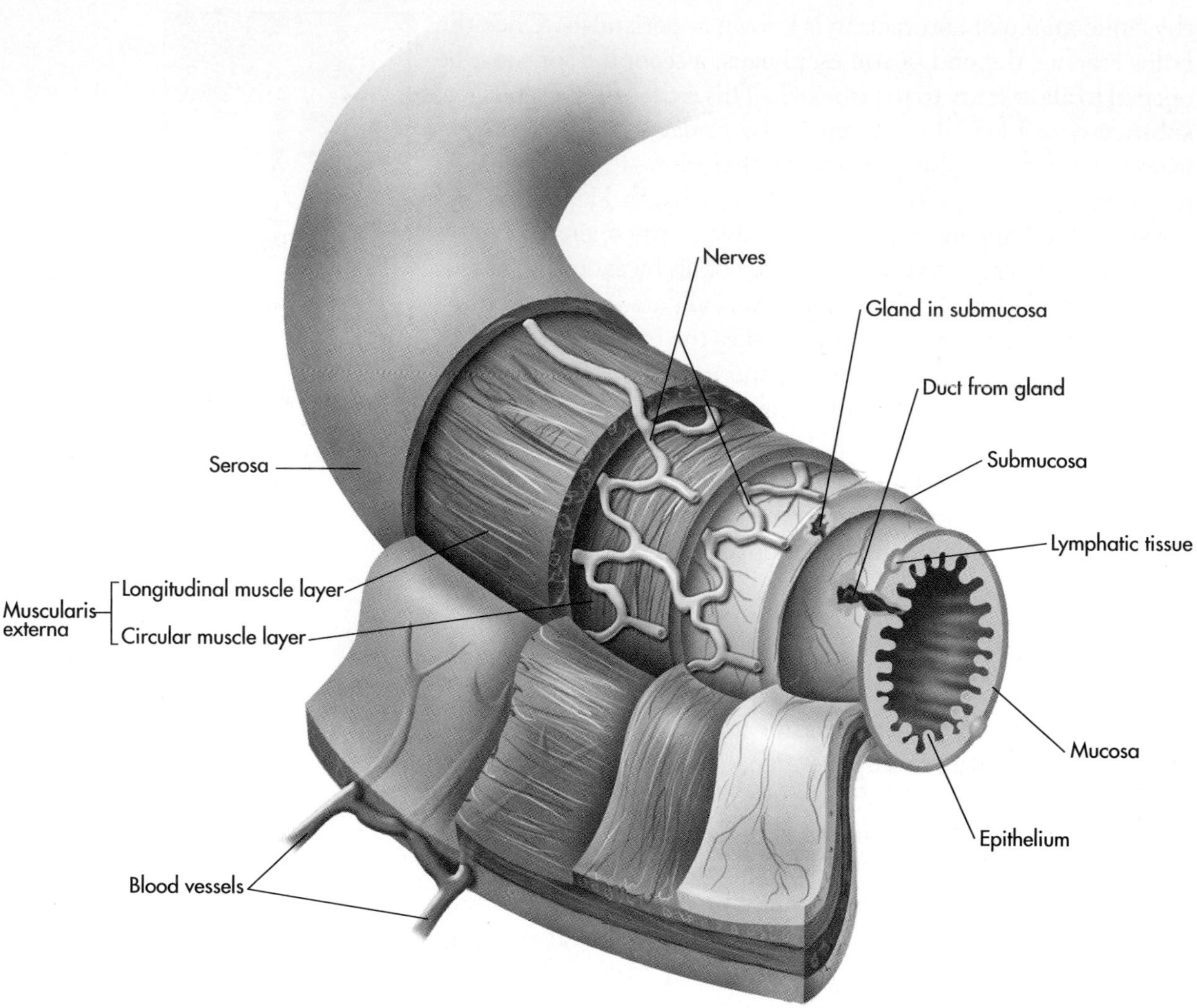

FIGURE 15–6

Basic tissue types of the alimentary canal.

TEST YOUR KNOWLEDGE 15-1

Choose the best answer:

1. The digestive tract is also called the
   a. elementary canal
   b. integumentary canal
   c. alimentary canal
   d. panama canal

2. A ball-like mass of food is called a
   a. bolus
   b. wad
   c. chyme
   d. mastion

3. What is the punching bag–shaped object dangling from the soft palate?
   a. tonsil
   b. uvula
   c. labia
   d. incisor

4. Which of the following is *not* a salivary gland?
   a. parotid
   b. sublingual
   c. submandibular
   d. substernal

Complete the following:

5. Externally, the three main structural parts of a tooth are the _____, _____, and _____.

STOMACH

The stomach is located in the left side of the abdominal cavity under the diaphragm and is covered almost completely by the liver. This organ is approximately 10 inches (25 centimeters) long with a diameter that varies, depending on how much you eat at any given time. Although the stomach can hold up to 4 liters (about a gallon) when totally filled, it can expand or decrease in diameter thanks to deep folds, called **rugae,** in the stomach wall that allow for these size changes. As the stomach receives food from the esophagus, it performs several functions:

rugae *(ROO gay)*

- acts as a temporary holding area for the received food
- secretes gastric acid and enzymes, which it mixes with the food, causing chemical digestion
- regulates the rate at which the now partially digested food (a thick, heavy, creamlike liquid called **chyme**) enters the small intestine
- absorbs small amounts of water and substances on a very limited basis (although the stomach does absorb alcohol)

chyme *(KIME)*

It takes about four hours for the stomach to empty after a meal. Liquids and carbohydrates pass through fairly quickly. Protein takes a little more time, and fats take even longer, usually between 4 to 6 hours.

The stomach is divided into four regions. Located near the heart, the *cardiac region* surrounds the lower esophageal sphincter (see Figure 15–7 ■). The **fundus,** which is actually lateral and slightly superior to the cardiac region, temporarily holds the food as it first enters the stomach. The *body* is the midportion and largest region of the stomach. The funnel-shaped, terminal end of the stomach is called the **pylorus.** Most of the digestive work of the stomach is performed in the pyloric region. This is also the region where chyme must pass through another door, the **pyloric sphincter,** in order to travel on to the small intestine. Two other points of interest are the concave curve called the *lesser curvature* and the larger convex curve to the left of the lesser curve called the *greater curvature*.

fundus *(FUN duss)*

pylorus *(pye LOR uss)*

pyloric sphincter *(pye LOR ik SFINK ter)*

The muscular action of the stomach works much like a cement mixer and is achieved by the three layers of muscle found in its walls. One layer is *longitudinal*, one is *circular*, and the third is *oblique* in orientation. This arrangement of muscles enables the stomach to churn food as it mixes with gastric juices excreted by *gastric glands* from *gastric pits* in the columnar epithelial lining of the stomach as well as to work the food toward the pyloric sphincter through the muscle activity, peristalsis. With the combined efforts of muscle and gastric juices, both physical and chemical digestion occur in the stomach.

Gastric juice is a general term for a combination of *hydrochloric acid* (HCl), *pepsinogen*, and *mucus*. About 1,500 milliliters of gastric juice is produced each day by gastric glands. Pepsinogen is secreted by the *chief cells*, and HCl is secreted by *parietal cells*. These two cell types have a special relationship in that once pepsinogen makes contact with HCl, the chief digestive enzyme, **pepsin,** is formed. Pepsin is needed to break down proteins (like the ones found in pepperoni). Even though it doesn't actually digest food by itself, HCl does break down connective tissue in meat (our pepperoni, again). HCl must be

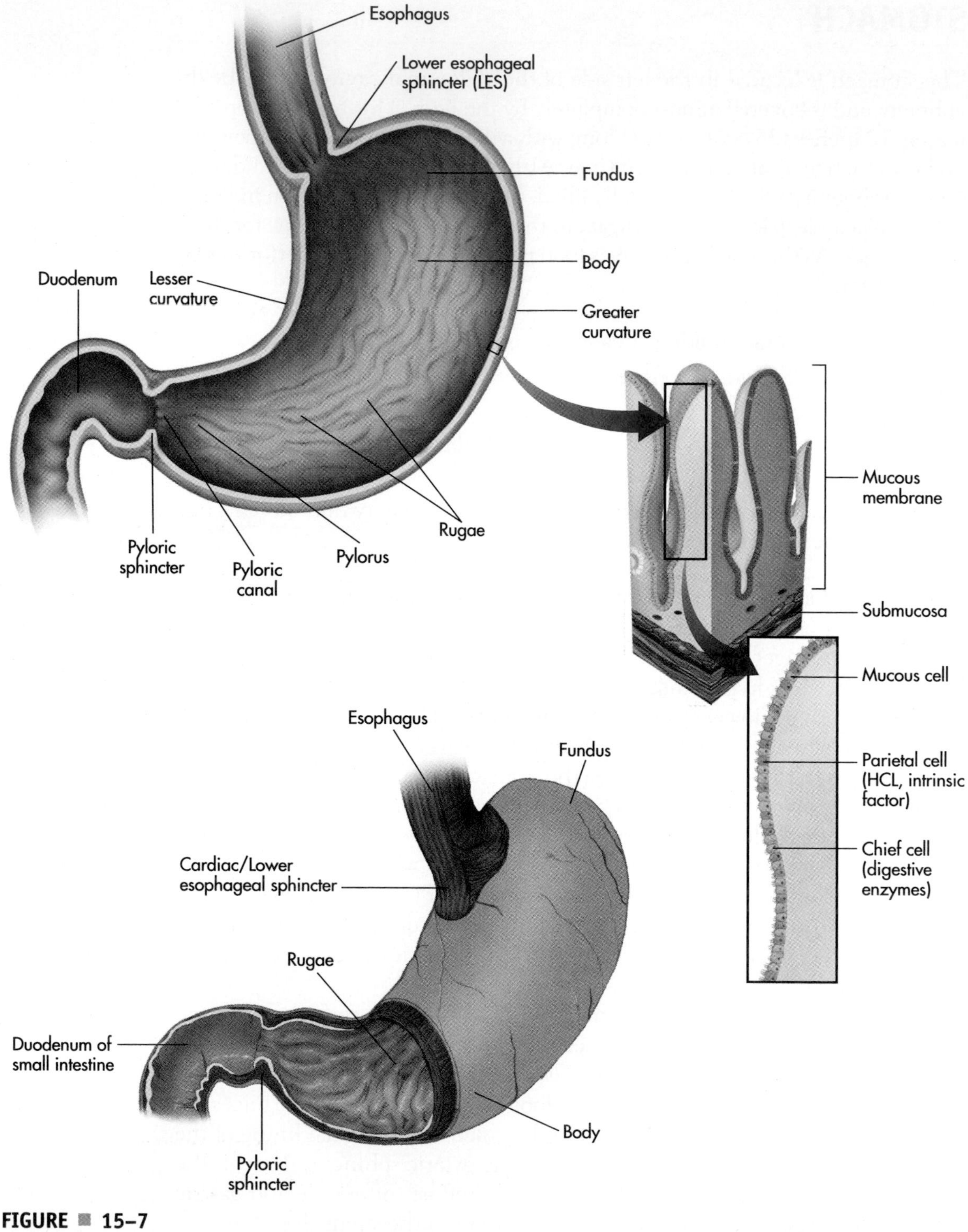

FIGURE ■ 15–7

The stomach.

very strong to work. Normally, it has a very acidic pH of 1.5 to 2. This highly acidic environment plays another important role: killing off most pathogens that enter the stomach. Why doesn't the stomach digest itself you may wonder. A healthy stomach is protected by *mucous cells*, which generate a thick layer of mucus to shield the stomach lining from the effects of HCl! Other specialized cells secrete what is known as *intrinsic factor*, which is needed for absorption of vitamin B_{12}. See Table 15–1, which describes gastric glands and their functions.

The stomach's activity is controlled by the parasympathetic nervous system, particularly the *vagus nerve*. Once the vagus nerve is stimulated, the stomach's *motility* (churning action) increases, as does the secretory rates of the gastric glands.

The three distinct phases of gastric juice production are illustrated in Figure 15–8 ■. The *cephalic phase* occurs as a result of sensory stimulation such as the sight or smell of food. This sensory input stimulates the parasympathetic nervous system (via the medulla oblongata) and the release of the hormone **gastrin** is increased. Once gastrin travels through the blood and reaches the stomach, gastric gland activity is increased. So, the sight or smell of that pizza literally does get your gastric juices flowing.

gastrin *(GAS trin)*

This leads us to the *gastric phase* in which over two thirds of the gastric juices are secreted as the food moves into the stomach. As the food moves in, the stomach begins to distend. As the stomach distends, it sends signals back to the brain, which fires a reply to the gastric glands to step up their work. As chyme is formed, it is passed through the pyloric sphincter to the first part of the small intestine, the **duodenum.**

duodenum *(doo ODD eh num)*

This begins the *intestinal phase* of gastric juice regulation. As the duodenum distends and senses the acidity of chyme, intestinal hormones are released that cause the gastric glands in the stomach to decrease gastric juice production. The brain is also signaled and sends a message to inhibit gastric juice secretion because it is no longer needed now that the food bolus (now called chyme) has left the stomach. Once the chyme begins its movement through the duodenum and on to the rest of the small intestine, those inhibitory responses are halted so gastric juice production can continue once again when a new bolus of food enters the stomach.

TABLE 15–1 Gastric Glands and Their Functions

DIGESTIVE CELLS	SECRETION TYPE	FUNCTION
chief cells	pepsinogen	begins digestion of protein
parietal cells	HCl	kills pathogens, activates pepsinogen, breaks down connective tissue in meat
mucous cells	alkaline mucus	protects stomach lining
endocrine cells	the hormone gastrin	stimulates gastric gland secretion

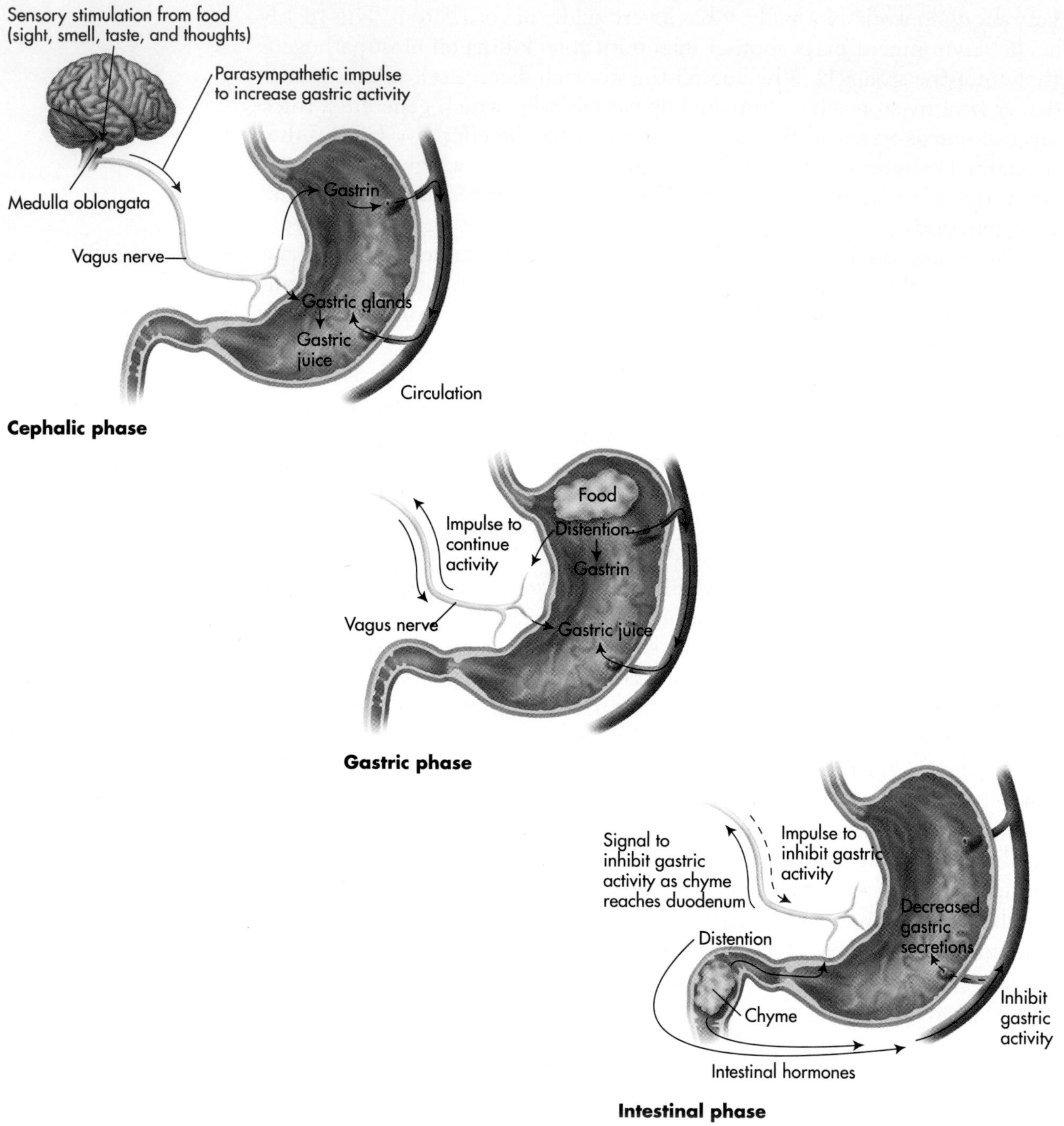

FIGURE ■ 15–8

Phases of gastric secretions.

Interestingly, the rate of the movement of chyme is very important. If it moves too slowly and slowly empties from the stomach, the rate of nutrient digestion and absorption is decreased and may allow the acidity of the chyme to cause erosion of the stomach lining. If chyme passes too quickly through the stomach, the food particles may not be sufficiently mixed with gastric juices, leading to insufficient digestion. Chyme that is not given time to be neutralized may lead to acidic erosion of the intestinal lining.

SMALL INTESTINE

Located in the central and lower abdominal cavity the small intestine is, surprisingly, *the* major organ of digestion. It is where most food is digested (see Figure 15–9 ■). The small intestine is small in diameter, not in length. Beginning at the pyloric sphincter, the small intestine is also the longest section of the alimentary canal, with a length up to 20 feet (up to 6 meters) and a diameter ranging from 4 centimeters where it connects with the stomach to 2.5 centimeters where it meets the large intestine.

pancreas *(PAN kree ass)*
jejunum *(jee JOO num)*
ileum *(ILL ee um)*

The walls of the small intestine secrete several digestive enzymes important for the final stages of chemical digestion and two hormones that stimulate the pancreas and gallbladder to act and that control stomach activity.

In the small intestine, almost 80 percent of the absorption of usable nutrients takes place when chyme comes in contact with the mucosal walls. Amino acids, fatty acids, ions, simple sugars, vitamins, and water are all absorbed here. Some of the remaining 20 percent was already absorbed by the stomach, with the rest being absorbed by the large intestine. Any residue that cannot be utilized is sent on to the large intestine for removal from the body.

> *Learning Hint*
>
> **EMULSIFIERS**
>
> Think about what Italian Salad dressing is like before you shake it. Emulsifiers allow the oil and vinegar to blend together.

There are three regions of the small intestine. The duodenum is approximately 25 centimeters long and is located near the head of the **pancreas.** The duodenum gets it name from *duo* (two), and *denum* (ten), which equal 12, the number of fingerwidths long that this organ is (10 inches)!

The **jejunum** is the middle section and is approximately 2.5 meters (8 feet) long.

The terminal end of the small intestine is the **ileum.** This 2 meter (6 to 7 feet) section attaches to the large intestine at the *ileocecal valve*.

The previously discussed pyloric valve is important in allowing small portions of chyme to enter the first part of the small intestine (duodenum) because the small intestine can process only small amounts of food at a time. At the duodenum, additional secretions are added from the pancreas and gallbladder. The pancreas provides pancreatic juices and the gallbladder provides bile. Bile *emulsifies* fat; that is, it makes fat able to disperse in water making the fat found in the cheese of the pizza easier to breakdown. Pancreatic juice contains enzymes and sodium bicarbonate, which neutralizes the acidic chyme. The pancreas is stimulated to secrete as a result of the hormone *secretin* that is produced by the small

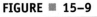

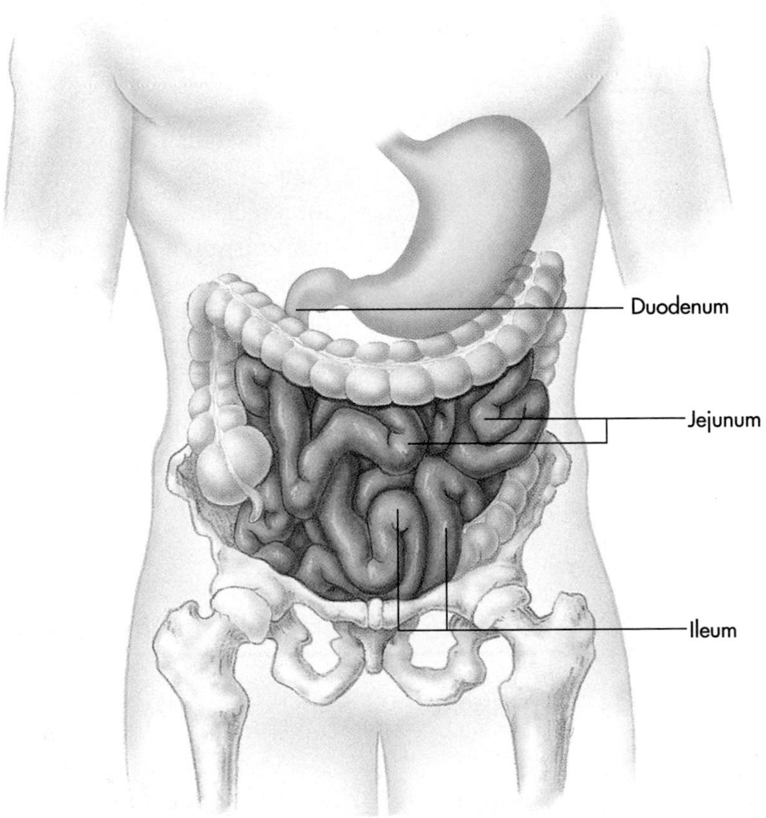

FIGURE ■ 15–9

The small intestine.

intestine. Gallbladder activity is caused by the hormone **cholecystokinin,** also known as **CCK,** which is also produced by the small intestine. Two types of muscular action occur in the small intestine. **Segmentation** is the muscle action that mixes chyme and digestive juices, working much like a cement mixer. Peristalsis also occurs, moving undigested food remains toward the large intestine. See Table 15–2 for the hormones active in the digestive process.

As previously stated, the small intestine also produces digestive enzymes that are needed to complete chemical digestion. These enzymes (and mucus) are produced by exocrine cells. *Lactase*, *maltase*, and *sucrase* are needed for the digestion of double sugars called *disaccharides* that are contained in starches (such as in the pizza crust). *Peptidase* is needed to digest portions of the protein structure called peptides. Internal *lipase* is needed for digestion of certain fats. It is interesting to note that the secretion of these substances is mainly due to the presence of chyme in the small intestine! Because of the acidity of chyme, both chemical and mechanical irritation occur. This irritation plus the distention of the intestinal wall causes the localized reflex action that results in the release of the enzymes and the two hormones.

Dieticians provide valuable information on nutrition and specialized diets. To view a video and obtain more information, visit your website for this chapter.

Learning Hint

THE ENDING *ASE*

Enzymes end in *ase* and break substances down.

15-3 For an interactive drag-and-drop labeling exercise of the digestive system, visit your CD for this chapter.

villi *(VILL eye)*

The structure of the wall of the small intestine is rather interesting. The wall possesses circular folds called *plicae circulares* and fingerlike protrusions into the lumen called **villi** (see Figure 15–10 ■). The villi also have outer layers of columnar epithelial cells, which possess microscopic extensions known as *microvilli*. These villi are tightly packed, giving a velvety texture and appearance. The purpose of the microvilli, villi, and circular folds is to provide an incredible increase in the surface area of the small intestine. This area, almost the surface area of a tennis court, increases the efficiency of the absorption of nutrients.

lacteal *(LACK te al)*
chyle *(KILE)*

Each villus (singular form of villi) contains a network of capillaries and a lymphatic capillary called a **lacteal.** Intestinal glands are located between villi. The capillaries absorb and transport sugars (the result of carbohydrate digestion)

TABLE 15–2 Hormones in the Digestive Process

HORMONE	SECRETING ORGAN	ACTION
gastrin	stomach	stimulates release of gastric juice
secretin	duodenum	stimulates release of bicarbonate and water from pancreas and bile from liver; slows stomach activity
cholecystokinin (CCK)	duodenum	stimulates digestive enzyme release from pancreas and bile release from gallbladder; slows stomach activity

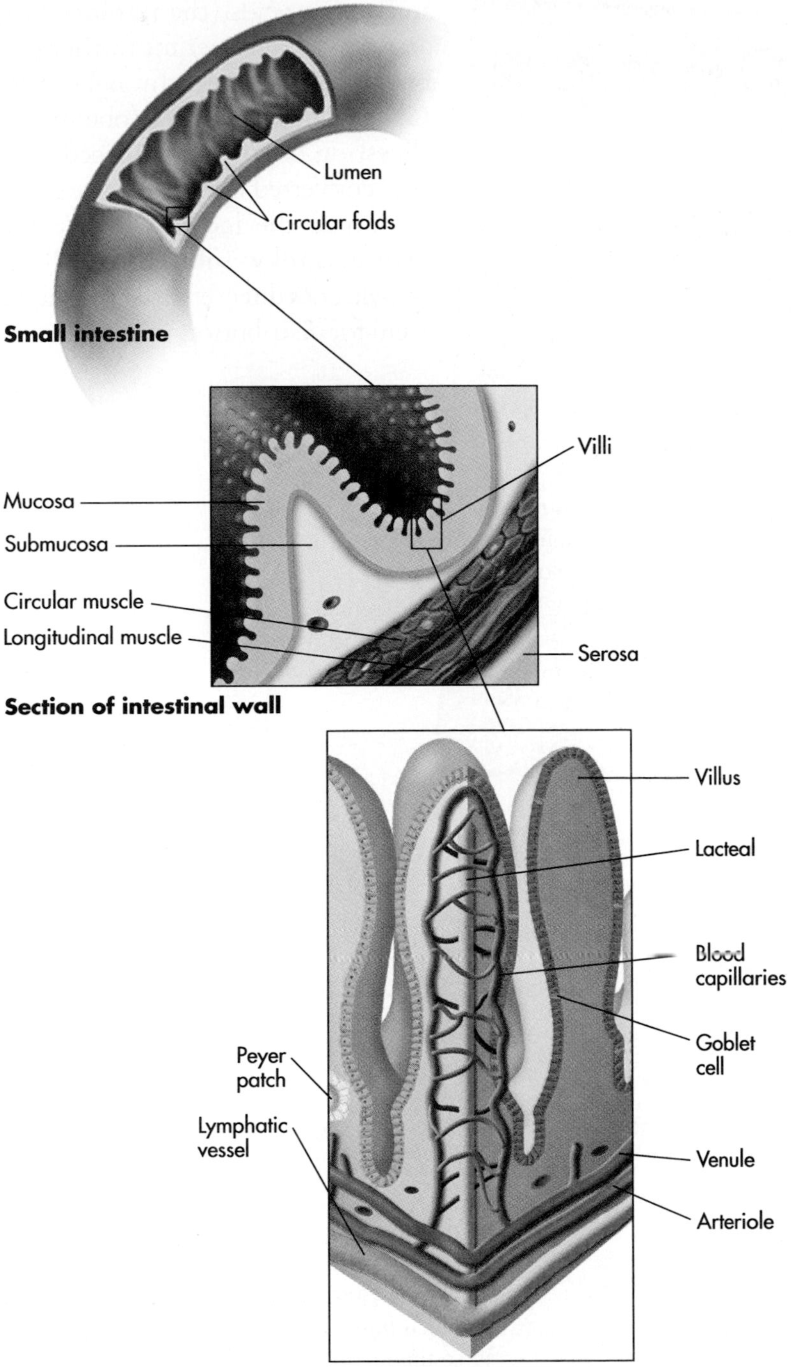
Lumen
Circular folds
Small intestine
Villi
Mucosa
Submucosa
Circular muscle
Longitudinal muscle
Serosa
Section of intestinal wall
Villus
Lacteal
Blood capillaries
Goblet cell
Peyer patch
Lymphatic vessel
Venule
Arteriole

FIGURE ■ 15–10

Villi.

and amino acids (the result of protein digestion) to the liver for further processing before they are sent throughout the body. Glycerol and fatty acids (obtained from the digestion of fat) are absorbed by the villi and converted into a lipoprotein that travels on to the lacteal where it is now a white, milky substance called **chyle.** Chyle goes directly into the lymphatic system for distribution throughout the body.

Clinical Application

LACTOSE INTOLERANCE

This unfortunate condition is the inability to digest the sugar (lactose) found in milk and dairy products such as cheese and ice cream. A person with lactose intolerance has a deficiency of lactase, an intestinal enzyme. As a result, lactose is not sufficiently digested. Normal bacteria found in the intestine utilizes those undigested sugars with gas production as a byproduct. This is what causes that "bloated feeling" you see on TV advertisements. In addition, the undigested lactose prevents normal water absorption by the small intestine, so diarrhea is formed. So the cheese pizza in our example would not be the meal of choice for these individuals who are lactose intolerant.

Interestingly, it seems that there is a genetic basis for this condition. In some populations, lactase production continues throughout their entire lives. Approximately 15 percent of the Caucasian population develops lactose intolerance, while 80 to 90 percent of the African American and Asian populations develop this condition to some degree.

To avoid this situation, individuals must either avoid milk and other dairy products or take an oral form of the enzyme lactase before consuming such products.

TEST YOUR KNOWLEDGE 15-2

Choose the best answer:

1. The deep folds of the stomach wall that allow for size changes of the stomach are called
   a. rugby
   b. sphincter
   c. rugae
   d. glottal folds

2. The final "door" of the stomach that needs to open for chyme to travel to the small intestine is located at the end of the
   a. fundus
   b. pylorus
   c. epiglottis
   d. adventitia

3. This chief digestive enzyme is needed to break down protein:
   a. guafinesin
   b. pepsin
   c. pylorin
   d. rugelin

4. A full two thirds of the gastric juices secreted in the stomach happen as food passes through this gastric juice production phase:
   a. cephalic phase
   b. intestinal phase
   c. gastric phase
   d. pharyngeal phase

Complete the following:

5. The stomach's activity is controlled by the _____ nervous system.

LARGE INTESTINE

Beginning at the junction with the end of the small intestine (*ileocecal orifice*) and extending to the **anus,** the **large intestine** almost totally borders the small intestine (see Figure 15–11 ■). The large intestine is responsible for

- water reabsorption
- absorption of vitamins produced by normal bacteria in the large intestine
- packaging and compacting waste products for elimination from the body.

Since there are no villi in the walls of the large intestine, little nutrient absorption occurs here.

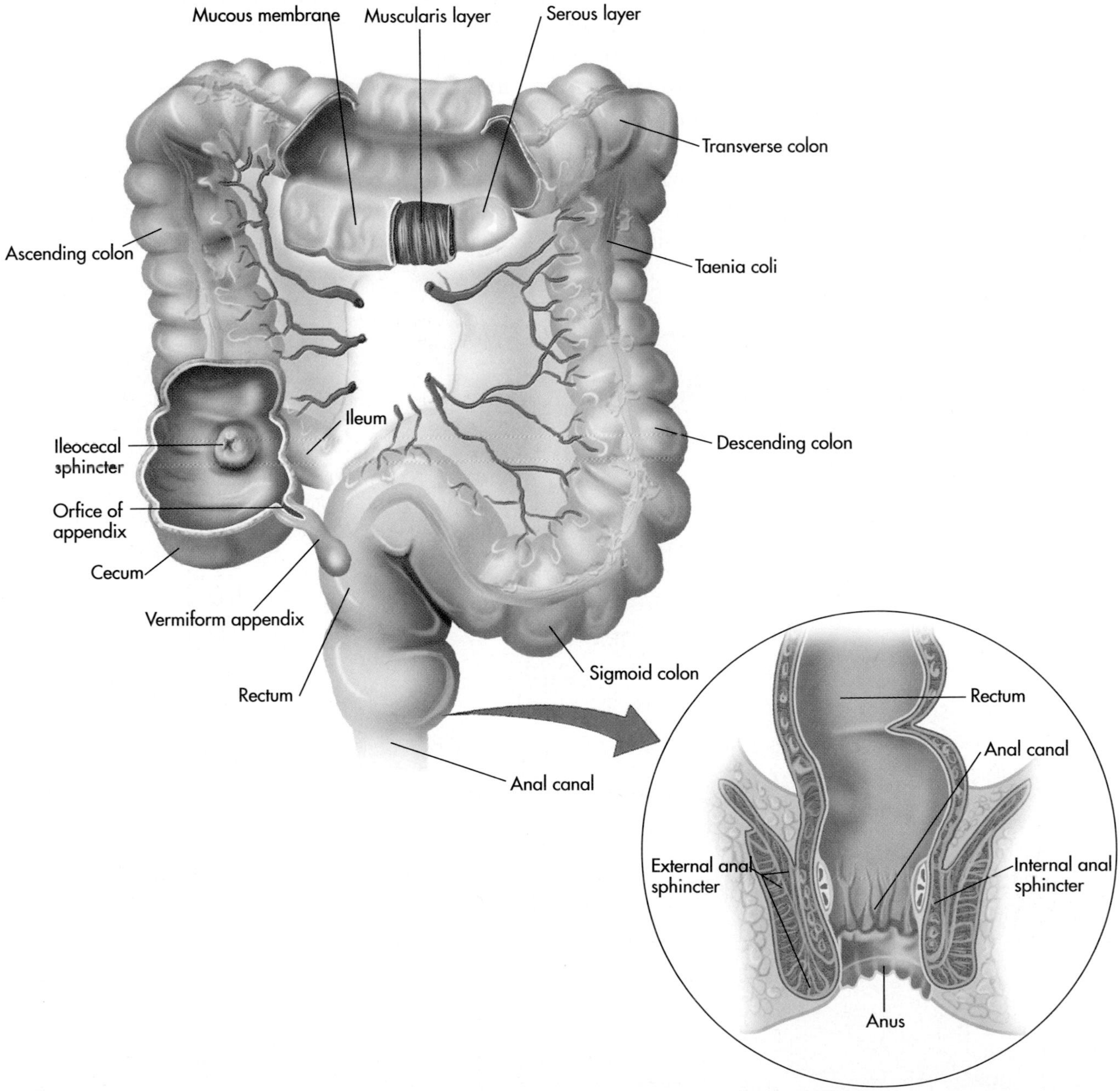

FIGURE ■ 15–11

The large intestine.

cecum *(SEE kum)*

Approximately 1.5 meters (5 feet) long and 7.5 centimeters (2.5 inches) in diameter, the large intestine is divided into three main regions: the **cecum, colon,** and **rectum.** The large intestine is large in diameter, not in length.

A pouch-shaped structure, the cecum receives any undigested food (such as cellulose) and water from the ileum of the small intestine. The infamous appendix is attached to the cecum. About 9 centimeters (3 inches) long, the appendix is a slender, hollow, dead-end tube lined with lymphatic tissue. Since it is wormlike in appearance, it is often called the *vermiform* appendix. There is no current reason why we have an appendix. It is considered a *vestigial organ*—an organ whose size and function seem to have been reduced as humans evolved. Researchers feel that because it possesses lymphatic tissue, it somehow fights infection. Ironically, if the appendix becomes blocked, inflammation can occur, causing **appendicitis.** Treatment for this is either antibiotics or the surgical removal of the appendix (*appendectomy*).

vermiform = *worm like*

appendicitis *(ah pen dih SIGH tiss)*

Some of the water (used in digestion) and electrolytes are reabsorbed by the cecum and the ascending colon, which we discuss momentarily. Although this is a relatively small amount of water reabsorption, it is crucial in maintaining the proper fluid balance in the body.

The colon can further be divided into four sections: ascending, transverse, descending, and sigmoid. The *ascending* colon travels up the right side of the body

Clinical Application

COLOSTOMY

Sometimes a portion of the colon must be bypassed because of disease to allow for healing and/or surgical repair. A new opening needs to be made, and this procedure is called a colostomy. A colostomy can be temporary or permanent depending on the condition. The sites where this procedure is formed are shown in Figure 15–12.

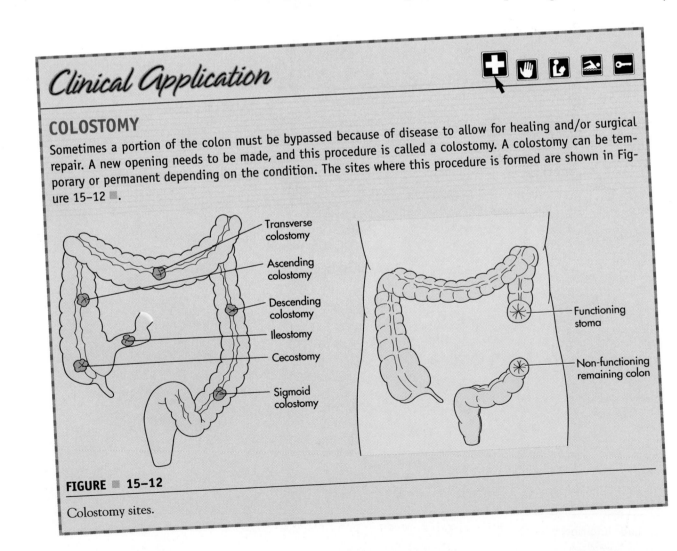

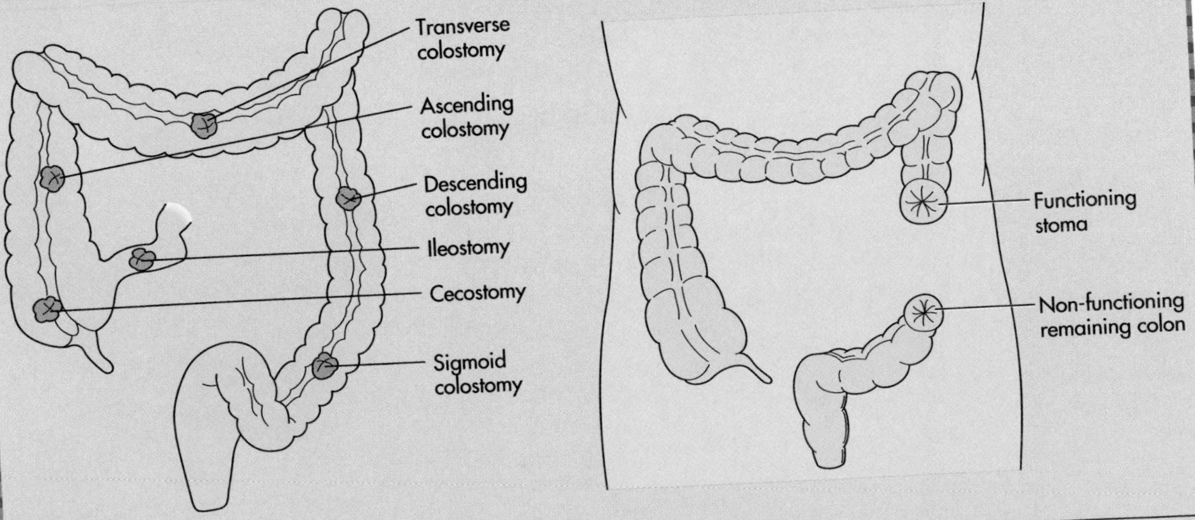

FIGURE 15–12

Colostomy sites.

to the level of the liver. The *transverse* colon travels across the abdomen just below the liver and the stomach. Bending downward near the spleen, the *descending* colon goes down the left side, where it becomes the *sigmoid* colon. The sigmoid ("S" shaped) colon extends to the rectum. The rectum opens to the anal canal, which leads to the anus that relaxes and opens to allow the passage of solid waste (feces).

sigmoid = *S-shaped*

Peristalsis continues in the large intestine but at a slower rate. As these slower, intermittent waves move fecal matter toward the rectum, water is removed, turning feces from a watery soup to a semisolid mass. As the rectum fills with feces, a defecation reflex occurs, which causes rectal muscles to contract and the anal sphincters to relax. If fecal material moves through the large intestine too rapidly, not enough water is removed and diarrhea occurs. Conversely, if fecal matter remains too long in the large intestine, too much water is removed and constipation occurs.

Bacteria found in the large intestine play two important roles: the bacteria help to (1) further break down indigestible materials and (2) produce B complex vitamins as well as most of the vitamin K that we need for proper blood clotting.

Here is a case where bacteria in the right place keeps us healthy. If that same bacteria left the intestinal wall and entered the blood stream, it could be fatal.

ACCESSORY ORGANS

In addition to the salivary glands of the mouth, other accessory organs are necessary for digestion: the liver, gallbladder, and pancreas.

Liver

Weighing in at approximately 1.5 kilograms (3.3 pounds) and located inferior to the diaphragm, the liver is the largest glandular organ in the body *and* the largest organ in the abdominopelvic cavity. This organ performs many functions that are vital for survival. As you can see in Figure 15–13 ■, the liver is divided into a larger right lobe and a smaller left lobe (remember, this is from the patient's perspective). The right lobe also has two smaller, inferior lobes.

The liver receives about 1.5 quarts of blood *every minute* from the hepatic portal vein (carrying blood full of the end products of digestion) and hepatic (referring to liver) artery (providing oxygen-rich blood).

Although this chapter is on the digestive system and the liver plays a central role in regulating the metabolism of the body, it is important to understand *all* of the functions that this amazing organ performs. Here is a list of what the liver does!

- Detoxifies (removes poisons) the body of harmful substances such as certain drugs and alcohol.
- Creates body heat.
- Destroys old blood cells and recycles their usable parts while eliminating unneeded parts such as the pigment *bilirubin*. Bilirubin is eliminated in bile and gives feces its distinctive color.
- Forms blood plasma proteins, such as *albumin* and *globulins*.

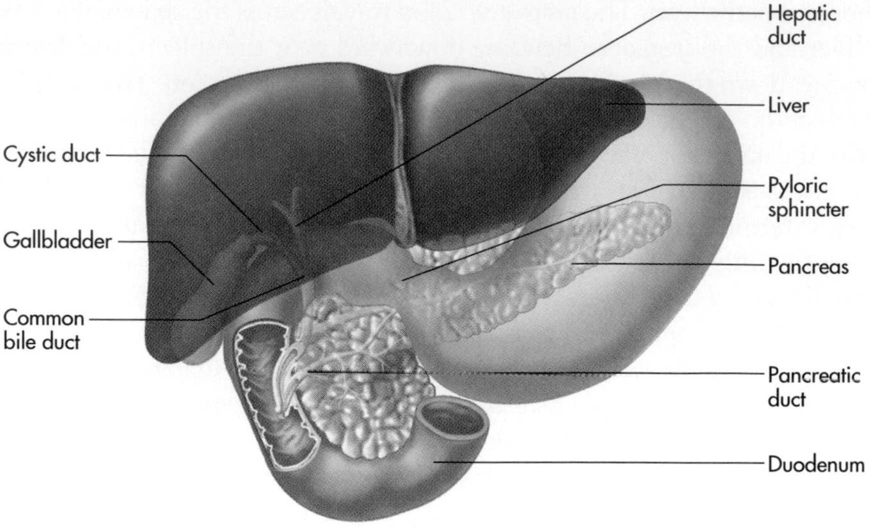

FIGURE ■ 15–13

The liver.

- Produces the clotting factors *fibrinogen* and *prothrombin*.
- Creates the anticoagulant *heparin*.
- Manufactures *bile*, which is needed for the digestion of fats.
- Stores and modifies fats for more efficient usage by the body's cells.
- Synthesizes *urea*, a byproduct of protein metabolism, so it can be eliminated by the body.
- Stores the simple sugar *glucose* as *glycogen*. When the blood sugar level falls below normal, the liver reconverts glycogen to glucose and releases enough of it into the bloodstream to bring blood sugar back to an acceptable concentration.
- Stores iron and vitamins A, B_{12}, D, E, and K.
- Produces cholesterol.

Stimulated into action by the duodenum's secretion of the hormone *secretin*, bile production is a critical liver digestive function. The salts found in bile act like a detergent to break up fat into tiny droplets that make the work of digestive enzymes easier. This mechanical action of breaking up fat into smaller particles is called **emulsification** and provides more surface area for the enzymes to do their job of chemically digesting fat.

emulsification
(ee mull sih fih KAY shun)

In addition, bile helps in the absorption of fat from the small intestine and transports bilirubin and excess cholesterol to the intestines for elimination. Once produced by the liver's cells, bile leaves the liver via the **hepatic duct** and travels through the cystic duct to the gallbladder where it is stored until needed by the small intestine.

Gallbladder

The gallbladder is a sac-shaped organ approximately 7.5 to 10 centimeters (3 to 4 inches) long and is located right under the liver's right lobe. Again, please refer to Figure 15–13. While it is storing the bile, your gallbladder also concentrates it by reabsorbing much of its water content. This makes the bile 6 to 10 times more concentrated than it was in the liver. This is a bit of a balancing act: if too much water is reabsorbed and the bile is constantly too concentrated, bile salts may solidify into gall stones.

When fatty foods enter the duodenum, the duodenum releases the hormone CCK (cholecystokinin). This release causes the smooth muscle walls of the gallbladder to contract and squeeze bile into the cystic duct and on through the common bile duct and then into the duodenum.

Pancreas

Although discussed in the endocrine chapter, your pancreas also plays an extremely important role in digestion. This 15 centimeter (6 to 9 inch) long organ is located posterior to the stomach and extends laterally from the duodenum to the spleen (see Figure 15–14 ■). The exocrine portion of this organ secretes buffers and digestive enzymes through the *pancreatic duct* to the duodenum. The buffers are needed to neutralize the acidity of the chyme in the small intestine. With a pH ranging from 7.5 to 8.8, the chyme is neutralized, saving the intestinal wall from damage. This secretory action is activated by the release of hormones by the duodenum.

> **15-4** For an interactive drag-and-drop exercise on the intestinal wall of the digestive system, please go to your CD-ROM for this chapter.

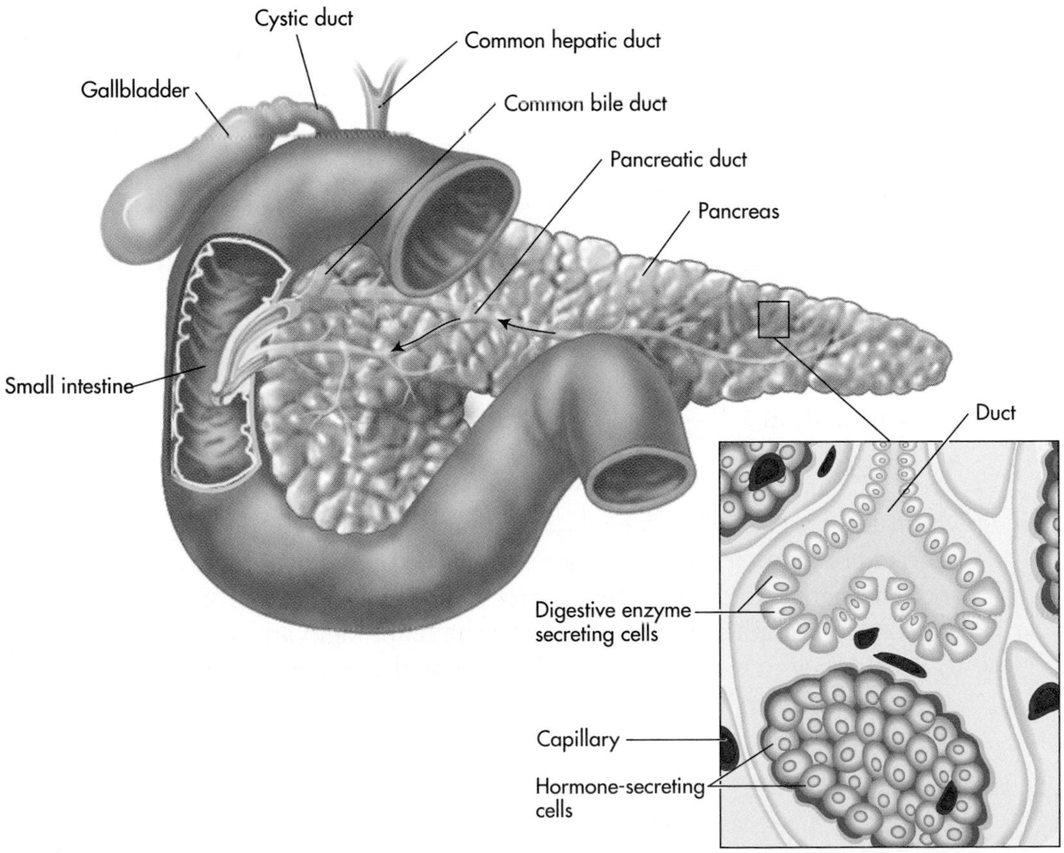

FIGURE ■ 15–14

The pancreas.

Clinical Application

CHOLECYSTITIS AND PANCREATITIS

As we previously discussed, stones can form from substances in the bile while it is stored in the gallbladder. This condition is called **cholelithiasis.** These stones, which are most often formed from cholesterol, can range in size from grains of sand to marble-size and larger. This condition can worsen if the stones lodge in the bile ducts, causing extreme pain, which, surprisingly, often radiates to the right shoulder. If inflammation develops, the condition is called **cholecystitis.**

If the bile backs up into the liver, the disease *obstructive jaundice* can occur. In this scenario, bilirubin is reabsorbed back into the blood, giving the victim a yellowish tint to the skin and eyes.

The problem must be resolved by unblocking the bile ducts. This can done by dissolving the stone through medication, using shock waves to smash the stones (*lithotripsy*), or surgically removing them.

Problems can also occur with the pancreas when the bile duct becomes blocked. In some cases, the pancreatic enzymes back up into the pancreas. As a result, those enzymes begin to inflame and destroy the pancreas. This condition is known as **pancreatitis** and can be caused by excessive alcohol consumption, gallbladder disease, or some irritation that causes an abnormally high rate of pancreatic enzyme activation. If this situation is not stopped, death can eventually occur.

cholecystitis
(koh lee siss TYE tiss)
chole = *gall*
cyst = *bladder*
lith = *stone*
itis = *inflammation*
tripsy = *to rub*
cholelithiasis
(KOH lee lith EYE ah siss)

The general digestive enzymes excreted by the pancreas are *carbohydrases* that work on sugars and starches, *lipases* that work on lipids (fats), *proteinases* that break down proteins, and *nucleases* that break down nucleic acids.

COMMON DISORDERS OF THE DIGESTIVE SYSTEM

Symptoms of digestive disorders generally include one or more of the following:

- vomiting
- diarrhea
- constipation
- abdominal pain

dia = *through*
rrhea = *flow; literally diarrhea means "flow through," which is exactly what happens*

Vomiting is a protective means of ridding the digestive tract of an irritant or overload of food. Sensory fibers are stimulated by the irritant or overdistention and send signals to the vomiting center (yes, you have a vomiting center) in the brain. Motor impulses are then sent to the diaphragm and abdominal muscles to contract, which squeezes the sphincter at the esophageal opening, and the contents are *regurgitated*.

Diarrhea results when the fluid contents in the small intestines are rushed through the large intestines before they can adequately reabsorb the water. Proper absorption of electrolytes and nutrients is also prevented, which can cause serious problems.

15-5 Please go to your CD to view videos on anorexia and bulimia, eating disorders, and diabetes.

Constipation is the opposite of diarrhea; the feces travels so slowly through the colon that too much water is reabsorbed and the stool becomes hard and dry and difficult to push through the system.

One of the more common diseases sometimes blamed on our fast-paced society is peptic ulcer disease (PUD), which can affect the lining of the esophagus, stomach, or duodenum. The most commonly affected region is the upper part of the small intestine, or duodenum. It is caused by an imbalance in the juices of the stomach that produce excess acid and erodes the mucosal lining of the digestive tract. It is believed the majority of the ulcers are caused by the bacteria *Helicobacter pylori*, which opens a wound in the lining that is made worse by exposure to digestive juices and stomach acids. See Figure 15–15 ■.

There are a host of diseases associated with the digestive system. Please see Table 15–3 for some of the more common ones.

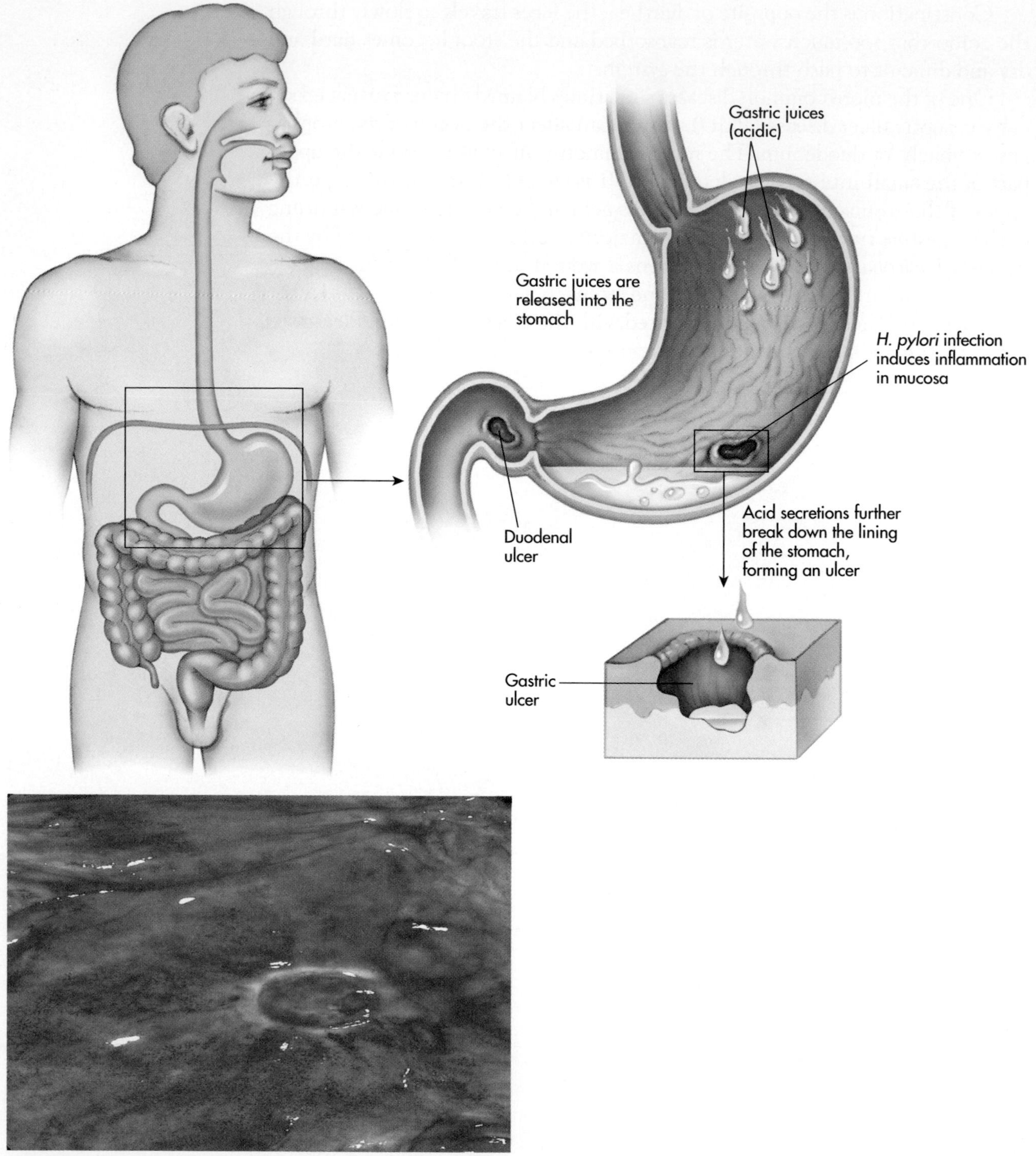

FIGURE ■ 15–15

Peptic ulcer disease (PUD).

TABLE 15–3 Pathology of the Digestive System

abscess (AB sess)	Swelling of soft tissues and the release of pus as a result of infection.
anorexia (an oh REK see ah)	Loss of appetite that can accompany other conditions such as a gastrointestinal (GI) upset.
bulimia (boo LIM ee ah)	Eating disorder that is characterized by recurrent binge eating and then purging of the food with laxatives and vomiting.
caries (KAIR eez)	Also known as a dental cavity, this is the gradual decay of teeth that can result in inflamed tissue.
cholecystitis (koh lee sis TYE tis)	Inflammation of the gallbladder.
cholelithiasis (koh lee lih THIGH ah sis)	Formation or presence of stones or calculi in the gallbladder or common bile duct.
cirrhosis (sih ROH sis)	Chronic disease of the liver.
cleft (CLEFT) lip	Congenital anomaly in which the upper lip fails to come together. Often seen along with a cleft palate. Corrected with surgery.
cleft palate (CLEFT PAL at)	Congenital anomaly in which the roof of the mouth has a split or fissure. Corrected with surgery.
Crohn's disease (KROHNZ dih ZEEZ)	Form of chronic inflammatory bowel disease affecting the ileum and/or colon. Also called *regional ileitis.* Named for Burrill Crohn, an American gastroenterologist.
diverticulitis (dye ver tik yoo LYE tis)	Inflammation of a diverticulum or sac in the intestinal tract, especially in the colon.
enteritis (en ter EYE tis)	Inflammation of only the small intestine.
esophageal stricture (eh soff ah JEE al STRIK chur)	Narrowing of the esophagus that makes the flow of fluids and food difficult.
esophageal varices (eh soff ah JEE al VAIR ih seez)	Enlarged and swollen veins in the lower end of the esophagus; they can rupture and result in serious hemorrhage.
fissure (FISH er)	Crack-like split in the rectum or anal canal.
gastritis (gas TRY tis)	Inflammation of the stomach that can result in pain, tenderness, nausea, and vomiting.
gastroenteritis (gas troh en ter EYE tis)	Inflammation of the stomach and small intestines.
gingivitis (jin jih VIGH tis)	Inflammation of the gums that is characterized by swelling, redness, and a tendency to bleed.
gum disease	Inflammation of the gums, leading to tooth loss, which is generally due to poor dental hygiene.

TABLE 15–3 Pathology of the Digestive System (*continued*)

hemorrhoids (HEM oh roydz)	Varicose veins in the rectum.
hepatitis (hep ah TYE tis)	Inflammation of the liver.
hiatal hernia (high AY tal HER nee ah)	Protrusion of the stomach through the diaphragm and extending into the thoracic cavity; reflux esophagitis is a common symptom.
ileitis (ill ee EYE tis)	Inflammation of the ileum.
impacted (im PAK ted) wisdom tooth	Wisdom tooth that is tightly wedged into the jaw bone so that it is unable to erupt.
inflammatory bowel disease (IBD) (in FLAM ah tor ee BOW el dih ZEEZ)	Ulceration of the mucous membranes of the colon of unknown origin. Also known as *ulcerative colitis*.
inguinal hernia (ING gwi nal HER nee ah)	Hernia or outpouching of intestines into the inguinal region of the body.
intussusception (in tuh suh SEP shun)	Result of the intestine slipping or telescoping into another section of intestine just below it. More common in children.
irritable bowel syndrome (IBS) (EAR it ah bul BOW el SIN drohm)	Disturbance in the functions of the intestine from unknown causes. Symptoms generally include abdominal discomfort and an alteration in bowel activity.
malabsorption syndrome (mal ab SORP shun SIN drohm)	Inadequate absorption of nutrients from the intestinal tract. May be caused by a variety of diseases and disorders, such as infections and pancreatic deficiency.
peptic ulcer (PEP tik ULL sir)	Ulcer occurring in the lower portion of the esophagus, stomach, and duodenum thought to be caused by the acid of gastric juices.
periodontal disease (pair ee oh DON tal dih ZEEZ)	Disease of the supporting structures of the teeth, including the gums and bones.
polyposis (pall ee POH sis)	Small tumors that contain a pedicle or footlike attachment in the mucous membranes of the large intestine (colon).
pyorrhea (pye oh REE ah)	Discharge of purulent material from dental tissue.
reflux esophagitis (REE fluks eh soff ah JIGH tis)	Acid from the stomach backs up into the esophagus causing inflammation and pain.
ulcerative colitis (ULL sir ah tiv koh LYE tis)	Ulceration of the mucous membranes of the colon of unknown origin. Also known as *inflammatory bowel disease (IBD)*.
volvulus (VOL vyoo lus)	Condition in which the bowel twists upon itself and causes an obstruction. Painful and requires immediate surgery.

SUMMARY

Snapshots from the Journey

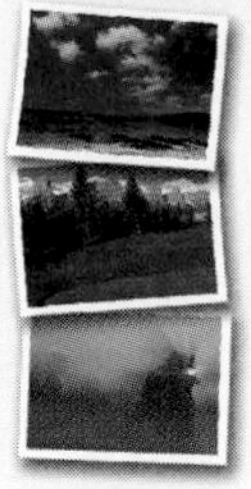

- The digestive tract is a hollow tube extending from the mouth to the anus. It contains a variety of structures that allow the digestion of food and the absorption of nutrients necessary for life.
- Food is processed mechanically and chemically to efficiently break it down to usable substances.
- Following are the main components of the digestive system and their functions:

Organ	Digestive Activity	Substance Digested	Required Digestive Secretions
Mouth, or oral cavity	Chews food and mixes it with saliva; forms food into a *bolus,* and swallows	starch	salivary amylase
Esophagus	Moves bolus to the stomach through *peristalsis*	not applicable	not applicable
Stomach	Stores food, also churns food while mixing in digestive juices	proteins	hydrochloric acid, pepsin
Small intestine	Secretes enzymes, receives secretions from the pancreas and liver, neutralizes the acidity in chyme, absorbs nutrients into the bloodstream and lymphatic system	carbohydrates, fats, nucleic acid, proteins	intestinal and pancreatic enzymes, bile from the liver
Large intestine	Creates and absorbs fat-soluble vitamins, reabsorbs water, forms and eliminates feces	vitamins B_{12} and K	not applicable

- Enzymes are formed by special cells and act as a catalyst that speeds up chemical reactions.
- The bulk of the digestive process and the absorption of most nutrients occur in the small intestine.
- Although not *directly* a part of the gastrointestinal system, the accessory organs (liver, gallbladder, and pancreas) are needed for proper and efficient functioning of the digestive process.
- The rate of speed that food travels through the gastrointestinal system affects the acidity of the digesting food, the absorption of nutrients, and the quality of the feces.
- Diseases of the gastrointestinal system can be a result of heredity, the type and amount of food consumed, substance abuse, or emotions.

Case Study

A patient presents in the emergency department around 3 a.m. with a severe burning sensation in his chest. The patient is anxious and thinks he is having a heart attack. All vital signs are within normal limits, and no other pain or discomfort is noted in other regions of the body. He states he ate a large bowl of spicy spaghetti around 11:30 p.m. Before falling asleep, he was uncomfortable and felt his large volume of food hadn't digested. He also states this burning sensation has happened in the past after eating, especially at night and when laying on his right side.

Do you think this is a heart attack?

What do you think the problem is?

What physiologic process is malfunctioning?

Why is the position of the patient important?

What suggestions would you make to the patient to prevent future episodes?

REVIEW QUESTIONS

Multiple Choice

1. Which of the following is not a responsibility of the large intestine?
   a. production of vitamin K
   b. absorption of water
   c. digestion of carbohydrates
   d. elimination of feces

2. Starches begin to be digested in the
   a. oral cavity
   b. esophagus
   c. stomach
   d. large intestine

3. This structure prevents food and liquid from entering the lungs:
   a. larynx
   b. pharynx
   c. epiglottis
   d. glottis

4. The liver receives approximately this much blood every minute:
   a. 500 milliliters
   b. 1 gallon
   c. 2 units
   d. 1.5 quarts

5. Which of the following is *not* a colon segment?
   a. transverse
   b. ascending
   c. descending
   d. absorbing

Fill in the Blank

1. _____________ is the muscle action that mixes chyme with digestive juices, while _____________ is the muscular action that moves food through the digestive system.

2. This vermiform structure is attached to the large intestine and is considered a vestigial organ: _____________.

3. The exocrine portion of this important organ secretes buffers needed to neutralize the acidity of chyme and also secretes several digestive enzymes: _____________.

4. _____________ is the mechanical breaking up of fat into smaller particles that can more readily be acted upon by digestive enzymes.

5. The end result of fecal matter remaining in the large intestine too long, with too much water being removed from it, is _____________.

Short Answer

1. Explain the difference between *chyme* and *chyle*.

2. Explain the importance of bacteria in the large intestine.

3. Discuss the importance of the liver in the digestive process.

4. Could you live without a gallbladder? Defend your answer.

Suggested Activities

1. Nutrition is a very important consideration when planning a healthy lifestyle. Research the different food groups and the daily recommended amounts that you should consume. List your daily consumption of food for a week and compare what you eat to what you should eat. List suggestions for changes that you should make in your diet, if any.

2. Although it is felt that most stomach ulcers are a result of bacteria, research ways that you can help to prevent their formation.

15-6

Now that you have completed your journey through this chapter, please go to the CD-ROM for interactive games and puzzles concerning the medical terms and concepts contained in this chapter. By playing the games you will reinforce your learning of medical terminology in a fun way.

Greetings from THE URINARY System

Filtration and Fluid Balance

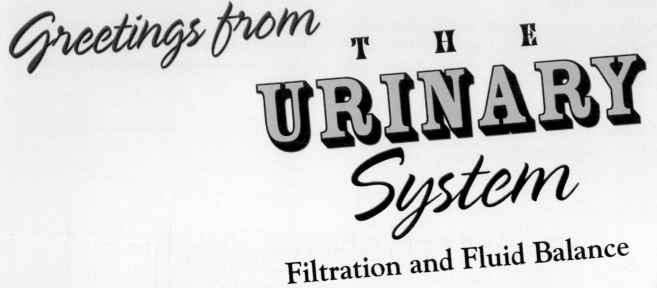

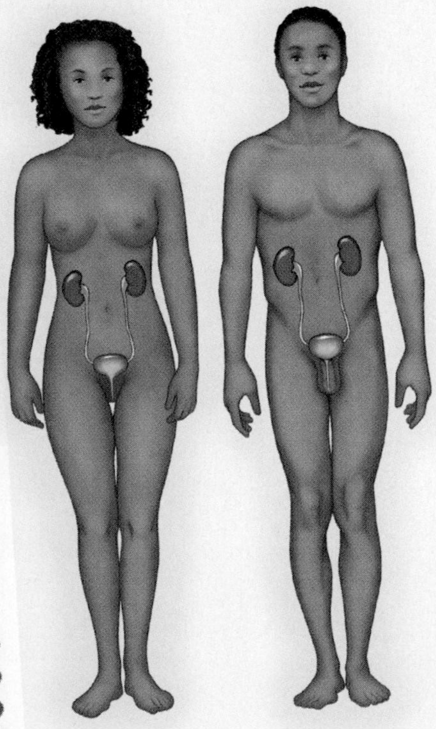

A city must have a safe, reliable water supply, usually obtained by pumping water from a reservoir or diverting a river. Sometimes cities have a series of wells to supply drinkable water. In desert areas, there are even special water treatment plants to remove salt from seawater to make fresh water for human consumption. In any case, there must be a way to clean the water. Water purification plants remove chemicals and debris and disinfect the water before it ever gets to your faucet. You are completely unaware of the activities of your city's water purification plant, but if it stopped working, you would be extremely unhappy. Imagine a glass full of muddy, bacteria-laden water. Yum!

Your body also must have a purification plant for its fluid—blood. Your liver does some of the purification, but your urinary system is responsible for controlling the electrolyte (ion) and fluid balance of your body. The kidneys filter blood, reabsorb and secrete ions, and produce urine. Without them, fluid and ion imbalance, blood pressure irregularities, and nitrogen waste buildup would cause death in a matter of days.

Chapter 16

LEARNING OBJECTIVES

Upon completion of your journey through this chapter, you will be able to:

- Present an overview of the organs and functions of the urinary system
- Describe the internal and external anatomy and physiology of the kidneys
- Discuss the importance of renal blood flow
- Describe the process of urine formation
- Trace the pathway of reabsorption or secretion of vital substances
- List and discuss the importance of hormones for proper kidney function
- Describe the anatomy and physiology of the bladder and urine removal from the body
- Discuss several common disorders of the urinary system

MULTIMEDIA APPLICATIONS

CD-ROM Interactive Exercises

- 3-D animation of the urinary system, 16.1
- Interactive labeling exercise for the kidney, 16.2
- Animation of renal blood flow, 16.3
- Animation of hypovolemic shock, 16.4
- Video of ultrasound procedure, 16.5
- Drag-and-drop exercise on labeling the urinary bladder, 16.6
- Videos on renal failure and kidney stones, 16.7
- Interactive puzzles and games, 16.8

www.prenhall.com/colbert

- Professional Profile
  - Ultra Sound Technician
- Related Links
- Additional Review Questions

Pronunciation Guide

Correct pronunciation is important in any journey so that you and others are completely understood. Here is a "see and say" Pronunciation Guide for the more difficult terms to pronounce in this chapter.

afferent arterioles (AFF er ent ahr TEE ree ohlz)

aldosterone (al DOSS ter ohn)

antidiuretic hormone (ADH) (AN tye dye yoo RET ik)

atrial natriuretic peptide (AY tree al nay tree your RET ick PEP tide)

calyx, calyces (KAY licks, KAY leh seez)

cortical nephron (CORE tih cull NEFF rahn)

efferent arterioles (EFF er ent ahr TEE ree ohlz)

external urethral sphincter (EKS ter nal yoo REE thral SFINK ter)

glomerulus (gloh MAIR yoo luss)

glomerular capsule (gloh MAIR you ler CAP sell)

juxtaglomedullary nephron (JUX ta glo MED DULL lair ee NEFF rahn)

juxtaglomerular cells (JUX ta gla MARE you ler)

renal hilum (REE nal HIGH lum)

renal medulla (REE nal meh DULL lah)

renin-angiotensin-aldosterone (REE nen-an gee oh TEN sen-al DOSS ter ohn)

ureter (yoo REE ter)

urethra (yoo REE thrah)

SYSTEM OVERVIEW

ureter *(yoo REE ter)*

urethra *(yoo REE thrah)*

The urinary system (see Figure 16–1 ■) consists of two **kidneys,** bean-shaped organs located in the superior dorsal abdominal cavity, and accessory structures that filter blood and make urine. A **ureter** is a tube that carries urine from each kidney to the single **urinary bladder,** located in the inferior ventral pelvic cavity. The urinary bladder is basically an expandable sac that holds the urine. The **urethra** is the tubing that transports urine from the bladder to the outside of the body.

16-1 To view a 3-D animation of the urinary system, please go to your CD-ROM for this chapter.

The job of the urinary system is to make urine, thereby controlling the body's fluid and electrolyte (ion) balance, and eliminating waste products. To make urine, three processes are necessary: **filtration, reabsorption,** and **secretion.** Filtration involves filtering the blood to a filtrate (that which is allowed to pass through the filter). This filtrate, which contains various substances, can then be either reabsorbed back into the bloodstream or secreted from the body as urine. Keep in mind the part of the filtrate that is reabsorbed is conserved and brought back into the bloodstream, while the part that is secreted is eliminated from the body. You'll learn how this process occurs as you journey through this chapter.

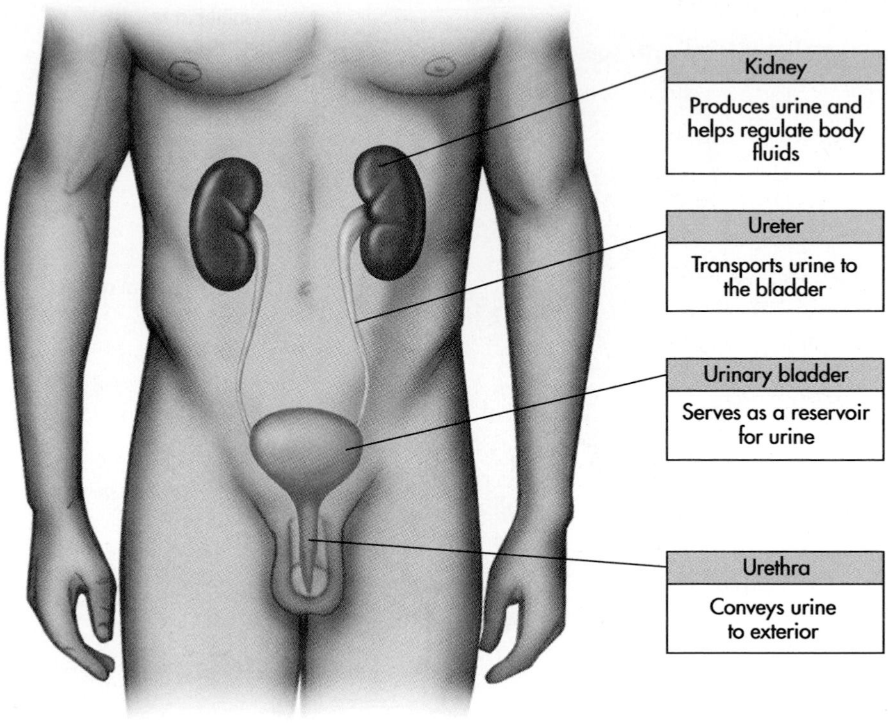
Kidney
Produces urine and helps regulate body fluids
Ureter
Transports urine to the bladder
Urinary bladder
Serves as a reservoir for urine
Urethra
Conveys urine to exterior

FIGURE ■ 16–1

Anatomy of the urinary system.

THE ANATOMY OF THE KIDNEY

The kidney is a very intricate filtration system. Though you have two kidneys, you can actually function well with only one healthy kidney. That is why someone can donate a kidney while he or she is alive.

External Anatomy

The external anatomy of the kidney is relatively simple. The kidney is covered by a fibrous layer of connective tissue called the **renal capsule.** The indentation that gives the kidney its bean-shaped appearance is called the **renal hilum.** At the hilum, renal arteries bring blood into the kidneys to be filtered. Once filtered, the blood leaves the kidney via the renal vein. The ureter is also attached at the hilum to transport the urine away from the kidney to the bladder (see Figure 16–2 ■).

renal capsule *(REE nal CAP sell)*
renal hilum *(REE nal HIGH lum)*
hilum = *root*

Internal Anatomy

The internal anatomy of the kidney (Figure 16–2) is considerably more complicated than its external anatomy. The kidney can be divided into three layers. The outer layer is the **renal cortex,** the middle layer is the **renal medulla,** and the innermost layer is the **renal pelvis.** Adding the word *renal* is important here. Remember that the brain and the adrenal gland both have a medulla and

renal cortex *(REE nal CORE tex)*
renal medulla *(REE nal meh DULL lah)*
renal pelvis *(REE nal PELL vis)*

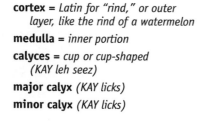

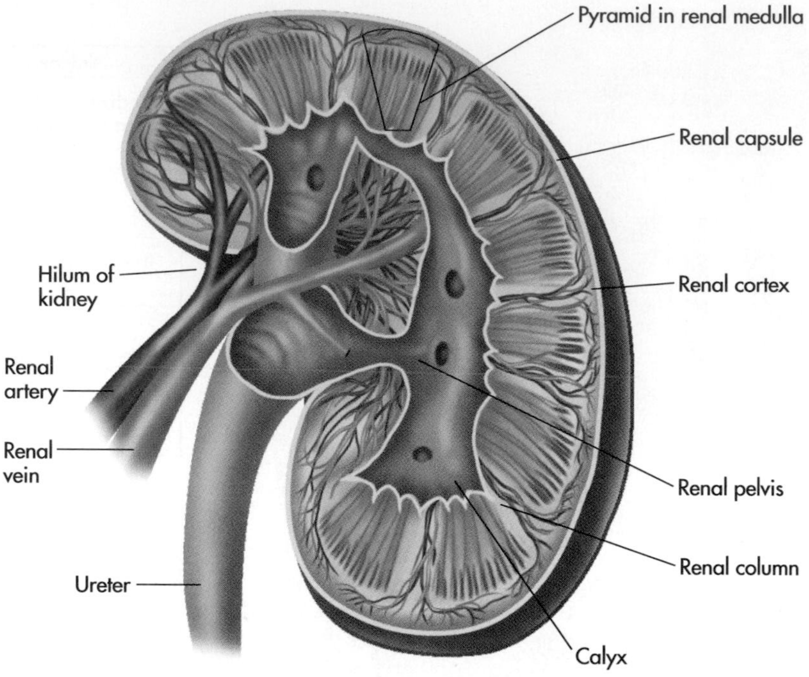

FIGURE 16–2

The internal and external anatomy of the kidney.

a cortex. Also keep in mind that the body also has more than one pelvis, as in the bony pelvis. The renal cortex is grainy in appearance and has very little in obvious structure to the naked eye. The renal cortex is where the blood is actually filtered.

cortex = *Latin for "rind," or outer layer, like the rind of a watermelon*
medulla = *inner portion*
calyces = *cup or cup-shaped (KAY leh seez)*
major calyx *(KAY licks)*
minor calyx *(KAY licks)*

The renal medulla contains a number of triangle-shaped striped areas called **renal pyramids.** The renal pyramids are composed of collecting tubules for the urine that is formed in the kidney. Adjacent pyramids are separated by narrow **renal columns,** which are extensions of the cortical tissue.

The renal pelvis is a funnel. The funnel is divided into two or three large collecting cups, called **major calyces.** Each major calyx is divided into several **minor calyces.** The calyces form cup-shaped areas around the tips of the pyramids to collect the urine that continually drains through the pyramids. The kidney is essentially a combination of a filtration and collection system. The blood is filtered by millions of tiny filters in the cortex, the filtered material flows through tiny tubes in the medulla, and the resulting urine is collected in the renal pelvis. The renal pelvis, which is simply the enlarged proximal portion of the ureter, empties into the ureter tube. The ureter then carries the urine to the urinary bladder where it is stored and eventually eliminated from the body (again, see Figure 16–2).

16-2 To perform an interactive labeling exercise for the kidney, please go to the CD-ROM for this chapter

BLOOD VESSELS

Because the kidney's job is to filter blood, the blood must reach every part of the kidney. To accomplish this filtration process there is a network of blood vessels throughout kidney tissue. A single **renal artery** enters each

Arcuate vein
Arcuate artery
Interlobular vein
Interlobular artery
Renal column
Lobar artery
Segmental artery
Cortex
Renal artery
Renal vein
Renal pelvis
Major calyx
Ureter
Minor calyx
Interlobar artery
Renal capsule
Interlobar vein
Renal pyramid

Renal artery → Segmental arteries → Lobar arteries → Interlobar arteries → Arcuate arteries →
Interlobular arteries → Afferent arterioles → Glomerulus → Efferent arterioles → Peritubular
capillaries → Interlobular veins → Arcuate veins → Interlobar veins → Lobar veins → Renal vein

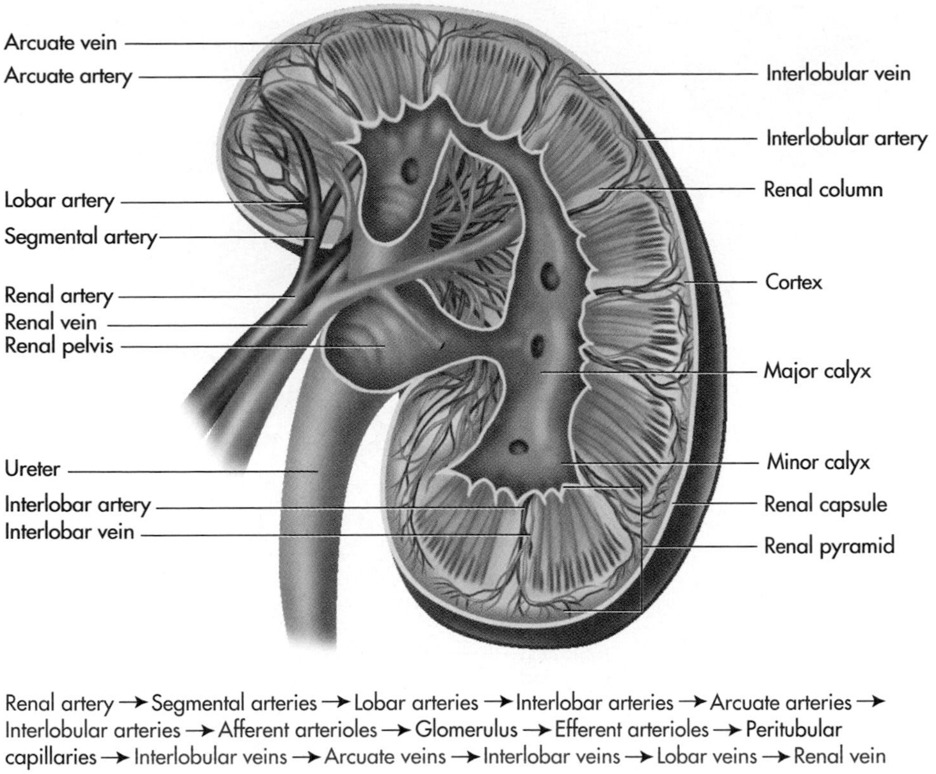

FIGURE ■ 16–3

Renal blood vessels and the pathway of blood through the renal system.

kidney at the hilum (see Figure 16–3 ■). The renal artery then branches into five segmental arteries. The segmental arteries branch into lobar arteries. The lobar arteries branch into interlobar arteries, which pass through the renal columns. Arcuate arteries originate from the interlobar arteries. The *arcuate* arteries are so named because they arch around the base of the pyramids in the renal medulla. Many tiny interlobular arteries branch from the arcuate arteries, supplying blood to the renal cortex. These interlobular arteries give rise to numerous **afferent arterioles.**

Each afferent arteriole leads to a ball of capillaries called a **glomerulus. Efferent arterioles** then leave from the glomerulus and travel to a specialized series of capillaries called the **peritubular capillaries** and *vasa recta* (straight, collecting tubes) that are associated with the **renal nephron,** the functional unit of the kidney. The peritubular capillaries wrap around the tubules of the nephron. You have seen a situation like this in the lungs, where the pulmonary capillaries

Learning Hint

VISUALIZING THE PERITUBULAR SYSTEM

Think of the peritubular capillaries as red yarn wrapped around plastic pipe, which represents the actual tubular system. You will soon learn that the filtrate that stays in the pipe eventually becomes urine and the filtrate that is reabsorbed into the red yarn (peritubular capillaries) is brought back into the body.

afferent arterioles
 (AFF er ent ahr TEE ree ohlz)
glomerulus *(gloh MAIR yoo luss)*
efferent arterioles
 (EFF er ent ahr TEE ree ohlz)
peritubular *(per ee TUBE you ler)*

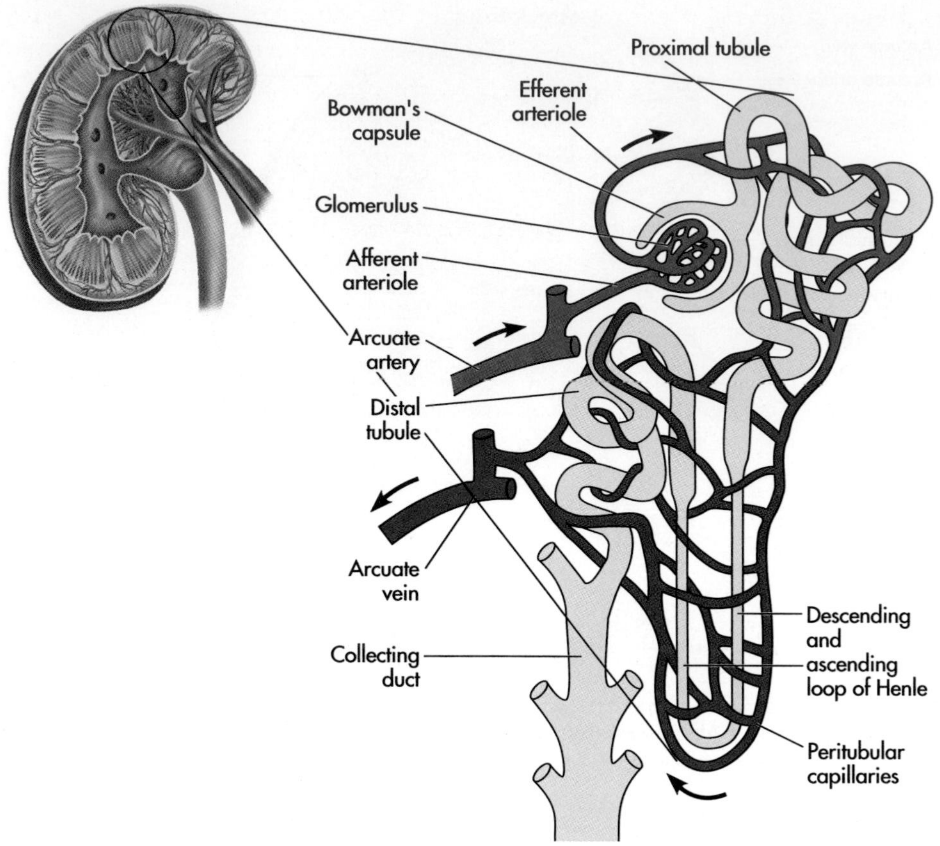

FIGURE ■ 16–4

The nephron.

surround the alveoli. Having blood vessels close to the nephron allows efficient movement of ions between blood and the fluid in the nephron, just as having pulmonary capillaries near the alveoli allows efficient diffusion of respiratory gases between the alveoli and the bloodstream.

From each set of peritubular capillaries, blood flows out the interlobular veins. From there, the blood flows out a series of veins that are the direct reverse of the arteries, with one exception. There are no segmental veins. The blood finally leaves the kidney via the **renal vein.** Please see Figure 16–3 for a diagram of the renal blood vessels.

16-3 To see an animation of the blood flow through the kidneys, please go to the CD-ROM for this chapter.

Microscopic Anatomy of the Kidney: The Nephron

nephron *(NEFF rahn)*
renal corpuscle *(REE nal KOR puss el)*

So far we have looked at an overview of the kidneys structure and function. Now let's take a closer look at what actually happens within the kidneys. The business end of the kidney, the part that performs the real functions of the kidney, consists of millions of microscopic funnels and tubules. These fundamental functional units of the kidney are called **nephrons** (see Figure 16–4 ■). The nephron is divided into two distinct parts: the **renal corpuscle** and the **renal tubule.** The renal corpuscle is a filter, much like a window screen or coffee filter.

Blood enters the renal corpuscle via the **glomerulus,** a capillary ball. Surrounding the glomerulus is a double-layered membrane called the **glomerular capsule** (Bowman's capsule). The layers of the glomerular capsule are similar to the layers of a serous membrane like the pleura or pericardium. The inner layer of the glomerular capsule, the visceral layer, surrounds the glomerular capillaries. The visceral layer is made of specialized squamous epithelial cells called **podocytes.** The combination of podocytes and the simple squamous epithelium making up the walls of the glomerular capillaries make a very effective filter.

glomerulus *(gloh MAIR yoo luss)*

glomerular capsule *(gla MARE you ler CAP sell)*

The outer or parietal layer of the glomerular capsule is simple sqamous epithelium and completes the container for the filter. Blood flows into the glomerulus and everything *but* blood cells and a few large molecules, mainly proteins, are pushed from the capillaries across the filter and into the glomerular capsule. The material filtered from the blood into the glomerular capsule is called **glomerular filtrate.** Can you see why blood cells or excessive protein found in urine may indicate a kidney filtration problem?

glomerular filtrate *(gla MARE you ler FILL trate)*

The rest of the nephron is series of tubes known as the *renal tubule*, sort of like a Habitrail system for a gerbil or hamster (see Figure 16–5 ■). Just like the water filtration system in our towns and cities, the water (glomerular filtrate) travels through a network of pipes (tubules) where the impurities remain in the pipes to be discharged while the filtered water is collected (peritubular capillaries) and recycled back into the city's water supply.

Now back to the kidney. Glomerular filtrate flows from the glomerular capsule into the first part of the renal tubule, the **proximal tubule.** The wall of the proximal tubule is made of cuboidal epithelium with microvilli. From the proximal tubule, glomerular filtrate flows into the **nephron loop** (also called the loop of Henle). The nephron loop consists of two segments, the **descending loop,** with a structure similar to the proximal tubule, and the **ascending loop,** with a wall made of simple cuboidal epithelium without microvilli. From the nephron loop, the glomerular filtrate flows into the **distal tubule.** The wall of the distal tubule is like that of the ascending branch of the nephron loop.

From the distal tubule, glomerular filtrate flows into one of several **collecting ducts** also made of cuboidal epithelium. The collecting ducts lead to the minor calyces, then to the major calyces, renal pelvis, and ureter. At this point, the glomerular filtrate is urine. Again, if you refer to our previous learning hint, what stays in the tubular system (plastic pipe) eventually gets eliminated as urine.

Clinical Application

TRAUMA, ISCHEMIA, AND KIDNEY DAMAGE

The kidney is obviously very well vascularized. Each nephron is literally surrounded by blood vessels, and the flow of blood around the nephron is controlled by flow through the afferent arteriole. Ischemia is a condition of tissue injury resulting from too little oxygen delivery to tissues, usually caused by decreased blood flow. When blood flow to the nephrons decreases for a period of time, oxygen delivery to the nephron decreases and ischemia can result. Decreased blood flow to the kidney results from anything that causes prolonged constriction of the afferent arterioles. Probably the most common cause of prolonged vasoconstriction in the kidney is any number of hormonal mechanisms used to increase blood pressure, such as after severe blood loss.

For example, a young boy runs into a storm door, puncturing his femoral artery, which begins to bleed profusely. As his blood volume falls, so does his blood pressure. His body fights desperately to bring his blood pressure back to normal, causing widespread vasoconstriction. The afferent arterioles, under the influence of sympathetic hormones and other vasoconstrictors, get smaller and smaller, greatly decreasing blood supply to the nephrons. If the situation continues long enough, the tissues will become ischemic and eventually begin to die. Even if the boy survives the initial blood loss from the wound, his kidneys may be damaged, resulting in temporary or permanent renal failure. It is not uncommon for trauma patients to survive the initial trauma only to become the victim of organ damage due to ischemia.

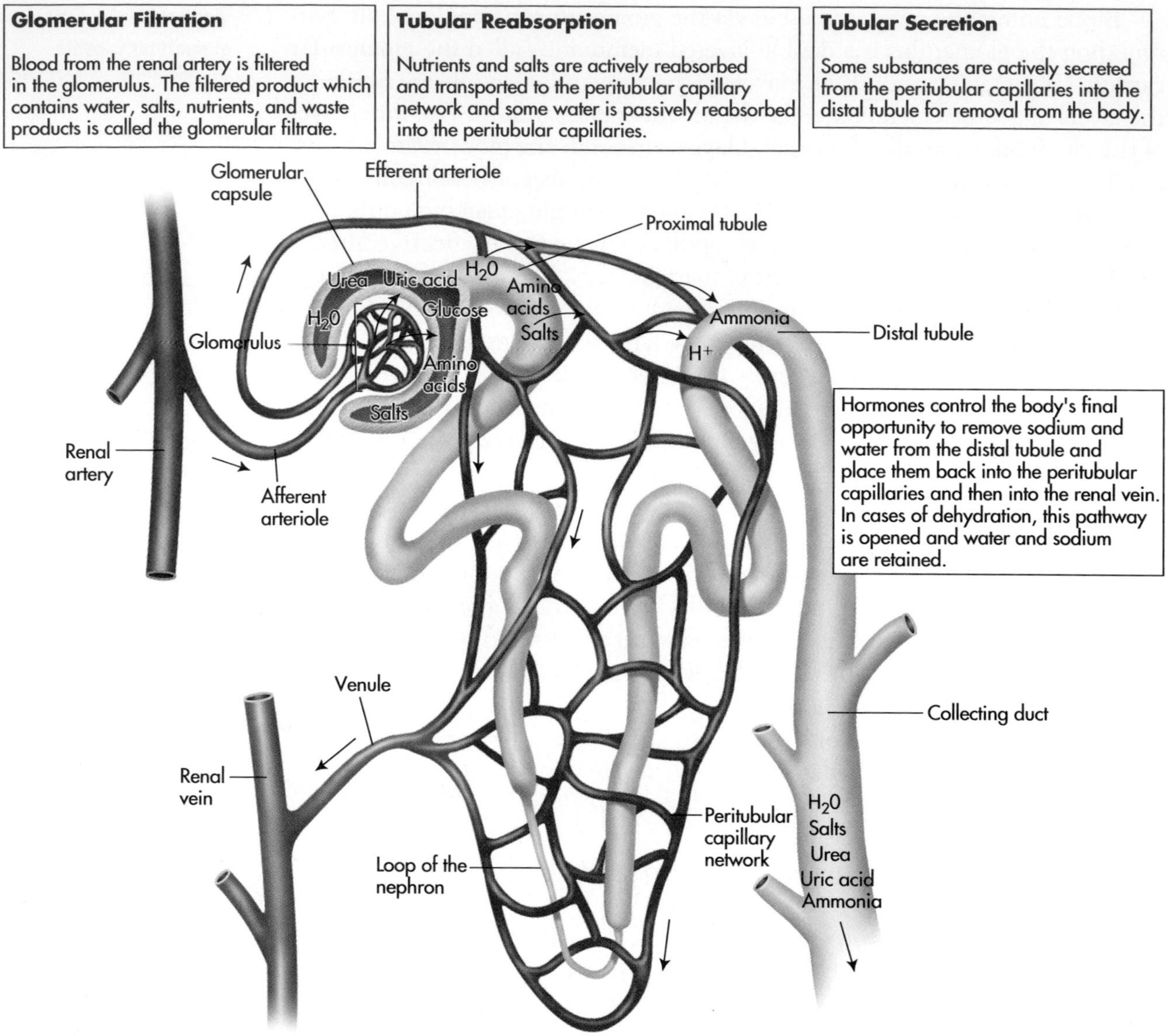
Glomerular Filtration
Blood from the renal artery is filtered in the glomerulus. The filtered product which contains water, salts, nutrients, and waste products is called the glomerular filtrate.
Tubular Reabsorption
Nutrients and salts are actively reabsorbed and transported to the peritubular capillary network and some water is passively reabsorbed into the peritubular capillaries.
Tubular Secretion
Some substances are actively secreted from the peritubular capillaries into the distal tubule for removal from the body.
Glomerular capsule
Efferent arteriole
Proximal tubule
Urea
Uric acid
H_2O
Amino acids
Glucose
Salts
Glomerulus
Ammonia
H^+
Distal tubule
Hormones control the body's final opportunity to remove sodium and water from the distal tubule and place them back into the peritubular capillaries and then into the renal vein. In cases of dehydration, this pathway is opened and water and sodium are retained.
Renal artery
Afferent arteriole
Venule
Collecting duct
Renal vein
Peritubular capillary network
Loop of the nephron
H_2O
Salts
Urea
Uric acid
Ammonia

FIGURE ■ 16–5

The renal tubule.

efferent arteriole
(EFF er ent ahr TEE ree ohlz)

As you might expect, blood vessels are in close proximity to the nephrons because certain substances within the filtrate must be brought back into the bloodstream. Blood approaches the nephron via the afferent arteriole. Blood flows from the afferent arteriole into the glomerulus, a capillary ball surrounded by the glomerular capsule. Blood flows from the glomerulus via the **efferent arteriole** into the peritubular capillaries and vasa recta, a series of blood vessels surrounding the renal tubules (or the red yarn from the learning hint). These surrounding blood vessels allow for reabsorption back into the bloodstream from the filtrate that is within the tubular system. Blood then leaves the area of the nephron via the interlobular veins.

16-4 To view an animation on hypovolemic shock, please go to your CD-ROM for this chapter.

TEST YOUR KNOWLEDGE 16-1

Choose the best answer:

1. What carries urine from the kidneys to the bladder?
   a. urethra
   b. ureter
   c. vagina
   d. all of the above

2. The renal _____ is the outer layer of the kidney.
   a. medulla
   b. pelvis
   c. hilum
   d. cortex

3. These vessels carry blood into the glomerulus:
   a. peritubular capillaries
   b. afferent arterioles
   c. segmental arteries
   d. none of the above

4. The fundamental functional unit of the kidney is the
   a. renal corpuscle
   b. renal pelvis
   c. nephron
   d. pyramid

5. Glomerular filtrate flows from the _____ into the _____.
   a. proximal tubule, distal tubule
   b. ascending loop, descending loop
   c. glomerular capsule, proximal tubule
   d. proximal tubule, collecting duct

URINE FORMATION

As the body's water purification system, the job of the kidneys is to control fluid and electrolyte balance by carefully controlling urine volume and composition. The kidneys also filter nitrogen-containing waste and other impurities from blood. In order to form urine, the nephron must perform three processes: **glomerular filtration, tubular reabsorption,** and **tubular secretion.** Please see Figure 16–6 ■ for a diagram of these three processes.

During glomerular filtration, fluid and molecules pass from the glomerular capillaries into the glomerular capsule, across a filter composed of the wall of the capillaries and the podocytes of the glomerular capsule. The filtrate flows into the renal tubule where the composition of the filtrate is controlled by reabsorption and secretion. Substances that are reabsorbed pass from the renal tubule into the peritubular capillaries and will not end up in urine but stay within the body. Substances that are secreted pass from the peritubular capillaries into the renal tubule and eventually leave the body via the urine. The combination of all three processes is necessary for the formation of urine. Filtration moves fluid and chemicals into the nephron from blood and reabsorption and secretion control the concentration of chemicals and volume of urine. Glomerular filtrate is chemically similar to blood, while urine is chemically very different. Some substances, like glucose, are completely reabsorbed, and other substances, like the metabolic waste products urea and creatinine, are secreted such that urea and creatinine are much more concentrated in urine than in blood. See Table 16–1 for a comparison of plasma, glomerular filtrate, and urine chemistry.

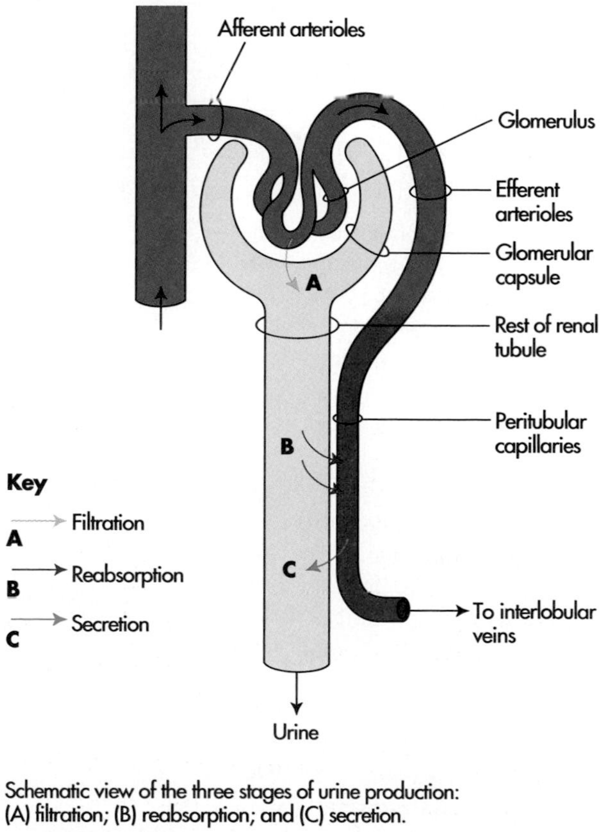

FIGURE ■ 16–6

The processes involved in urine formation.

TABLE 16–1 Kidney Fluid Chemistry

SUBSTANCE	PLASMA	GLOMERULAR FILTRATE	URINE
Protein	3,900–5,000	none	none
Glucose	100	100	none
Sodium	142	142	128
Potassium	5	5	60
Urea	26	26	1,820
Creatinine	1.1	1.1	140

All concentrations in mg/100ml

Control of Filtration

Think for a moment about filters you are familiar with. What controls these filters? What force drives filtration? What determines whether a substance passes through the filter or stays on one side? The example you are most familiar with is a window screen. Why do you have window screens in your windows? To keep out the bugs. Without screens, every insect in the neighborhood would be in your bedroom eating you alive, right? So what determines whether something gets through the screen? The most obvious answer is the size of the mesh in the screen. Dust gets through the screen, but most bugs don't. Imagine a screen with holes twice the size of a typical screen. You would spend all night swatting mosquitoes! The screens would be pretty much useless. Filter size determines what gets through the filter. All filters are *selective:* only some substances pass through, mainly depending on the size of the openings in the filter (see Figure 16–7 ■).

Can you think of a situation where something might get through a window screen? Leaving behind the bugs, let's think about a screen porch. During a gentle snow storm, snow doesn't come through the screen. But in a high wind, the inside of the porch is covered in snow. The high winds force the snow through the screen. Substances are moved through a filter by differences in pressure across the filter. Pressure pushes stuff through the holes. The

nephropathy *(neff ROPP ah thee)*
nephro = *kidneys*
pathy = *disease*

Clinical Application

DIABETIC NEPHROPATHY

Diabetes mellitus is a condition characterized by abnormally high blood glucose. This hyperglycemia, caused by production of too little insulin or by insensitivity to insulin, wreaks havoc with blood chemistry, including osmotic balance. One of the functions of your kidney is to remove all that extra glucose from your blood. When the blood glucose is high, the kidneys must work that much harder to remove it. Patients with elevated glucose eliminate a much greater volume of urine than do patients with healthy levels of blood glucose because their kidneys try to excrete the excess blood glucose.

Prolonged high blood glucose causes a type of kidney damage known as diabetic nephropathy. It begins with a thickening of the filter surface of the glomerular capsule and eventually leads to a complete breakdown of that tissue. Once the tissue is damaged, the selectivity of the filter is destroyed. Substances that usually would not pass through the filter and into glomerular filtrate, like proteins and blood cells, begin to appear in urine. The efficiency of filtration is compromised and kidney function begins to deteriorate. Protein and blood cells in the urine are early indicators of renal failure. Diabetics can help prevent the onset of kidney damage by keeping blood sugar levels as tightly controlled as possible, preventing high blood pressure, and reducing blood cholesterol to safe levels. Diabetic nephropathy is the leading cause of kidney failure in the United States.

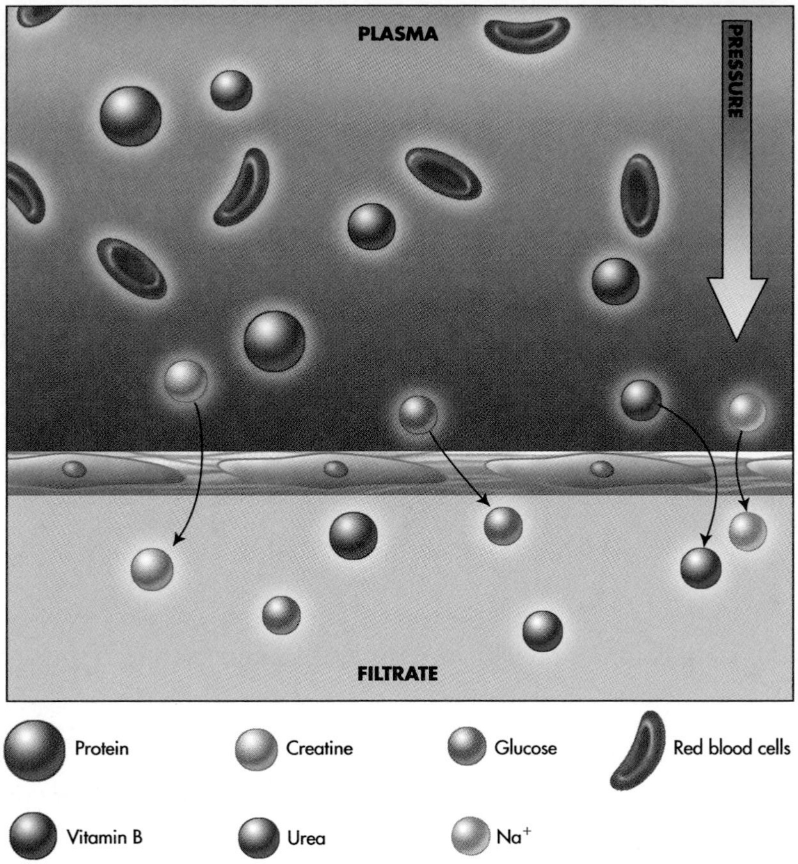

FIGURE 16–7

Filter selectivity.

higher the pressure on one side of the filter compared to the other side, the faster substances are filtered.

This combination works great in coffee makers. The filters have holes too small to let any but the tiniest coffee grounds pass through. The pressure of the water on top of the filter pushes the water, and the chemicals that make coffee grounds into drinkable coffee, through the filter, but the grounds stay on the other side.

> *Amazing Body Facts*
>
> **GLOMERULAR FILTRATION**
>
> The millions of tiny filters in your kidneys perform a truly Herculean task. Average glomerular filtration rate is 110 milliliters per minute, or 160 liters per day. That's more than 40 gallons filtered every 24 hours!

The glomerulus and glomerular capsule work in much the same way. Like most filters, the podocytes and capillary walls of the renal corpuscle create a filter with fixed openings. Plasma and many of the substances dissolved in plasma pass through the filter, but red and white blood cells, platelets, and some large molecules, like proteins, do not pass through the filter, in a healthy kidney, but remain in the bloodstream. What passes through the filter is predetermined by the size of the openings. This explains why protein in urine is a sign of kidney damage. Under normal circumstances, protein molecules are too large to fit through the glomerular filter, so proteins do not get into the renal tubule or into the urine. Only when the

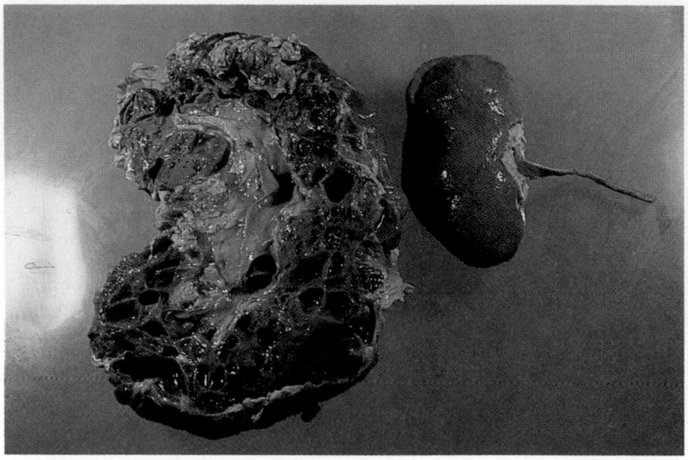

FIGURE ■ 16–8

Comparison of damaged and healthy kidneys.

filter is damaged can protein pass into the filtrate and then into the urine (see Figure 16–8 ■).

Clinical Application

KIDNEY STONES

Kidney stones are exactly what their name implies: hard bodies (stones) in the kidney. Kidney stones result when substances in the urine crystallize in the renal tubule, often because the concentration of the molecule is higher than normal in the renal tubule. However, sometimes the cause of kidney stones is a mystery. Stones can be made of many different chemicals, including calcium or uric acid, or can be caused by kidney infection. Some individuals appear to be more susceptible to stones than others, and once you have had a kidney stone, you are more susceptible to kidney stones in the future. Many kidney stones pass through the kidney unnoticed. However, larger or irregularly shaped stones may lodge in the kidney tubules, obstructing flow and irritating nearby tissues. Most patients diagnosed with kidney stones are driven to seek treatment because of blood in their urine (hematuria) or excruciating lower back pain. Patients with kidney stones often describe the pain as the worst they have ever felt. Even painful stones will often pass on their own without medical intervention. Patients are treated for pain and sent home with instructions to drink lots of water and wait for the stone to pass. (Often, they are asked to save the stone as it passes so it can be sent for chemical analysis!) Twenty years ago, the only treatment for a stone too large to pass on its own was surgery to remove the stone. Today, however, a noninvasive technique called lithotripsy, which uses shock waves applied to the outside of the body, can often break up the stone so it is small enough to pass through the kidney, allowing the patient to avoid surgery.

FILTRATION RATE

Filtration rate, however, can be controlled by changing the pressure difference across the filter. The most obvious way to control the pressure is to change the pressure of the blood in the glomerular capillaries. Higher pressure in the glomerulus will increase filtration, lower pressure will decrease filtration. You might think that every minor change in systemic blood pressure would affect glomerular filtration rate. That would be the logical conclusion. However, the glomerulus is protected from minor changes in blood pressure by a mechanism called **autoregulation.** As systemic blood pressure increases, the afferent arterioles leading into the glomerulus constrict, decreasing the amount of blood getting into the glomerulus. If less blood gets into the glomerulus, the pressure doesn't rise. Autoregulation protects the delicate filter from repeated rapid changes in blood pressure caused, for example, by walking up steps.

Autoregulation can be overridden in situations when blood pressure must be regulated. Because the kidney controls fluid volume, it is often part of mechanisms, along with the cardiovascular system, that regulate systemic blood pressure. For example, if there is a decrease in systemic blood pressure or volume, such as during severe blood loss, glomerular filtration decreases dramatically in an attempt to conserve fluid volume by producing less urine.

> **16-5** Ultrasound technicians help to view the kidneys for diagnostic purposes. They also perform diagnostic images on other body organs. To view a video on ultrasound procedures, please go to your CD-ROM for this chapter.

Remember that flight-or-fight response includes decreased urine production. The sympathetic nervous system and the hormones of the adrenal medulla, epinephrine and norepinephrine, decrease glomerular filtration by causing dramatic vasoconstriction of the afferent arterioles. This prevents blood from flowing to the glomerulus, decreasing glomerular filtration rate. Small changes in systemic blood pressure do not affect glomerular filtration, because autoregulation keeps glomerular pressure relatively constant, but during shock, for example, glomerular filtration decreases significantly. This is one of the reasons that urine output is monitored in trauma and surgery patients. Remember when we discussed blood vessels, one serious complication of severe blood loss is permanent kidney damage due to decreased blood flow and subsequent death of kidney tissue.

The reverse is also true: if blood volume is elevated, sympathetic output to the afferent arterioles decreases, the arterioles dilate, and glomerular filtration rate increases, allowing the kidneys to get rid of excess fluid.

CONTROL OF TUBULAR REABSORPTION AND SECRETION

Glomerular filtration controls the speed of filtration and ultimately the amount of urine formed. Tubular reabsorption and secretion control the chemistry and volume of the urine. Substances that are reabsorbed move from the tubule back to the bloodstream via the peritubular capillaries and stay in the body. Substances that are secreted stay in the tubule and eventually leave the body via the urine. Thus, anything that affects reabsorption and secretion affects urine chemistry.

The first thing that affects tubular reabsorption and secretion is tubule permeability. Each portion of the tubule can reabsorb and secrete different substances. Remember that molecules can move across membranes via several different methods. *Diffusion* is the movement of molecules from high to low concentration. *Osmosis* is the movement of water across a semipermeable membrane. Some molecules can only move across membranes by being carried across by proteins. This type of movement is called *active transport*. Differences in tubule permeability result in dramatic differences in which molecules are reabsorbed or secreted in each part of the tubule. See Table 16–2 for a list of substances reabsorbed or secreted in each part of the tubule.

> *Amazing Body Facts*
>
> **TUBULAR REABSORPTION**
>
> You already know about the amazing ability of your kidneys to filter blood. However, the ability of your renal tubule to reabsorb the fluid filtered by the glomerulus is just as incredible. Your kidneys filter 160 liters (40 gallons) per day, yet you only produce between 1 and 3 liters (less than 1 gallon) of urine per day!

The second factor that affects tubular reabsorption and secretion is a special type of circulation around the nephron loop,

TABLE 16–2 Individual Tubule Functions

TUBULE	SUBSTANCES REABSORBED OR SECRETED
proximal	potassium, chloride, sodium, magnesium, bicarbonate, phosphate, amino acids, glucose, fructose, galactose, lactate, citric acid, water, Hydrogen (H+), neurotransmitters, bile, uric acid, drugs, toxins, ammonia
descending loop	water
ascending loop	sodium, potassium, chloride
distal tubule	sodium, potassium, chloride, Hydrogen (H+), water
collecting duct	sodium, potassium, chloride, water

called **countercurrent circulation.** When ions move across cell membranes, they move from areas of high to low concentration. They are said to move "down their concentration gradient." In a solution, if there is a lot of solvent (water), there is less solute (dissolved substances), and vice versa, so you would expect that solute and solvent would move in opposite directions down their concentration gradients. Figure 16–9 ■ shows two solutions separated by a diffusible membrane. In solution A, the solvent water is more concentrated and therefore it will move down its concentration gradient into B. The dissolved solutes, in this case ions, are more concentrated in solution B, so they move down their concentration gradient into A. As always in the body, this is an attempt to maintain the homeostatic balance.

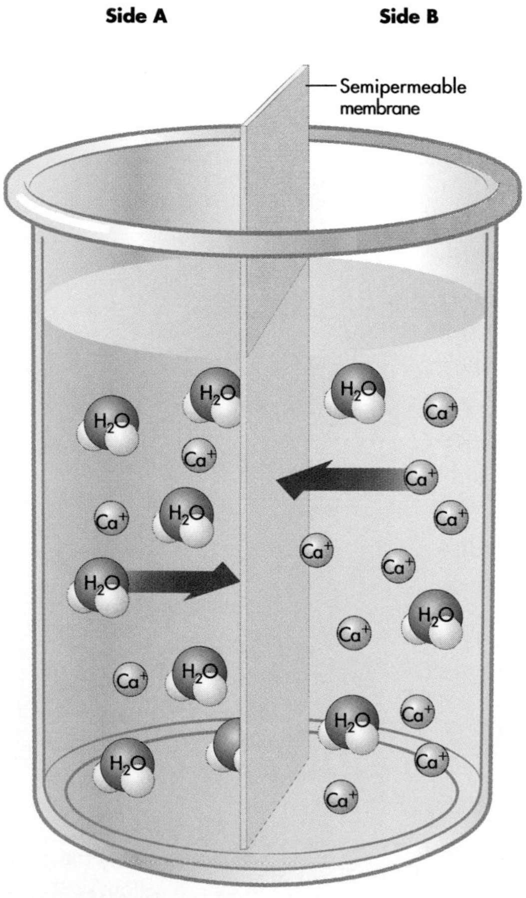

FIGURE ■ 16–9

Movement of solute (ions) and solvent (water) down their concentration gradient.

Because of the tendency for water and ions to move in opposite directions, as shown in Figure 16–9, the kidney could not reabsorb both ions and water without the special selective environment around the nephron loop. One would be reabsorbed and one would be secreted if it weren't for selected areas of the nephron being impermeable to one or the other. The characteristics of the nephron that make the countercurrent circulation work include the concentration gradient in the fluid surrounding the nephron, with low ion concentration at the beginning of the descending loop and high concentration at the tip of the loop, and the differences in permeability between the descending loop (water) and ascending loop (ions).

As filtrate flows into the *descending loop*, *water* is reabsorbed, and the concentration of ions in the loop increases as water leaves the tubule. As the filtrate turns the corner and enters the *ascending loop*, much of the water has left and the fluid is extremely concentrated. The ascending loop is permeable only to ions, so *ions* are reabsorbed from the ascending loop. Water and ions that leave the renal tubule enter the capillaries and go back to the bloodstream (see Figure 16–10 ■).

The third set of factors that affect reabsorption and secretion are several hormones that regulate blood pressure. You were introduced

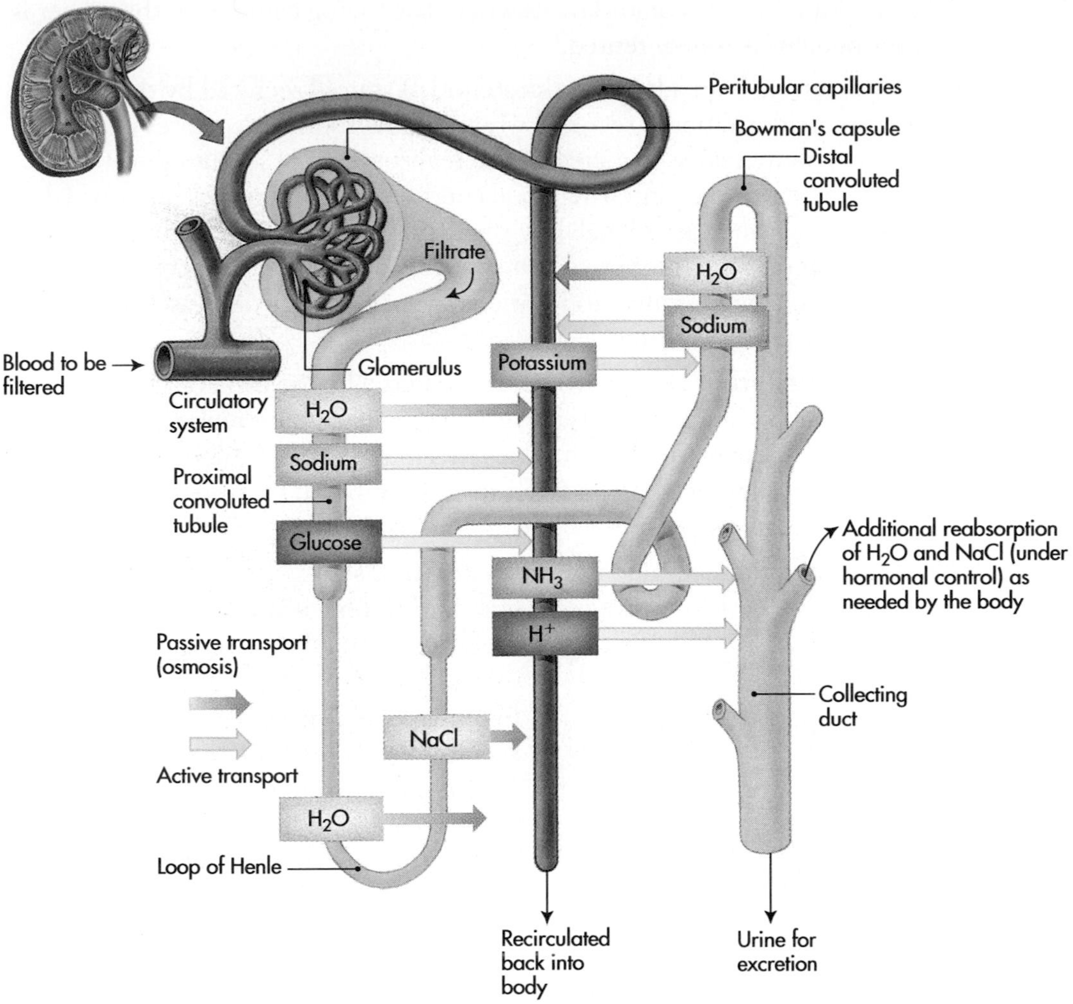

FIGURE ■ 16–10

Sites of tubular reabsorption and secretion.

to these mechanisms when you learned about regulation of blood pressure. It should come as no surprise that these mechanisms affect kidney function, since the kidneys control ion and fluid balance.

The hormones secreted by the kidneys perform a variety of functions. You met some of these hormones during your visit to the cardiovascular and endocrine systems.

antidiuretic hormone *(ADH)* *(AN tye dye yoo RET ik)*

- **Antidiuretic hormone** (ADH) is made by the hypothalamus and secreted from the posterior pituitary when blood pressure decreases or blood ionic concentration increases. ADH increases the permeability of the distal tubule and the collecting duct so that more water is reabsorbed, thereby increasing the blood volume and blood pressure and diluting the ionic concentration. Less urine is produced as more water is reabsorbed, hence the name antidiuretic hormone. Alcohol or caffeine actually inhibit ADH from working and thus preventing the distal tubules and collecting duct from becoming permeable to water. The water then stays in the collecting tubules and is sent to the bladder, thereby increasing urination. The more beverages containing these substances that you drink, the more dehydrated you become. This is where the saying came from that "beer is not bought, it is only rented."

aldosterone *(al DOSS ter ohn)*

- **Aldosterone** is an adrenocorticosteroid, a steroid secreted by the adrenal cortex. Aldosterone is secreted when plasma sodium decreases or plasma potassium increases. It increases the reabsorption of sodium ions (thus bringing more back into the blood) and secretion of potassium ions (thus decreasing the plasma levels) by the distal tubule and ascending limb of the nephron loop. Because sodium is reabsorbed back into the bloodstream, so is more water, and urine volume therefore decreases under the influence of aldosterone.

atrial natriuretic peptide *(AY tree al nay tree your RET ick PEP tide)*

- **Atrial natriuretic peptide** (ANP) is secreted by the atria of the heart when blood volume increases. ANP decreases sodium reabsorption and therefore increases urination. Does this make sense? If blood volume has increased dramatically, how would you keep blood pressure constant? Would you get rid of water or keep more water?

renin-angiotensin-aldosterone *(REE nen-an gee oh TEN sen-al DOSS ter ohn*

juxtaglomerular *(JUX ta gla MARE you ler)*

- **Renin-angiotensin-aldosterone** system is a series of chemical reactions that regulate blood pressure in several different ways. When there is a decrease in blood flow to the kidney, a special group of cells near the glomerulus called the **juxtaglomerular** apparatus secretes renin into the bloodstream. Renin converts angiotensinogen, a protein made by the liver, into angiotensin I. Another enzyme made by the lungs, angiotensin converting enzyme (ACE), converts angiotensin I to angiotensin II. Angiotensin II (active angiotensin) has several different effects. It increases thirst, increases ADH secretion, increases aldosterone secretion, and causes vasoconstriction. Blood pressure is therefore increased either by increased fluid volume due to higher water intake or decreased urination caused by increased levels of ADH or aldosterone. Notice how the kidneys, lungs, and liver work together to regulate blood pressure. Many patients with high blood pressure may be given an ACE inhibitor, which inhibits all the previous effects and therefore lowers blood pressure.

Applied Science

ELECTROLYTES AND ACID BASE

The kidney maintains electrolyte balance by selectively excreting or reabsorbing the electrolytes within the tubular system. One very important interaction is the relationship of hydrogen ion (H^+) and bicarbonate ions (HCO_3^-). The relationship between these ions determine the blood's pH (level of acidity or alkalinity). This is referred to as the acid–base relationship. If too much acid is present in the blood, H^+, which causes acidity and the pH to drop, will be excreted to a greater level in the urine. At the same time, more bicarbonate ions (base that neutralizes acids) will be reabsorbed back into the acidic blood to bring the pH value back toward normal. The respiratory system also plays a role in maintaining the acid–base balance by increasing ventilation to "blow off" more acid in the form of exhaled carbon dioxide (carbonic acid) if the blood is too acidic.

Clinical Application

POLYCYSTIC KIDNEY DISEASE (PKD)

Polycystic kidney disease is a genetic disorder in which large cysts form in the kidneys. One form of PKD is so serious that some patients die in infancy. The more common form is an adult onset disorder characterized by decreasing kidney function as normal nephrons are displaced by the cysts. As more and more cysts develop, kidneys get very large. One polycystic kidney weighed 22 pounds! There is no cure for PKD except kidney transplantation. About half a million people in the United States have PKD.

TEST YOUR KNOWLEDGE 16-2

Choose the best answer:

1. Glomerular filtrate is most similar in composition to
   a. blood
   b. lymph
   c. urine
   d. none of the above

2. When substances move from the tubule into the bloodstream, this is known as
   a. secretion
   b. reabsorption
   c. filtration
   d. all of the above

3. Which of the following is usually completely reabsorbed in the proximal tubule?
   a. sodium
   b. urea
   c. glucose
   d. water

4. The descending nephron loop is permeable to _____, while the ascending is permeable to _____.
   a. water, ions
   b. ions, water
   c. water, water
   d. ions, ions

5. If blood pressure increases beyond normal range, what happens to glomerular filtration rate?
   a. it increases
   b. it decreases
   c. it stays the same
   d. none of the above

6. Which of the following is not typically found in urine?
   a. glucose
   b. protein
   c. blood cells
   d. all of the above

The Urinary Bladder and Urination Reflex

Glomerular filtrate flows out the collecting ducts into the minor calyces and then into the major calyces that form the renal pelvis. Once the glomerular filtrate leaves the collecting ducts, its concentration cannot be changed. At this point, filtrate is urine. Urine collects in the renal pelvis and flows down the ureters to the urinary bladder where it is stored.

The urinary bladder is a small, hollow organ posterior to the pubic symphysis and behind the peritoneum. It is lined with transitional epithelium, the only epithelium stretchy enough to expand as the bladder fills. The stretchiness of the bladder is enhanced by a series of pleats called *rugae*. The bladder has a muscular wall consisting of several layers of circular and longitudinal smooth muscle and is covered by connective tissue and parietal peritoneum (see Figure 16–11 ■).

As urine accumulates, the bladder fills and stretches. At some point, this stretch triggers urination, or voiding—the emptying of the bladder. For years, urination was thought to be a spinal cord reflex, influenced but not controlled by the brain. New research, however, suggests that the brain actually controls urination. When the bladder is full, signals are sent from the bladder to the spinal cord and then to the pons. The pons sends parasympathetic signals down the spinal cord that cause contraction of the muscular walls of the bladder, and the bladder empties.

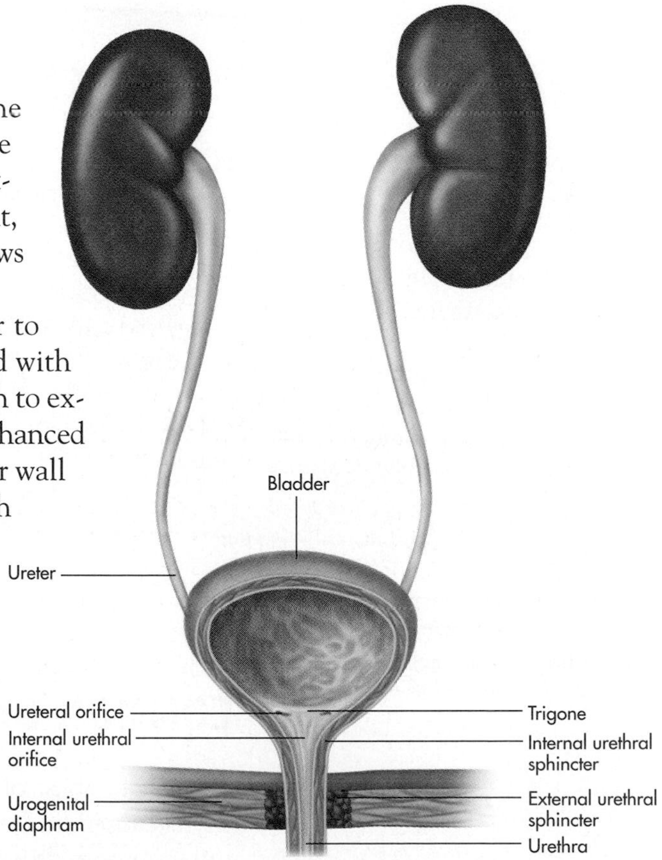

FIGURE ■ 16–11

The urinary bladder.

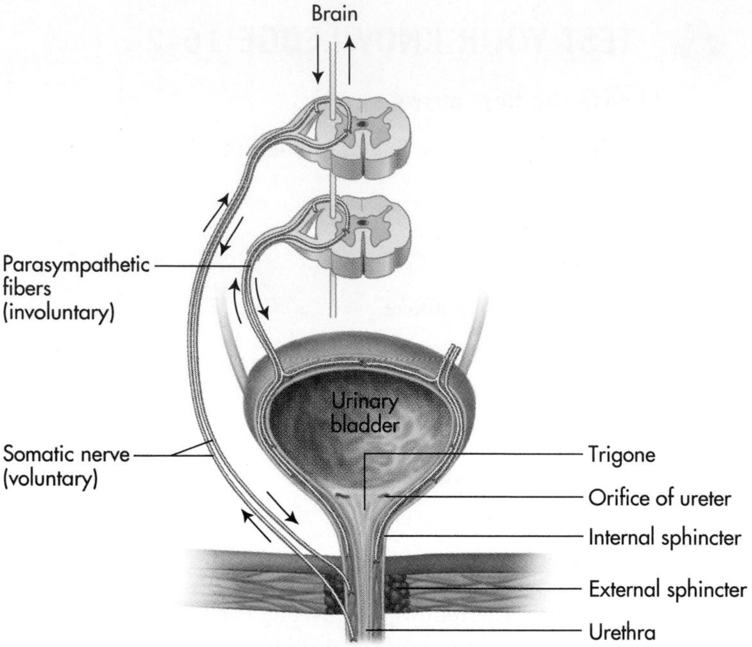

FIGURE ■ 16–12

Control of urination.

16-6 To perform an interactive exercise on labeling the urinary bladder, please go to your CD-ROM for this chapter.

Urine leaves the bladder via the urethra, a thin muscular tube lined with several different types of epithelium along its length. (For details on the anatomy of the urethra, including sexual differences, see Chapter 17.) Parts of the brain can inhibit urination by controlling the **internal urethral sphincter,** a valve at the junction of the bladder and the urethra, and the **external urethral sphincter,** a valve that is part of the muscles of the pelvic floor. Sympathetic stimulation of these sphincters prevents urine from leaving the body (see Figure 16–12 ■). Fortunately, although you have little control over contractions of the bladder wall, you have very good control over the sphincters.

Clinical Application

URINARY TRACT INFECTION (UTI)

Urinary tract infection is caused by the movement of fecal bacteria into the urinary tract. Symptoms include frequent, painful urination. Sometimes the urine is bloody or cloudy or has an unusual odor. Urinary tract infections must be treated promptly because they can cause damage to the kidneys if the infection moves from the bladder up the ureter and into the kidneys. Urinary tract infections are more common in women than in men, probably because women's urethras are shorter than men's. Urinary tract infections may be prevented in susceptible individuals by drinking plenty of water and increasing the acidity of the urine by regular consumption of cranberry juice.

internal urethral sphincter *(IN ter nal yoo REE thral SFINK ter)*

external urethral sphincter *(EKS ter nal yoo REE thral SFINK ter)*

COMMON DISORDERS OF THE URINARY SYSTEM

Overuse or abuse of drugs can severely affect renal function. Analgesic nephropathy is caused by long-term use of pain relievers, particularly nonsteroidal anti-inflammatory drugs (NSAIDs) like ibuprofen and naproxyn, particularly when combined with caffeine or codeine or acetominophen. Even over-the-counter dosages can cause chronic kidney damage leading to kidney failure.

Chronic renal failure is an ongoing, progressive kidney disease. Often, the progression can be controlled by treating the underlying cause of the damage or controlling blood pressure and blood cholesterol. Chronic kidney failure may lead to end-stage renal failure. End-stage renal failure is the final stage of renal failure. Patients in end-stage renal failure can only be treated with kidney dialysis or transplantation.

Diabetes insipidus is an endocrine disorder characterized by too little ADH or insensitivity of the kidney to ADH. Without normal ADH activity, copious amounts of urine are produced. Even as the patient gets dehydrated, the production of urine cannot be slowed. A rarer form of the disorder is caused by abnormalities of the thirst mechanism, in which patients drink uncontrollably. Patients with uncontrollable thirst actually drink so much water that they have water toxicity (dangerously low blood sodium because of large volume of water dilution), which can cause brain damage or death.

> 16-7 To view videos on renal failure and kidney stones, please go to your CD-ROM for this chapter.

Glomerulonephritis is inflammation of the glomerulus. Glomerulosclerosis is scarring of the glomerulus. Both cause damage to the delicate filter apparatus. When the filter is damaged, blood cells and blood proteins enter the filtrate and eventually appear in the urine. Removal of waste products is decreased and electrolyte balance is generally abnormal because of the change in urine chemistry. There are many causes of glomerulonephritis and glomerulosclerosis, including bacterial infection, diabetic nephropathy, systemic lupus erythematosus, and genetic disorders such as Alport syndrome and Goodpasture's syndrome.

> **Amazing Body Facts**
>
> **URINE**
>
> In a healthy renal system, the urine produced is sterile. The urea found in urine is the same substance that is used to melt ice in the winter. Urea is also a component in plant fertilizer: although nitrogen is a waste product for humans, it is an essential product for plant growth. Finally, pain from a jellyfish sting can be alleviated by the application of urine.

Hemolytic uremic syndrome is a disorder caused by an infection with the bacteria *E. coli*, typically from eating undercooked meat. The bacteria infect the digestive tract and release toxins that destroy red blood cells. The damaged red blood cells lodge in the blood vessels in the kidney, blocking them and preventing blood flow to the nephrons. Without treatment, permanent kidney damage may result.

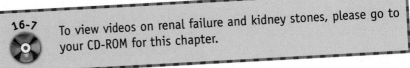

SUMMARY

Snapshots from the Journey

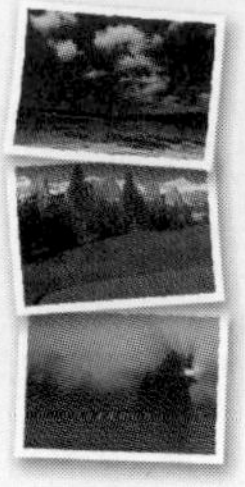

- The urinary system consists of paired kidneys and paired ureters, which carry urine to the single urinary bladder. The urethra transports urine from the bladder to outside the body. The function of the urinary system is control of fluid and electrolyte balance and elimination of nitrogen-containing waste.
- The kidney is bean-shaped and covered in a capsule. It has an indentation known as the renal hilum and an interior cavity known as the renal sinus. The kidney can be divided into three layers: renal cortex, renal medulla, and renal pelvis. The renal pelvis is a funnel that is divided into large pipes, the major calyces. Each major calyx is divided into several minor calyces. The renal pelvis empties into the ureter.
- The kidney is very well vascularized. Blood is supplied to each kidney by a renal artery. The blood vessels split into smaller and smaller branches until there are millions of tiny arterioles, the afferent arterioles. The afferent arterioles supply millions of nephrons, the functional unit of the kidney, with blood. Blood leaves the kidney by a series of veins and ultimately returns to circulation via the renal vein.
- The nephron is the functional unit of the kidney. There are millions of nephrons in each kidney. The nephron is divided into two parts. The renal corpuscle, consisting of the glomerulus (capillaries) and the glomerular capsule, filters blood and produces glomerular filtrate. The renal tubule, consisting of the proximal tubule, nephron loop, distal tubule, and collecting ducts, control the concentration and volume of urine by reabsorbing and secreting water, electrolytes, and other molecules. The walls of the nephron are made of epithelium. The type of epithelium changes depending on the specific function of each part of the nephron.
- Urine is formed by a combination of three processes: glomerular filtration, tubular reabsorption, and tubular secretion. The selectivity of the glomerular filter is determined by the size of the openings in the filter and the difference between the blood pressure of the glomerulus and the pressure in the glomerular capsule. The size of the filter does not change unless the glomerulus is damaged. Protein, for example, cannot pass through the filter. However, the filtration rate will change if the pressure in the glomerulus changes. Most of the time, autoregulation, control of the diameter of the afferent arteriole, keeps glomerular pressure and glomerular filtration rate constant. But sympathetic stimulation can regulate (in this case decrease) glomerular filtration and urine output due to constriction of afferent arterioles.
- Tubular reabsorption and secretion is controlled by differences in tubular permeability. The proximal tubule is the most versatile, reabsorbing dozens of different molecules. The nephron loop is part of an elaborate countercurrent mechanism, with the descending loop permeable to water and ascending loop permeable to ions. The distal tubule and collecting ducts reabsorb water. The permeability of the renal tubule can be regulated by a number of hormones that control blood pressure. These hormones, aldosterone, ADH, atrial natriuretic peptide, and others, regulate blood pressure by regulating urine volume and ion secretion. Changes in urine volume change total body fluid volume and thereby change blood pressure.
- The urinary bladder is a collecting and storage device for urine and is located in the pelvic cavity. It has a muscular wall. Contractions of the muscle result in voiding (urination), emptying the bladder. Urination is a reflex controlled by parasympathetic neurons in the pons. Signals from a full bladder reach the pons. The neurons in the pons then send signals for the bladder to contract. Sympathetic neurons control two valves, the internal and external urethral sphincters, which allow significant conscious control of the urination reflex.

Case Study

Jane has recently developed very annoying symptoms. She has to go to the restroom several times a day. Sometimes it seems that she spends every waking moment in there. She hasn't slept through the night in more than a week. She goes to see her doctor, who orders a series of tests to differentiate between several disorders that cause frequent urination: diabetes mellitus, overactive bladder, and urinary tract infection.

Jane's test results:

Urine bacteria	no
Blood	no
Leukocytes	no
Glucose	normal
Proteins	no

What is your diagnosis and why?

REVIEW QUESTIONS

Multiple Choice

1. The function of this part of the renal tubule is filtration of blood:
   a. renal calyx
   b. renal corpuscle
   c. renal cortex
   d. renal colums

2. The collecting ducts are found in this part of the kidney:
   a. renal cortex
   b. renal capsule
   c. renal pelvis
   d. renal pyramids

3. This tube leads from the urinary bladder to the outside:
   a. collecting ducts
   b. distal tubule
   c. ureter
   d. none of the above

4. The ion responsible for causing acidic blood is
   a. Na^+
   b. H^+
   c. K^+
   d. HCO_3^-

5. The renal hormone secreted by the hypothalamus when blood pressure decreases to promote the reabsorbtion of water is
   a. aldosterone
   b. atrial natriuretic peptide
   c. antidiuretic hormone
   d. epinephrine

Fill in the Blank

1. Most substances are reabsorbed or secreted in this part of the renal tubule: ______________.

2. This part of the renal tubule has an elaborate countercurrent mechanism for reabsorption of sodium and water: ______________.

3. This hormone is released by the heart when fluid volume increases: ______________.

Short Answer

1. List and explain the activity of three regulators of kidney function.

____

____

____

____

2. Explain the three processes that are necessary for urine formation. In which part of the nephron are these functions performed?

3. Describe the structure of the wall of the urinary bladder.

4. Explain the control of urination reflex.

Suggested Activities

1. Grab a partner and trace the flow of a particular substance from blood through the kidney. What happens to hydrogen ions or vitamin C? Use the Internet to help you find the answers.

2. Quiz yourself. Do you know what happens in each part of the nephron? Do you know the difference between plasma, glomerular filtrate, and urine chemistry?

3. There are many different disorders that affect the kidneys. Use the Internet to research one of these diseases. How does it cause the changes in kidney function?

16-8 Now that you have completed your journey through this chapter, please go to the CD-ROM for interactive games and puzzles concerning the medical terms and concepts contained in this chapter. By playing the games you will reinforce your learning of medical terminology in a fun way.

Greetings from THE REPRODUCTIVE System

Replacement and Repair

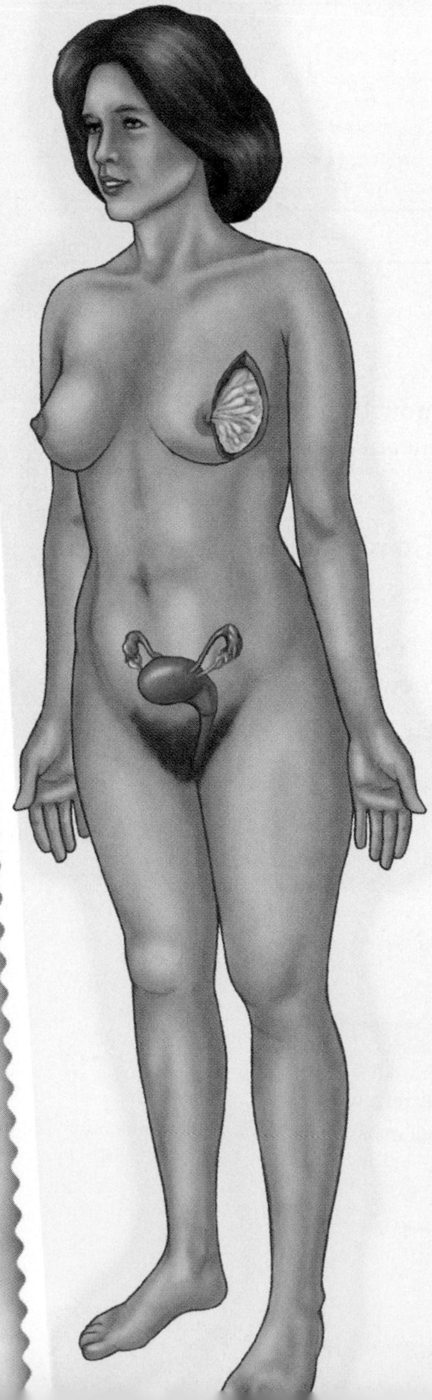

In order for a city to run smoothly, it must have an infrastructure, buildings, roads, playgrounds, schools, and more. All of these structures must be repaired on a regular basis, or if damaged beyond repair, they must be replaced. As a city grows along with its population, it needs the resources and means to expand. The same is true of your body. Cells and tissues get damaged or simply wear out. Damaged or worn-out cells and tissues must be repaired or replaced. Asexual reproduction, or mitosis, the process by which cells make exact copies of themselves, is absolutely necessary to maintain a healthy body. Mitosis was discussed in Chapter 3. Ultimately, cellular reproduction leads to the complicated process by which humans produce new humans: sexual reproduction. Without this ability, the human species would die out and the journey would end for the human race. Thankfully, all the splendid diversity of the human race is passed on for generations to come, who will also get to enjoy this amazing journey called "life."

Chapter 17

LEARNING OBJECTIVES

Upon completion of your journey through this chapter, you will be able to:

- Differentiate mitosis from meiosis
- Locate and describe the male and female reproductive organs
- Describe the function of the male and female reproductive organs
- Discuss the phases of the menstrual cycle
- Discuss the effects of hormonal control on the male and female reproductive systems
- Describe the stages of labor and delivery
- Relate common disorders of the male and female reproductive systems

MULTIMEDIA APPLICATIONS

CD-ROM Interactive Exercises

- Animation on cellular division, 17.1
- Animation of fertilization of the sperm and egg cell, 17.2
- 3-D animation of the female reproductive system with drag-and-drop labeling exercise, 17.3
- Animation on oogenesis with drag-and-drop labeling exercise, 17.4
- 3-D animation of the male reproductive system with drag-and-drop labeling exercise, 17.5
- Animation on spermatogenesis with drag-and-drop labeling exercise, 17.6
- Videos on the vasectomy procedure, fetal lie, labor, infant delivery, the placenta, and postpartum assessment, 17.7
- Movies on preclampsia, PMS, EDD, and breast cancer, 17.8
- Interactive games and puzzles, 17.9

www.prenhall.com/colbert

- Professional Profiles
  - Doula or Midwife
- Related Web Sites
- Additional Review Questions

Pronunciation Guide

Correct pronunciation is important in any journey so that you and others are completely understood. Here is a "see and say" Pronunciation Guide for the more difficult terms to pronounce in this chapter.

bulbourethral gland (BUHL boh yoo REE thral)
clitoris (KLIT oh riss)
corpus luteum (KOR pus LOU tee um)
cytokinesis (SIGH toe kih NEE suss)
endometrium (EHN doh MEE tree um)
epididymis (ep ih DID ih miss)
eukaryotic cell (you care ee AH tic sell)
fimbria (FIM bree ah)
follicle-stimulating hormone (FALL ih kle stim you LAY ting HOR mohn)
gametes (ga MEETS)
genitalia (jen ih TALE ya)
gonadotropin-releasing hormone (GO nad oh TROH pin)
human chorionic gonadotropin (HUE man core ee AH nik GO nad oh TROH pin)
labia majora (LAY bee ah mah JOR ah)
labia minora (LAY bee ah mih NOR ah)
luteal phase (LOO tee al faze)
luteinizing hormone (LOO tee ah NIZE ing)
meiosis (my OH sis)
menses (MEN seez)
menstruation (MEN stroo AY shun)
myometrium (MY oh MEE tree um)
oocyte (OH oh site)
oogenesis (OH jenn eh siss)
perimetrium (pair ee MEE tree um)
primordial follicles (pry MORE dee all FALL ih klz)
progesterone (proh JESS ter ohn)
pudendal cleft (PEW den dall cleft)
seminal vesicles (SEM ih nal VESS ih klz)
seminiferous tubules (SEM ih NIF er uss TOO byoolz)
sertoli cells (sir TOW lee sells)
spermatocytes (sper MAT oh sites)
spermatids (sper MAT ids)
spermatogonia (sper MAT oh GO nee ah)
spermatozoa (sper MAT oh ZOE ah)
testis, testes (TESS tiss, TESS teez)
testicles (TESS tih klz)
testosterone (tess TOSS ter ohn)
urethra (yoo REE thrah)
uterus (YOO ter uss)
vagina (vah JYE nah)
vas deferens (VAS DEFF er enz)
vulva (VULL vah)
zygote (ZIGH goht)

TISSUE GROWTH AND REPLACEMENT

Although mitosis was discussed in the Chapter 3, we will briefly review that form of cellular reproduction in this chapter. Cellular reproduction is the basis for *all* more complex reproduction, so this is a good starting point.

Mitosis

Cellular reproduction is the process of making a new cell. It is also known as **cell division,** because one cell divides into two cells when it reproduces. Cells can only come from other cells. When cells make *identical* copies of themselves *without the involvement* of another cell, the process is called **asexual reproduction.** Most cells can reproduce themselves asexually, whether they are animal cells, plant cells, or bacteria.

a *= without*

The cells that make up the human body are a type of cell known as a **eukaryotic cell.** Eukaryotic cells have a nucleus, cellular organelles, and usually several chromosomes in the nucleus. (Reminder: the genetic material of the cell, DNA, is bundled into "packages" of chromatin known as chromosomes.) Since chromosomes carry all the instructions for the cells, all cells

eukaryotic cell
(you care ee AH tic sell)

must have a complete set after reproduction. These instructions include how the cell is to function within the body and blueprints for reproduction. No matter whether a cell has one chromosome, like bacteria, or 46 chromosomes, like humans, all the chromosomes must be copied before the cell can divide.

Now let's go to the more complex form of cellular reproduction. Eukaryotic cells, like yours, must go through a more complicated set of maneuvers in order to reproduce. Not only do your cells have to duplicate all 46 of their chromosomes, they have to make sure that each cell gets all of the chromosomes and all of the right organelles. The process of sorting the chromosomes so that each new cell gets the right number of copies of all of the genetic material is called **mitosis.** Mitosis is the only way that eukaryotic cells can reproduce asexually. For a quick review on mitosis, go back to Chapter 3.

17-1 Go to your CD-ROM to view an animation on cellular division.

mitosis *(MY toe sis)*

MITOSIS IN THE BODY

Mitosis, asexual cellular reproduction, serves many purposes in your body. Any time your cells must be replaced, mitosis is the method used to replace them. Many of your tissues, such as bone, epithelium, skin, and blood cells, are replaced on a regular basis. Repair and regeneration of damaged tissue is accomplished by mitosis as well. If you cut your hand, the skin is replaced, first by collagen, but eventually by the original tissue. Mitosis increases in cells near the injury so that the damaged or destroyed cells can be replaced. A broken bone is replaced in much the same way.

Growth is also accomplished by mitosis. Lengthening of bones as you grow, increases in muscle mass due to exercise, indeed, most ways that tissue gets bigger, are due to mitosis of cells in the tissues or organs. Without mitosis, your body would not be able to grow or replace old or damaged cells.

SEXUAL REPRODUCTION

Thus far we have discussed cell division for growth and repair, but we must also be able to perpetuate the species. This requires sexual reproduction.

gametes *(ga MEETS)*

Reduction Division: Meiosis

Many animals reproduce sexually; that is, they produce, with the aid of another individual, offspring that are not identical to themselves. Sexual reproduction involves the union of a cell from one organism with a cell from another organism of the same species. In animals, females produce **eggs** and males produce **sperm** for the purpose of reproducing sexually. These special cells are known as **gametes.**

Learning Hint

MITOSIS VERSUS MEIOSIS

These words sound and look alike and are therefore often confused. Remember, meiosis produces gametes or sexual cells, which contain half of the chromosomes because the sexual union of male and female will contribute the other half. Mitosis (I reproduce myself) is asexual and produces exact copies of the cell and the full complement of chromosomes because no union is needed.

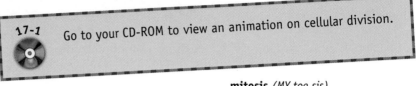

meiosis *(my OH sis)*

Gametes are produced by a specialized type of cell division known as **meiosis,** or **reduction division.** Meiosis is called reduction division because the daughter cells produced at the end of meiosis have half as many chromosomes as the original mother cell. (Note: the cells are called mother cells and daughter cells even when we are talking about the process in males.) These daughter cells must have half as many chromosomes because they will fuse together during sexual reproduction. In humans, the total number of chromosomes in a cell is 46. If the gametes did not lose half of their chromosomes somewhere along the way, then the cell that resulted from sexual reproduction would have twice as many chromosomes (92 chromosomes) as necessary. It is absolutely necessary to control the number of chromosomes in a cell. Cells with too few or too many chromosomes often die.

The fact that you were produced by the fusion of an egg from your mother and a sperm from your father means that your 46 chromosomes can be thought of as being 23 *pairs* of chromosomes. Each pair of chromosomes consists of one from your father and one from your mother. They can be thought of as pairs because they can be matched based on size, shape, and which genes they carry. For example, you get a chromosome 1 from your father and a chromosome 1 from your mother, the same for chromosome 2, 3, 4, and up to 22.

The 23rd "pair" of chromosomes is a set of sex chromosomes. These are called sex chromosomes because their identity determines the sex of a baby. XX is female, XY is male (see Figure 17–1 ■). The female always contributes an X, but the male can contribute either an X or Y chromosome. The male actually determines the sex of the baby by either contributing an X chromosome for a girl or a Y chromosome for a boy.

Clinical Application

DOWN'S SYNDROME

Down's syndrome is a relatively common birth defect that causes short stature, heart defects, increased risk of leukemia, Alzheimer's disease, and mental retardation. Down's syndrome is caused by the presence of an extra chromosome 21 in a person's cells. Some time during meiosis, usually in the mother, chromosomes fail to separate, leaving some daughter cells without a chromosome 21 and others with two copies of chromosome 21. If the egg with the extra chromosome is fertilized, the resulting fetus will have three copies of chromosome 21 instead of two.

The possibility of having a baby with Down's syndrome increases dramatically in women over 35 years old. Down's syndrome is one of very few disorders resulting from abnormal chromosome numbers, probably because most fertilized eggs with abnormal numbers of chromosomes do not develop normally enough to survive.

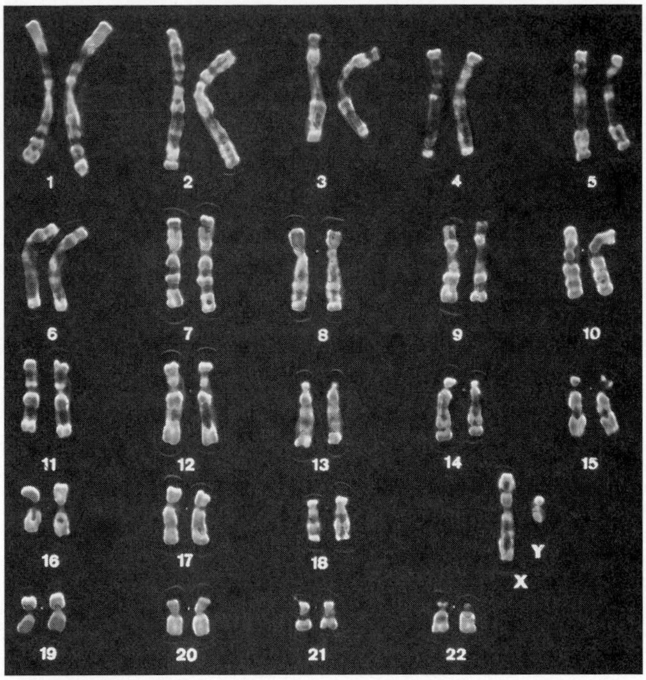

FIGURE ■ 17–1

Photo of human chromosome profile: Both an X and a Y chromosome appear in the image; therefore, this is a male sample. (Source: CNRI/SPL, Photo Researchers, Inc.)

THE HUMAN LIFE CYCLE

Both mitosis and meiosis are absolutely necessary parts of human life. Without them, cells could not be replaced, injuries could not be repaired, new humans could not be produced. The relationship between mitosis and meiosis and their importance can be easily explained by looking at human life as a cycle (see Figure 17–2 ■). Eggs and sperm, with only half as many chromosomes as other cells, are produced by meiosis in specialized organs known as the **gonads.** The male gonads are called **testes.** The female gonads are the **ovaries.** During sexual reproduction, the gametes (egg and sperm) unite and combine their genetic material. This union and combination of genetic material is called **fertilization.** The fertilized egg is known as a **zygote.** Unlike gametes, which have only 23 chromosomes, the zygote has the typical number of chromosomes for a human cell, 46. The zygote undergoes millions of rounds of mitosis and development within the female to change from an *embryo* to a *fetus* (the infant that is not born yet). The rest of this chapter is devoted to describing sexual reproduction in humans.

gonad *(GO nad)*

testis, testes *(TESS tiss, TESS teez)*

ovary, ovaries *(OH vah ree, OH vah reez)*

zygote *(ZIGH goht)*

17-2 Please go to your CD-ROM for an animation of fertilization of the sperm and egg cell.

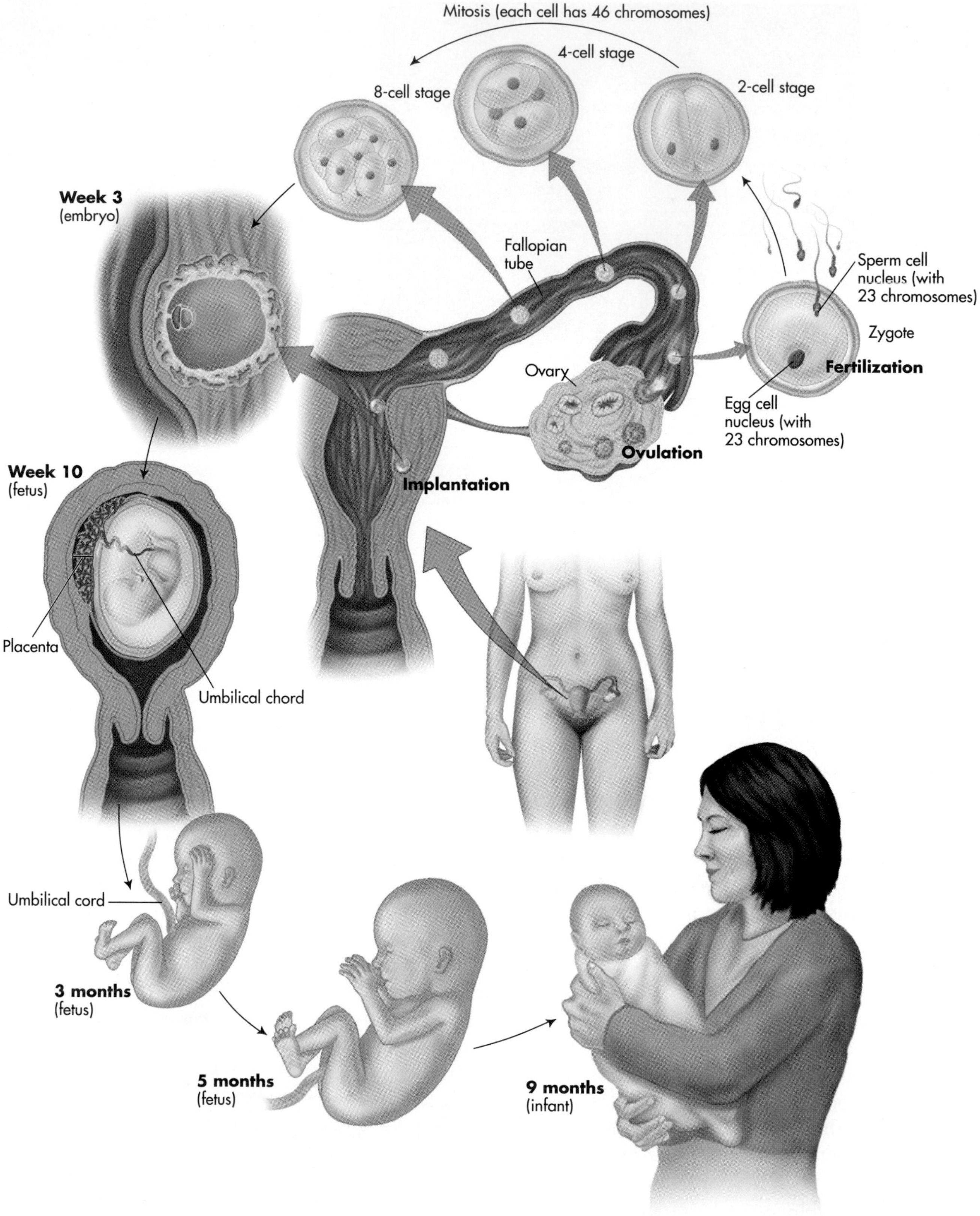

FIGURE ■ 17–2

The early stages of the human life cycle.

TEST YOUR KNOWLEDGE 17-1

Choose the best answer:

1. Cells with half the number of chromosome used for sexual reproduction are known as
   a. zygotes
   b. daughter cells
   c. gametes
   d. half cells

2. Organs that produce sperm and egg are called
   a. gametes
   b. gonads
   c. zygotes
   d. chromosomes

3. After _____, the egg is called a _____ and has 46 chromosomes.
   a. reproduction, gamete
   b. meiosis, daughter cell
   c. mitosis, zygote
   d. fertilization, zygote

THE HUMAN REPRODUCTION SYSTEM

Reproductive organs are called **genitalia.** The primary genitalia are the gonads, which produce the gametes. The secondary genitalia are all the other structures that aid in the reproductive process. In this section, we will first discuss female anatomy and physiology and then male anatomy and physiology.

genitalia *(jen ih TALE ya)*

Female Anatomy

In females, the primary genitalia are the ovaries. The secondary genitalia are the **uterine tubes** (also known as **oviducts** or **fallopian tubes**), the **uterus,** the **vagina,** and the external genitalia, called the **vulva.**

uterus *(YOO ter uss)*
vagina *(vah JYE nah)*
vulva *(VULL vah)*

The primary genitalia, or ovaries, are paired structures, about 3 centimeters long, in the peritoneal cavity. There is one ovary on each side of the uterus. Several ligaments suspend or anchor each ovary. The *mesovarium* suspends the ovary, the *suspensory ligament* attaches the ovary to lateral pelvic wall, and the *ovarian ligament* anchors the ovary to the uterine wall. Blood vessels, the ovarian artery, and the ovarian branch of the uterine artery travel through the mesovarium and suspensory ligament, supplying the ovary with oxygenated blood. Please see Figure 17–3 ■ for a diagram of internal reproductive anatomy.

THE OVARY

The ovary is covered by a fibrous capsule called the *tunica albuginea* made of cuboidal epithelium. The interior of the ovary is divided into the cortex, which contains the eggs, and the medulla, which contains blood vessels, nerves, and lymphatic tissue surrounded by loose connective tissue. The anatomy of the cortex is relatively complicated and will be described during our discussion of physiology.

THE UTERINE TUBES

The uterine tubes, also known as oviducts or fallopian tubes, are the passageway for the egg to get to the uterus. The uterine tubes begin as a large funnel, the *infundibulum*, surrounded by ciliated projections, the **fimbria.** The in-

fimbria *(FIM bree ah)*

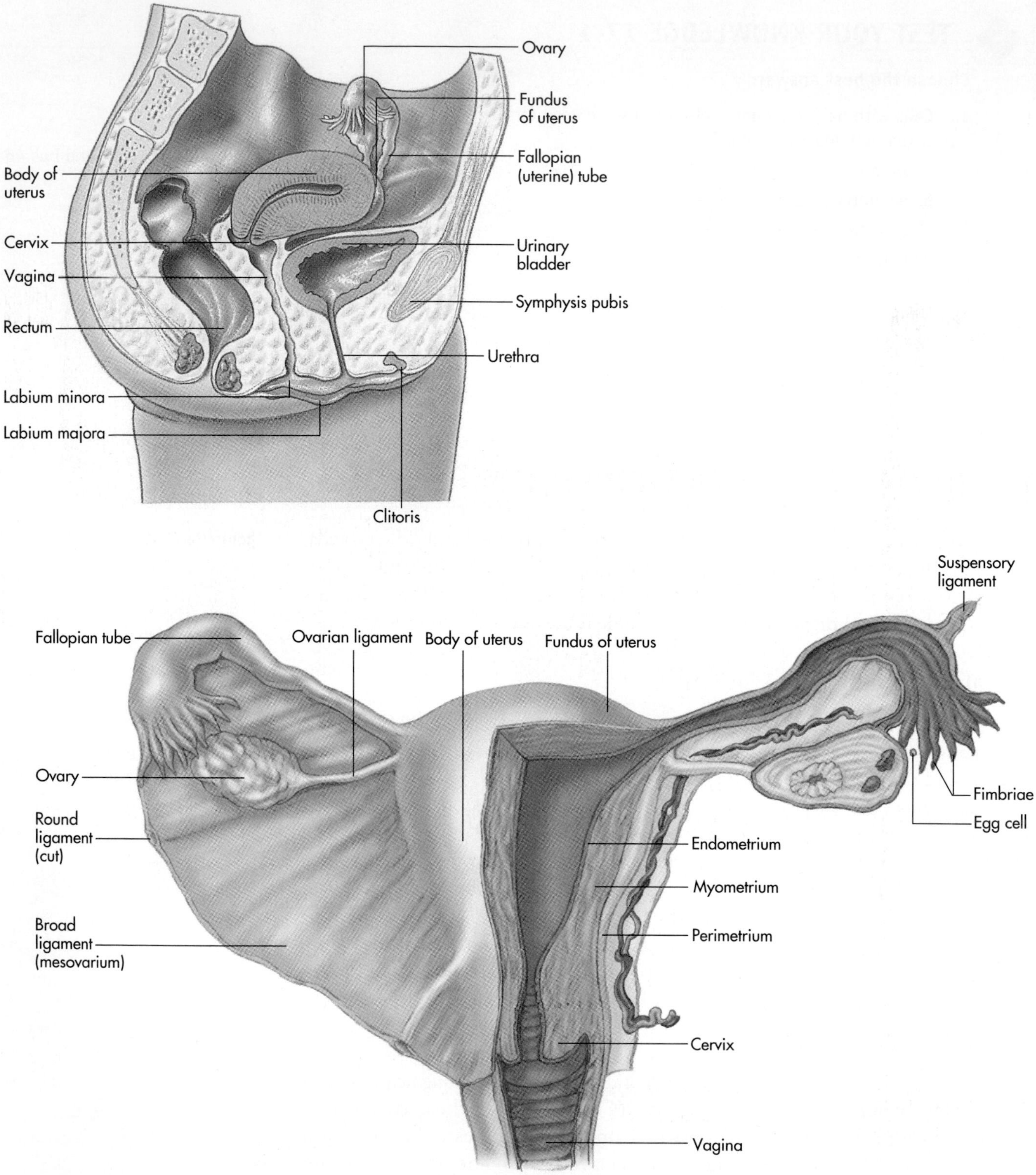

FIGURE ■ 17–3

Internal female reproductive organs.

fundibulum leads to a widened area, the *ampulla*, followed by a longer, narrower portion known as the *isthmus*. The uterine tubes are connected to the superior portion of the uterus. The tube is constructed of sheets of smooth muscle lined with highly folded, ciliated, simple columnar epithelium. The outside of the tube is covered by the visceral peritoneum and suspended by a mesentery known as the *mesosalpinx*.

Clinical Application

ENDOMETRIOSIS

Each month, women of child-bearing age shed and replace the endometrium, the lining of the uterus. In many women, this endometrial tissue escapes the uterus and implants in the abdominal and pelvic cavities. There, the tissue responds to the woman's hormonal cycles, continuing to build up and decay each month. Unfortunately, the continued proliferation and decay and bleeding of endometrial tissue in the abdominal and pelvic cavities can cause scarring and damage to the organs. Many women who have endometriosis have no noticeable symptoms, while other women experience severe abdominal and back pain around the time of their period. Untreated, endometriosis can cause adhesions on the intestines and urinary bladder, which can be extremely painful and must be removed surgically. Endometriosis is the most common cause of infertility, blocking the uterine tubes and therefore blocking the journey of the egg and scarring the ovaries and uterus.

THE UTERUS

The uterus is in the pelvic cavity, posterior and superior to the urinary bladder and anterior to the rectum. The major portion of the uterus is called the body. The rounded superior portion between the uterine tubes is the fundus, and the narrow inferior part is the isthmus. The **cervix** is a valve-like portion of the uterus that protrudes into the vagina while the cervical canal connects with the vagina. Like the ovaries, the uterus is suspended and anchored by a series of ligaments. The *mesometrium* attaches the uterus to the lateral pelvic walls. (The combination of the mesometrium and mesovarium is called the *broad ligament*.) The lateral cervical ligaments attach the cervix and vagina to the lateral pelvic walls. The uterus is anchored to the anterior wall of the pelvic cavity by the round ligaments.

cervix *(SER viks)*

Like most of the hollow organs or tubes we have visited, the walls of the uterus consist of three layers, the **perimetrium,** the outermost layer, is also the visceral peritoneum. (Just like the outermost layer of the heart is the visceral pericardium.) The **myometrium** consists of smooth muscle, and the **endometrium,** or inner lining, is a mucosa layer of columnar epithelium and secretory cells. The mucosa has two divisions. The **basal layer** is responsible for regenerating the uterine lining each month. The **functional layer** sheds about every 28 days when a woman has her period.

perimetrium *(pair ee MEE tree um)*

myometrium *(MY oh MEE tree um)*
endometrium *(EHN doh MEE tree um)*

The endometrium is highly vascular. (No big surprise to any woman of child-bearing age.) Blood is supplied by the uterine arteries that branch from the internal iliac arteries on each side. The uterine arteries split into arcuate arteries, which supply the myometrium, and radial arteries, which supply blood to the endometrium. As you might expect, since the endometrium has two separate divisions, there are two different types of radial arteries. Straight radial arteries supply the basal layer. Spiral radial arteries supply the functional layer. The spiral arteries actually decay and regenerate every month, as part of the menstrual cycle, and undergo spasms that contribute to the shedding of the endometrium each month. (For more on control of the menstrual cycle see the section "Hormonal Control" later in this chapter.) Blood returns to circulation via a network of venous sinuses.

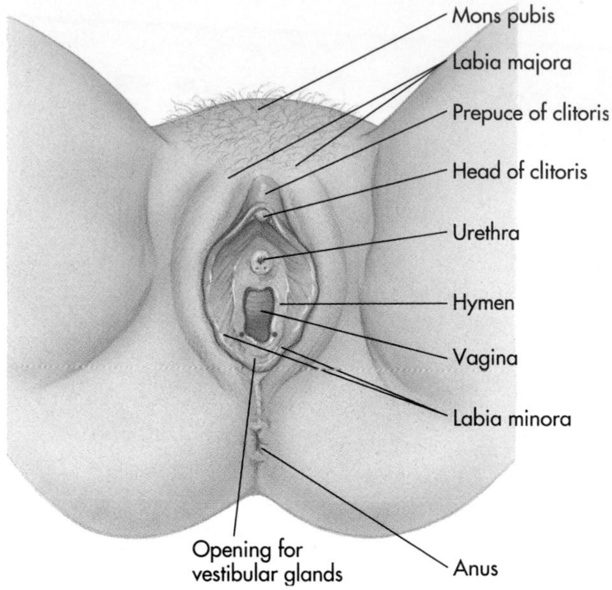

FIGURE ■ 17–4

The external female genitalia (vulva).

THE VAGINA

The vagina is a tube, approximately 10 centimeters long, which runs from the uterus to the outside of the body. Its purpose is to receive the penis during intercourse and to allow for the passage of menstrual fluid out of the uterus. The vagina is also known as the birth canal, since its primary function is to allow the movement of a baby out of the uterus during childbirth. The external opening of the vagina may be covered by a perforated membrane called the hymen. A torn hymen was once thought to "prove" that a woman had had intercourse. However, many hymens are highly perforated and easily ruptured by day-to-day activities such as riding a bicycle or jogging. An intact hymen is no longer considered a litmus test for virginity; however, some cultures still hold this erroneous belief to be true.

THE EXTERNAL GENITALIA

vulva *(VULL vah)*

labia majora *(LAY bee ah mah JOR ah)*

The external genitalia (Figure 17–4 ■), collectively known as the **vulva,** while not perhaps as obvious as the male external genitalia, are a complex and important part of reproduction. The vulva is surrounded on each side by two prominences called the **labia majora.** The labia majora are rounded fat deposits that meet and protect the rest of the external genitalia. The labia majora meet anteriorly to form the mons pubis. Both the mons pubis and the labia majora are covered by pubic hair.

pudendal cleft *(PEW den dall cleft)*

labia minora *(LAY bee ah mih NOR ah)*

prepuce *(PREE pewce)*

Between the two halves of the labia majora is an opening known as the **pudendal** cleft. Within the pudendal cleft lies the **vestibule,** a space into which the urethra (anterior) and vagina (posterior) empty. (Unlike the male reproductive system, the female urinary system is completely separate from the reproductive system.) The lateral border of the vestibule is formed by the thin **labia minora,** which meet anteriorly to form the **prepuce.** Several glands surround the vestibule, helping to keep it moist.

clitoris *(KLIT oh riss)*

Just posterior to the prepuce, and anterior to the vestibule, is the **clitoris.** The clitoris is a small erectile structure, 2 centimeters in diameter. Like the penis (see "Male Anatomy" in this chapter), the clitoris has a shaft, or body, and a glans (tip), and it becomes engorged with blood during sexual arousal. However, the clitoris increases in diameter, but not in length.

MAMMARY GLANDS

mammary glands *(MAM ah ree)*

There is another set of external accessory sexual organs in the female, far removed from the pubic area, the **mammary glands.** The mammary glands are milk production glands housed in the breasts (see Figure 17–5 ■). In young children, mammary tissue is virtually identical in boys and girls. At puberty, estrogen and progesterone stimulate breast development in girls. In adult females, the breasts consist of 15 to 20 lobes, which are glandular,

> 17-3 Please go to your CD-ROM to view a 3-D animation of the female reproductive system along with a drag-and-drop interactive labeling exercise.

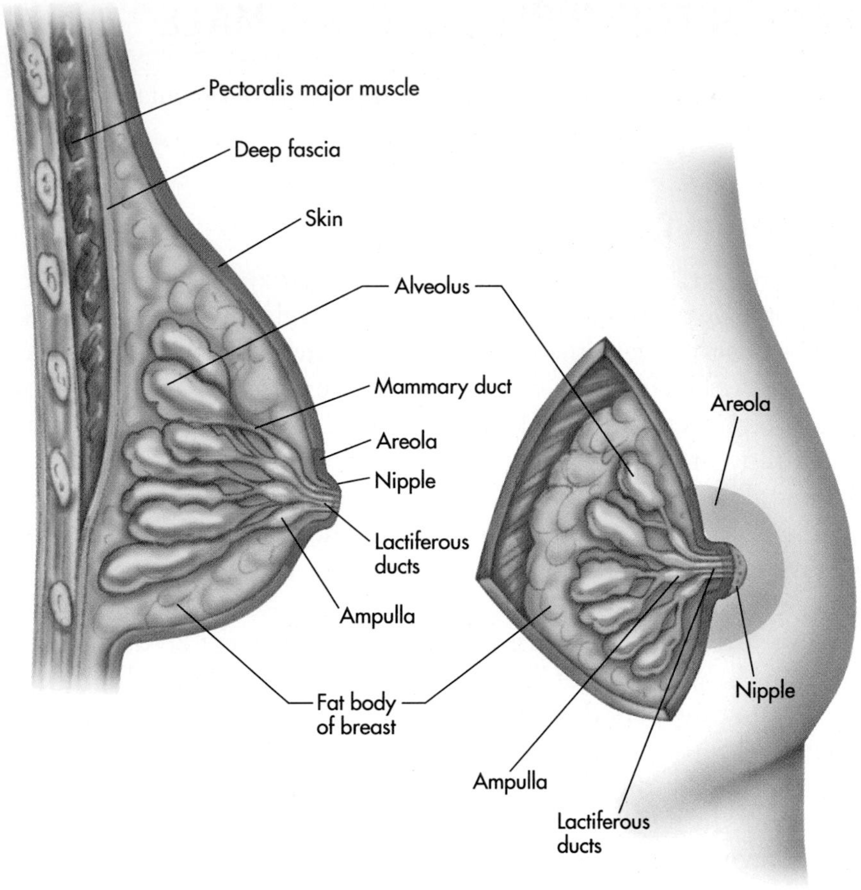

FIGURE ■ 17–5

The mammary glands.

and lots of adipose tissue. Each lobe is divided into smaller lobules, which house milk-secreting sacs called alveoli, when a woman is lactating (producing milk). Milk, made in the alveoli, travels through a series ducts and sinuses, eventually reaching the areola or nipple. Milk production is controlled by the hormone prolactin.

TEST YOUR KNOWLEDGE 17-2

Choose the best answer:

1. The _____ is also known as the birth canal.
   a. ovary
   b. uterus
   c. uterine tubes
   d. vagina
2. The inner lining of the uterus that is shed each month is the
   a. perimetrium
   b. endometrium
   c. myometrium
   d. all of the above
3. This part of the female reproductive system is erectile.
   a. ovary
   b. labia majora
   c. clitoris
   d. penis

REPRODUCTIVE PHYSIOLOGY: FEMALE

The female reproductive physiology is closely tied to a regulated cycle. This cycle is normally regulated by hormonal control.

The Menstrual Cycle

menstrual cycle *(MEN stroo al)*
ovarian cycle *(oh VAIR ee an)*
uterine cycle *(YOO ter in)*

Female reproduction is organized around an approximately 28-day cycle involving both the ovaries and the uterus, collectively known as the **menstrual cycle.** The **ovarian cycle** involves the monthly maturation and release of eggs from the ovary. The **uterine cycle** consists of the monthly build-up, decay, and shedding of the uterine lining. The cycles begin during a woman's teen years at the beginning of puberty and end during her 40s or 50s, with the end of menopause. The ultimate goal of the cycle is to release an egg that might be fertilized and to prepare the uterus to receive and nourish the fertilized egg should pregnancy result. If pregnancy does not occur, the uterine lining sheds and the cycle begins again.

menses *(MEN seez)*

menstruation *(MEN stroo AY shun)*

The menstrual cycle, occurring approximately every 28 days in sexually mature women who are not pregnant, begins with the first day of **menses.** Menses is the time period when the uterine lining is shed. You are probably more familiar with the term **menstruation.** Menstruation is the actual shedding of the endometrium, while menses is the time during which a woman is menstruating. In more common terms, menses is the time during which a woman is having her "period," and menstruation is the "period" itself. Menses typically lasts 4 to 5 days but can be longer or shorter in different women and can even vary month to month in the same woman.

ovulation *(OV yoo LAY shun)*

oocyte *(OH oh site)*

follicular *(fa lik YOU ler)*
proliferative *(pro LIFF er ah TIV)*

luteal *(LOO tee al)*

Once menses is over, the endometrium begins to proliferate, or build up, readying itself for the egg that is about to be released from the ovary, during **ovulation.** From day 1 to day 14, the ovary is also busy. In the ovary, an egg cell, or **oocyte,** is undergoing a number of developmental changes getting ready for ovulation on day 14. Ovulation is the release of a mature egg from the ovary. The egg travels from the ovary to the uterus, which has been getting ready to receive the egg. If the oocyte has been fertilized by a sperm, it will implant in the thickened endometrium. If the egg does not implant within a few days, the endometrium will begin to decay and menstruation will occur about two weeks after ovulation. The time between the end of menses and ovulation is known as the **follicular** or **proliferative phase,** because the endometrium is proliferating and the follicles are maturing in the ovary. Follicle is the term used to refer to an egg and associated helper cells. The time between ovulation and menses is known as the **luteal phase** or **secretory phase,** because of the development of a structure called the *corpus luteum* in the ovary and the beginning of secretion in the uterus.

Sounds simple enough, right? The cycle is deceptively simple when described without details or information about control of the cycle. Now that you understand the cycle itself, let's get down to the nitty gritty. Just how does an egg mature, and how is the cycle controlled?

OOGENESIS, FOLLICLE DEVELOPMENT, AND OVULATION

The process by which eggs are produced is called **oogenesis.** Oogenesis begins with the birth of **oogonia,** or egg stem cells, in the ovary. The oogonia undergo mitosis, producing millions of **primary oocytes.** This happens very early in a woman's life. There are millions of primary oocytes produced in a fetus. That's right: women have all the eggs they will ever have five months before they are born!

oogenesis *(oh oh JENN eh siss)*

oocyte *(OH oh site)*

Primary oocytes, since they are born via mitosis, still have all 46 chromosomes. In order to become gametes, they must undergo meiosis to cut their chromosome number to 23. Remember, gametes must have only 23 chromosomes in order for fertilization (successful combining of sperm and egg) to produce a cell with the normal number or 46 chromosomes. So, primary oocytes begin meiosis. However, they do not fully complete their development. The primary oocytes stay in a kind of suspended animation until puberty when they finish developing! (That's at least 10 years!)

These primary oocytes eventually are surrounded by helper cells, called *granulosa cells*. Once surrounded by granulosa cells, the primary oocyte and surrounding cells are known as **primordial follicles.** These primordial follicles stay dormant until puberty. Hormonal signals during puberty cause some primordial follicles to enlarge and increase the number of granulosa cells. These enlarged cells are then called **primary follicles** (see Figure 17–6 ■).

primordial *(pry MORE dee all)*

Once a girl reaches puberty, one primary follicle will become a **secondary follicle.** The secondary follicle will not complete its development unless it is ovulated and fertilized. Just before ovulation, the secondary follicle fills with fluid and moves toward the surface of the ovary, where it becomes a visible lump. The

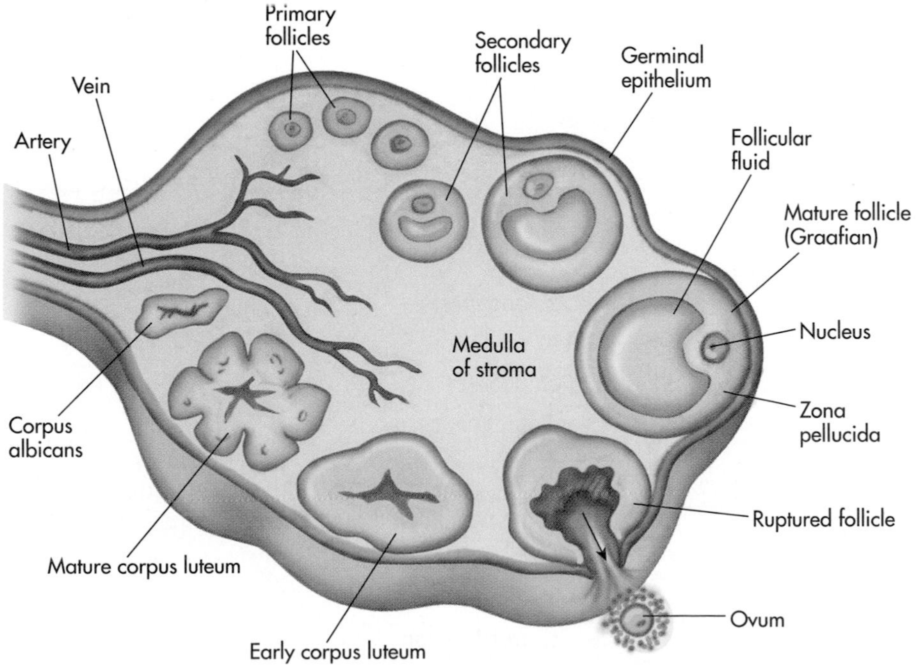

FIGURE ■ 17–6

Maturation of follicle.

fimbria of the uterine tubes brush the surface of the ovary, causing the follicle to rupture. When the follicle ruptures, the egg (now an oocyte) is released into the peritoneal cavity. The fimbria then pulls the egg toward the funnel, drawing it into the uterine tube.

zygote *(ZIGH goht)*

corpus luteum *(KOR pus LOU tee um)*

As the egg travels down the uterine tube (also called the oviduct or fallopian tube), it either will or will not be fertilized. If sperm are present in the uterine tube and all the conditions are right, the sperm will penetrate the egg, fertilizing it and triggering the rest of the egg development. The successfully fertilized egg has 46 chromosomes and is now called a **zygote.** When the zygote enters the uterus, the newly proliferated endometrium is ready for it. If the zygote successfully implants in the uterus, pregnancy will result and the woman will not menstruate. The ruptured follicle left behind in the ovary during ovulation will become the **corpus luteum** (remember the luteal phase?) and secrete hormones to help maintain the thickened endometrium, which will serve to nourish the growing fetus.

If there is no sperm in the uterine tube, conditions are not right, or something goes wrong after fertilization, the zygote will not implant in the uterus. If there is no implantation within a few days, the uterine lining will begin to degenerate and the woman will have her period. The corpus luteum will become a corpus albicans and eventually disappear (see Figure 17–7 ■).

17-4 Please go to your CD-ROM to view an animation on oogenesis and fertilization and for an interactive drag-and-drop labeling exercise on oogenesis.

TEST YOUR KNOWLEDGE 17-3

Choose the best answer:

1. The time from the end of menses to ovulation is what phase?
   a. luteal phase
   b. follicular phase
   c. mitotic phase
   d. ovarian phase

2. The union of an egg and a sperm is called
   a. sex
   b. fertilization
   c. oogenesis
   d. ovulation

3. The act of the egg being expelled from the ovary is called
   a. oogenesis
   b. ovulation
   c. puberty
   d. pregnancy

4. If _____ does not occur, the endometrium will decay and a woman will menstruate.
   a. sex
   b. ovulation
   c. fertilization
   d. oogenesis

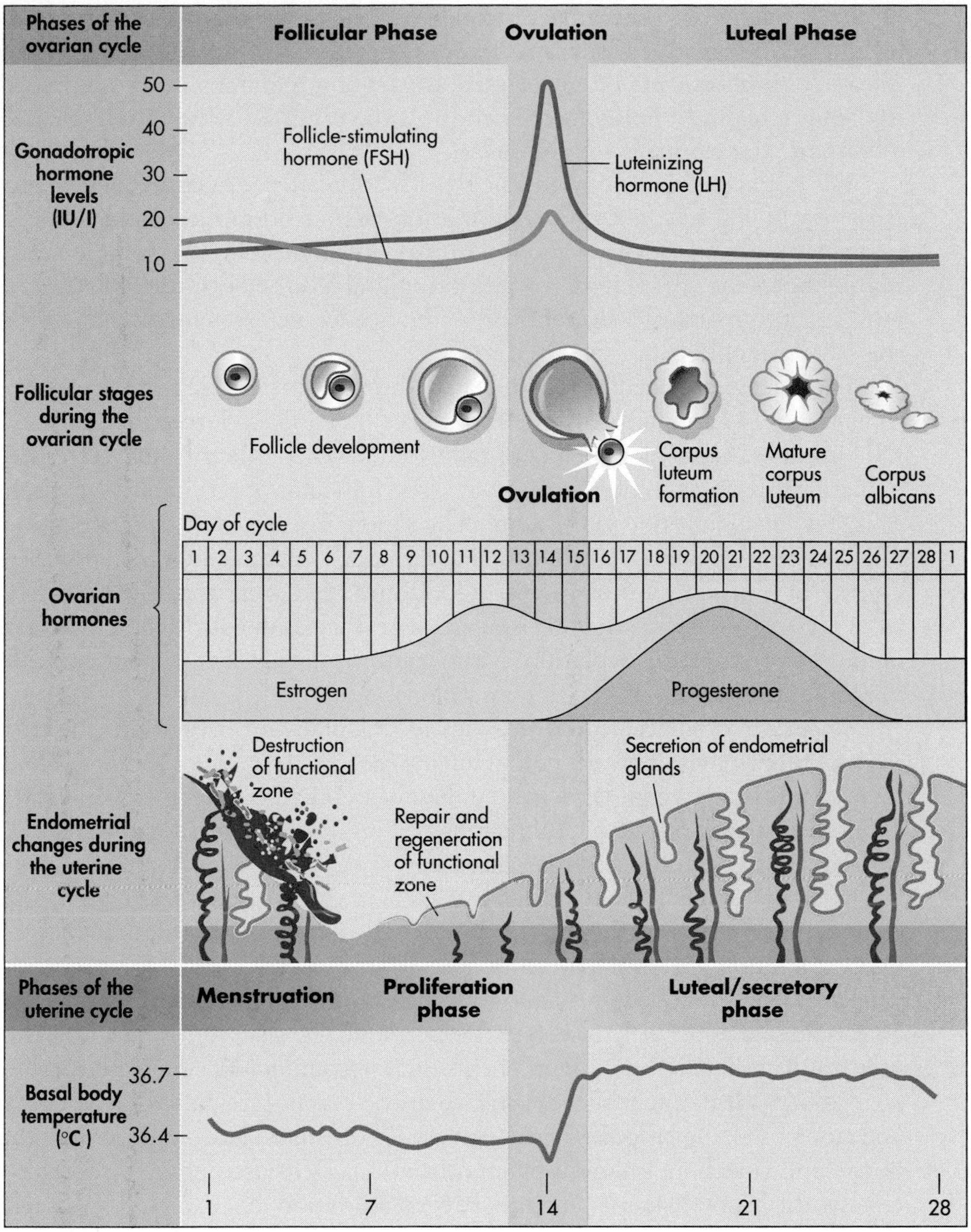

FIGURE ■ 17–7

The menstrual cycle.

HORMONAL CONTROL

It seems obvious that something must control the complex cyclic changes in the female reproductive system. The control system that keeps the uterus and ovaries in synch is the endocrine system, specifically hypothalamic, pituitary, and ovarian hormones.

Remember that hormones are chemical signals released by one organ into the bloodstream to control another organ or tissue some distance away.

progesterone *(proh JESS ter ohn)*
luteinizing hormone *(LOO tee ah NIZE ing)*
follicle-stimulating hormone *(FALL ih kle stim you LAY ting HOR mohn)*
gonadotropin-releasing hormone *(GO nad oh TROH pin)*

Hormone levels are generally controlled by negative feedback. As hormone levels rise, the organ releasing the hormone decreases the amount of hormone released. Hormones are often released as part of a hierarchy, with the hypothalamus releasing a hormone that controls the pituitary, which then releases a hormone that controls another organ.

The hormones controlling female reproduction are no exception. The menstrual cycle is controlled by a combination of four hormones: **estrogen** and **progesterone** from the ovary and **luteinizing hormone** (LH) and **follicle-stimulating hormone** (FSH) from the pituitary gland. At the beginning of puberty, estrogen and progesterone secretion from the ovaries increases greatly, increasing the secretion of LH and FSH.

The release of **gonadotropin-releasing hormone** (GnRH) from the hypothalamus causes an increase in the secretion of LH and FSH from the pituitary. FSH initiates the development of primary follicles each month, and LH triggers ovulation. During this part of the cycle (the follicular or proliferative phase), estrogen levels continue to rise as more and more is secreted by the developing follicle. Estrogen exerts a positive influence on the hypothalamus, increasing secretion of GnRH and thus increasing LH and FSH secretion. This positive feedback loop increases the levels of LH and FSH, stimulating follicle development and triggering ovulation. Rising estrogen levels also stimulate proliferation of the uterine lining (endometrium).

Once ovulation occurs, the feedback loop actually reverses itself! The leftover ruptured follicle, now the corpus luteum, begins to secrete progesterone and secretes a little estrogen. Under the influence of progesterone, estrogen exerts negative feedback on the hypothalamus and pituitary, decreasing GnRH, LH, and FSH secretion. Progesterone also exerts negative feedback on the hypothalamus and pituitary. Thus, during the luteal or secretory phase, LH, FSH, and estrogen levels drop while progesterone levels rise. These hormonal changes prevent another egg from maturing.

For about 10 days after ovulation, progesterone levels remain high as the corpus luteum continues to secrete the hormone. Progesterone's effect on the uterus is to *maintain* the buildup of the endometrium and to decrease uterine contractions. If no pregnancy results, then the corpus luteum will degenerate and stop producing progesterone. Decreased progesterone causes degeneration of the endometrium, followed by menstruation. Decreased progesterone also releases the hypothalamus and pituitary from inhibition. FSH and LH levels rise and the cycle begins again (again see Figure 17–7).

human chorionic gonadotropin *(HUE man core ee AH nik GO nad oh TROH pin)*

If pregnancy does result, the implanted fertilized egg secretes a hormone called **human chorionic gonadotropin** (HCG). HCG stimulates the corpus luteum, which keeps secreting progesterone and a little estrogen to maintain the uterine lining. At about three months gestation (pregnancy), the placenta begins to secrete its own progesterone and estrogen, thereby becoming an endocrine organ. For a list of hormones and functions related to pregnancy, please see Table 17–1.

TABLE 17–1 Hormones Controlling Pregnancy

HORMONE	WHERE SECRETED	CAUSES
human chorionic gonadotropin	implanted fertilized egg	maintains the function of corpus luteum; this is what gives a positive pregnancy test
estrogen and progesterone	corpus luteum for first two months of pregnancy; then by the placenta	both stimulate development of uterine lining and mammary glands; progesterone prohibits uterine contractions during pregnancy; estrogen relaxes the pelvic joints; once labor begins, estrogen negates the effects of progesterone on uterine contractions and makes the myometrium sensitive to oxytocin
prolactin	anterior pituitary gland	stimulates milk production by breasts
oxytocin	posterior pituitary gland	uterine contractions to begin labor; stimulates the release of milk from the breasts (see Figure 17–8 ■)

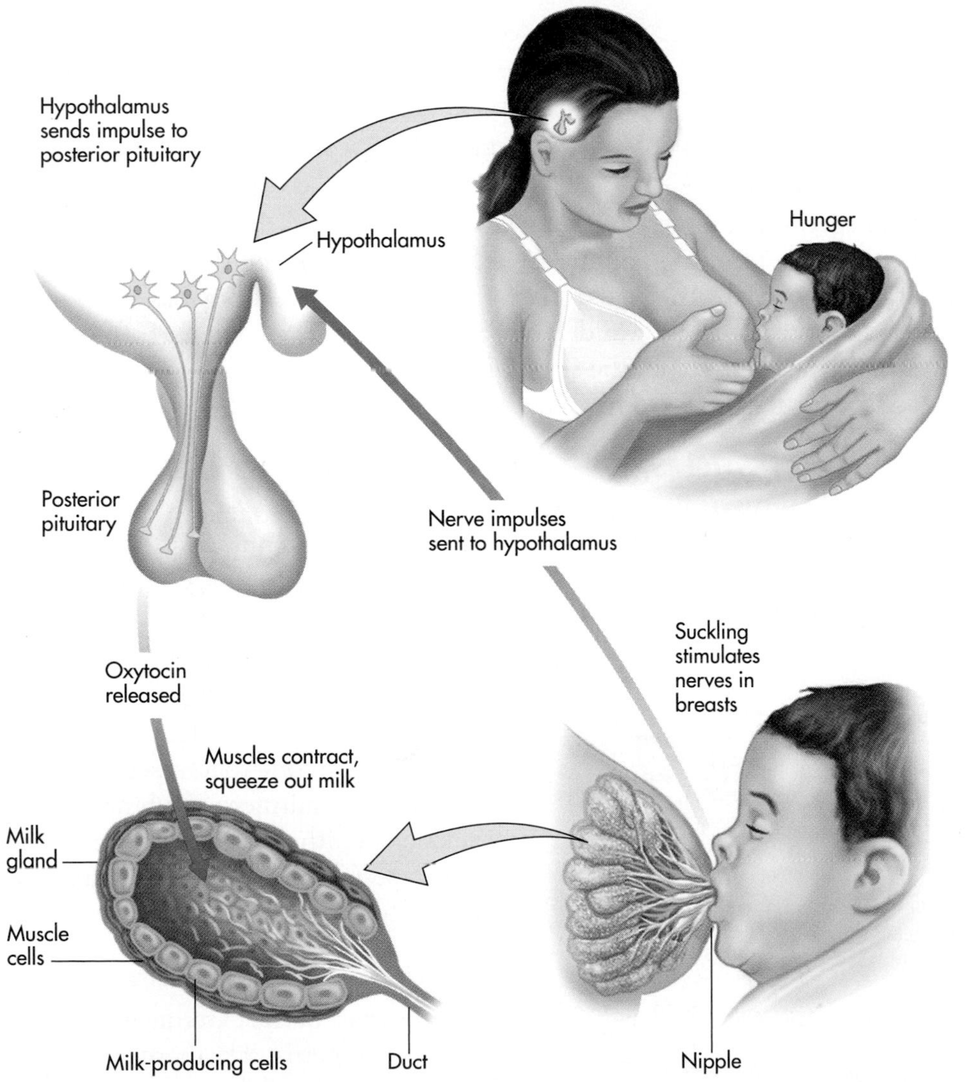

FIGURE ■ 17–8

Oxytocin and breast feeding.

TEST YOUR KNOWLEDGE 17-4

Choose the best answer:

1. At puberty, the ovaries begin to secrete
   a. FSH
   b. LH
   c. estrogen
   d. all of the above

2. These hormones stimulate follicle maturation and ovulation:
   a. estrogen and progesterone
   b. estrogen and GnRH
   c. LH and FSH
   d. FSH and progesterone

3. Before ovulation, estrogen _____ the secretion of FSH and LH.
   a. decreases
   b. increases
   c. not enough information
   d. there is no relationship between estrogen, FSH, and LH

4. The role of progesterone is
   a. to promote ovulation
   b. to keep the endometrium from shedding
   c. to enhance fertilization
   d. to increase FSH and LH levels

Male Anatomy

epididymis *(ep ih DID ih miss)*
vas deferens *(VAS DEFF er enz)*
urethra *(yoo REE thrah)*
seminal vesicles *(SEM ih nal VESS ih klz)*
bulbourethral gland *(BUHL boh yoo REE thral)*

Like the female reproductive system, the male reproductive system has a pair of primary genitalia, or gonads, called the *testes*. The testes produce the male gamete or sperm that must travel along its journey to find the egg. Unlike the female, the male primary genitalia are external. In addition, the male has many secondary genitalia—the **penis,** an external sperm-delivery organ; several sperm ducts; the **epididymis;** the **vas deferens;** and the **urethra**—and several accessory glands, the **prostate gland,** the **seminal vesicles,** and the **bulbourethral glands.** Please see Figure 17–9 ■ for the anatomy of the male reproductive system.

THE TESTES (TESTICLES)

seminiferous tubules *(SEM ih NIF er uss TOO byoolz)*
sertoli cells *(sir TOW lee sells)*

The primary genitalia, the testes (or testicles), are paired glands suspended in a sac called the **scrotum.** The testicles are external genitalia, one hanging on either side of the penis. (Viable sperm cannot be made at normal human body temperature.) Each testis is surrounded by a serous membrane, called the tunica vaginalis, which originates from the peritoneum. The inside of the testes are divided into 250 to 300 wedges called lobules, each of which contain one to four **seminiferous tubules.** The seminiferous tubules, which are made of epithelium and areolar tissue, contain sperm stem cells and sperm helper cells (**sertoli cells** or nurse cells).

Amazing Body Facts

BOXERS OR BRIEFS?

Normal human body temperature is too warm for healthy sperm development. The testes are on the outside of the body because sperm development is extremely temperature sensitive and sperm could not develop normally inside the pelvic cavity. Indeed, there is some speculation that very tight clothing might contribute to male infertility by holding the gonads too close to the body and raising their temperature. In addition, there is a testes–blood barrier to prevent the immune system from destroying sperm, which the white blood cells would recognize as invaders.

THE PENIS

The other part of the external genitalia in males is the penis. The penis, from the Latin word for "tail," is a sperm-delivery organ that transfers sperm from male to female. The attached portion of the penis

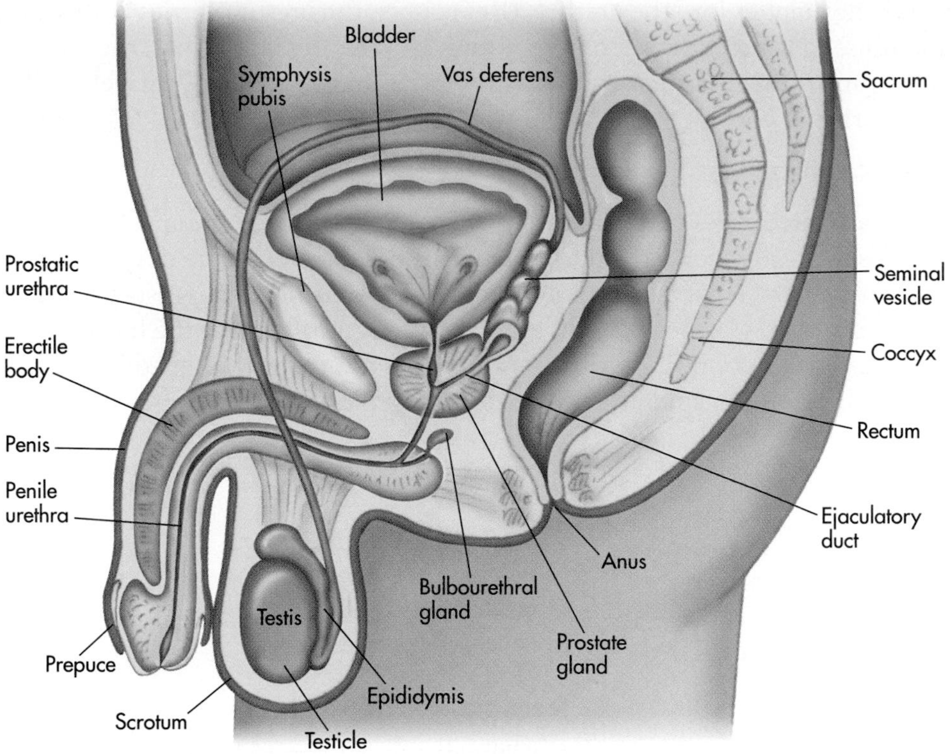

FIGURE ■ 17–9

Male reproductive anatomy.

is called the root, while the freely moving portion is the shaft or body. The tip of the penis, the glans penis, is covered by a loose section of skin called the foreskin, unless a man has been circumcised. Internally, the penis contains the urethra, which is a transport passage for both sperm and urine. (But not at the same time!) In addition, the penis has three erectile bodies, tubes with a spongelike network of blood sinuses.

THE EPIDIDYMIS

There are several ducts in the male reproductive system. The epididymus is a comma-shaped duct on the posterior and lateral part of the testes. (It looks something like a stocking cap for each gonad.) The tube is highly coiled. If unraveled, it would be 6 meters long! It is made of pseudostratified ciliated epithelium and smooth muscle. Sperm mature here.

THE VAS DEFERENS

The vas deferens is a short tube, only 45 centimeters long. It is lined with ciliated pseudostratified epithelium, like the epididymus, but has a thick smooth muscle layer and is surrounded by a connective tissue layer called the *adventitia*. The vas deferens runs from the scrotum to the penis via a relatively complicated pathway. The vas deferens runs from the anterior part of the scrotum as a pair of tubes, one on each side, into the abdominal wall (through the inguinal canal) and pelvic cavity, medially over the urethra and along the posterior bladder wall. Posterior to the bladder, the vas deferens joins the seminal vesicle to form the **ejaculatory duct.** The ejaculatory duct then passes through the prostate gland and empties into the urethra. (Remember, the urethra carries both sperm and urine in males.) Between the scrotum and the inguinal canal, the vas deferens runs through a tube, with blood vessels and nerves, collectively called the **spermatic cord.**

ACCESSORY GLANDS

There are three accessory glands in the male reproductive system. The seminal vesicles are highly coiled glands posterior to the bladder, made of pseudostratified epithelium, smooth muscle, and connective tissue. The prostate gland is a chestnut-sized gland surrounding the urethra just inferior to the bladder. It is a dense mass of connective tissue and smooth muscle with embedded glands. The bulbourethral glands are pea-sized glands inferior to the prostate.

TEST YOUR KNOWLEDGE 17-5

Choose the best answer:

1. The _____ are the gonads, where sperm are made.
   a. vas deferens
   b. testes
   c. scrotum
   d. penis
2. After passing the seminal vesicles, the vas deferens becomes the
   a. prostate gland
   b. urethra
   c. penis
   d. none of the above
3. Sperm mature in the
   a. epidiymis
   b. testes
   c. scrotum
   d. penis

17-5 Please go to your CD-ROM to view a 3-D animation of the male reproductive system along with a drag-and-drop labeling exercise.

REPRODUCTIVE PHYSIOLOGY: MALE

Unlike female reproduction, male reproductive physiology is not organized around a tightly controlled monthly cycle. Let's explore the physiologic processes of the male reproductive system.

Spermatogenesis

Sperm production, in the testes, is a continuous process beginning when a boy reaches puberty and usually continuing until death. As such, the control of spermatogenesis, sperm production, is much less complicated than control of oogenesis.

spermatogonia *(sper MAT oh GO nee ah)*
spermatocytes *(sper MAT oh sites)*
spermatids *(sper MAT ids)*
spermatozoa *(sper MAT oh ZOE ah)*

The **spermatogonia,** sperm stem cells, undergo mitosis to form **primary spermatocytes.** Unlike primary oocytes, the primary spermatocytes do not wait to go through meiosis. Primary spermatocytes form two **secondary spermatocytes.** Secondary spermatocytes complete meiosis to form **spermatids,** and spermatids go through a period of development to form immature **spermatozoa** (**sperm**). All of this takes place in the testes inside the seminiferous tubules. The distribution of the different stages of sperm development is predictable. Spermatogonia line up against the walls of the tubules, and mature sperm cluster near the lumen of the tubules (see Figure 17–10 ■). Sperm then travel from the seminiferous tubules to the epididymis, where the sperm spend about two weeks maturing and gaining the ability to swim.

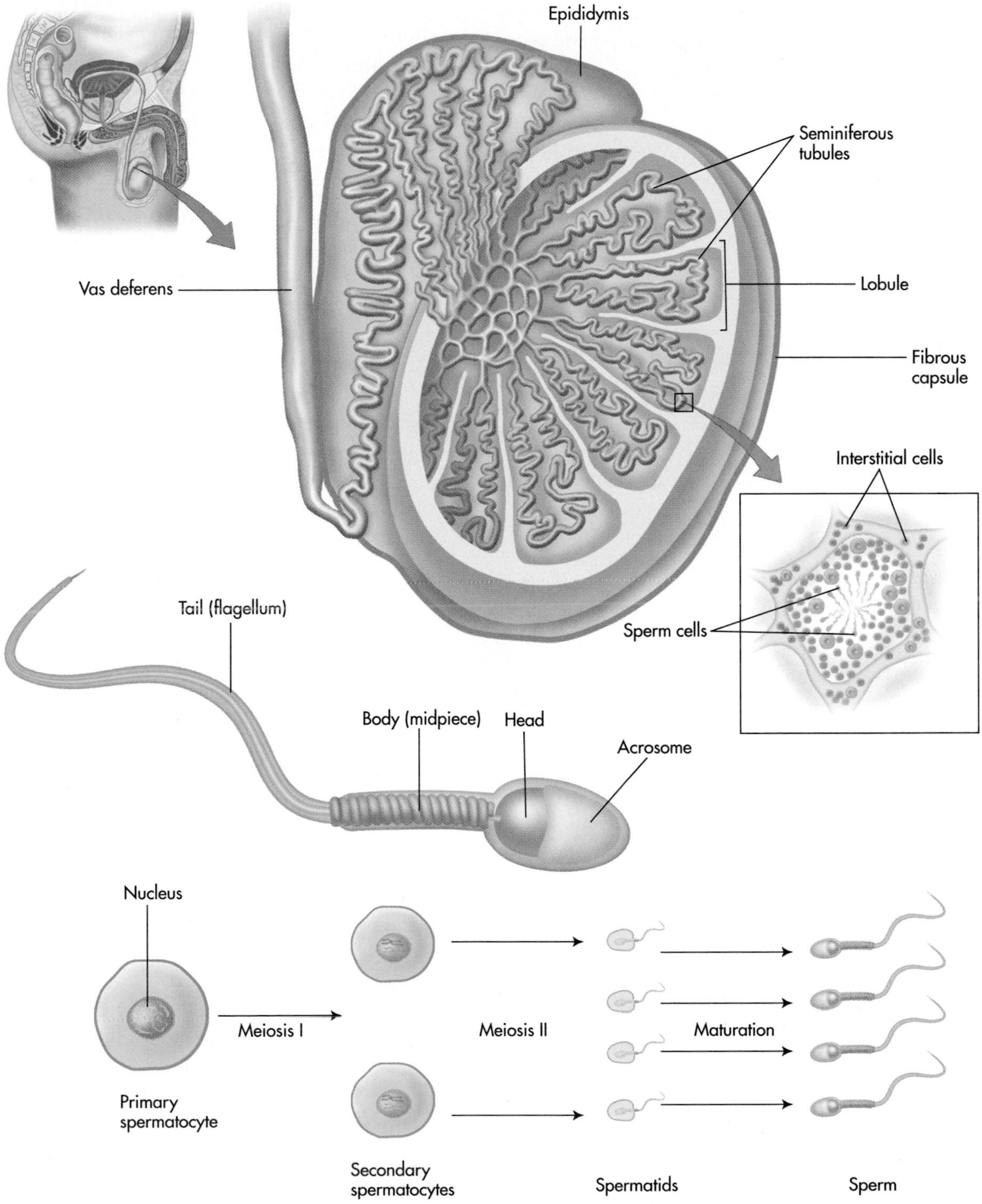

FIGURE ■ 17–10

Spermatogenesis.

HORMONAL CONTROL OF MALE REPRODUCTION

testosterone *(tess TOSS ter ohn)*

Testosterone is arguably the most important male sex hormone. Before birth, HCG secreted by the placenta causes the embryonic (still developing) testes to secrete testosterone, masculinizing the fetus. (Fetuses not exposed to testosterone or insensitive to testosterone look female.) After birth, there is little testosterone secreted until puberty. At puberty, two hormonal changes occur that signal the beginning of sexual maturity. First, testosterone secretion by the testes increases dramatically. Second, there is a change in the relationship between testosterone and GnRH, LH, and FSH. (Yes, the same hormones that control female reproduction control male reproduction!) Before puberty, the small amount of testosterone that is secreted by the testes inhibits GnRH secretion. After puberty, testosterone does not inhibit GnRH secretion. So after puberty, GnRH and therefore FSH and LH secretion increase. In addition, FSH and LH also enhance testosterone secretion in a major positive feedback loop, but only after the onset of puberty. Testosterone secretion at puberty is also responsible for the obvious physical changes of the male secondary sexual characteristics, including body, facial, and pubic hair growth; deepening of the voice; and increased muscle and bone mass.

> 17-6 Please go to your CD-ROM to view an animation on spermatogenesis and an interactive drag-and-drop labeling exercise on spermatogenesis.

> *Clinical Application*
>
> **ANDROGEN INSENSITIVITY SYNDROME**
>
> Testosterone secretion *in utero* is important for masculinizing a male fetus. Males who are not sensitive to testosterone will not respond to the masculinizing effects and will not develop normal male reproductive systems. Androgen insensitivity is a genetic disorder that can result in a broad range of malfunctions of the male reproductive system, from complete lack of external or internal male genitalia (testicular feminization—individuals look female though they are genetically male) to patients with ambiguous genitalia to patients who have typical male genitalia but are sterile. Treatment for the disorder depends of the severity of the genital malformation.

LH and FSH affect males exactly as they do females. They stimulate gamete development. They are controlled in the same way in males as in females. GnRH is released from the hypothalamus, which stimulates LH and FSH secretion from the pituitary.

ERECTION AND EJACULATION

When a man is sexually aroused, the erectile bodies in the penis (remember the spongelike tissue with blood spaces?) become engorged with blood, stiffening and expanding the penis. The change in shape of the penis is called **erection.**

semen *(SEE men)*

In order for sperm to leave the male reproductive system, ejaculation must occur. **Ejaculation** is the expulsion of **semen** (sperm and assorted chemicals) from the urethra. Smooth muscle contracts throughout the ducts and glands of the male reproductive system and propels the sperm from the epididymis into the vas deferens, which then carries the sperm into the pelvic cavity. As the sperm passes the seminal vesicles, sugar and chemicals are added to the sperm. The sperm and chemicals then enter the ejaculatory duct. As the ejaculatory duct passes through the prostate gland, prostatic fluid is added, liquefying the semen and protecting sperm from the acid environment of the vagina by the secretion of an alkaline substance. The semen then passes by the bulbourethral glands, which add mucus to the semen. The semen then enters the urethra and is carried outside of the body.

If a man is engaged in sexual intercourse with a woman and ejaculates, the sperm enter the vagina and make their way to the uterus and into the uterine tubes. The female reproductive system is not particularly hospitable to sperm, and many sperm do not survive the journey to the uterine tubes. If there is an egg waiting to be fertilized in the uterine tubes, sperm will find the egg and attempt to penetrate it and fertilize it. New research suggests that the egg is not a passive participant in fertilization, but may actually engulf the sperm and even choose which sperm to allow inside. One sperm and only one sperm will fertilize the egg. If the egg is fertilized, and all other conditions are met, a pregnancy will result.

Amazing Body Facts

HORMONES

Did you know that females have some natural testosterone and males have natural estrogen? It's true. The balance between the hormones—not the presence or absence of the hormones—is what is important.

TEST YOUR KNOWLEDGE 17-6

Choose the best answer:

1. The stiffening and expanding of the penis is known as
   a. ejaculation
   b. erection
   c. emulsification
   d. erectile dysfunction

2. The combination of sperm, sugars, chemicals, and mucus is
   a. semen
   b. urine
   c. spermatozoa
   d. all of the above

3. Male secondary sexual characteristics, masculinization of the body, and enhancement of FSH and LH levels are cause by
   a. LH
   b. FSH
   c. estrogen
   d. testosterone

PREGNANCY

Pregnancy occurs when an egg is fertilized by the sperm and implants in the female reproductive system. The period of time during which the developing baby grows within the uterus is called the gestational period, approximately 40 weeks. A baby born before 37 weeks gestational period is termed a premature infant.

From the time the egg is fertilized by a sperm and implants in the uterine wall until the eighth week, the developing infant is referred to as an embryo. During the embryonic period, the organs and systems are fundamentally formed. Beyond the eight-week period until the birth, the developing infant is called a fetus.

Doulas and midwives assist the mother through the labor and delivery process. To learn more about these professionals, visit the website for this chapter.

The growing fetus is nourished by a spongy structure called the placenta, which is attached to the fetus and the mother via the umbilical cord. The fetus is encased in

Clinical Application

CONTRACEPTION

The prevention of pregnancy is termed contraception ("against conception") and can be accomplished by a number of means such as an intrauterine devices (IUDs), spermicidal agents, birth control pills, or shields such as a condom.

Sterilization of the male can be accomplished through a vasectomy. The vas deferens are the tubes that carry the sperm into the urethra, and tying off these tubes prevents the sperm from traveling out of the penis during sexual intercourse. Females may be sterilized via tubal ligation. The fallopian tubes are cut or tied shut, preventing the egg from traveling from the ovary to the uterus.

a membranous sac called the *amnion*, which contains the amniotic fluid in which the fetus floats. Labor is the actual process whereby the fetus is delivered from the uterus through the vagina and into the outside world.

Labor consists of three stages. In the dilation stage, the uterine smooth muscle begins to contract, thereby moving the fetus down the uterus and causing the cervix to begin to dilate. When the cervix is completely dilated (10 centimeters), the second stage (expulsion) begins during

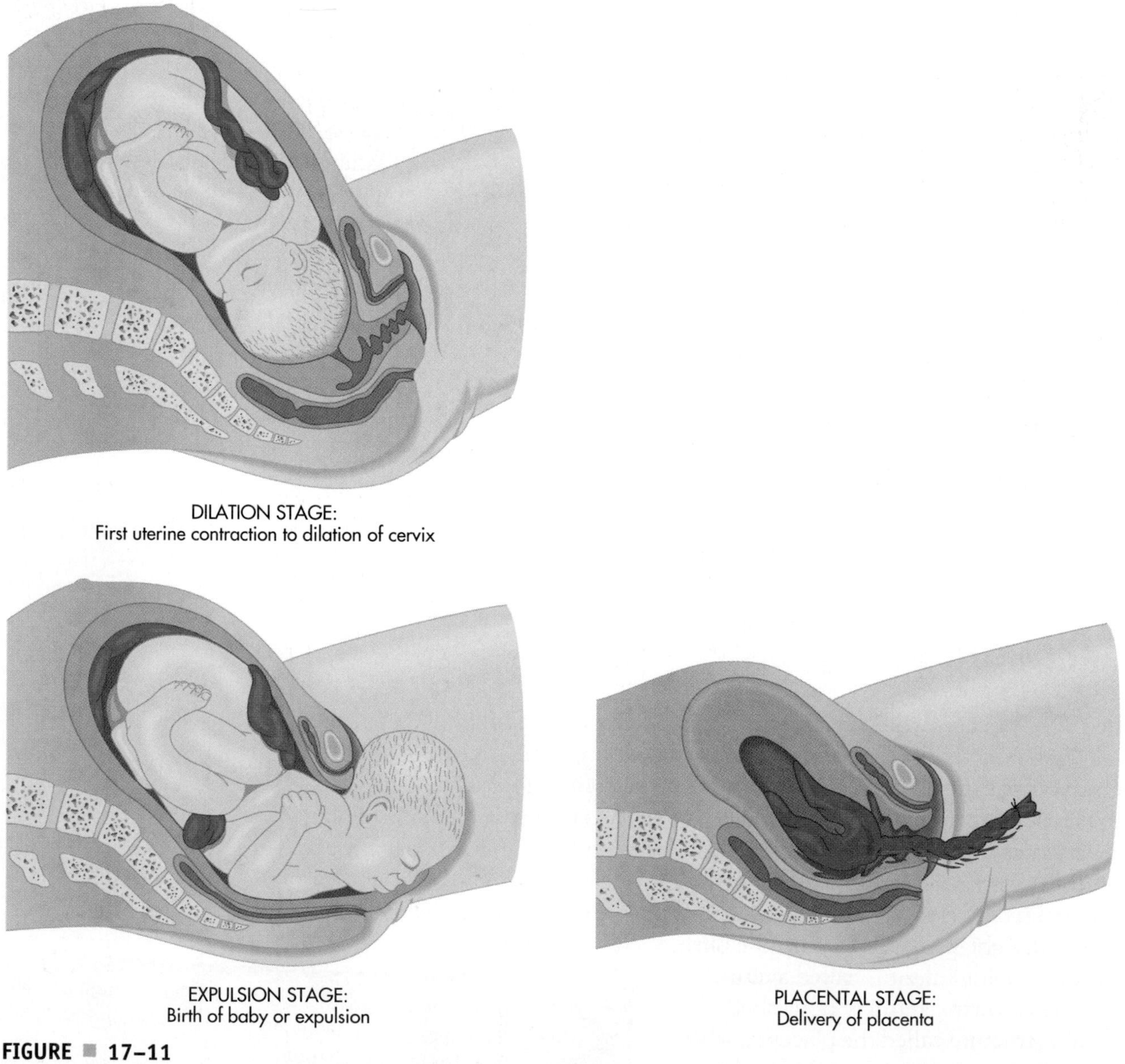

FIGURE ■ 17–11

Stages of labor.

which the baby is actually delivered. Generally, the head presents first, which is called crowning, and this is when the baby's mouth should be suctioned before the baby takes its first breath to prevent aspiration of fluid into the baby's lung. Sometimes, the baby is turned around and the buttocks appear first in a breech presentation, which makes the delivery difficult. The last stage of labor is the placental stage in which the placenta or afterbirth is delivered due to final uterine contractions (see Figure 17–11 ■).

17-7 For videos on the vasectomy procedure, fetal lie, labor, infant delivery, the placenta, and postpartum assessment, please go to your CD-ROM for this chapter.

COMMON DISORDERS OF THE REPRODUCTIVE SYSTEM

Both male and female reproductive systems are susceptible to many disorders. Common to both systems are sexually transmitted diseases (STDs). However, each system has its own specific disorders tied to anatomical and physiologic differences of the sexes.

Diseases of the Female Reproductive System

The first menstrual period is referred to as *menarche*, and *menopause* represents the ending of menstrual activity, both of which are normal cycles in the female reproductive system. However, this normal cycle can be disrupted. **Amenorrhea** is the absence of menstruation and can be a result of pregnancy, menopause, or other factors such as emotional distress, extreme dieting, or poor health. **Dysmenorrhea** is difficult menstruation usually resulting in painful cramping.

amenorrhea *(ah MEN oh REE ah)*
a = *absence*
dysmenorrhea *(DISS men oh REE ah)*
dys = *difficult*

Premenstrual syndrome (PMS) occurs several days prior to the onset of menstruation. This is characterized by effects on many systems of the body, including the emotional realm. These symptoms vary among individuals and usually subside near the onset on menstruation. For a list of the multisystem effects, please see Figure 17–12 ■.

Like any system, the reproductive system can become infected. **Vaginitis** is the inflammation of the vagina that is usually caused by a microorganism such as bacteria or yeast. Vaginitis is often not a result of sexually transmitted diseases. Sexually transmitted diseases represent a large number of infections found in both male and female reproductive systems and can be bacterial, viral, or fungal.

vaginitis *(vaj ih NYE tiss)*

The cervix is the area where a Pap smear (named after George Papanicolaoua) is taken that examines scrapings from the cervical cells to detect the presence of cancer. Regular Pap smears allow for early detection, which increases the likelihood of successful treatment.

In some cases of pregnancy, the fertilized egg implants in the fallopian tubes and does not make the full trip down to the uterus. This is an **ectopic** or **tubal pregnancy,** which requires surgical intervention. **Abruptio placentia** is an emergency situation in which the placenta tears away from the uterine wall before the 20th week of pregnancy.

ectopic pregnancy *(ek TOP ik PREG nan see)*
abruptio placentia *(ah BRUP tee oh plah SEN shah)*

Postpartum depression is a serious psychological state that can occur after childbirth, and mothers should be monitored for signs and symptoms because it can lead to harm to the mother or baby or both.

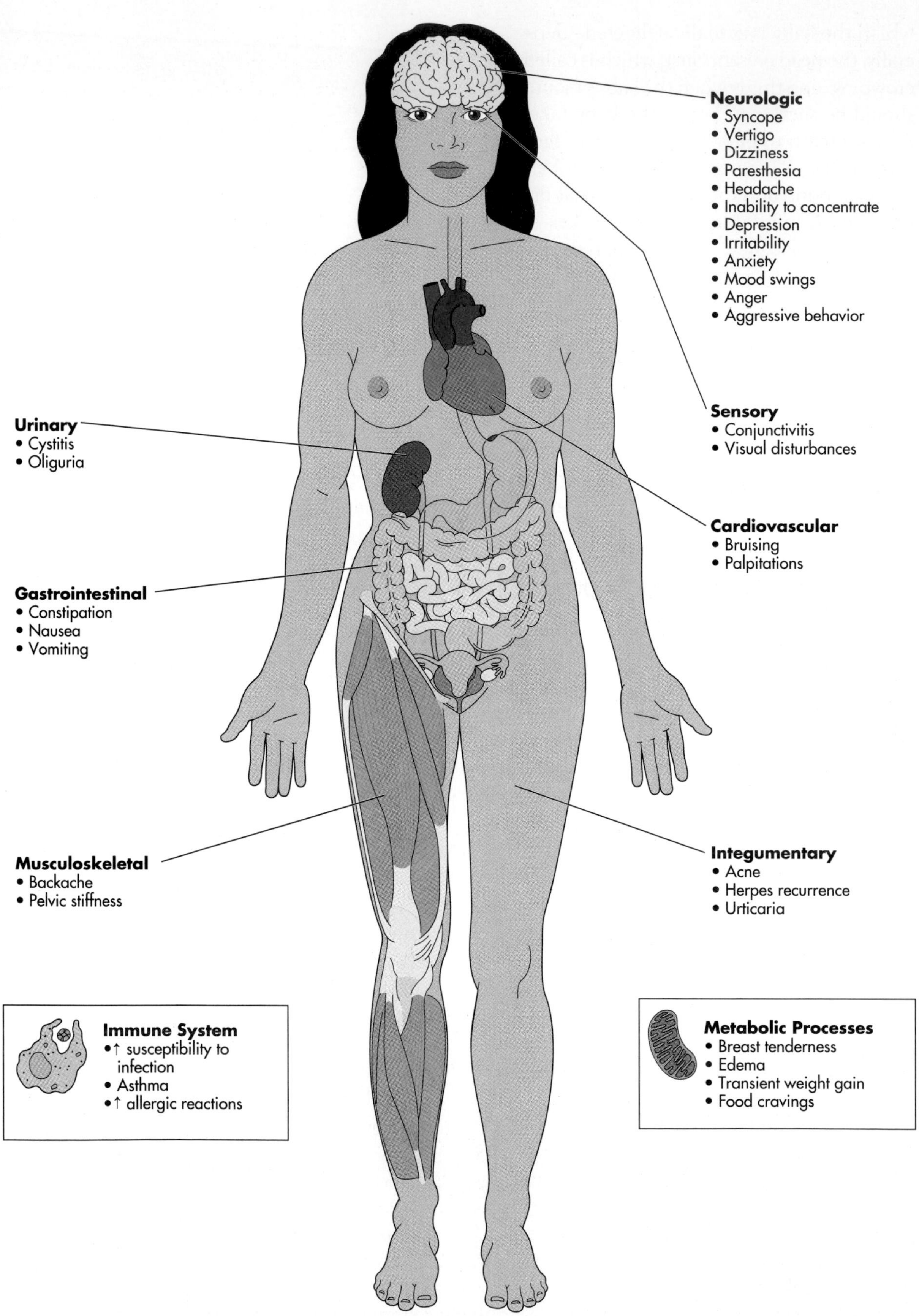
Neurologic
• Syncope
• Vertigo
• Dizziness
• Paresthesia
• Headache
• Inability to concentrate
• Depression
• Irritability
• Anxiety
• Mood swings
• Anger
• Aggressive behavior
Sensory
• Conjunctivitis
• Visual disturbances
Urinary
• Cystitis
• Oliguria
Cardiovascular
• Bruising
• Palpitations
Gastrointestinal
• Constipation
• Nausea
• Vomiting
Musculoskeletal
• Backache
• Pelvic stiffness
Integumentary
• Acne
• Herpes recurrence
• Urticaria
Immune System
• ↑ susceptibility to infection
• Asthma
• ↑ allergic reactions
Metabolic Processes
• Breast tenderness
• Edema
• Transient weight gain
• Food cravings

FIGURE ■ 17–12

Multisystem effects of premenstrual syndrome.

Mastitis is inflammation of the breast, which can occur at any age and in both male and females, but is usually associated with lactating females. **Breast cancer** is one of the leading causes of death in woman between the ages of 32 and 52 and kills about 46,000 women a year. Men can also get breast cancer but at a lower rate, and it was estimated that there were about 1,000 cases of male breast cancer in 2003 compared to 182,000 female cases. Cancer of the breast may require a full or partial *mastectomy*, but the earlier it is detected, the better chance for a positive outcome. Please see Figure 17–13 ■, which shows the steps for a breast self-examination.

mastitis *(mass TYE tiss)*
mast = *breast*
ectomy = *removal of*

WHY DO THE BREAST SELF-EXAM?

There are many good reasons for doing a breast self-exam each month. One reason is that it is easy to do and the more you do it, the better you will get at it. When you get to know how your breasts normally feel, you will quickly be able to feel any change, and early detection is the key to successful treatment and cure.

REMEMBER: A breast self-exam could save your breast – and save your life. Most breast lumps are found by women themselves, but in fact, most lumps in the breast are not cancer. Be safe, be sure.

WHEN TO DO BREAST SELF-EXAM

The best time to do breast self-exam is right after your period, when breasts are not tender or swollen. If you do not have regular periods or sometimes skip a month, do it on the same day every month.

NOW, HOW TO DO BREAST SELF-EXAM

1. Lie down and put a pillow under your right shoulder. Place your right arm behind your head.

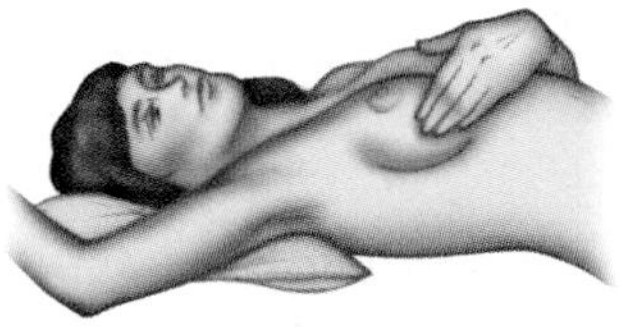

2. Use the finger pads of your three middle fingers on your left hand to feel for lumps or thickening. Your finger pads are the top third of each finger.

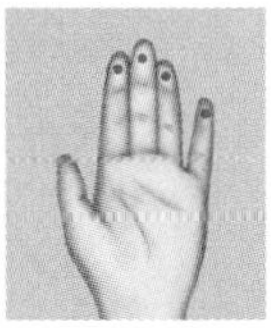

3. Press firmly enough to know how your breast feels. If you're not sure how hard to press, ask your health care provider. Or try to copy the way your health care provider uses the finger pads during a breast exam. Learn what your breast feels like most of the time. A firm ridge in the lower curve of each breast is normal.

4. Move around the breast in a set way. You can choose either the circle (A), the up and down line (B), or the wedge (C). Do it the same way every time. It will help you to make sure that you've gone over the entire breast area, and to remember how your breast feels.

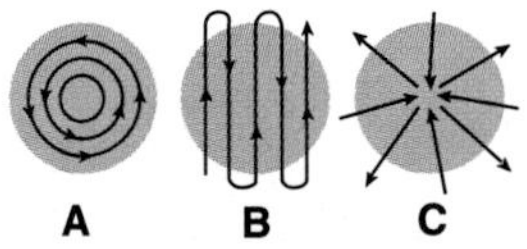

5. Now examine your left breast using your right hand finger pads.

6. If you find any changes, see your doctor right away.

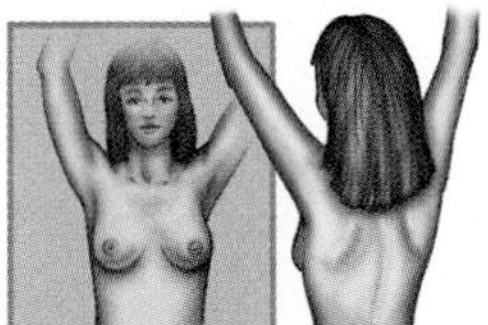

FOR ADDED SAFETY:

You should also check your breasts while standing in front of a mirror right after you do your breast self-exam each month. See if there are any changes in the way your breasts look: dimpling of the skin, changes in the nipple, or redness or swelling.

You might also want to do a breast self-exam while you're in the shower. Your soapy hands will glide over the wet skin, making it easy to check how your breasts feel.

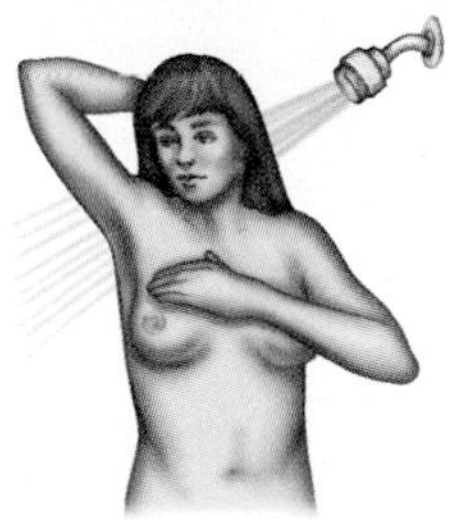

FIGURE ■ 17–13

Breast Self-examination.

17-8 Go to your CD-ROM to view movies on preclampsia, PMS, EDD, and breast cancer.

Diseases of the Male Reproductive System

In **erectile dysfunction disorder,** or **EDD,** the penis cannot attain full erection. Medication can help to increase blood flow to the penis and thus treat some forms of erectile dysfunction. The inability to develop an erection is often referred to as impotency.

cryptorchidism *(kript OR kid izm)*

The failure of the testes to descend into the scrotal sac is termed **cryptorchidism** and may require surgical intervention. If the testes remain undescended, the male may become sterile because of the body heat destroying the sperm. A **hydrocele** is an abnormal collection of fluid within the testes.

hydrocele *(HIGH droh seel)*

Amazing Body Facts

A MILLION TO ONE SHOT

The adult male produces 200 million sperm daily but it takes only one sperm to fertilize the egg.

Impotency is often confused with the inability to conceive children due to low sperm counts. This is incorrect. To determine male fertility, a semen analysis must be performed. Semen is collected 3-5 days after abstaining from sexual activity. The semen is analyzed for the shape, number and swimming strength of the sperm. This is also used to determine the effectiveness of a vasectomy where the blocking of the vas deferens should result in no sperm in the semen sample 6 weeks postoperatively

benign prostatic hypertrophy *(bee NINE pross TAT ik high PER troh fee)*

Benign prostatic hypertrophy, or **BPH,** is the enlargement of the prostrate gland and is commonly seen in males over 50 years old (see Figure 17–14 ■). **Prostate cancer** is a slow-growing cancer that also affects males within this age group and can be treated effectively if detected early. A PSA test (prostate-specific antigen) can aid in early detection.

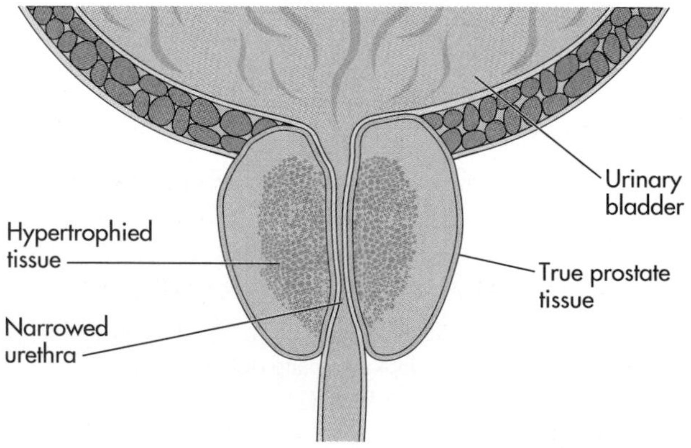

FIGURE ■ 17–14

Benign prostatic hyperplasia.

SUMMARY

Snapshots from the Journey

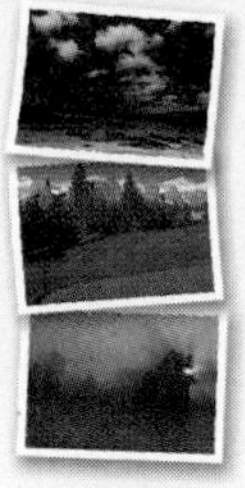

- Tissues grow, are replaced, and are repaired by asexual reproduction. Cells make identical copies of themselves. Asexual reproduction takes place all over the body as tissues grow or are repaired. Some tissues, like epidermis, blood, and bone, replace themselves continually, always by asexual reproduction.
- Asexual reproduction in eukaryotic cells is accomplished by a relatively complex process called mitosis.
- If an organism is going to reproduce sexually, it must use specialized cells called gametes with only half the typical number of chromosomes for that organism. (It must have half as many chromosomes because, during fertilization, the gametes will fuse and combine their genetic material.)
- In humans, the gametes are eggs and sperm. Eggs and sperm are produced by a special type of cell division called meiosis, or reduction division. Reduction division produces four daughter cells, each with only 23 chromosomes. These cells are not identical to each other or to the mother cell.
- Cells undergoing meiosis go through two divisions. The chief difference between mitosis and meiosis is the pairing of homologous chromosomes (alike in size shape and genetic content) during meiosis.
- Human reproduction can be described as a cycle, known as the human life cycle. Adult humans have specialized organs called gonads (ovaries and testes), which produce gametes via meiosis. Gametes get together during sexual reproduction in a process known as fertilization. The fertilized egg is called a zygote. The zygote undergoes many rounds of mitosis, eventually becoming an embryo, a fetus, a baby, a child, and finally an adult.
- The female reproductive system consists of several internal genitalia. The gonads (ovaries) produce eggs (gametes). The uterine tubes provide a passageway for the egg to get to the uterus. The uterus is an incubator for the fertilized eggs. The vagina is the birth canal, connecting the uterus with the outside world. The external genitalia include the external opening of the vagina and several protective structures.
- Female reproductive physiology is relatively complicated, organized around a monthly cycle of changes in both the ovaries and the uterus, collectively known as the menstrual cycle. The cycle begins with menstruation, the shedding of the uterine lining. After the lining, the endometrium, has finished shedding, it begins to build up again in a process called proliferation. As the endometrium is proliferating, an egg (follicle) is maturing in the ovary. Eventually, the follicle will be released from the ovary (ovulation) and travel to the uterus. If fertilization occurs, then the fertilized egg will implant in the thickened endometrium and pregnancy will result. If the egg is not fertilized, the endometrium will degenerate and menstruation will occur.
- Control of the menstrual cycle is accomplished by four hormones: estrogen, progesterone, follicle-stimulating hormone (FSH), and luteinizing hormone (LH). During puberty, the ovaries begin to secrete larger amounts of estrogen and progesterone, which cause the development of female secondary sexual characteristics and set the cycle in motion.
- The cycle works this way: The hypothalamus releases gonadotropin-releasing hormone (GnRH) that causes the pituitary to increase secretion of FSH and LH. FSH and LH cause follicles to develop and eventually trigger ovulation. Estrogen levels continue to rise as the developing follicles secrete more

and more estrogen. Estrogen causes positive feedback to the hypothalamus and pituitary, which increases the levels of FSH and LH. This positive feedback loop continues right up until ovulation.

- At ovulation, the ruptured follicle (left behind after ovulation) begins to secrete progesterone and backs off on estrogen secretion. Under the influence of progesterone, the feedback loop between estrogen and the hypothalamus and pituitary reverses itself, becoming a negative feedback loop. Thus, LH and FSH levels drop. Progesterone levels continue to rise, maintaining the thickened endometrium in case fertilization occurs. If fertilization does not occur, progesterone decreases, the endometrium decays, and the cycle begins all over again.
- The male reproductive system has somewhat more obvious external genitalia, the penis, and the testes. Internal genitalia include a series of ducts, the vas deferens, ejaculatory duct and urethra, and a series of glands, the seminal vesicles, prostate, and bulbourethral glands.
- Male reproductive physiology is not cyclic and is therefore a bit less complicated than female reproduction. Sperm, like eggs, develop via meiosis under the control of LH and FSH in the testes. Sperm mature in the epididymis. When a man is sexually aroused, the penis becomes engorged with blood, and an erection occurs. If arousal continues, ejaculation, the movement of sperm from the testes to the penis and out of the man's body, may occur. During ejaculation, sperm move from the epididymis through the vas deferens, ejaculatory duct, and out the urethra. Along the journey, the seminal vesicles, prostate, and bulbourethral glands add sugar, chemicals, and mucus to the sperm to form semen.
- Testosterone is the chief male hormone. It is secreted by the testes and is responsible for masculinizing male fetuses, triggering LH and FSH production, and the development of male secondary sexual characteristics.

Case Study

Maria and her husband Trey have been planning a family for many years. Now that the time seems right, she cannot seem to get pregnant. After two years of trying, they have decided to consult their family physician for a referral to a fertility specialist. Before making the referral, their family doctor runs some tests herself.

Here are the results:

Trey is producing sperm at normal levels, and the sperm are healthy and mobile.

Maria's hormone levels and all other blood tests are normal. She has a more or less regular menstrual cycle, but she has always had cramps during the middle of her cycle. On further questioning, she admits to the doctor that in the last few years, the pain seemed to get worse but she thought that was just normal for her. She also admits to some low back pain and some urinary disturbances, particularly around her period.

To prevent exploratory abdominal surgery, can you think of any other diagnostic tests?

What should Maria's doctor be looking for given the timing of the pain during the cycle and the inability to get pregnant?

REVIEW QUESTIONS

Multiple Choice

1. In each lobule of the testes are several ______________, tubes in which the sperm are made and develop.
   a. seminal vesicles
   b. seminiferous tubules
   c. bulbourethral glands
   d. all of the above

2. The female primary genitalia are the
   a. ovaries
   b. uterus
   c. vagina
   d. testes

3. This division of the endometrium sheds each month:
   a. horny layer
   b. basal layer
   c. menstrual layer
   d. none of the above

4. This hormone stimulates ovulation:
   a. estrogen
   b. progesterone
   c. LH
   d. FSH

5. Which of the following in *not* a function of asexual reproduction (mitosis)?
   a. making gametes
   b. tissue growth
   c. tissue repair
   d. all are functions of asexual reproduction

Fill in the Blank

1. The stiffening of the penis is known as ______________, and the actual movement of sperm out of the penis is ______________.

2. In the male reproductive system the ______________ is posterior to the bladder, and the ______________ gland is inferior to the bladder.

3. ______________ is the type of cell division that produces egg and sperm.

4. After ovulation, estrogen and progesterone send ______________ (positive or negative) feedback to the pituitary and hypothalamus.

5. The union of sperm and egg is called ______________.

Short Answer

1. Trace the journey of a sperm from its birth through fertilization.

____

____

____

____

2. Explain the role of hormones in controlling the female reproductive cycle.

3. Contrast mitosis and meiosis.

Suggested Activities

1. List all the hormones involved in reproduction. Describe what they do.

2. Describe the human life cycle in detail. How much do you know about your own reproductive system?

3. With a partner, list the similarities and differences between male and female reproduction. How many can you list?

17-9 Now that you have completed your journey through this chapter, please go to the CD-ROM for interactive games and puzzles concerning the medical terms and concepts contained in this chapter. By playing the games you will reinforce your learning of medical terminology in a fun way.

Greetings from THE JOURNEY'S End

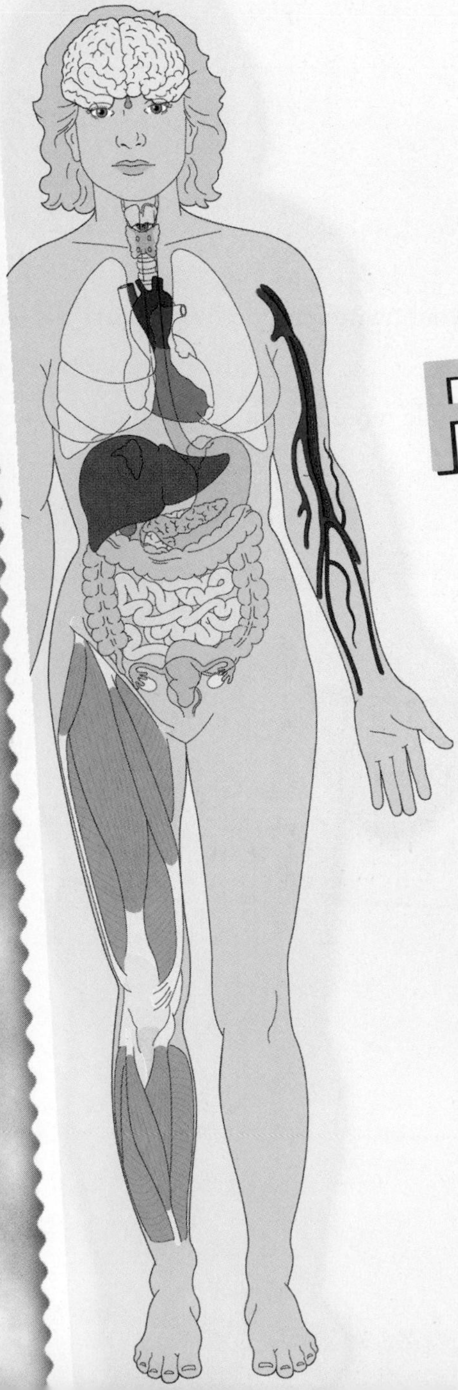

Now What?

For any of you who have ever taken a memorable journey or have lived through a significant event, you know that you have been changed to some degree forever. We hope that this book in some positive way has also changed you.

At the risk of sounding like one of those bad graduation speakers, your study of anatomy and physiology has only just begun. The basics that you have learned will act as a foundation of understanding for many things that you will encounter in your life. So go forth and make your mark in the world! Plant a tree, perfect a rose, look for the best in mankind, gain the respect of intelligent people, and—sorry, got a little carried away.

Anyhow, the following topics are just a small sampling of how anatomy and physiology plays an important role in many areas. We have added a whole section of Amazing Facts so you can impress friends, family, and the old boyfriend or girlfriend who dumped you back in high school. They'll be sorry now! Enjoy the chapter!

Chapter 18

LEARNING OBJECTIVES

Upon completion of your journey through this chapter, you will be able to:

- Discuss the relationship between forensic science and anatomy and physiology
- Relate anatomy and physiology changes to the process of aging
- Describe the concept of wellness and personal choices
- List and describe wellness concepts for each body system
- Discuss cancer prevention and treatment
- Dazzle your friends with amazing anatomy and physiology facts

MULTIMEDIA APPLICATIONS

CD-ROM Interactive Exercises

- Animation of the cause and effect of lead poisoning, 18.1
- Animations and movies on mental health disorders such as bipolar disorder, schizophrenia, dissociative disorders (multiple personalities), and autism, 18.2
- Video on carpal tunnel syndrome, 18.3
- Video on skin cancer, 18.4
- Video on audiology, 18.5
- Video on eating disorders such as anorexia and bulimia, 18.6
- Video on AIDS, 18.7
- Interactive games and puzzles, 18.8

www.prenhall.com/colbert

- Professional Profiles
  - Criminalist
  - Mental Health Professionals
  - Physician Assistant
- Related Web Sites
- Additional Review Questions

Pronunciation Guide

Correct pronunciation is important in any journey so that you and others are completely understood. Here is a "see and say" Pronunciation Guide for the more difficult terms to pronounce in this chapter.

anhidrosis (an HIGH droe sis)
bacilli (bah SILL eye)
Chlamydia trachomatis (klah MID ee ah TRAY koh mah tis)
forensic science (fa REN sik)
geriatric (jair ee AT rik)
herpes simplex virus 2 (HER peez)
human papilloma virus (pap ih LOW ma)
incontinence (in KAH tih nens)
Neisseria gonorrhoeae (nye SEE ree ah gon ah REE ah)
spina bifida (SPY nah BIFF ih dah)
thallium (tha LEE um)
Treponema pallidum (trep eh NEE ma PAL ih dum)

FORENSIC SCIENCE

forensic science *(fa REN sik)*

We've all watched movies or TV shows featuring super-sleuths solving such crimes as murders or disappearances using some amazing scientific technology. Some of the methods used seem pretty far-fetched, as though invented just for entertainment purposes. Actually, much of the **forensic** science we see on TV is very close, if not "dead on," to the actual technologies that are applied to solve crimes. It is important to note that this kind of investigation can be extremely tedious and take longer than a 46-minute TV show to solve. Most forensic scientists don't look like supermodels or drive $50,000 SUVs either. This section deals with just a sampling of how anatomy and physiology is used to help solve crimes and explain historical mysteries.

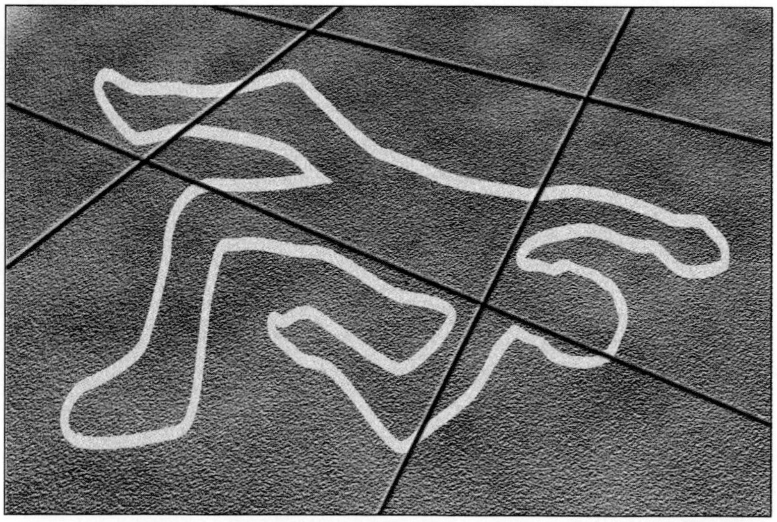

So what exactly is forensic science? Simply put, forensic science is the application of science to law. A forensic scientist often searches for and examines physical traces that can be useful in establishing or excluding some association between a victim and an individual suspected of committing a crime. It is interesting to note that both physical science and social science are used when solving crime. The physical science of anatomy and physiology often play a key role in solving a crime or identifying the remains of a victim.

Applied Science

TOMATOES WERE ONCE THOUGHT POISONOUS

For several hundreds of years, it was believed that tomatoes were poisonous. This erroneous fact occurred because during the Middle Ages, the wealthier people ate from pewter plates that contained high levels of lead. The acidic tomatoes leached out the lead, which was consumed and resulted in lead poisoning.

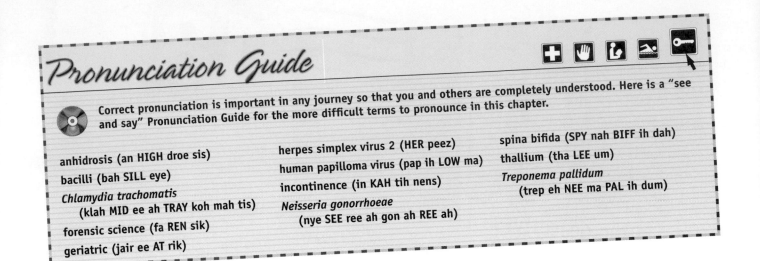

Disease Detection

Forensic science has unlocked ancient mysteries and allowed us to learn something about the health of ancient people. Proof that the ancient Egyptians were stricken with tuberculosis was discovered by examining their skeletons. We normally think of tuberculosis as a lung disease, but tuberculosis thrives in areas of the body that possess high levels of oxygen. These include the lungs, brain, kidneys, and *the ends of long bones!* Since the organs were long ago decomposed, the only thing left to examine were the skeletal remains, particularly the ends of the long bones such as the femur. On examination of these bones, bone scouring that is typically caused by tuberculosis was discovered. Bone scouring is the destruction of the smooth bone surface as a result of colonization by the tuberculosis **bacilli.**

bacilli *(bah SILL eye)*

Primitive Surgery

Forensic scientists have discovered evidence of primitive surgery. A skull fragment found in a 400-year-old trash dump at the site of the Jamestown, Virginia, settlement provided evidence that skull surgery had been performed on a patient. The circular marks on the fragment indicated that there was an attempt to drill a hole in the skull probably to relieve pressure on the brain due to a skull fracture that may have been caused by a tomahawk blow to the head or an accident. Scientists analyzing the fragment were able to determine that the patient was a European male on the basis of the fragment's shape and thickness *and* because the bone contained traces of lead that was absorbed by the body from using lead-glazed pottery and/or eating off of pewter plates!

Remains Identification

Nazi Josef Mengele, the "Angel of Death," was responsible for the death of at least 400,000 humans during World War II. As the war ended, Mengele escaped to South America and avoided capture. There were numerous reported sightings throughout the years but none produced the war criminal. Then, in 1979, an elderly Wolfgang Gerhard drowned and was buried in a Brazilian cemetery. Suspicions that this was Mengele prompted the Brazilian government to exhume the body. Analysis of the bones revealed a right-handed male Caucasian between 60 and 70 years old with a height approximated within a half centimeter of Mengele's. Having a pile of bones, a shattered skull, and no current medical information or dental records, the forensic anthropologists turned to a technique called video skull–face superimposition. After reconstructing the shattered skull, the experts marked it with pins at 30 specific structural landmarks. The same thing was done with a picture of Mengele that

18-1 For an animation of the cause and effect of lead poisoning, please go to your CD-ROM for this chapter.

Applied Science

FORENSICS AND HISTORY

DNA fingerprinting techniques are used extensively to clear up mysteries. For example, it is now standard to use this technology to solve rape and murder cases. DNA fingerprinting also helped determine that Thomas Jefferson did actually father children of his slave Sally Hemmings. It was also used to identify many of the victims of the World Trade Center, Pentagon, and Flight 93 in Shanksville, Pennsylvania, after 9/11.

Applied Science

IF BONES COULD SPEAK

Skeletal remains can also assist in telling the sex of an individual. The female pelvis is shaped like a basin and is wider than the male to allow for the larger birth canal. In general, it is broader and lighter than the male pelvis, and the pubic angle is 100 degrees or greater (see Figure 18–1). The male pelvis is more funnel shaped and is heavier and stronger, with a pubic angle of 90 degrees or less.

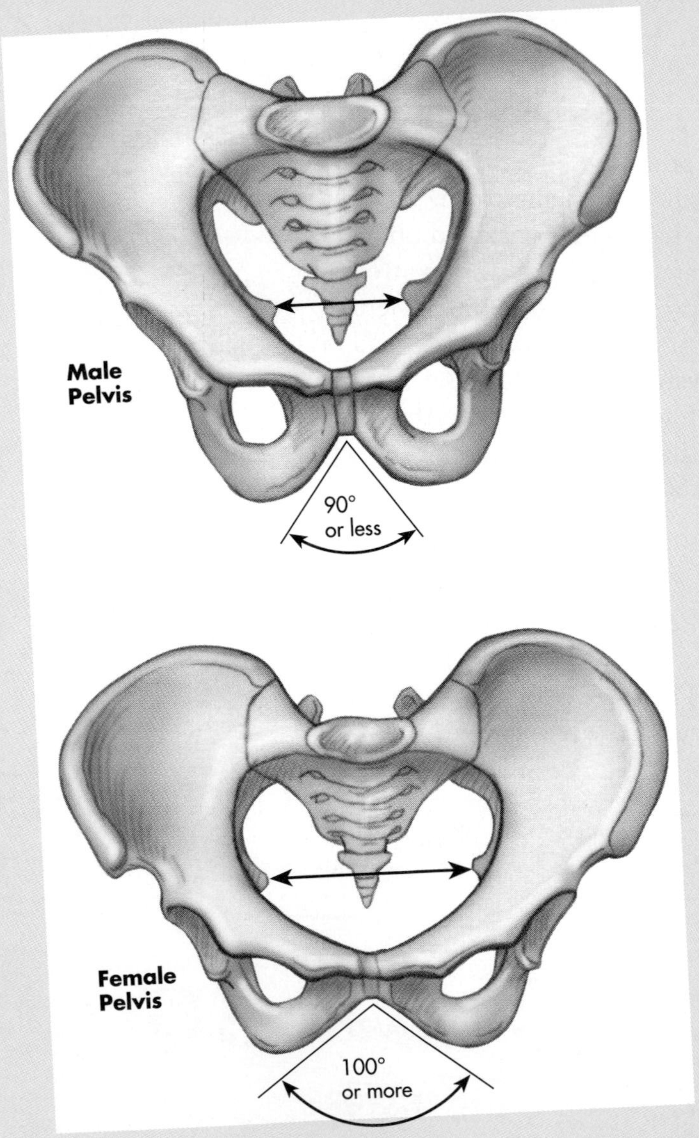

FIGURE 18–1

The male pelvis and female pelvis.

was scaled to match the size of the skull. Compared side by side, the pins matched up. Photo images of the skull and picture were then superimposed and the points matched up. They had their man. Later, when his old dental records were found, it was again a match, as was a later DNA analysis. More recently, an updated similar procedure was used to determine the actual facial structure of Tutankhamen (King Tut), the Boy Pharaoh of Egypt.

Murder Most Foul!

Although it possesses no vocal chords, your hair speaks volumes about your health and your habits! Hair can reveal the race of an individual, whether the hair was cut or pulled out from the body, or if it was dyed. If the hair shaft has its follicle still attached, genetic information such as DNA or blood type can also be discerned. Hair samples can place an individual at the scene of a crime.

Even though hair is technically dead, just like your fingernails and toenails, it acts like a library (as do your nails), storing information about substances you have ingested or have been exposed to. Since hair grows relatively slowly, it can contain a *timeline* of substances that an individual ingested or was exposed to. In an interesting case of thallium poisoning, a man's wife was convicted of murder partially on the basis of hair samples of the victim. The victim's hair was long enough that it provided a record of ingestion of thallium for approximately 330 days. During that period of time, the spikes in concentration of thallium in sections of his hair matched the times the victim was with his wife. Drops in the level of thallium in other sections of his hair coincided with the times he was away from his wife or in the hospital for other illnesses. There was a massive spike in thallium concentration a few days before he died, which was indicative of premeditated poisoning. In a plea bargain, it was revealed that victim's wife had been feeding him rat poison that contained thallium in order to collect on a life insurance policy!

Fingerprints

Even with all the new advances, fingerprints are still a time honored crime-solving method (see Figure 18–2 ■). Like snowflakes, no two prints are exactly alike. Fingerprints are actual *friction ridges* that form a pattern on the anterior surface of the hands and also on the planar surface of the feet. They are especially prominent on the skin covering the tips of the fingers and toes. Fingerprints are made inside the womb in response to the pull of the elastic fibers in the dermal papillary layer upon the epidermis. As the name applies, the friction ridges help prevent slippage when grasping or holding objects. Interestingly, even identical twins who have the same DNA configuration will not have identical fingerprints.

Interest in fingerprints have been around for a long period of time (see Figure 18–2). Their uniqueness was discovered in the 1600s. They were described and studied for many years, and then in 1880, Dr. Henry Faulds wrote the first article suggesting that fingerprints may be used to solve crimes. In 1886, he began trying to convince Scotland Yard to adopt a fingerprinting identification system.

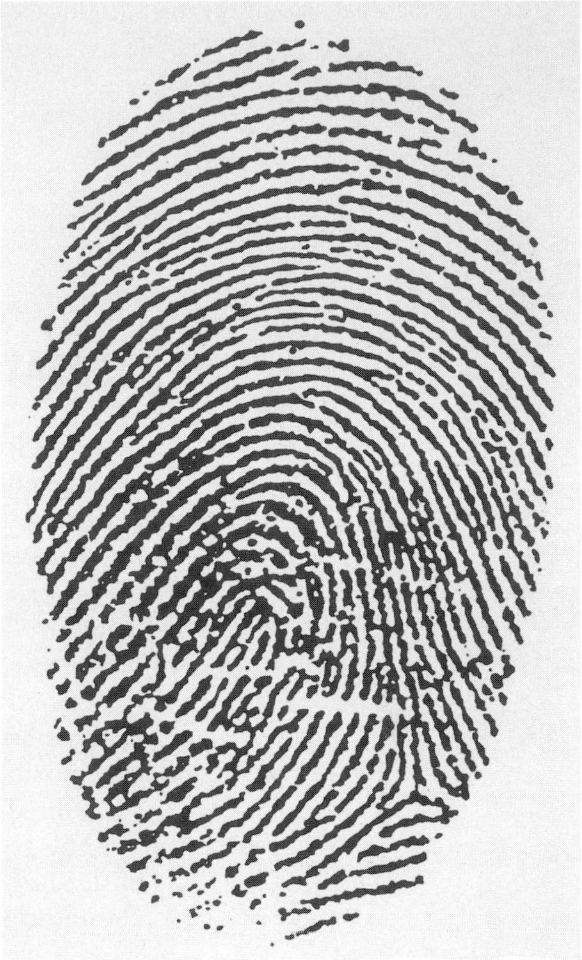

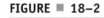

FIGURE ■ 18–2

The fingerprint. (Source: Dorling Kindersley Media Library.)

DNA Fingerprinting

Forensic scientists may also use DNA, the molecule found in the nucleus of our cells, to identify unknown individuals. DNA can be sampled at a crime scene from body fluids, such as blood or semen, or can be extracted from skeletal or even very tiny soft tissue remains. During the process of DNA fingerprinting (which has nothing to do with actual fingerprints), DNA molecules are split into pieces and separated using electrical currents. These pieces can be compared to pieces of a known DNA sample from a relative of a victim, from hair samples off a comb or mouth cells from a toothbrush, or can be compared to a suspect in a criminal case.

The criminalist is responsible for analyzing the evidence at a crime scene and is one member of the forensic team. To view a video about this profession, please visit the companion Web site for this chapter.

TEST YOUR KNOWLEDGE 18-1

Choose the best answer:

1. This part of your body acts as a library and provides a timeline to record substances that you have ingested or have been exposed to:
   a. heart
   b. lungs
   c. hair
   d. spinal cord

2. This metal has been detected in the bones of medieval skeletons and can be traced to eating off of pewter plates:
   a. silver
   b. gold
   c. kryptonite
   d. lead

3. Proof that ancient Egyptians had tuberculosis was discovered by examining their
   a. tombs
   b. bones
   c. hair
   d. mommy's

4. The difference between male and female skeletal remains can be determined by examining the angle of the
   a. skull
   b. vertebrae
   c. sternum
   d. pelvis

GERIATRICS

geriatric *(jair ee AT rik)*

Many regions in the United States are exhibiting a major change in patient demographics. In general, we are seeing an older population due to safer workplaces, healthier lifestyles, effective vaccines and medications, and opportunities to access health care. As a result, you probably will deal with a high number of **geriatric** patients in the health care profession that you choose (even the maternity departments may have 50- to 60-year-old mothers in the future, as witnessed by several recent news reports!).

Geriatric patients differ in many ways from other patient age groups, so it is important to recognize these differences in order to provide the best health care possible for this patient population. Here are some general tidbits to get you started.

The general use of the term *elderly* when describing patients is somewhat misleading. Currently, this patient group can be divided into the following classifications.

- Age 65 to 75: younger old
- Age 76 to 84: older old
- Age 85 and older: elite old

Using the vague term *aging* as a way to generally describe a patient is interesting in that an individual's body does not age uniformly. For example, an individual may look older due to aging skin but may have a cardiovascular system of a person 10 to 15 years younger than his or her chronological age. With that said, there is the general "1 percent rule" in which we see a 1 percent decrease in the function of most body systems each year beginning around the age of 30.

So what general characteristics or tendencies do we see in an aging patient? The hallmark sign of aging is a decrease in the ability to maintain homeostasis. These individuals may have normal baselines but will begin exhibiting a decrease in the ability to adapt to stressors. Often, disease processes along with aging will accelerate the loss of body reserves that younger patients take for granted, such as recovery

Amazing Body Facts

YOU'RE NOT GETTING OLDER, YOU'RE GETTING SMARTER

There are a lot of misconceptions about the brain and aging. In the absence of disease, your brain continues to mature up to the age of 50. Interestingly, we have better overall brain function and decision-making skills at age 60 than at age 30! Even though an older patient may lose up to 1,000 neurons a day, you have to realize that we all started out with several billion! This is why you may not see a decrease in brain function until the age of 75.

time or complications following an accident or surgery. In addition, you may have increased difficulties in evaluating these patients because of decreases in their vision, hearing, and possibly their mental abilities.

General Body Changes

Let's take a general look at the aging process of the body. There is a decrease in the total body water for both males and females. The clinical significance of this is that they have a tendency to dehydrate more rapidly, which can potentially affect the excretion rate of medications they are on.

From ages 20 to 70, we see a loss of lean body mass due to up to a 30 percent loss in the number of muscle cells, atrophy of remaining muscle cells, and a general decrease in muscle strength. Conversely, we see an increase to total body fat, which slowly increases between the ages of 25 and 45, peaking at 40. This trend can continue up to age 70. The fat accumulated is a "deeper" fat, meaning that it is more abdominal fat and found more in the viscera than subcutaneously.

Bone density usually reaches its greatest peak around age 35. Contrary to what you see on TV, loss of bone mass occurs both in women *and* men. For women, during the first 5 years postmenopause, 1 percent to 2 percent bone loss per year can occur. In general, we see a 1 percent loss per year between the ages of 55 and 70. After that, it is approximately 0.5 percent per year.

So in general, as an individual ages, he or she loses muscle mass, gains fat, and loses bone density. This varies among individuals and can be affected by lifestyle choices. Later in this chapter, we discuss steps that can be taken to slow (or even reverse) this process.

Gustatory Changes

Sensory changes can also occur in this patient group. The senses of taste and smell begin to deteriorate as a natural process of aging. The number of taste buds decreases by about 50 percent as the body reaches the geriatric stage. Sweet versus bitter tastes becomes less discernable. The acuity of salt and bitter tastes decline. Orange juice may taste metallic. Patients on oxygen via a nasal cannula may have a decrease in their ability to taste. These changes are clinically significant because they may make it more difficult to insure a properly balanced diet for good health and activity. This is also a concern coupled with the additional functional and physiologic difficulties affecting grocery shopping and food preparation. It is estimated that 33 percent of this patient group lives alone. These and other sensory impairments affect activities of daily living (ADLs), and as a result, we see approximately 5 percent to 15 percent of this population exhibiting protein and calorie malnutrition.

Additional barriers to proper nutrition include a loss of teeth, difficulties in swallowing, and decreases in salivary secretion. In addition, there are decreases in digestive juices acidity and secretion, nutrient absorption, and bowel function.

The Brain and Nervous System

The main problem with the aging process and the nervous system is the slower reaction time that occurs. As a result, there are increased chances for motor vehicle accidents, falls, burns, and so forth.

Pain is something usually associated with the aging process. Even though the authors of this book are young in spirit, vibrant, and good looking, they have occasional creaking joints and stiff, sore muscles! Untreated pain can lead to an overall decrease in the quality of a person's life, including impaired sleep, a decrease in socialization, confusion, depression, malnutrition, polypharmacy (use of multiple medications), and impaired ambulation. If any of these conditions were occurring before the pain was introduced, the pain may cause these conditions to worsen.

Often, geriatric patients are undermedicated for pain. This may be because patients who are debilitated, cognitively impaired, or have a history of substance abuse are sometimes unable to effectively relate how they feel. Sometimes, it is a result of the ignorance of health care professionals who cannot recognize indicators of pain.

Clinically, these are some of the potential behavioral changes related to pain:

- changes in personality such as becoming agitated, quiet, withdrawn, sad, confused, depressed, grumpy
- loss of appetite
- screaming, swearing, name calling, grunting, noisy breathing
- crying, rocking, fidgeting
- splinting or rubbing a sore area, wincing
- cold, clammy, and pale skin

The Cardiovascular System

Within the cardiovascular system, we see changes such as calcification of the heart valves, which decreases their efficiency. We also see a lessening in the flexibility of the blood vessels, which leads to clogging. This makes them less able to deal with blood pressure changes, so increased blood pressure is common.

(Source: Arthur Tilley/Getty Images, Inc.—Taxi.)

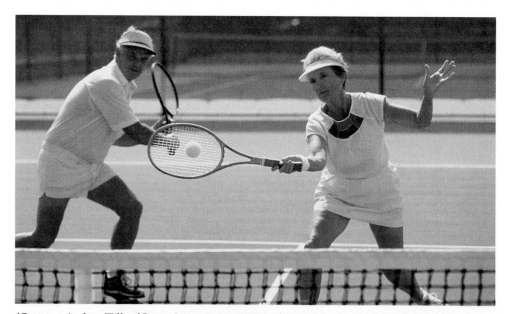

There is also a decrease in cardiac output and an approximate 25 percent decrease in the maximum heart rate

The Genitourinary System

Between the ages of 20 and 80, we lose about 50 percent of our renal function. This is clinically significant when you consider the amount of drugs used by the geriatric population that are excreted by the kidneys. Therefore, a drug taken by someone with impaired renal (and/or liver) function can lead to the drug not being metabolized at the expected rate. This can lead to an accumulation of the drug in the body at harmful or toxic levels. There is also an increase in **incontinence** (loss of bladder control) in this group.

incontinence *(in KAH tih nens)*

The Integumentary System

Here we see a loss in skin elasticity, increased skin delicacy, multiple skin lesions, and incidences in skin cancer. While many of these problems could have been reduced by limiting sun exposure and not smoking earlier in their lives, the use of medications such as systemic corticosteroids does accelerate many of these conditions.

Polypharmacy

Polypharmacy, the administration of many drugs at the same time, is a major concern for this patient group. Contributing factors to this problem include the fact that these patients typically see several specialists for a variety of diseases, often with one doctor not knowing what the other is prescribing. These multiple diseases have competing therapeutic needs, and the combinations of utilized drugs can cause life-threatening situations. Aging also can affect the rates of drug absorption, drug distribution throughout the body, metabolism of the drugs, as well as their excretion from the body.

As a result, here are some clinical considerations. Review the drugs that the individual is taking, looking for possible drug interactions or medications that are no longer needed. Look at your patient's liver and kidney functions. They will affect the rate of removal of medications from the body and resultant drug blood levels. When medicating with opioids, dose by age, not by body weight. Remember, opioids slow the gastrointestinal tract. In general, when considering an *equal* dose given to a geriatric patient compared to a middle-aged patient, analgesics are stronger and last longer in elderly patients. So, start low and go slow.

For example, allied health professionals working in a physician's office or in home care might remind patients to bring all of the drugs they're taking to each appointment. It is also important that they are instructed to keep an updated list of their drugs and dosages in case they have to make a trip to the emergency department.

TEST YOUR KNOWLEDGE 18-2

Choose the best answer:

1. There is a ______________ decrease in the function of most body systems each year beginning around the age of 30.
   a. 10%
   b. 20%
   c. 5%
   d. 1%

2. The hallmark sign of aging is the decrease in the ability to maintain
   a. cardiac enzymes
   b. exercise potential
   c. homeostasis
   d. sense of humor

3. ______________ is a term used for the administration of many drugs at the same time.
   a. addiction
   b. polypharmacy
   c. multimeds
   d. overdose

4. In the absence of disease, your brain continues to mature up to the age of
   a. 50
   b. 35
   c. 75
   d. 10

WELLNESS

One of the most important personal choices you will ever make will be the decision on what kind of lifestyle you want to live. Choices you make now may have a *profound* effect on your future health and lifespan. Will you eat properly, exercise within reason, smoke, do drugs and/or alcohol, live or work in a dangerous environment, have risky behaviors?

Individual accountability and *informed choices* are two key concepts in deciding your lifestyle. It is amazing that individuals have sued fast-food companies for making their food too appealing and, as a result, making the "victim" get fat. People don't force other people to smoke cigarettes. In each of these cases, the individual made a conscious choice to eat more than necessary and to begin smoking.

Yes, peer pressure is real, but it is too often looked at from the negative side. What about peers and influential people who promote good, healthy lifestyles? Think about it. Do you know people or have friends who do healthy things? Once again, it is a conscious choice to surround yourself with the type of friends you want.

Read and critically analyze what you read. Utilize multiple reliable sources. Even though the Internet is a wonderful source of information, there is a lot of "junk" science that is more opinion than fact.

Let's take a quick review of the body systems that we covered and briefly discuss some ways to improve your health. While there are always some controversial issues in wellness, we have chosen the more commonly held beliefs.

Nervous System

Let's talk a little bit about stress. First of all, stress is a natural part of life. Stress is also good and necessary: it is a motivator, it helps you to protect yourself. The problem occurs when stress becomes chronic and you can no longer effectively deal with it. The high cost of stress is that it can affect some or all of your body's various systems to varying degrees. A poor stress response can lead to an assortment of disorders such as eating and digestive disorders, decreased immune response, decreased memory and work capacities, sleep problems, joint and muscle aches, heart problems, and personality changes. Some of these problems can be life threatening. For an extensive review of a healthful stress management system, remember to consult your Study Companion Guide found in the back of your textbook.

> **18-2** To view animations and videos on mental health disorders such as bipolar disorder, schizophrenia, dissociative disorders (multiple personalities), and autism, please go to your CD-ROM for this chapter.

> The mind and body cannot be separated. There are a host of mental health professionals trained in diagnosing and treating mental health issues. For a review of these various professions, please go to our Web site for this chapter.

Often, when dealing with a patient, we focus specifically on the presenting illness and fail to realize we should look at the whole person. The "whole person" includes not only other systems of the body but also the mental and spiritual aspects of the person. Too often in the past, dealing with mental health has had a negative image. We don't hide the fact that we have the flu or a broken arm, so why should we hide the fact that we may be sad for long periods of time (depression) and need help to resolve that condition?

> **18-3** To view a video on carpal tunnel syndrome, please go to your CD-ROM for this chapter.

Skeletal System

Diet is extremely important in the growth and protection of your bones. A diet rich in calcium and vitamins helps to maintain good bone growth and development. Weight-bearing exercise has also been shown to be beneficial in maintaining healthy bones over a lifetime.

One common occupational condition related to repetitive motion, such as typing on a keyboard , playing a piano, or hammering, is known as carpal tunnel syndrome. While this syndrome is caused by damage to the median nerve, it is the result of the *skeletal* structure of the wrist being too restrictive during extended periods when the wrist is kept in an upward bent position. See Figure 18–3 ■, which illustrates the structures that affect this repetitive syndrome.

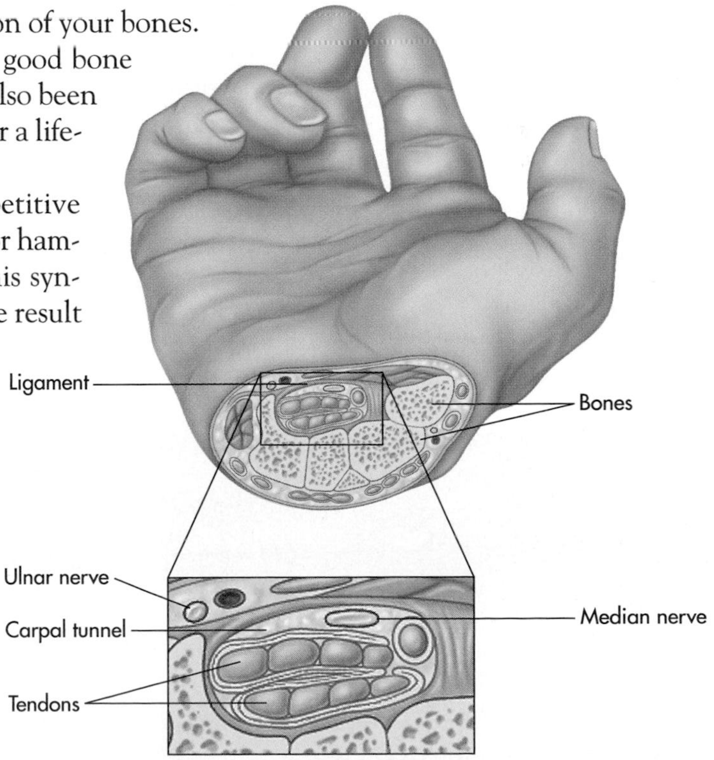

FIGURE ■ 18–3

Anatomical structures affecting carpal tunnel syndrome.

Muscular System

Again, proper exercise and diet will help to develop and maintain properly functioning muscles. While there are many types of muscle-training programs, you need to investigate which type is best for you depending on your needs or desired outcomes. See Figure 18–4 ■, which presents the Activity Pyramid as a possible guide.

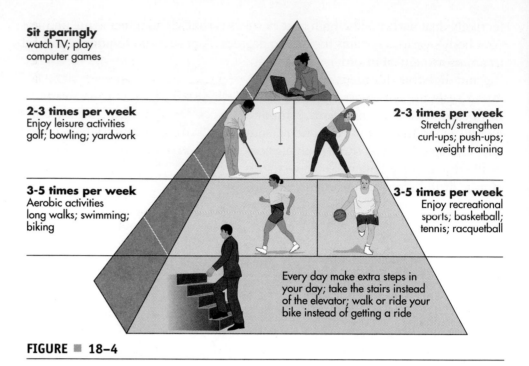

FIGURE ■ 18–4

The Activity Pyramid.

Be careful of muscle enhancement drugs: many are dangerous and have serious side effects. Again, careful critical investigation is the best rule to follow.

Integumentary System

Proper diet and hydration is important for the functioning of the integumentary system. This is why it is important to drink *at least* eight glasses of water a day. Other fluids such as caffeinated coffee and alcohol are diuretics and can cause a net water loss. Smoking also affects this system by causing premature aging of the skin.

> **18-4** To view a video on skin cancer, please go to your CD-ROM for this chapter.

While sun exposure is important for the production of vitamin D in your body, limiting the amount of sun exposure to prevent skin cancer is equally important. While some forms of skin cancer are treatable, others can be lethal. The effect of the sun is cumulative, and severe sun burns as a child can have severe consequences in adulthood. There are several ways to prevent excessive sun exposure. First, minimize your time in the sun between 10 a.m. and 4 p.m. because this is when the sun's rays are most intense. Wear long-sleeved shirts when possible, brimmed hats, sunglasses (preferably wraparounds), and, of course, sun screen.

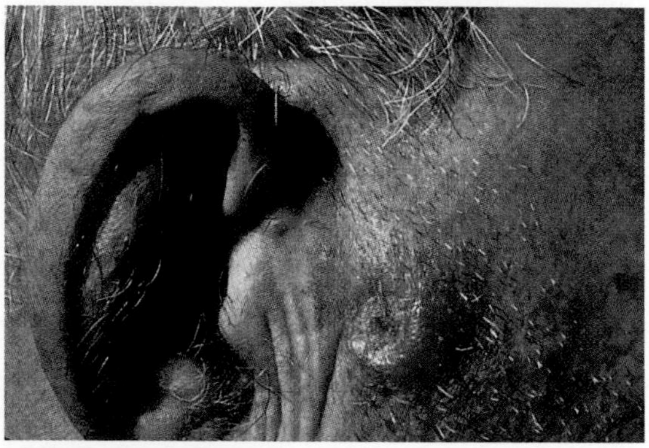

Squamous cell cancer.

Cardiovascular System

A heart-healthy diet low in saturated fats (remember, we all need some fat for proper function) and high in fiber, rich in fruit and vegetables, will help maintain an optimal cardiovascular system.

Diet alone is not sufficient for a healthy heart, and the proper level and regularity of exercise also helps condition heart for maximum functioning. This can be as simple as brisk walking for 30 minutes a day, three to four times a week. Of course, the level of your exercise program depends on many individualized factors. As always, consult your doctor before beginning any exercise program.

Smoking, alcohol, and other drugs can adversely affect the cardiovascular and other systems. For an illustration of the effects of chronic alcoholism on the cardiovascular, digestive, and nervous system, please see Figure 18–5 ■.

Respiratory System

Smoking is the number one preventable cause of respiratory diseases. Smoking can lead to damage of lung tissue and chronic diseases such as bronchitis, emphysema, and asthma. In addition, smoking increases the occurrence of lung infections and colds as well as sinus infections. Approximately 80 percent of all lung cancers can be traced to smoking. Smoking also affects the heart by reducing the availability of oxygen to the heart muscle.

Smoking along with alcohol consumption leads to an increase in stomach and mouth cancers.

What we breathe in, depending on where we live or work, can also affect the health of the respiratory system. Both outdoor and indoor pollution can lead to a number of respiratory problems.

Occupational hazards can occur when workers are exposed to dust or vapors. For example, coalminers exposed to coal dust without proper protection can develop black lung. The lung's initial response to an inhaled irritant is to close down or restrict the airway, thereby minimizing the inhalation of the substance. This can lead to severe breathing difficulties. See Figure 18–6 ■, which shows the constricted airway in an asthma attack.

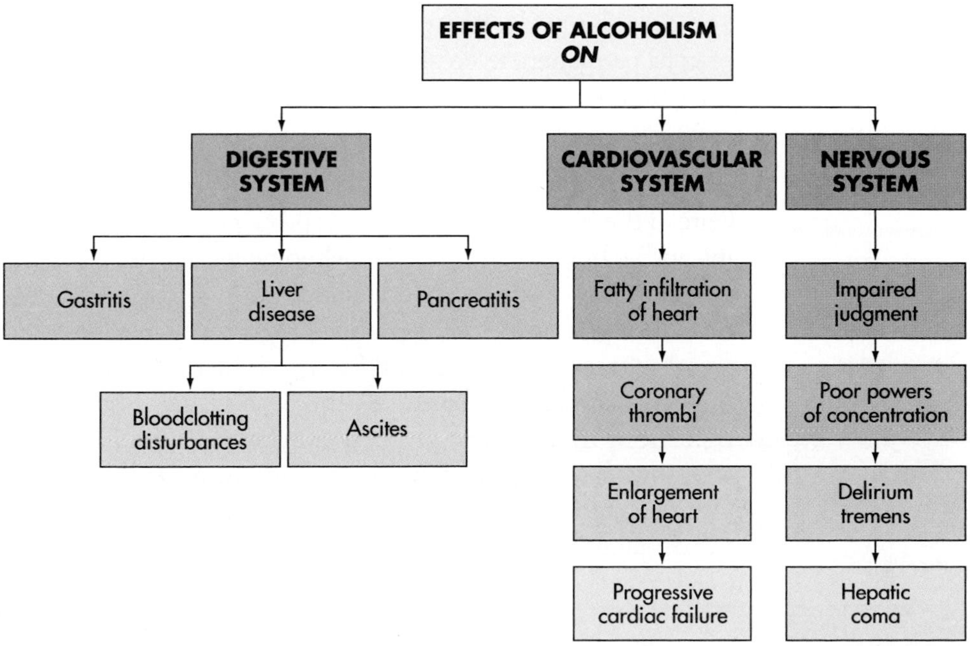

FIGURE ■ 18–5

The effects of alcoholism on the body systems.

Clinical Application

AGE- AND ACTIVITY-RELATED DIETS AND NUTRITIONAL NEEDS

At some time in our educational careers, we have seen the old food pyramid, which told us what portion of our diet should be dairy, what portion of our diet should be vegetables, and so forth. One of the problems with this pyramid was that it was designed to fit *everyone*. Unfortunately, not everyone is the same sex, height, shape, or age, nor has the same level of activity. Enter MyPyramid.gov. This is the USDA's newest spin on the food pyramid that takes into account your age, sex, and activity level when determining the best diet for YOU.

18-5 To view a video on audiology, please go to your CD-ROM for this chapter.

Gastrointestinal System

A proper diet is critical for growth, development, and health in general. Lack of a proper diet, which leads to undernourishment, can affect all the systems, as can be seen in Figure 18–7 ■. While most experts agree that the best source of vitamins and minerals comes from natural food sources, the responsible use of supplemental vitamins and minerals can play an important role in health. For example, excessive dosages of fat-soluble vitamins (A, D, E, and K) can actually harm the body because they can build up in toxic levels. See Table 18–1 for a list of some of the vitamins and the systems they assist.

Endocrine System

Again, proper diet and exercise assist the endocrine system. One of the areas of concern, in professional and even high school sports, is the use of performance-enhancement substances. For example, anabolic steroids are used to increase strength and endurance rapidly and to build muscle mass. Anabolic steroids are closely related to the male hormone testosterone. However, these steroids have *serious* side effects that include kidney damage, liver damage, increased risk of heart disease, irritability, and aggressive behavior. Woman taking steroids can develop facial hair and deeper voices. In men, these substances diminish sperm production. Some of these effects can be permanent even after ceasing the use of the drugs. The use of anabolic steroids is banned and is tested for in sports.

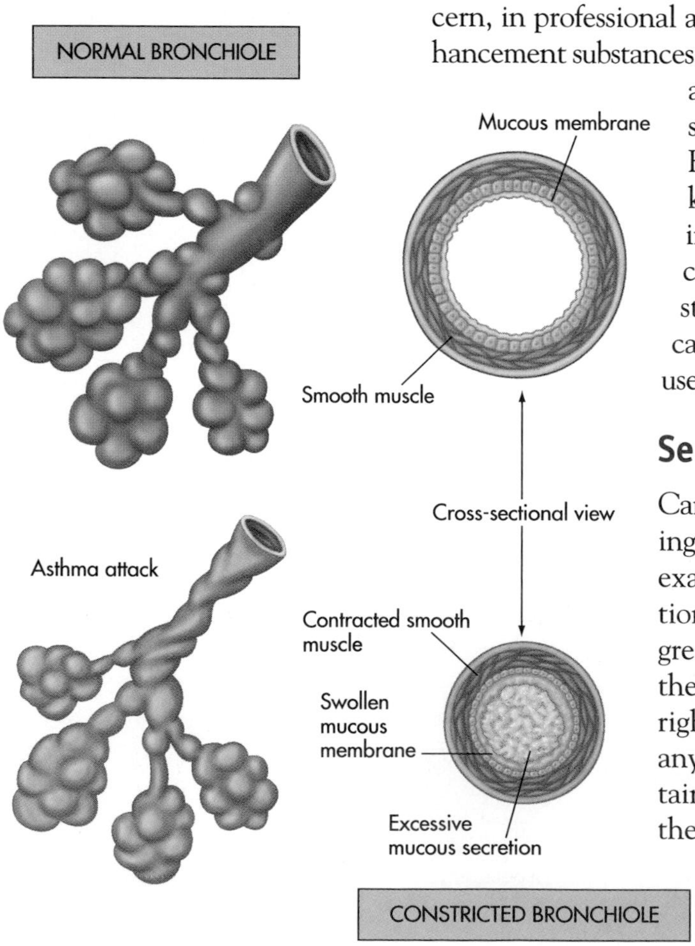

FIGURE ■ 18–6

The normal and constricted airway.

Sensory System

Care of the sensory system includes proper diet, wearing hearing and sight protective devices when necessary, and periodic examination of the eyes and ears. Wearing hearing protection during activities that produce high levels of noise will greatly extend the functional life of your hearing. Damage to the ear is cumulative, so there is no better time to start than right now. In addition, protective eyewear should be worn any time that the risk of eye injury can occur, such as in certain occupations, hobbies, and sports. Figure 18–8 ■ shows the Snellen Eye chart for determining visual acuity.

Immune System

Proper diet and exercise are needed for optimal functioning of the immune system. In addition, other factors can assist your immune system. One of the sim-

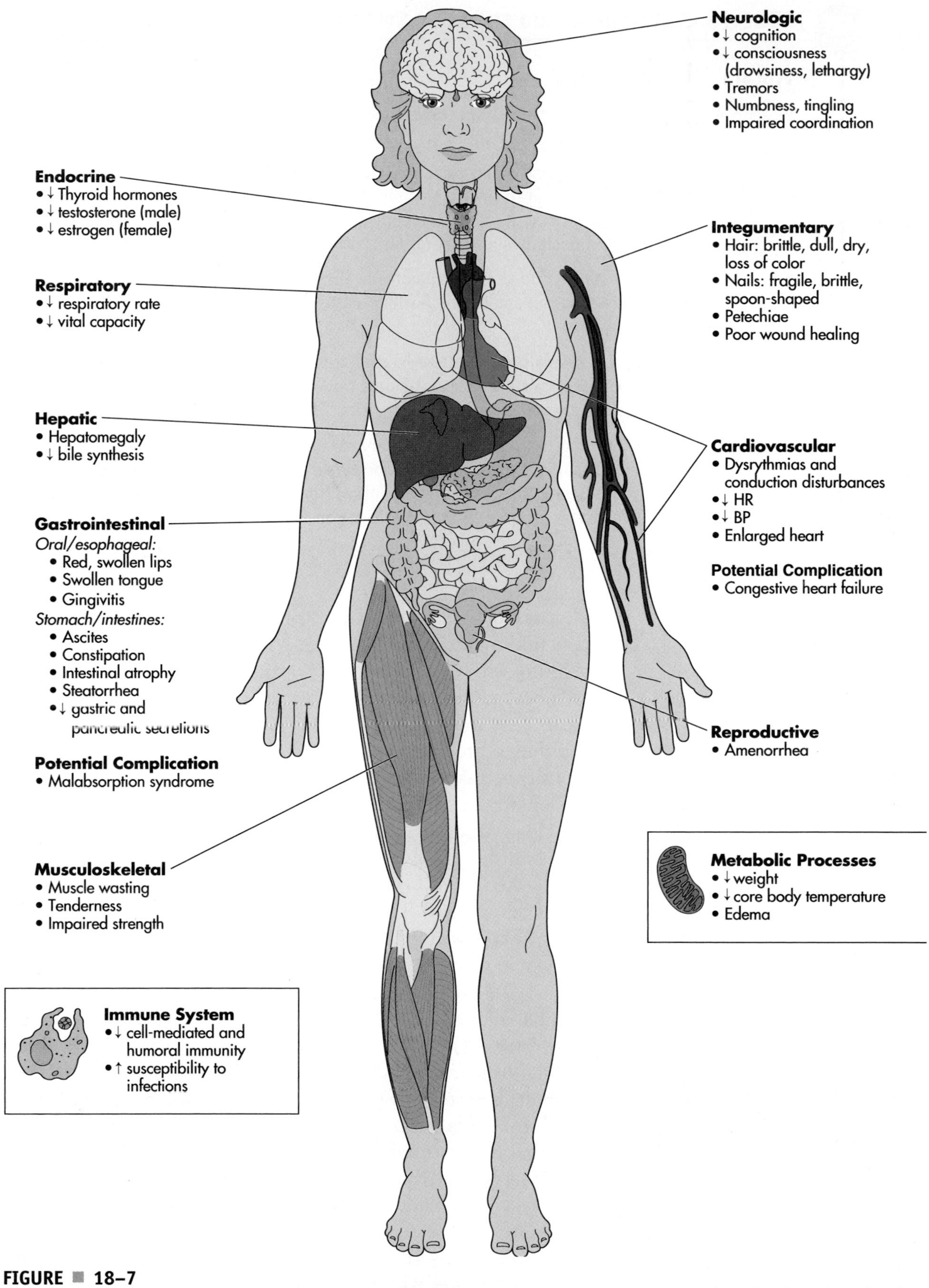
Neurologic
• ↓ cognition
• ↓ consciousness (drowsiness, lethargy)
• Tremors
• Numbness, tingling
• Impaired coordination
Endocrine
• ↓ Thyroid hormones
• ↓ testosterone (male)
• ↓ estrogen (female)
Integumentary
• Hair: brittle, dull, dry, loss of color
• Nails: fragile, brittle, spoon-shaped
• Petechiae
• Poor wound healing
Respiratory
• ↓ respiratory rate
• ↓ vital capacity
Hepatic
• Hepatomegaly
• ↓ bile synthesis
Cardiovascular
• Dysrythmias and conduction disturbances
• ↓ HR
• ↓ BP
• Enlarged heart
Potential Complication
• Congestive heart failure
Gastrointestinal
Oral/esophageal:
• Red, swollen lips
• Swollen tongue
• Gingivitis
Stomach/intestines:
• Ascites
• Constipation
• Intestinal atrophy
• Steatorrhea
• ↓ gastric and pancreatic secretions
Potential Complication
• Malabsorption syndrome
Reproductive
• Amenorrhea
Metabolic Processes
• ↓ weight
• ↓ core body temperature
• Edema
Musculoskeletal
• Muscle wasting
• Tenderness
• Impaired strength
Immune System
• ↓ cell-mediated and humoral immunity
• ↑ susceptibility to infections

FIGURE ■ 18–7

The effects of undernourishment on the body systems.

TABLE 18–1 Vitamins and the Body Systems

VITAMIN	DESCRIPTION
Vitamin A	proper night vision; proper development of bones and teeth; mucous membrane and epithelial cell integrity; helps resist infection
Vitamin B	B_2 promotes healthy muscular growth; B_{12} is needed for healthy blood cell development and to treat pernicious anemia; B_1 and B_{12} promote healthy function of nervous tissue; B_1 aids in carbohydrate metabolism, normal digestion, and appetite; niacin is necessary for fat synthesis and cellular respiration
Vitamin C	aids in absorption of iron; promotes healing of fractures, development of teeth and bone matrix, and wound healing; ensures capillary integrity; bolsters immune system
Vitamin D	promotes strong bones and teeth, regulates skeletal calcium reabsorption; aids in absorption of calcium and phosphorus from the intestinal tract; D_3 helps regulate release of parathyroid hormone
Vitamin E	promotes muscle growth; E_1 necessary for hemolytic resistance of red blood cell membranes; helps prevent anemia for proper reproductive system functioning; current research shows that consumption from *natural* sources may reduce the risk of Parkinson's disease; further investigation is needed
Vitamin K	needed for proper blood clotting

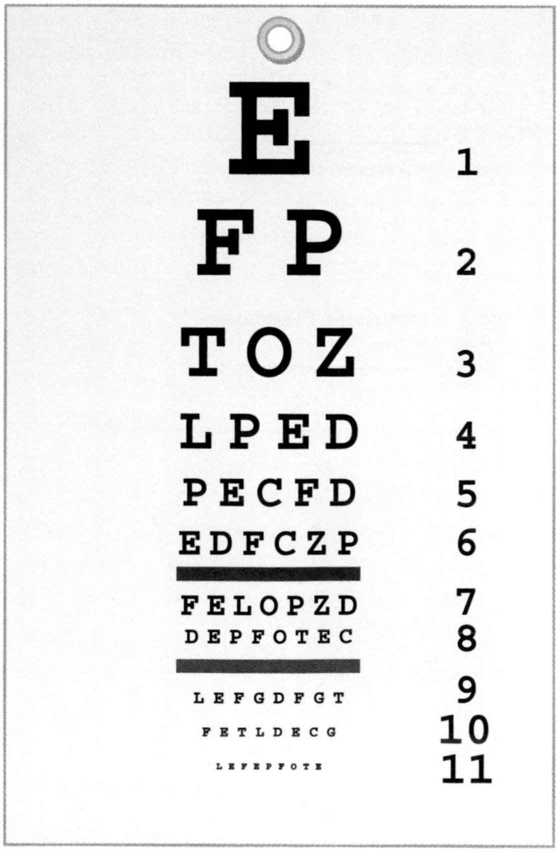

FIGURE ■ 18–8

The Snellen Eye Chart.

plest and most effective ways to protect not only yourself but your patients is hand-washing. Always wash your hands before and after working with each of your patients. Just because you are a staff member in a hospital or health care institution, you may still be a carrier of infectious organisms—in addition, you could be susceptible to becoming infected by hospital pathogens. As we previously discussed, correct washing of your hands goes a long way in stopping the spread of infection.

However, there is also another way to protect yourself and others from the spread of pathogens via body fluids, and this is accomplished by following the Universal Precautions Guidelines (see Figure 18–9 ■). These guidelines are standard precautions that are to be followed for every patient that you deal with.

Having current immunizations is important to assist the immune system in being prepared for certain pathogens. Immunization schedules are recommended by the Centers for Disease Control (CDC), the American Academy of Pediatrics (AAP), and the American Academy of Family Physicians (AAFP). Many individuals mistakenly believe immunizations only occur in childhood. Influenza vaccines are just one example of an immunization that is particularly important for the geriatric population.

A big issue is when and when not to take antibiotics. Most infections can be handled by the body's immune system in a few days. The overuse of antibiotics has led to several critical health issues. First, many viral infections are mistakenly treated with antibacterial agents, which do nothing to the virus and cause harm to normal bacteria such as in our intestinal system. Second, over-

Universal Precaution Guides

Procedure	Wash Hands	Gloves	Gown	Mask	Eyewear
Talking to patient					
Adjusting IV fluid rate or noninvasive equipment					
Assess patient without touching blood, body, fluids, mucous membranes	●				
Assess patient including contact with blood, body fluids, mucous membranes	●	●			
Drawing blood	●	●			
Inserting venous access	●	●			
Suctioning	●	●	If splattering is likely	If splattering is likely	If splattering is likely
Handling soiled waste, linen, other materials	●	●	If they are extensively soiled or splattering is likely	If they are extensively soiled or splattering is likely	If they are extensively soiled or splattering is likely
Intubation	●	●	●	●	●
Inserting arteriole access	●	●	●	●	●
Endoscopy	●	●	●	●	●
Operating and other procedures producing extensive splattering of blood or body fluids	●	●	●	●	●

FIGURE ■ 18–9

Universal Precaution Guides.

Applied Science

ANTIBIOTICS

The term antibiotics means "against life" and technically includes medications that inhibit or destroy any microorganism, including bacteria, viruses, and fungi. However, antibiotics in medicine has become associated only with antibacterial agents.

use does not allow the immune system of a child to properly develop and respond to future infections and can cause related disorders, such as asthma. Finally, many patients do not properly take their antibiotics. For example, they do not take the full dose for the full length of time but discontinue when they "feel better." However, often there are still surviving bacteria that are left that represent a stronger, drug-resistant strain, and they are now free to reproduce stronger drug-resistant offspring. This has led to small epidemics of drug-resistant infections.

Reproductive System

Don't smoke! Smoking mothers tend to have babies of lower birth weights, tendency toward premature births, and a higher rate of SIDS (sudden infant death syndrome). And while we're talking about babies and children, don't forget about the hazards of second-hand smoke in the home. In homes that have at least one smoking parent, kids have slower than normal lung development and are predisposed to increased incidences of bronchitis, asthma, and ear infections (otitis media).

18-6 To view videos on eating disorders such as anorexia and bulimia, please go to your CD-ROM for this chapter.

The physician's assistant is trained in the diagnoses and treatment of all the body systems. To learn more about this profession and to view a video, please go to the Web site for this chapter.

DIET

As the old saying goes, when you are pregnant you are now eating for two! This doesn't mean that mom should pig out at every chance she gets. What it means is that diets should be followed that provide important vitamins, minerals, and nutrients for the developing fetus and to maintain the health of the mother. Think about it. If the diet is lacking in calcium, where does the fetus get calcium for bone development? It has to take it from the bones and teeth of the mother, thus decreasing the integrity of her system. The congenital condition of **spina bifida** can be prevented by a dietary supplement of a member of the vitamin B complex, folic acid. The elimination of alcohol during pregnancy is also important to assure the best chances of normal spinal cord and nervous system development.

spina bifida *(SPY nah BIFF ih dah)*

SEXUALLY TRANSMITTED DISEASES (STDS)

STDs are a growing problem and can have serious effects on the reproductive system and lethal effects on the body. There are various types of diseases and organisms that can be transmitted through unprotected sex (including oral sex). Please see Table 18–2 for a list of sexually transmitted diseases.

CANCER PREVENTION AND TREATMENT

All the body systems can be ravaged by cancer. Cancer is the runaway reproduction and spreading of abnormal cells and is a very complicated disorder. Each type of cancer, named for the location or the type of cells that are running amok

TABLE 18–2 Sexually Transmitted Diseases

DISEASE	ORGANISM	SYMPTOMS
Herpes	Herpes simplex virus 2	Male: fluid-filled vesicles on penis
		Female: blisters in and around vagina
Gonorrhea	*Neisseria gonorrhoeae*	Male: purulent discharge from urethra, dysuria, and urinary frequency
		Female: purulent vaginal discharge, dysuria, urinary frequency, abnormal menstrual bleeding, abdominal tenderness; can lead to sterility
Chlamydia	*Chlamydia trachomatis*	May be asymptomatic
		Male: mucopurulent discharge from penis, burning and itching in genital area, dysuria, swollen testes; can lead to sterility
		Female: mucopurulent discharge from vagina, inflamed bladder, pelvic pain, inflamed cervix; can lead to sterility
Syphilis	*Treponema pallidum*	Systemic disease that can lead to lesions, lymph node enlargement, nervous system degradation, chancre sores
Genital Warts	Human papilloma virus (HPV)	Cauliflower-like growths on penis and vagina

herpes simplex virus 2 *(HER peez)*

neisseria gonorrhoeae *(nye SEE ree ah gon ah REE ah)*

chlamydia trachomatis *(klah MID ee ah TRAY koh mah tis)*

Treponema pallidum *(trep eh NEE ma PAL ih dum)*

human papilloma virus *(pap ih LOW ma)*

(for example, colon cancer, prostate cancer, squamous cell carcinoma), has its own unique characteristics. However, in the past few years, medical science has learned a number of things about cancer that have made great improvements in cancer prevention and treatment.

Any number of triggers can make a cell cancerous, including genes, radiation, sunlight exposure, smoking, fatty foods, viruses, and chemical exposure. Some of these triggers, like genes or some viruses, are difficult to avoid. But others, like smoking, sunlight, radiation exposure, and fatty foods, can be pretty easily avoided by eating right, avoiding smoking, and wearing sunscreen. Many types of cancer can be prevented or managed with a healthy diet and exercise. Even genetic susceptibility to cancer does not make cancer unavoidable. Testing, such as mammograms (for breast cancer), colonoscopy (for colon cancer), and Pap smears (for cervical cancer), can improve survival by catching cancers early, before they have spread, or even allowing the removal of abnormal cells before they become cancerous.

> 18-7 To view a video on AIDS, please go to your CD-ROM for this chapter.

Treatments for cancer typically involve removal of the cancerous cells, if possible, and some form of treatment to kill any cells remaining in the body. Chemotherapy is the treatment of cancer with chemicals that kill rapidly dividing cells. Radiation uses energy waves to shrink tumors. Biological or immunotherapy targets the cancer by manipulating the immune system to hunt down and kill the cancer cells. New treatments are constantly under development to treat cancers that are difficult to fight. Research has made great strides in the treatment of cancer.

Let's use the skin cancer, melanoma, as an example. Melanoma is the most deadly form of skin cancer. It is formed by the runaway reproduction of melanocytes, the pigment-forming cells of the skin. People at the highest risk of melanoma are those with fair skin and light eyes or hair, who have been exposed to lots of sun during their lifetime. However, new evidence indicates that even people who tan easily may develop melanoma if they get enough sun exposure. Melanoma risk is higher for those living near the equator, but people in the northern parts of the United States are not without risk. Exposure to sunlight, particularly sunburns, even as an adult, is the key risk factor for melanoma. Genetic factors are involved in some cases of melanoma.

Melanoma can be easily prevented by decreasing exposure to UV light. Aside from staying indoors all the time, which isn't very practical, sunscreen is the best way to protect yourself from melanoma. Individuals at risk should have a skin screening on a regular basis.

Standard treatment for melanoma in early stages (stage I, no spread) has been the "watch and wait" approach. The melanoma is removed, and the patient is monitored for several years. Patients with more advanced melanomas often have lymph nodes sampled and removed to prevent further spread. This more extensive surgery was deemed unnecessary for patients in very early-stage disease. However, a 2005 study has shown that even patients with no obvious spread of their cancer benefit from having lymph nodes sampled and removed if they contain cancer cells. Patients who had the procedure, called a sentinel lymph node mapping and biopsy, were 26 percent less likely to have their cancer return within 5 years than patients who only had the tumor removed. See Figure 18–10 ■ for the possible causes and warning signs of cancer.

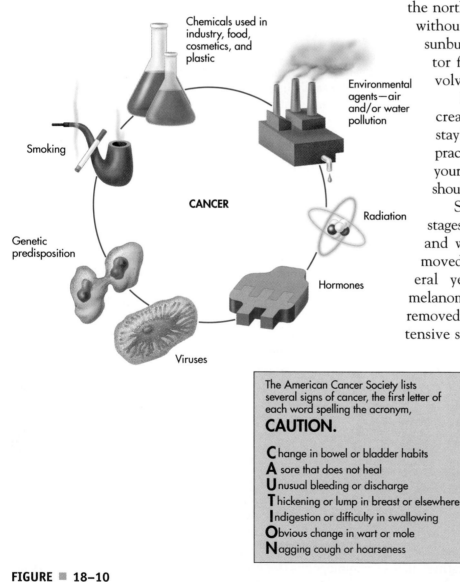

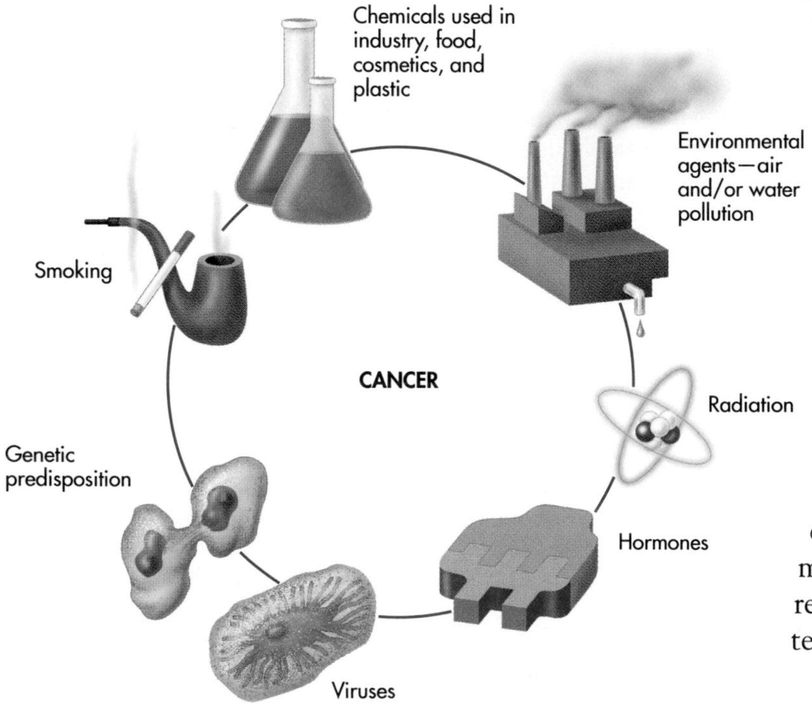

The American Cancer Society lists several signs of cancer, the first letter of each word spelling the acronym,

CAUTION.

Change in bowel or bladder habits
A sore that does not heal
Unusual bleeding or discharge
Thickening or lump in breast or elsewhere
Indigestion or difficulty in swallowing
Obvious change in wart or mole
Nagging cough or hoarseness

FIGURE ■ 18–10

Possible causes and warning signs of cancer.

TEST YOUR KNOWLEDGE 18-3

Choose the best answer:

1. This vitamin is needed for proper blood clotting:
   a. A
   b. B
   c. C
   d. K
2. The abuse of this substance can have side effects such as facial hair and deeper voices in women, kidney and liver damage, and aggressive behavior.
   a. antidepressants
   b. aspirin
   c. anabolic steroids
   d. chocolate
3. The ______________ eye chart is used to determine normal vision.
   a. Snellen
   b. Seymour
   c. See Clear
   d. Optical
4. The guidelines that help prevent the spread of disease by contact with body fluids are the
   a. barrier reef
   b. splash guard
   c. universal precautions
   d. body shield

MORE AMAZING FACTS

Remember those amazing facts we promised you at the beginning of the chapter? True to our word, here is a list of a few to amaze your friends and family.

- Senior citizens are more prone to food poisoning not only because of decreases in their senses of smell and taste but because their digestive juices are not as acidic as they used to be and so cannot always efficiently destroy all of the food-borne pathogens they ingest.
- Nerve impulses can travel up to 426 feet per second!
- Approximately 450,000 people die in the United States annually because of smoking-related diseases. That is about equivalent to a jumbo jet full of passengers crashing *each day with no survivors*.
- On average, a healthy kidney filters about *180 quarts of fluid* every day. What makes this amazing is that the kidney is only about 4 inches long, 2 inches wide, and 1 inch thick!
- Hair grows about a quarter inch each month and grows faster during the day than at night. Hair also grows faster in the summer than in the winter.
- You use a little over a half pint of oxygen each minute when you are at rest.
- Everyone has one nare that is larger than the other. If you don't believe it, take a look at people next time you go out to the mall or out to eat.
- Talk about a busy worker! Your heart beats over *36 million* times a year!
- You possess over *16,000 miles* of capillaries!
- Because viruses are continuously mutating, your immunity to influenza will not last a lifetime.

- More hair facts! You have from 110,000 to 150,000 hairs just on your head! Each strand of hair can support approximately 100 grams of weight, so, at least in theory, a full head of hair could support the weight of two African elephants!
- Vitamins, natural or in pill form, which is best? Research appears to indicate that vitamins and minerals from natural food sources are better utilized than synthetic pills. But the pills are better than nothing!
- The horns of a bull are composed of the same material that makes up your fingernails and toenails.
- You have about a quarter million sweat glands on your feet.
- Based on current research of fibroblasts' doubling ability before they can no longer accurately divide, we have the *potential* to live to 120 years of age.
- Your eyes can see approximately 7 *million* shades of color.
- Due to its sterile nature, urine can be used to clean out a wound when no antiseptic is available!
- The ability to roll your tongue into a tube is inherited, not everyone can do it (or cares to do it).
- Cavities and poor oral hygiene can lead to diabetes and heart attacks. In fact some health experts believe that daily flossing can add 6.4 years to your life! That's because bacteria that grows in the mouth of an individual with poor oral hygiene can escape into the bloodstream and travel throughout the body, causing problems. As a result, in worst-case scenarios, that individual may be at a four times greater risk for stroke and at a 14 times greater risk for heart attack. The risk for diabetes is also increased.
- Current research indicates that stomach cancer, which affects 24,000 Americans annually, may originate from bone marrow cells that enter the stomach to repair damage to the stomach lining.
- Walking uphill or downhill may make a difference in your desired health outcomes. A recent study showed that individuals who walked uphill cleared fats (especially triglycerides) from their blood faster, while downhill hiking reduced blood sugars more readily and improved glucose tolerance. Hiking either way removed LDL, or bad cholesterol. This information may be applicable for exercise regimens for diabetics who may have trouble with aerobic exercises.

anhidrosis *(an HIGH droe sis)*

- CIPA (congenital insensitivity to pain with **anhidrosis**) is a rare genetic disorder that affects the development of the small nerve fibers that transmit the sensations of pain, heat, and cold to the brain. There are only 17 cases known in the United States. Patients with this untreatable condition receive bruises without knowing they are hurt. Since these patients can't sense extreme cold or heat, they don't sweat! Biting through their tongue while eating is a distinct possibility.

SUMMARY SNAPSHOTS FROM THE JOURNEY

Snapshots from the Journey

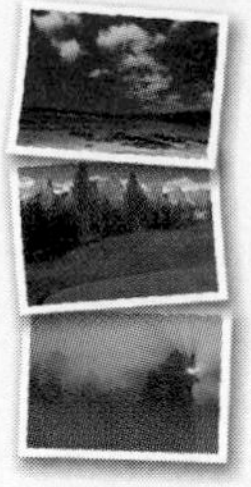

- Forensic science is the application of science to law. Natural sciences (including anatomy and physiology) and social sciences are used when solving crimes.
- Forensic science is not only used to solve current mysteries but has been used to solve ancient mysteries as well.
- The uniqueness of fingerprints were written about as early as the 1600s.
- DNA fingerprinting is a form of identifying individuals from small samples of body fluid or tissues.
- The geriatric population is the fasting growing population in the United States.
- The hallmark sign of aging is the decreased ability to maintain homeostasis.
- Our bodies don't age evenly, and certain systems age more rapidly than others.
- The loss of mental capacities is not directly related to aging until age 75, when it is still minimal unless disease is present.
- Due to changes in the gastrointestinal, renal, and hepatic systems, geriatric patients respond differently to many medications.
- Polypharmacy is the use of many drugs at the same time and often is the result of seeing many specialists at the same time.
- The most important personal choice you will make is a healthy lifestyle.
- To maintain a healthy lifestyle, it is important to eat properly, exercise, manage stress, and avoid bad habits.
- Some cancers, such as skin and lung cancer, can be highly preventable. Limiting the amount and intensity of sunlight exposure and not smoking are two ways that can help prevent cancer.

Case Study

Riga and Mortis Smith are suspects in the murder of their rich aunt. They are identical twins. Tissue samples taken from under the fingernails of the aunt reveal the DNA of the murderer. The police know that Riga and Mortis are identical twins and that one can only be the murderer because one has a rock-solid alibi with reliable witnesses—but the witnesses do not know which twin it was.

Will the DNA testing prove who the real murderer is?

What other crime-solving forensics can tell for sure who the real murderer is?

REVIEW QUESTIONS

Multiple Choice

1. The pelvic angle of the female is
   a. less than 90 degrees
   b. 100 degrees or greater
   c. 75 degrees
   d. greater than 180 degrees

2. From ages 20 to 70, there is up to a ______________ percent loss of lean body mass.
   a. 10
   b. 20
   c. 30
   d. 50

3. This vitamin is needed for strong bones and teeth and calcium absorption:
   a. A
   b. B
   c. C
   d. D

4. The overuse of this classification of drugs has caused drug-resistant strains of bacteria:
   a. steroids
   b. antibiotic
   c. diuretics
   d. pain killers

5. The congenital condition of spina bifida can be prevented by the addition of what vitamin during pregnancy?
   a. A
   b. folic acid
   c. niacin
   d. K

Fill in the Blank

1. The new food pyramid takes into account your ______________, ______________, and ______________ when determining the best diet for you.

2. The fat soluble vitamins are ______________, ______________, ______________, and ______________.

3. Cauliflower-like growths on the penis and vagina are ______________ ______________.

4. The test for cervical cancer is called the ______________ ______________.

Short Answer

1. Discuss various ways to prevent skin cancer.

____

____

____

____

2. List and discuss way to prevent STDs.

3. Discuss ways to protect yourself and your patient from the spread of infection.

4. Discuss ways that forensic science can be used in solving crimes.

Suggested Activities

1. Discuss the various aging processes you have seen in your parents and grandparents.

2. Be old for a day by changing your senses. This can be experienced by covering your eyes or your glasses with clear plastic wrap. Wear thin cotton gloves or surgical gloves (if you are not allergic to latex). Gently plug your ears with cotton balls (not cotton swabs). During the next class period, discuss the difficulties you had doing simple, everyday activities.

3. List the foods you've eaten for three days. Share the list with your classmates and determine whether or not it is a healthy diet. Discuss ways to improve it.

4. Make poster presentations on one of the following topics or choose your own: STDs, passive smoking, hazards of smoking, healthy lifestyles, forensic science, aging process, proper diet, healthy pregnancy.

18-8

Now that you have completed your journey through this chapter, please go to the CD-ROM for interactive games and puzzles concerning the medical terms and concepts contained in this chapter. By playing the games you will reinforce your learning of medical terminology in a fun way.

Greetings from

THE STUDY SUCCESS *Companion*

The Key to Your Successful Journey

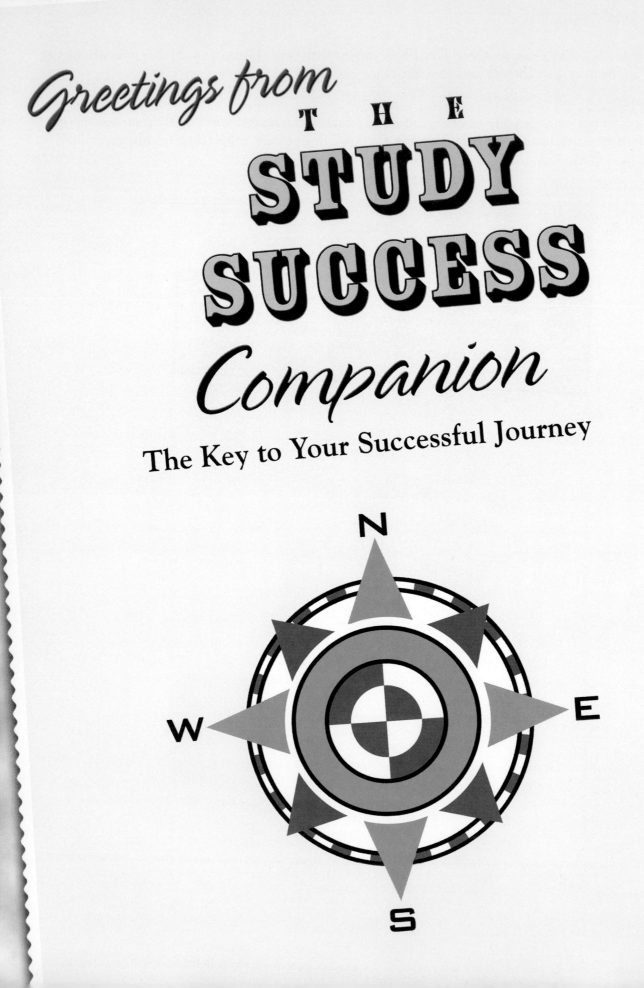

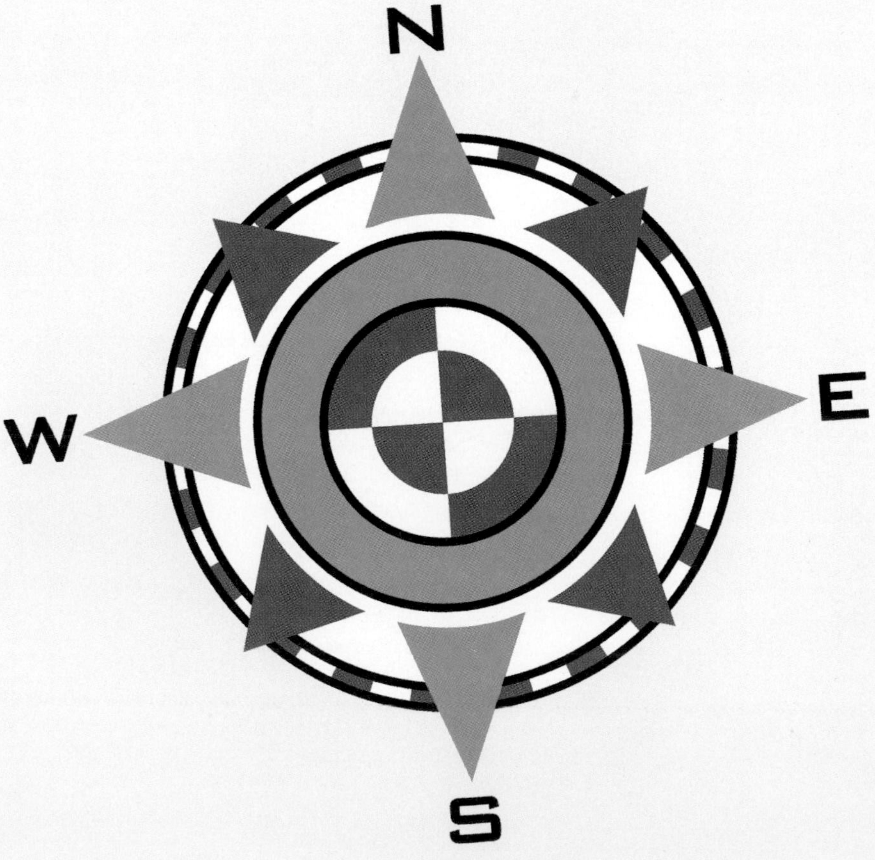

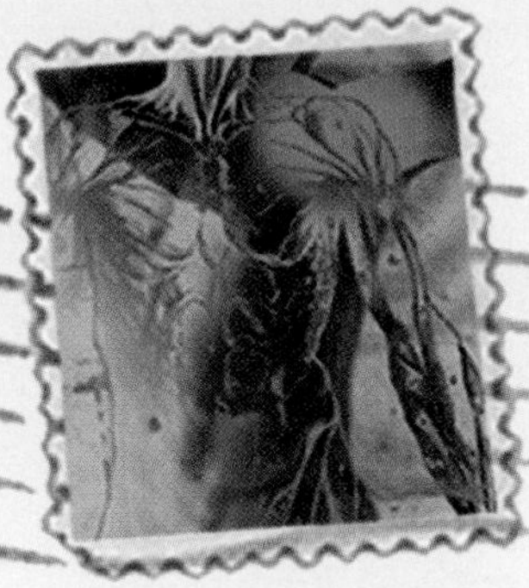

WHY USE THIS STUDY SUCCESS COMPANION?

On any journey, a well written travel guide can make the experience positive, less stressful, and more productive. This is the main reason for including this guide along with your textbook.

Anatomy and Physiology (A&P) can be a tough course to navigate. Students interested in the health professions who are taking an Anatomy and Physiology course may feel like this is a very long and arduous journey. In reality, this should be a very fascinating journey, for the human body is the vehicle in which we will all travel through life. This guide is devoted to helping you make the most of this journey.

Effective study strategies will be given, along with a simple and effective stress management system to help you through the rough parts of this journey and even throughout the rest of your life. In addition, this guide will help with "need to know concepts" such as the metric system which is usually not covered in an A&P course due to time constraints. However, knowing the metric system is critical because it is the mathematical language of Anatomy and Physiology and of medicine in general. Besides, every other country in the world uses the metric system and we do want you to have an international education!

In summary, the *Study Success Companion* covers the following areas:

- Study Skills
- Stress Management
- The Metric System

"The difference between ordinary and extraordinary is that little ***extra.***"
Author unknown

STUDY SKILLS

While you may have had courses on study skills, it can never hurt to review the fundamentals. We have chosen the top three general study skills we feel are critical, not just for Anatomy and Physiology, but for all the current and future courses you will ever take. And the top three choices are:

Clinical Application

CLASSICAL CONDITIONING

Throughout the textbook you will notice instances of the mind-body connection. The psychological term *classical conditioning* illustrates this concept and actually has impact upon study skills. The term came from an experiment performed on dogs by the Russian scientist, Ivan Pavlov. In this experiment, a bell was rung and dogs were then fed meat. The meat stimulated the dogs to salivate in anticipation of beginning the digestive process. Repeatedly, experimenters would ring a bell and feed the dogs. The dogs soon learned to connect the ringing of the bell to the arrival of meat. Eventually, the scientists only had to ring a bell and the dogs would salivate like crazy, even if they didn't receive meat.

So what's the purpose of telling you this story other than making you hungry or grossing you out? When you study in bed and then go to sleep repeatedly, you soon connect studying to sleeping. Every time you begin to study (even in mid-afternoon), you may begin to yawn and not be focused. You are conditioning yourself to connect studying to sleeping. Simply avoid studying in bed because you will not be as focused and therefore less effective. Besides, studying in bed may interfere with your ability to get a good night's sleep. Classical conditioning can also be used to your advantage in health care. Repeated, positive interactions and therapies with clients will "classically condition" them to feel good each time they see you.

1. Select a Good Time and Place to Study

As with any trip, there is NO substitute for good planning and preparation. Successful preparation includes developing a daily schedule that includes proper study time. Don't be discouraged if your first few schedules don't work well; just make sure to build in some flexibility. Be sure to schedule relaxation and recreational time, as these are important. Studies show that you learn more in three 30 minute sessions than in one marathon 2 hour session. Therefore, studying notes over shorter periods of time at more frequent intervals is more effective than long cramming sessions. We suggest using 30–45 minutes as your *maximum* study time without a break. A good way to check if you are studying efficiently is to periodically ask yourself questions about what you have just read. If you can't answer these questions, you probably are losing interest and need to take a short break and become more focused.

The actual time of day you choose to study is very important. It may not be the same time for everyone. Some people are "morning people" while others are not. We all have different biological clocks, and this physiologic concept is elaborated upon in the endocrine system. The message for now is to schedule study times when you are most alert and focused.

The place you choose to study is also very important. Ideally, it should be the same place each time so you "connect" this place to studying and consequently become focused. It should have minimal or no distractions and good lighting. The table or desk should have the needed study tools such as pen, paper, calculator, computer, etc.

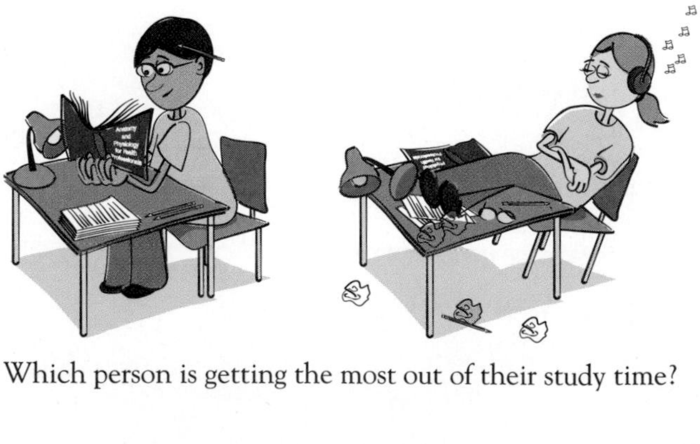

Which person is getting the most out of their study time?

TEST YOUR KNOWLEDGE 1

Assess your current place of study by answering the following questions. Be critical and honestly circle the response that best answers the question.

1. Do you have a dedicated study area?
   a. Sometimes
   b. Always
   c. Rarely
2. Is it quiet where you study?
   a. Sometimes
   b. Always
   c. Rarely
3. Are the conditions and lighting comfortable?
   a. Sometimes
   b. Always
   c. Rarely
4. Do you have all the tools (pencils, paper, electronic tools, etc.) you need to study at this place?
   a. Sometimes
   b. Always
   c. Rarely

How well did you do? For now, it doesn't matter as long as you were honest. Remember, this is an assessment of where you are now. Your eventual goal should be to have all your responses be "Always." If they are now—great! If not, you need to develop an action plan to make all the responses "Always" in the near future.

2. Use Good Study Habits

Take good, accurate, legible notes. Remember that the purpose of taking notes is to get key points from textbooks and lectures and not to write down every word that is said or written. Instead of highlighting the chapter, outline your chapters so you can make the connection from your brain to the pencil. This is what you'll need to do on the test. Outlining may *initially* take longer than highlighting, but you will learn the material better. Outlining will actually save you studying time in the long run. Review your lecture and outline notes frequently.

Also, make diagrams and pictures to help visualize concepts within your outline. The more you can "see it" the better you can understand relationships or how it all fits together. Use the Web and CD visualizations to help reinforce the concepts in your mind's eye.

Anatomy and Physiology is a great subject to study with a friend or study group. An excellent method to help truly learn the material is to explain concepts to each other. Each time you explain something, the oral recitation reinforces your understanding. *You'll soon learn that there is no better way to learn something than to teach it to someone else.*

Applied Science

HOW WE LEARN

A quick generalization of learning theory is as follows:

WE LEARN:
10% of what we read
20% of what we hear
30% of what we see
50% of what we both see and hear
70% of what is discussed with others
80% of what we experience
95% of what we TEACH to someone else

While some may argue the percentages, the general concepts are true to what the research on learning has shown. The more senses you can get involved in the learning process the more internalized the learning becomes. Therefore, the text illustrations and the CD and Web site animations and videos enhance the learning process. Lab experiences and interactive games and exercises will also increase learning. Group or study discussions are highly beneficial and if you have to teach the group your concept, you will really learn what it is all about.

Clinical Application

AIDING YOUR MEMORY

To succeed, it is important to truly "learn" the material and use critical thinking and problem-solving skills. One who knows how to obtain information and understand it, is much better off than someone who merely memorizes for short term storage.

Say, for example, you memorize the steps to cardio-pulmonary resuscitation (CPR) but you truly don't understand why you need to establish an open airway, or even how to actually do it. You may be able to repeat the steps on a pen and paper test and receive a good grade, but what if, in 6 months, you are in a situation where you need to perform CPR on an individual in need? You don't want to say, "I had that six months ago and I really didn't learn the material."

While the purpose of education is to encourage thinking skills rather than memorization, you do have to recognize that memory is vital. Memory is used as an index of success because most of the techniques used to measure learning rely on it. Therefore, a good memory is an asset that you should definitely develop. Try to memorize only when you are well rested. Also, use memorization techniques such as the use of mnemonics. Mnemonics are words, rhymes, or formulas that aid your memory. Acronyms are one type of mnemonics. An acronym is a word made from the first letters of other words. For example, the ABC's of CPR remind you that **A** = establish **A**irway, **B** = rescue **B**reathing, and **C** = establish **C**irculation. This helps you to better remember the steps and their proper order in a critical situation.

You can also use rhymes or formulas to assist your memory. For example, "spring forward, fall back", helps us to adjust our clocks accordingly for daylight savings time. You can also make up silly stories to help remember facts. In fact, often, the sillier the story, the easier it is to remember.

Other good study habits include taking personal responsibility for your success. Go to class and read the assigned readings *prior* to class. This will also help you to begin to develop professional responsibility skills that are crucial in health care. Good study habits will greatly reduce the test anxiety you may feel because you will have properly prepared. However, it is normal to have some anxiety about taking an exam no matter how well you have prepared.

Here are some other hints on test taking that may help to further reduce the anxiety and increase your performance. Know what type of test you are taking. With an objective exam (multiple choice, true/false) be sure you understand all directions first. With objective exams, usually your first idea about the answer is your best. If it is an essay exam (short answer), survey the questions, plan your time, and give time to questions in proportion to their value.

Some people develop their own test taking strategies. For example, they may do all the easy questions first and then return to the more difficult ones. Make sure you mark the questions you skipped or you may forget to return to them. Finally, do not destroy your old exams—keep them and learn from them!

3. Take Care of Yourself

Learning requires a healthy mind, body, and attitude. It is important to exercise your brain to stay mentally fit, but it is also important to stay physically fit. A poor physical condition can distract the mind and minimize your mental focus. Eating right, exercising several times a week, and staying free of drugs will make you feel better and enhance your ability to learn. There may be times you must study when sick or tired. Begin these study sessions with slow rhythmic breathing. This can help you relax and, in turn, your concentration may improve. Remember to get sufficient rest, especially before exams. Learning to manage your stress level is so important to both your mental and physical fitness that the next section is devoted to this topic. Taking time for hobbies, music, or doing things you like to do is important to help refresh your mind.

TEST YOUR KNOWLEDGE 2

A portion of Chapter 18, the final chapter in your textbook, will be devoted to proper exercise, nutrition, and healthy living habits. However, for now, circle the answer to the following general questions and make an action plan for each "yes" answer.

1. Do you feel tired during the day when studying?
   a. Yes
   b. No
2. Do you take any mood altering drugs? Remember alcohol and cigarettes are included in this category.
   a. Yes
   b. No
3. Do you skip your exercise sessions during the week?
   a. Yes
   b. No
4. Do you eat a diet that is heavy in fats and "junk food?"
   a. Yes
   b. No

STRESS MANAGEMENT

Stress Misconceptions

The major misconception about stress is that all stress is bad for you. This is certainly not true. As you are reading this text, your body is probably in a room that is between 20 and 25 degrees centigrade. This may feel comfortable to you, but it is actually causing stress within your body. In order to survive, the body must maintain a core temperature of around 36 degrees centigrade and therefore it is continually working on a level we are not consciously aware of to sense and adapt to an externally stressful environment. This response is vital and needed for our survival.

Here is another example of good stress: in the nervous system chapter you learn about the sympathetic system and the fight or flight response in more detail. Picture for a moment the first time you are called upon to do CPR on a cardiac arrest victim. This is going to be a stressful event in your life and may stimulate your sympathetic nervous system. Even though you practiced and trained hard, you are still uncertain of how it will be in a real life-and-death situation. This is normal. Your physical and psychological symptoms may include:

- increased adrenalin levels for more energy to perform better
- faster heart rate (**tachycardia**) to supply more oxygen to muscles
- increased blood pressure to get more blood flow to the brain
- pupil dilation to bring in more light to see better
- faster breathing (**tachypnea**) to bring in more oxygen
- heightened state of awareness to focus on the job at hand
- mild level of anxiety to keep you sharp and not take the situation too lightly

These can all be helpful reactions that enhance your performance. However, they can go too far and lead to a "bad stress" situation where you can't perform at your peak level. Therefore, you can have "good stress" and "bad stress." The key, again, is balance or moderation. A little stress will get you "up" for the task at hand. However, if you let stress get out of hand and panic, you now have bad stress and your anxiety level rises to the point where you perform poorly or may be even not at all.

Applied Science

TEST YOURSELF—HOW MANY STRESS SIGNALS DO YOU HAVE?

How many of the following signals do you have on a regular basis (once every week or two)? If you checked 2 or less signals, you're doing pretty good and need minor improvement. Three or more means you need to work hard on how you're handling stress.

_____ Headaches
_____ Shortness of breath
_____ Fast or irregular pulse
_____ Nausea
_____ Insomnia
_____ Difficulty eating
_____ Sadness
_____ Chronic fatigue
_____ Irritability
_____ Diarrhea
_____ Feeling overwhelmed
_____ Difficulty concentrating
_____ Neck or back pain

What Causes Physical and Emotional Stress?

To be able to manage and harness stress to your advantage, you must first understand what stress is all about. First, it is important to realize that no situation or event by itself causes us stress. Rather it is how we "perceive" a situation that causes stress. It is our learned, internal response to external stimuli.

For example, two individuals can volunteer to give blood. They will both undergo the same procedure with the same technician in the same environment. Yet one individual may not feel any stress or anxiety and the other may be highly stressed at the thought of giving blood. Stress occurs as a result of how we *interpret* and *react* to a situation or event. It can be either positive or negative depending on our reaction.

Stress can have many definitions. For now, we will define **stress** as "how our mind and body react to an environment that is largely shaped by our perceptions of an event or situation." Notice that mind and body connection. Have you ever heard any of the following sayings?

I lost my breath.
My heart was pounding.
My brain is fried.
My stomach was twisted in knots.

Clinical Application

SADNESS VERSUS DEPRESSION

It's important to differentiate between depression and sadness. If someone is sad following a painful disappointment or the loss of a loved one, this is a normal part of the grieving process. However, if the sadness remains for a prolonged period of time and interferes with the ability to go about your daily business, it becomes depression.

Stress can also relate to time. We all have temporary stressors in our lives. However, when a stressor becomes constant and negative it has serious effects upon our body and mind. Continual or constant negative stress can lead to:

- high blood pressure, heart attack, or stroke
- stomach ulcers
- lack of sleep, or insomnia
- decreased immune system functioning
- depression and personality changes
- poor academic and job performance

However, good or positive stress can actually help us to perform better. Indeed, any time you try something new or meet a new challenge, stress can be a powerful friend. This is how we grow and develop. Continual uncontrolled negative stress will exact a price on our minds and bodies. So the key is learning how to maintain good stress in your life and avoid bad stress.

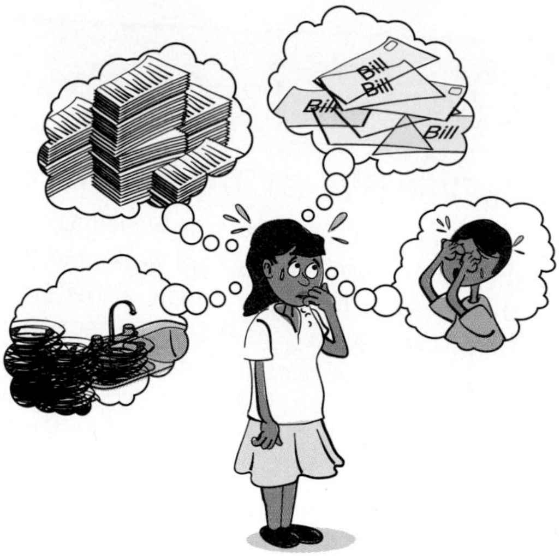

A Stress Management System

The first step in treating a patient is good assessment. This is also the first step in a good personal stress management system. First, recognizing your own stressors and the symptoms they cause can help you determine when your stress is out of balance or, in other words, when you have entered your bad stress zone. These signals can be valuable to your good health and positive attitude. They represent a "wake up call" that says you need to cope with what's going on in your life before it overtakes you.

As already stated, a certain amount of stress is normal. We need it to develop and grow. This good stress can make you feel energized, focused, and "up" for the event: so you can ace your Anatomy and Physiology exams, for example. However, going beyond your good stress zone and "losing it" by entering your bad stress zone can be harmful. You need to determine when you are losing balance. The best way is to look for physical and emotional signs or indicators that the stress is too much. See Table 1 for some physical and emotional changes that signal too much stress.

Looking at the list of stress signs should paint a pretty good visual picture of what high levels of stress can cause. It's no wonder that individuals who can't handle stress have more accidents, poorer attendance, and are unable to study and learn.

TABLE 1 Physical and Emotional Signs of Stress

PHYSICAL CHANGES	EMOTIONAL CHANGES
headaches	lack of concentration
shortness of breath (SOB)	irritability
increased pulse rate (tachycardia)	hopeless feelings
nausea	mood swings
insomnia	overreaction
fatigue	depression
neck or back pain	eating disorders
dermatological problems (acne)	anxiety
chronic constipation/diarrhea	low self image

Clinical Application

PREVENTIVE MEDICINE AND EARLY INTERVENTION

In recent years preventive medicine has gained much focus versus the traditional Disease Model where we *waited* until the individual got sick and then treated them. The signals in the previous table are all late signals that mean you have been in your bad stress zone for quite some time. If you can pick up earlier signals and perform a healthy intervention, you can prevent many of these from happening. One hint is that nervous habits such as biting fingernails, pulling your hair, shaking your leg, clicking your pen, etc. are early signs you have just entered your bad stress zone. If you intervene then and there you can prevent more serious problems. This awareness is often difficult because many of these habits are so automatic that we aren't aware of them. So, if you catch yourself shaking your leg and intervene, you can prevent the subsequent muscle tightness, upset stomach, and headache from occurring.

Effective Coping Strategies

Remember, the most important aspect of stress is that it is individually determined. Its meaning lies within us. Therefore, we are the ones to determine what is stressful and whether we are going to use stress to our advantage or let it use us. It should logically follow, if WE determine the level of stress, WE should be able to control it.

Someone once said you don't get ulcers from what you eat, but rather from what's eating you. It's important to cope with stress before you suffer from stress overload or burnout. There are two basic ways you can cope with stress. The first is to effectively cope with the emotional side of stress. The second way is to deal with its physical side. Keep in mind the key is to recognize when you are stressed out and intervene as early as possible.

Effective Physical Strategies

You can't separate the mind and body. If we mentally feel bad it affects our physical well-being. If we don't take care of our physical bodies, we lack energy and focus, can't sleep, and do not reach our full intellectual potential. Therefore, you must balance emotional and physical strategies. Indeed, you'll see that some of these techniques help both our physical and emotional health.

Let's discuss some of the major points you should consider in reducing physical stress. Handling stress "physically" can be broken down into the following four areas:

- Rest and leisure
- Exercise
- Nutrition
- Relaxation techniques

REST AND LEISURE

Adequate sleep is a must for us to function at our peak and handle stress. Research has shown that lack of sleep (sleep deprivation) makes you more susceptible to illness. Of course, lack of sleep also makes you more irritable and less able to focus. Experts recommend that most adults get between seven and nine hours of sleep a night.

Taking leisure time for yourself can also help restore your ability to deal with stress. Even if that leisure time is only fifteen minutes, it can help greatly. Sometimes the more you focus on a major problem, the more stress it causes. When this happens it is good to take a break and get away from the problem by doing something else. In many cases, the solution will then just come to you as if by magic. It's not magic, just your subconscious mind working for you.

EXERCISE

Physical exercise and sports are a great way to work off the tensions of everyday life. If done properly they help you to gain both a physical and mental focus. Any type of aerobic activity which gets your heart beating will exercise your muscles and relieve mental tension. Vigorous walking, jogging, running, bicycling, and lifting weights are all things you can do by yourself. Of course, you can find a good workout partner or play team sports also. Vigorous exercise also releases a group of hormones known as endorphins. These are our body's natural painkillers. They also are mood elevating chemicals that give us a healthy, natural high.

Remember to properly warm up and stretch before any vigorous exercise. This not only helps prevent injuries, but stretching helps to relieve muscular tension and lower blood pressure. Never rush through the stretches by bouncing or using fast, jerky movements that could strain or tear muscles. Stretch slowly until you feel mild tension and then hold the position for 10 to 30 seconds.

NUTRITION

Good nutrition is a must for our growth and development. It also aids us in fighting off stress and disease. In addition, it is a good idea to drink plenty of water. Water makes up the majority of the body. Water aids in digestion, absorption of nutrients, and removal of waste products. While water is found in most foods, you should drink 6–8 glasses each day for good health.

Cut down on caffeine which is found in coffee, tea, and many sodas. Caffeine is a potent central nervous system stimulant. Large amounts can make you anxious, nervous, and unable to get a good night's sleep. Eating a well balanced diet in moderation is important in maintaining nutritional health.

RELAXATION TECHNIQUES

Practicing relaxation techniques will help to clear your mind and make you sharper. Most people will find a million excuses why they can't take the time to relax. Do you see the illogical thinking? If they are *that busy*, then they need to take the time to relax and restore the body and mind. This time also allows you to listen to your body. Two types of relaxation techniques that are very effective are breathing relaxation and meditation.

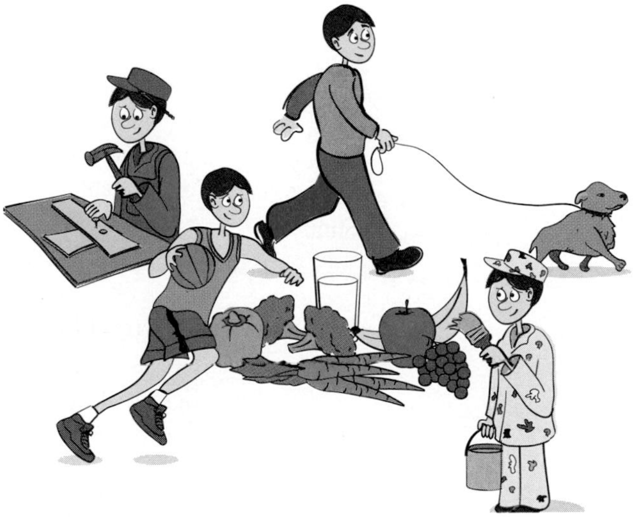

Slow, deep breathing serves several purposes. First, it increases oxygen to your brain and your body. It also slows down your thinking to help clear your head and relax your muscles.

Finally, don't forget to have a good laugh. The average four-year-old laughs every few minutes. Laughter helps bring you back in to perspective and besides, it feels good. Laughter also helps you physically by lowering blood pressure, releasing endorphins, and stimulating the pleasure centers of the brain. Table 2 lists some dos and don'ts, when stress is getting the better of you.

TABLE 2 The Dos and Don'ts of Stress Management

DO	DON'T
appropriately confront a problem	think it will resolve itself
discuss calmly	fight or yell
exercise	be a couch potato
accept responsibility	blame others
use relaxation techniques	use alcohol or drugs
accept/learn from your mistakes	be perfectionistic
follow good nutrition	over- or under-eat
be concerned and take action	worry and do nothing
live in the present	agonize over past or future
help others	avoid people

THE MATHEMATICAL LANGUAGE OF ANATOMY & PHYSIOLOGY AND MEDICINE

Why Learn the Metric System?

Whereas medical terminology represents the written and spoken language for understanding Anatomy and Physiology, the metric system is the "mathematical language" of Anatomy and Physiology. For example, blood pressure is measured in millimeters of mercury (mm Hg) and organ size is usually measured in centimeters (cm). Medications and fluids are given in milliliters (ml) or cubic centimeters (cc) and weight is often measured in kilograms (kg). What exactly does it mean when you are taught that normal cardiac output is 6 liters per minute? You can now see why one must be familiar with the metric system in order to truly understand A&P and medicine.

> **Learning Hint**
>
> Try to visualize the physical comparison between the metric and English system. For example, a meter is a little more than a yard and a liter is a little more than a quart. So a normal cardiac output of 6 liters per minute means that the heart is pumping out approximately 6 quarts of blood every minute.

In addition, you must be able to perform calculations to properly treat patients. For example, a particular drug may be ordered to be given at 5 milligrams/kilogram of body weight. In order to find the right amount to administer, you must first be able to convert the patient's body weight in pounds to kilograms. While it may seem complicated, it really isn't if you have a basic understanding of the following concepts:

- Exponential Powers of 10
- Systems of Measurement; in particular, the Metric System

Exponential Powers of Ten

The **Metric System of Measurement** is based upon the power of 10. Therefore, understanding the powers of 10 gives us a thorough knowledge of the base upon which the metric system is built.

To understand the powers of 10, we need to review some terminology. Consider the expression $\mathbf{b^n}$, where **b** is called the **base** and **n** the **exponent.** The **n** represents the number of times that **b** is multiplied by itself. See Figure 1 ■.

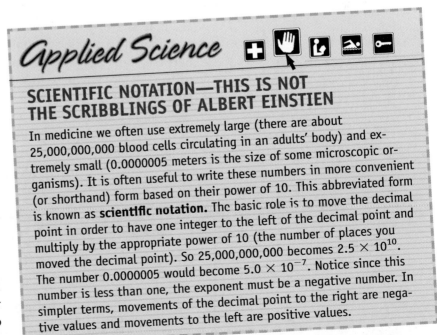

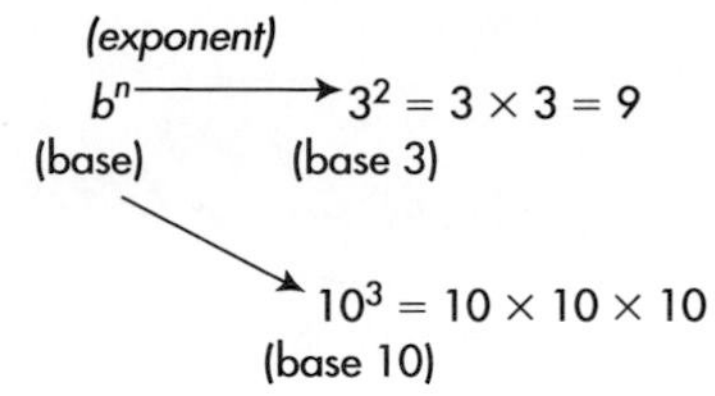

FIGURE ■ 1

The Exponential Expression

If we use 10 as the base we can develop an exponential representation of the powers of ten as follows:

$10^0 = 1$ (mathematically, any number that has an exponent of 0 = 1)
$10^1 = 10$
$10^2 = 10 \times 10 = 100$
$10^3 = 10 \times 10 \times 10 = 1{,}000$
$10^4 = 10 \times 10 \times 10 \times 10 = 10{,}000$
$10^5 = 10 \times 10 \times 10 \times 10 \times 10 = 100{,}000$
$10^6 = 10 \times 10 \times 10 \times 10 \times 10 \times 10 = 1{,}000{,}000$

Thus far, we have discussed positive exponents which result in numbers equal to or greater than 1. However, numbers that are less than one can also be represented in exponential notation. In this case we will use negative exponents. A negative exponent can be thought of as a fraction. For example,

$10^{-1} - 1/10 - .1$
$10^{-2} = 1/10 \times 1/10 = .01$
$10^{-3} = 1/10 \times 1/10 \times 1/10 = .001$
$10^{-4} = 1/10 \times 1/10 \times 1/10 \times 1/10 = .0001$
$10^{-5} = 1/10 \times 1/10 \times 1/10 \times 1/10 \times 1/10 = .00001$
$10^{-6} = 1/10 \times 1/10 \times 1/10 \times 1/10 \times 1/10 \times 1/10 = .000001$

Systems of Measurement

There are two major systems of measurement in our world today. The United States Customary System (USCS) is used in the United States and Myanmar (formerly Burma) and the System International (SI) is used everywhere else and especially in health care. The SI system is also known as the International or **Metric System.** The metric system is also the system used by drug manufacturers.

Applied Science

SCIENTIFIC NOTATION—THIS IS NOT THE SCRIBBLINGS OF ALBERT EINSTIEN

In medicine we often use extremely large (there are about 25,000,000,000 blood cells circulating in an adults' body) and extremely small (0.0000005 meters is the size of some microscopic organisms). It is often useful to write these numbers in more convenient (or shorthand) form based on their power of 10. This abbreviated form is known as **scientific notation.** The basic role is to move the decimal point in order to have one integer to the left of the decimal point and multiply by the appropriate power of 10 (the number of places you moved the decimal point). So 25,000,000,000 becomes 2.5×10^{10}. The number 0.0000005 would become 5.0×10^{-7}. Notice since this number is less than one, the exponent must be a negative number. In simpler terms, movements of the decimal point to the right are negative values and movements to the left are positive values.

Applied Science

The Apothecary System developed in the 1700's still has measurements used today. For example, the pint, quart, and gallon were derived from this system. Apothecary measurements for calculating liquid doses of drugs include the minim and fluid dram. Solids are measured in grams, scruples, drams, ounces, and pounds. Two unique features of the apothecary system are the use of Roman numerals and placement of the unit of measure before the Roman numeral. However, the metric system is now used to calculate drug dosages, since the apothecary system is less precise.

The USCS system is based on the British Imperial System and uses several different designations for the basic units of length, weight, and volume. We commonly call this the **English System.** For example, in the English system volumes can be expressed as ounces, pints, quarts, gallons, pecks, bushels, or cubic feet. Distance can be expressed in inches, feet, yards, and miles. Weights are measured in ounces, pounds and tons. This may be the system you are most familiar with, but it is not the system of choice used throughout the world nor within the medical profession. The reason is the English system is very cumbersome to use because it has no common base. It is very difficult to know the relationship between each of these units because they are not based, in an orderly fashion, according to the powers of 10 as in the metric system. For example, how many pecks are in a gallon? Just what is a peck? How many inches are in a mile? These all require extensive calculations and memorization of certain equivalent values, whereas in the metric system you simply move the decimal point the appropriate power of 10.

Most scientific and medical measurements utilize what is commonly referred to as the metric system. The metric system utilizes three basic units of measure for lengths, volume, and mass and these are the **meter, liter,** and **gram** respectively. While the term "mass" is commonly used for weight, weight is actually the force exerted on a body by gravity. In space, or zero gravity, all objects have mass but are indeed weightless. Since current health care is confined to earthly gravitational forces, we will use the term "weight." Table 3 gives you the metric designation for the three basic units of measure, along with an approximate English system comparison.

Again, notice that there are only three basic types of measures (meter, liter, and gram) and the metric system has only one base unit per measure. Because the metric system is a base 10 system, prefixes are used to indicate different powers of 10. Conversion within the metric system is done by simply moving the decimal point in the appropriate direction by the power of ten according to the prefix before the unit of measure. For example, the prefix kilo means 1000× or 10^3. Therefore, one kilogram is equal to 1000 grams. See Table 4 for the common prefixes and their respective powers of 10.

TABLE 3 Metric and English System Comparison

TYPE	UNIT	ENGLISH SYSTEM COMPARISON (APPROXIMATE SIZE)
length	meter	slightly more than a yard
volume	liter	slightly more than 1 quart
mass/weight	gram	about 1/40 of an ounce

TABLE 4 Common Prefixes of the Metric System

THOUSANDS	HUNDREDS	TENS	BASE UNITS	TENTH	HUNDREDTH	THOUSANDTH
KILO	HECTO	DECA	LITER, METER, OR GRAM	DECI	CENTI	MILLI
(K)	(H)	(Da)	(l) (m) (g)	(d)	(c)	(m)
10^3	10^2	10^1	10^0 or 1	10^{-1}	10^{-2}	10^{-3}

It can be seen from Table 4, that a kilometer would be 1000 or 10^3 meters. A centigram would be (.01) one-hundredth or 10^{-2} of a gram. Working with the metric system is easy because to change from one prefix to another you simply move the decimal point to the correct place. In other words, to convert within the system, simply move the decimal point for each power of 10 as indicated in the prefix.

EXAMPLE CALCULATION 1

In drug dosage calculations you often need to convert between grams and milligrams and liters and milliliters. A common conversion requirement might be something like: 500 milliliters is equal to how many liters? We know from Table 2 that 500 milliliters (mls) would be equal to 0.5 liters because you would simply move the decimal point 3 spaces (powers of 10) to the left for the equivalent value since you are starting with milliliters and going to the base unit of liters.

Learning Hint

Deci is associated with decade meaning ten years; centi is associated with cents or a hundred cents in a dollar; and milli is associated with a millipede with a thousand legs. Biological note: A millipede doesn't actually have a thousand legs, it just looks like it.

EXAMPLE CALCULATION 2

How many grams are equal to 50.0 kilograms? Start at kilograms on Table 4 and move to the unit you want to convert to, in this case grams. You would need to move the decimal point three places (powers of ten) to the right to give an equivalent answer of 50,000 grams.

This knowledge of the metric system will prove invaluable to you as you work within the medical profession and even if you travel outside the United States. That is of course, unless you go to Myanmar. One final note before leaving this part of the discussion on the metric system. It has been determined that one cubic centimeter (cc) would hold the approximate volume of one milliliter (ml). Therefore, 1 cc = 1 ml. See Figure 2 ■. You may hear someone say you have 500 cc of an intravenous (IV) solution on hand, while someone else may say you have 500 ml of solution; either way they are both saying the same thing. Efforts are being made to standardize between cubic centimeters and milliliters, making milliliters the preferred choice. However, you will see and hear both used in health care settings.

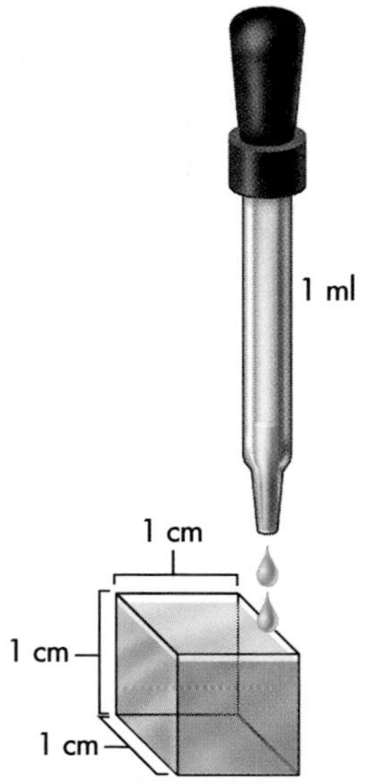

FIGURE ■ 2

1 cc = 1 ml

Learning Hint

Always check your answer to see if it makes sense. For example, a common mistake is moving the decimal point in the wrong direction. If you had done that in example calculation 1, you may have erroneously said that 500 milliliters is equal to 500,000 liters. If you visualize this you would know that 500 comparatively very small units (milliliters) in no way can equal 500,000 comparatively larger units (liters).

TEST YOUR KNOWLEDGE 3

Choose the best answer:

1. The metric system is based on the exponential power of:
   a. 100
   b. 10
   c. 2
   d. 15

2. Which of the following is not a basic unit of measure in the metric system?
   a. liter
   b. gram
   c. pound
   d. meter

Complete the following:

3. A cubic centimeter (cc) is equal to:

4. 500 grams is equal to how many kilograms?

5. 200 meters is equal to how many centimeters?

Conversion of Units

You should now be able to work comfortably within the metric system, but what if we need to take an English unit and convert it to a metric unit? For example, in the introduction of this chapter we said that a certain drug order read to give a patient 5 milligrams per kilogram of body weight. You would need to know the relationship between pounds in the English system and kilograms in the metric system to properly treat this patient.

The following is a method for changing units or converting between the English and metric system. This method is sometimes referred to as the **Factor-Label Method** or **Fraction Method.** This method allows your starting units to cancel or divide out until you reach your desired unit. There are two basic steps:

Step One: Write down your starting value with units over one. This places it in the form of a fraction, but since the number one is in the denominator it does not change the numerical value.

Step Two: Place the starting unit in the denominator of the next fraction to divide or cancel out and place the desired unit in the numerator along with the corresponding equivalent values. Since the values are equivalent, this is the same as multiplication by 1 which does not change the value of the quantity. This allows you to treat the units as in the multiplication of fractions and **"cancel" the units.** Notice that by carefully placing the units so that canceling is possible, the units can be converted.

EXAMPLE CALCULATION 3

How many inches are there in one mile?

First, put down what value is given as a fraction over 1.

$$\frac{1 \text{ mile}}{1}$$

Next, put miles in the denominator and the desired unit in the numerator with equivalent values. You know that 1 mile = 5,280 feet so:

$$1 \cancel{\text{mile}} \times \frac{5{,}280 \text{ ft}}{1 \cancel{\text{mile}}}$$

You've cancelled out miles, but need to go to inches. Just carry the process out until you reach your desired unit.

$$1 \cancel{\text{mile}} \times \frac{5{,}280 \cancel{\text{ft}}}{1 \cancel{\text{mile}}} \times \frac{12 \text{ inches}}{1 \cancel{\text{ft}}} = 63{,}360 \text{ inches}$$

EXAMPLE CALCULATION 4

How many seconds are there in 8 hours?

Step One: $\frac{8 \text{ hours}}{1}$

Step Two: $\frac{8 \cancel{\text{hours}}}{1} \times \frac{60 \cancel{\text{minutes}}}{1 \cancel{\text{hour}}} \times \frac{60 \text{ seconds}}{1 \cancel{\text{minute}}} = 28{,}800 \text{ seconds}$

TEST YOUR KNOWLEDGE 4

Complete the following:

1. How many days in 3 years?
2. How many inches in 4.5 yards?
3. How many quarts in 10.5 gallons?

Factor Label Method for Conversion Between Systems

One can attempt to memorize the hundreds of conversions between the English and metric systems, but that would be nearly impossible. All that is needed is to memorize one conversion in each of the three units of measure. This will allow a "bridging of the systems." These conversions are:

1 inch = 2.54 cm	used for units of lengths
2.2 lbs = 1 kg	used for units of mass or weights
1.06 qt = 1 L	used for units of volume

Clinical Application

BODY SURFACE AREA

A six foot man who weighs 240 lbs. may require a different dosage than a six foot man weighing 150 lbs. This is especially true with highly toxic agents such as those used in cancer chemotherapy. A method to determine the total body surface area (BSA) combines both height and weight in a single measurement to determine the true overall body size. Comparisons like this are called nomograms. See Figure 3 ■ for a nomogram used in determining BSA. Simply mark the patient's corresponding height and weight on the respective scale and either draw a straight line or use a ruler to find the intersection point to get the body surface area. Due to America's eating habits, the importance of BSA in relationship to the development of a form of diabetes is very important. Often that form of diabetes may improve with simple weight loss.

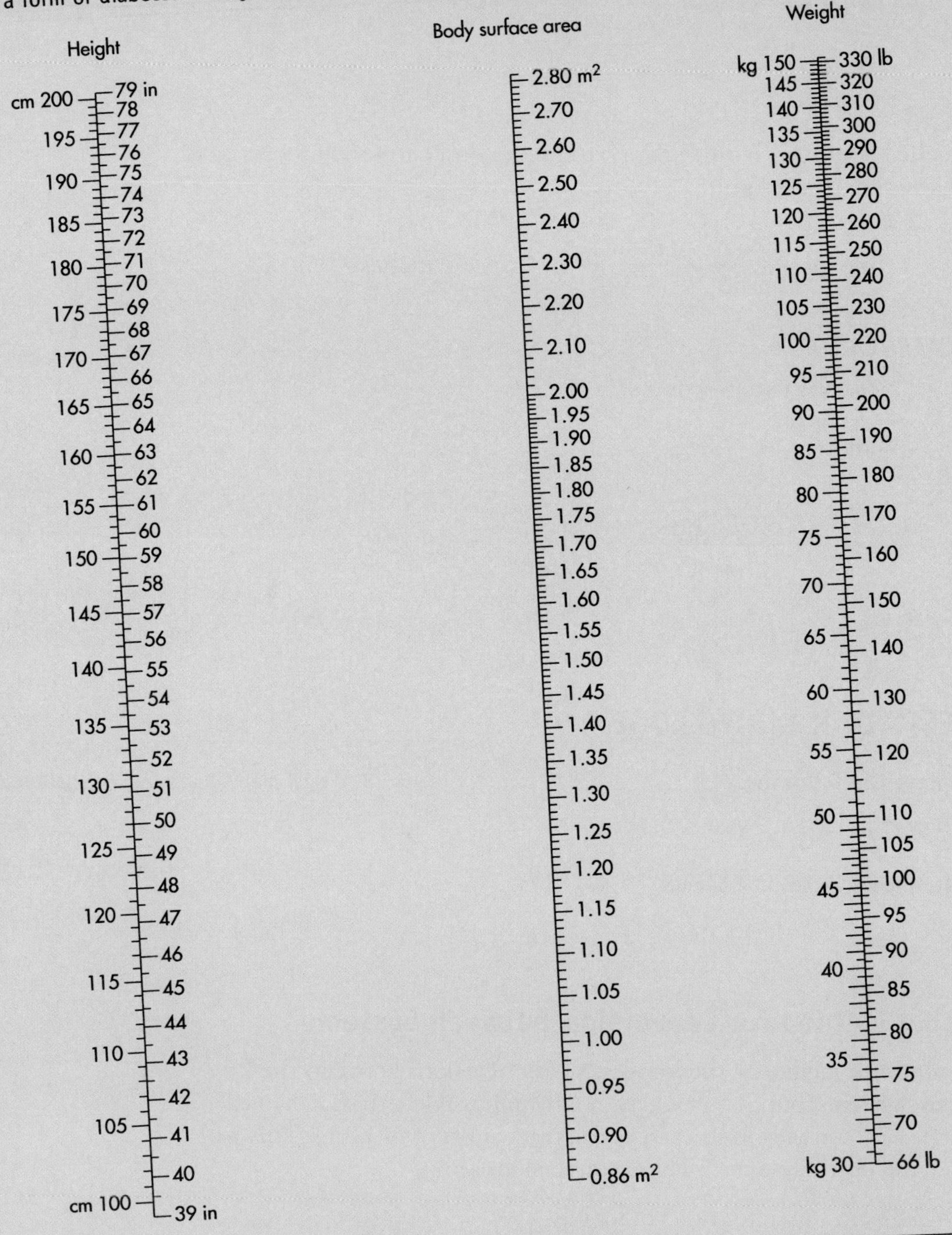

FIGURE ■ 3

Nomogram for Determining Body Surface Area (BSA)

EXAMPLE CALCULATION 5

If an individual weighs 150 pounds, how many kilograms does the patient weigh? First, you must change pounds to kilograms; therefore, write the given weight as a fraction over 1 (one). Then place the unit you want to cancel (pounds) in the denominator and the unit you want to convert to (kilograms) in the numerator of the next fraction.

$$\frac{150\ \cancel{\text{pounds}}}{1} \times \frac{1\ \text{kilogram}}{2.2\ \cancel{\text{pounds}}} = 68.18\ \text{kilograms}$$

EXAMPLE CALCULATION 6

The conversion will not always be as direct but it is no problem if you simply follow the system. For example, one foot is equal to how many centimeters? There is an equivalency somewhere for feet and centimeters, but you don't need to know that using the Factor Label Method and the conversion for distance.

Now, answer the question of how many centimeters are there in one foot. Remember, your unit conversion for length is 1 inch = 2.54 cm.

$$\frac{1\ \cancel{\text{foot}}}{1} \times \frac{12\ \cancel{\text{inches}}}{1\ \cancel{\text{foot}}} \times \frac{2.54\ \text{cm}}{1\ \cancel{\text{inch}}} = 30.48\ \text{cm}$$

TEST YOUR KNOWLEDGE 5

Choose the best answer:

1. The Body Surface nomogram compares what two units of measure?
   a. weight and sex
   b. height and sex
   c. surface area and length
   d. height and weight

Complete the following:

2. A quart of blood is equal to how many ml's?

3. If a patient voids (passes urine) 3.2 liters of urine in a day, what is the amount in ml's?

4. Convert 175 lbs to kilograms.

APPENDICES

Appendix A: Answers to Test Your Knowledge

Appendix B: Medical Terminology Word Parts and Singular and Plural Endings

Appendis C: Clinical Abbreviations

Appendix D: Lab Values

APPENDIX A: Answers to Test Your Knowledge

Chapter 1

Page 6, 1-1

1. G
2. M
3. M
4. G
5. M

Page 10, 1-2

1. blueness of the extremities
2. inflammation of the stomach
3. surgical repair of the nose
4. slow heart rate
5. recording or image of the breast
6. enlarged cell
7. nephritis
8. gastrectomy
9. cardiomegaly
10. osteopathy
11. neurologist

Page 13, 1-3

1. a. vital sign
   b. not a vital sign
   c. vital sign
   d. not a vital sign
   e. not a vital sign
   f. vital sign
   g. vital sign
2. c
3. a

Chapter 2

Page 26, 2-1

1. person should be standing face forward palms out as in Figure 2–1
2. a. prone
   b. fowler's
   c. fowler's
   d. supine

Page 30, 2-2

1. a. inferior
   b. anterior
   c. cephalic
   d. dorsal
   e. proximal
   f. internal
   g. deep
   h. central
   i. lateral
2. posterior
3. transverse or horizontal
4. mid-sagittal
5. superficial
6. proximal and distal
7. superior
8. lateral
9. peripheral

Page 31, 2-3

a. thoracic
b. spinal or dorsal
c. abdominal
d. thoracic
e. pelvic
f. cranial or dorsal

Page 37, 2-4

1. oral or buccal
2. axillary
3. umbilical
4. lumbar
5. patellar

Chapter 3

Page 49, 3-1

1. diffusion
2. low, higher
3. filtration
4. diffusion
5. facilitated diffusion

Page 51, 3-2

1. Phagocytosis is "cell eating" where a solid particle is engulfed. Pinocytosis is a form of endocytosis where liquid is brought into the cell or "cell drinking."
2. a. active
   b. passive
   c. passive
   d. active
   e. passive

Page 57, 3-3

a. nucleus
b. endoplasmic reticulum
c. mitochondria
d. golgi bodies
e. flagella or cilia

Page 59, 3-4

1. b
2. a
3. c
4. d

Chapter 4

Page 77, 4-1

1. squamous–flat or scale-like shaped, cuboidal–cubed shaped; columnar- column like; transitional- stretchy or variable shaped.
2. synovial
3. Because it is a support tissue for many other tissues.
4. Mucous is the adjective that describes the type of membrane while mucus is the noun or the actual substance produced by the membrane.

Page 91, 4-2

1. respiratory
2. urinary
3. skeletal
4. Nervous and sensory system
5. Immune
6. Cardiovascular
7. Digestive
8. Integumentary

Chapter 5

Page 103, 5-1

1.

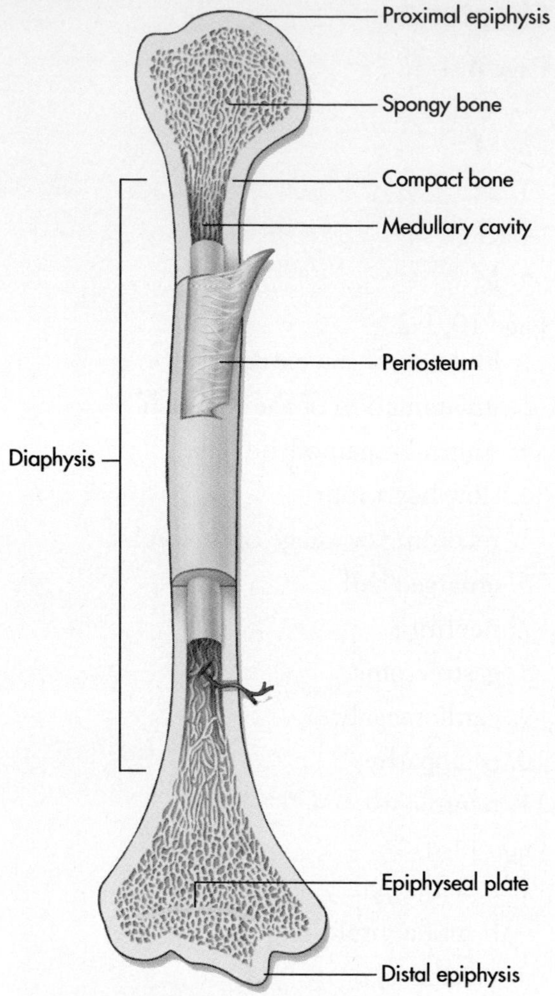

2. Found in the skull, clavicle, vertebrae of the spinal column, sternum, ribs, pelvis, and the epiphysis of the long bones and is needed for the production of red blood cells.
3. Provides support and allows for movement, protects organs, produces red blood cells and acts as storage for minerals and fats.
4. b
5. a

Page 107, 5-2

1. a
2. d
3. b
4. c
5. b
6. a

Page 117, 5-3

1. The axial skeleton is the central portion that protects and provides support for the organ systems in the dorsal and ventral cavities. The appendicular skeleton is the bones of the limbs.
2. d
3. c
4. flexion is the movement in the anterior-posterior plane that reduces the angle in articulated elements. Extension occurs in the same plane, but increase the angle like kicking a football.

Chapter 6

Page 128, 6-1

1. c
2. d
3. b

Page 135, 6-2

1. rotation
2. abduction
3. adduction
4. flexion
5. extension

Page 139, 6-3

1. sarcomere
2. myosin
3. actin
4. calcium and ATP

Chapter 7

Page 154, 7-1

1. a. epidermis
   b. dermis
   c. subcutaneous fascia
2. (any four)
   a. Protects from invasion of pathogens
   b. keeps you from drying out
   c. storage unit for fatty tissue
   d. produces vitamin D
   e. helps regulates body temperature
   f. helps to provide sensory input
3. d
4. c

Page 160, 7-2

1. b
2. c
3. b
4. d

Chapter 8

Page 177, 8-1

1. b
2. b
3. c
4. b

Page 183, 8-2

1. c
2. b
3. c
4. b
5. c

Page 190, 8-3

1. b
2. b
3. b
4. c

Chapter 9

Page 207, 9-1

1. d
2. c
3. c
4. c
5. d

Page 213, 9-2

1. a
2. b
3. b
4. d

Chapter 10

Page 227, 10-1
1. c
2. c
3. c

Page 231, 10-2
1. c
2. a
3. b

Page 235, 10-3
1. c
2. c
3. b
4. a

Chapter 11

Page 253, 11-1
1. a
2. c
3. d

Page 257, 11-2
1. c
2. c
3. pinna
4. cerumen
5. hammer
6. incus
7. stapes

Chapter 12

Page 277, 12-1
1. d
2. d
3. d
4. left ventricle
5. right

Page 283, 12-2
1. a
2. b
3. b
4. albumin
5. sino-atrial node

Page 291, 12-3
1. a
2. c
3. b
4. tunica interna, tunica media, tunica externa

Chapter 13

Page 311, 13-1
1. d
2. a
3. c
4. c
5. b

Page 315, 13-2
1. d
2. d
3. c
4. a

Page 321, 13-3
1. d
2. b
3. a
4. d
5. a
6. a

Page 325, 13-4
1. b
2. d
3. d
4. b

Chapter 14

Page 341, 14-1
1. d
2. d
3. c
4. b
5. b
6. d

Page 343, 14-2
1. b
2. d
3. c

Page 348, 14-3
1. d
2. c
3. d
4. d
5. c

page 353, 14-4
1. a
2. b
3. c
4. b

page 357, 14-5
1. c
2. c
3. a
4. c

Chapter 15

Page 376, 15-1
1. c
2. a
3. b
4. d
5. crown, neck and root

Page 384, 15-2
1. c
2. b
3. b
4. c
5. parasympathetic nervous system

Chapter 16

Page 409, 16-1
1. b
2. d
3. b
4. c
5. c

Page 417, 16-2
1. a
2. b
3. c
4. a
5. a
6. d

Chapter 17

Page 431, 17-1
1. c
2. b
3. d

Page 435, 17-2
1. d
2. b
3. c

Page 438, 17-3
1. b
2. b
3. b
4. c

Page 442, 17-4
1. d
2. c
3. b
4. b

Page 444, 17-5
1. b
2. d
3. a

Page 447, 17-6
1. b
2. a
3. d

Chapter 18

Page 463, 18-1
1. c
2. d
3. b
4. d

Page 468, 18-2
1. d
2. c
3. b
4. a

Page 479, 18-3
1. d
2. c
3. a
4. c

Study Success Companion

Page 500, 3
1. b
2. c
3. 1 milliliter
4. 0.5 kilogram
5. 20,000 centimeters

Page 501, 4
1. 1095 days
2. 162 inches
3. 42 quarts

Page 503, 5
1. d
2. 943 milliliters
3. 3200 milliliters
4. 79.55 kilograms

APPENDIX B: Medical Terminology, Word Parts, and Singular and Plural Endings

Word Parts Arranged Alphabetically and Defined

The word parts that have been presented in this textbook are summarized with their definitions for quick reference. The chapter numbers correspond to the first chapter in which the word part is described. Prefixes are listed first, followed by combining forms and suffixes.

Prefix	Definition
a-	without absence of
ad-	toward
an-	without, absence of
ana-	up, toward, apart
ante-	before
anti-	against, opposing
bi-	two
bin-	two
brady-	slow
di-	two
dia-	around, passing through
dys-	bad, abnormal
e-	to remove
en-	within, upon, on, over
endo-	within, inner, absorbing
ep-	upon, on, over
epi-	upon
eu-	normal, good
ex-	outside, away from
exo-	outside, away from
hemi-	one-half
homo-	same
hydro-	water
hyper-	excessive
hypo-	under, below normal
im-	not
inter-	between
intra-	within
macro-	large
meta-	after, change
micro-	small
mono-	single
multi-	many
my-	muscle
myo-	muscle
neo-	new
nulli-	none
ortho-	straight, normal
pan-	all, entire
para-	near, alongside; departure from normal
per-	through
peri-	around, about, surrounding
poly-	many
post-	after
pre-	before
pro-	forward, preceding
quad-	four
re-	back
sub-	beneath
sym-	together, joined
syn-	together, joined
tachy-	rapid, fast
tetra-	four
trons-	through, across, beyond
uni-	one

Combining Form	Definition
abdomin/o	abdomen, abdominal cavity
acou/o	hearing
acoust/o	hearing
acr/o	extremity, extreme
aden/o	gland
adren/o	adrenal gland
aer/o	air or gas
albumin/o	albumin
alvcol/o	alveolus (air sac)
amni/o	amnion, amniotic fluid
amnion/o	amnion, amniotic fluid
an/o	anus
andr/o	male
angi/o	blood vessel
ankyl/o	crooked
anter/o	front
aort/o	aorta
appendic/o	to hang onto, appendix
aque/o	water
arche/o	first, beginning

Combining Form	Definition
arter/o	artery
arteri/o	artery
arthr/o	joint
astheni/o	weakness
atel/o	imperfect, incomplete
ather/o	fat
atri/o	atrium
aud/o	hearing
audi/o	hearing
aur/i	ear
aut/o	self
azot/o	urea, nitrogen
bacter/o	bacteria
balan/o	glans penis
bi/o	life
bil/i	bile
blast/o	germ, bud
blephar/o	eyelid
bronch/i	bronchus (airway)
bronch/o	bronchus (airway)
burs/o	purse or sac; bursa
calc/i	calcium
cancer/o	cancer
carcin/o	cancer
card/o	heart
cardi/o	heart
carp/o	wrist
cartil/o	gristle, cartilage
caud/o	tail
cec/o	blind intestine, cecum
cel/o	hernia, protrusion
celi/o	abdomen, abdominal cavity
cephal/o	head
cerebell/o	cerebellum (little brain)
cerebr/o	cerebrum (brain)
cerumin/o	wax
cervic/o	cervix, neck
cheil/o	lip
chir/o	hand
chol/e	bile, gall
choledoch/o	common bile duct
chondr/o	cartilage
chori/o	membrane, chorion
chromat/o	color
clon/o	spasm
col/o	colon
colp/o	vagina
conjunctiv/o	to bind together, conjunctiva
cor/o	pupil
core/o	pupil
corne/o	horny, cornea
coron/o	crown, circle
cortic/o	tree bark, outer covering, cortex
cost/o	rib
cran/o	skull, cranium
crani/o	skull, cranium
crin/o	to secrete
crypt/o	hidden
culd/o	cul-de-sac
cutane/o	skin
cyan/o	blue
cyes/i	pregnancy
cyes/o	pregnancy
cyst/o	bladder, sac
cyt/o	cell
dacry/o	tear
dent/i	teeth
derm/o	skin
dermat/o	skin
diaphragmat/o	diaphragm
dipl/o	double
dips/o	thirst
dist/o	away
diverticul/o	small blind pouch, diverticulum
dors/o	back
duct/o	lead, move
duoden/o	twelve, duodenum
dur/o	hard
ech/o	sound
electr/o	electricity
embol/o	a throwing in
embry/o	embryo
encephal/o	brain
endocrin/o	endocrine
enter/o	small intestine
epididym/o	epididymis
epiglott/o	epiglottis
episi/o	vulva
eryth/o	red
erythr/o	red
esophag/o	gullet, esophagus
esthesi/o	sensation

Combining Form	Definition
eti/o	cause (of disease)
fasci/o	fascia
femor/o	thigh
fet/i	fetus
fet/o	fetus
fibr/o	fiber
fibul/o	clasp of buckle, fibula
fovea/o	small pit
gangli/o	ganglion
gastr/o	stomach
gen/o	formation, cause, produce
ger/o	old age
geront/o	old age
gingiv/o	gums
gli/o	glue, neuroglia
glomerul/o	little ball, glomerulus
gloss/o	tongue
gluc/o	glucose, sugar
glut/o	buttock
glyc/o	glycogen, sugar
glycos/o	sugar
gravid/o	pregnancy
gravidar/o	pregnancy
gyn/o	woman
gynec/o	woman
halat/o	breath
hem/o	blood
hemat/o	blood
hepat/o	liver
hern/o	protrusion, hernia
herni/o	protrusion, hernia
heter/o	other
hidr/o	sweat
hist/o	tissue
hom/o	sameness, unchanging
hormon/o	to set in motion
hydr/o	water
hymen/o	hymen
hyster/o	uterus
iatr/o	to heal
idi/o	person, self
ile/o	ileum of small intestine, to roll
ili/o	flank, groin, ilium of the pelvis
immun/o	exempt; immunity
infect/o	to enter, invade
infer/o	below
inguin/o	groin
ir/o	rainbow, iris
irid/o	rainbow, iris
isch/o	to hold back, deficiency, blockagestomach
ischi/o	haunch, hip joint, ischium
jejnun/o	empty, jejunum
kal/i	potassium
kerat/o	hard, horny; cornea
ket/o	ketone bodies
keton/o	ketone bodies
kinesi/o	motion
kyph/o	hump
labyrinth/o	labyrinth, internal ear
lacrim/o	tear
lact/o	milk
lamin/o	thin, lamina
lapar/o	abdomen, abdominal cavity
laryng/o	larynx
later/o	side
lei/o	smooth
leuk/o	white
lingu/o	tongue
lip/o	fat, lipid
lith/o	stone
lob/o	lobe
lord/o	bent forward
lumb/o	loin, lower back
lymph/o	clear water or fluid
lys/o	dissolution
mal/o	bad
mamm/o	breast
mast/o	breast
meat/o	opening
medi/o	middle
megal/o	abnormally large
melan/o	dark, black
men/o	month, menstruation
menstru/o	month, menstruation
mening/o	meninges, membrane
menisc/o	cresent-shaped moon, meniscus membrane
ment/o	mind
metr/o	uterus
mon/o	one
muc/o	mucus

Combining Form	Definition
my/o	muscle
myc/o	fungus
myel/o	bone marrow; spinal cord; medulla; myelin
myelon/o	bone marrow; spinal cord; medulla; myelin
myos/o	muscle
myring/o	membrane; eardrum
myx/o	mucus
nas/o	nose
nat/o	birth
natr/o	sodium
necr/o	death
nephr/o	kidney
neur/o	sinew or cord, nerve, fascia
noct/i	night
nucl/o	kennel, nucleus
nyct/o	night, nocturnal
nyctal/o	night, nocturnal
obstetr/o	midwife, prenatal development
ocul/o	eye
olig/o	few in number
omphal/o	umbilicus (navel)
onc/o	tumor
onych/o	nail
oophor/o	ovary
opt/o	eye, vision
opthalm/o	eye
or/o	mouth
orch/o	testis or testicle
orchi/o	testis or testicle
orchid/o	testis or testicle
organ/o	tool
orth/o	straight
oste/o	bone
ot/o	ear
ov/i	egg
ov/o	egg
ovari/o	ovary
ox/o	oxygen
pachy/o	thick
palat/o	roof of mouth, palate
pancreat/o	sweethread, pancreas
par/o	parturition or labor
parathyroid/o	parathyroid
pariet/o	wall

Combining Form	Definition
part/o	parturition or labor
patell/o	small pan, patella
path/o	disease
pector/o	chest
ped/o	child
pediatr/o	child
pelv/l	basin, pelvis
pen/o	penis
peps/o	digestion
perine/o	perineum
peritone/o	to stretch over, peritoneum
petr/o	stone
phac/o	lens
phag/o	eat, swallow
phak/o	lens
phalang/o	row of soldiers
pharyng/o	pharynx (throat)
phas/o	speech
phleb/o	vein
phot/o	light
physi/o	nature
physis/o	growth
plegi/o	paralysis
pleur/o	pleura
pneum/o	lung or air
pneumat/o	lung or air
pod/o	foot
poikil/o	irregular
polyp/o	polyp
poster/o	back
presby/o	old age
prim/i	first
proct/o	anus
prostat/o	prostate gland
proxim/o	near
pseud/o	false
psych/o	mind
pub/o	grown up
puerper/o	childbirth
pulmon/o	lung
py/o	pus
pyel/o	pelvis (renal)
pylor/o	pylorus
quad/o	four gate keeper
quadr/i	four
rachi/o	spine

Combining Form	Definition	Combining Form	Definition
radi/o	spoke of a wheel, radius	taxi/o	reaction to a stimulus
radic/o	nerve root	ten/o	to stretch out; tendon
radicul/o	nerve root	tend/o	to stretch out; tendon
rect/o	straight, erect, rectum	tendin/o	to stretch out; tendon
ren/o	kidney	test/o	testis, testicle
retin/o	net, retina	testicul/o	small testis, testicle
rhabd/o	rod	thalam/o	thalamus
rhin/o	nose	thel/o	nipple
rhytid/o	wrinkles	therm/o	heat
sacr/o	sacred, sacrum	thorac/o	thorax (chest)
salping/o	tube: eustachian tube; fallopian tube	thromb/o	clot
		thym/o	wart-like, thymus gland
sarc/o	flesh, muscle	thyr/o	shield, thyroid
scler/o	thick, hard; sclera	toc/o	birth, labor
scoli/o	curved	tom/o	cut, section
seb/o	sebum, oil	ton/o	tone, tension, pressure
semin/o	seed	toxic/o	poison
sept/o	wall, partition	trache/o	trachea
sial/o	saliva, salivary gland	trachel/o	neck, cervix
sigm/o	the letter "s" sigmoid colon	trich/o	hair
sinus/o	cavity	tubercul/o	little mass of swelling
somat/o	body	tympan/o	eardrum
somn/o	sleep	umbilic/o	navel
son/o	sound	ur/o	urine
sperm/o	seed	ureter/o	ureter
spermat/o	seed	urethr/o	urethra
sphygm/o	pulse	urin/o	urine
spin/o	spine or thorn	uter/o	womb, uterus
spir/o	breathe	uvul/o	grape, uvula
splen/o	spleen	vagin/o	sheath, vagina
spondyl/o	vertebra	valvul/o	little valve
staped/o	stapes	varic/o	dilated vein
staphyl/o	grape-like clusters (bacterium)	vas/o	blood vessel; duct
		vascul/o	little blood vessel
stasis/o	standing still	ven/o	vein
steat/o	fat	ventr/o	front, belly
sten/o	narrowness, constriction	ventricul/o	little belly or cavity, ventricle
stern/o	chest, sternum		
steth/o	chest	vers/o	turn
stigmat/o	point	vertebr/o	joint, vertebra
stomat/o	mouth	vesic/o	bladder, sac
strept/o	twisted or gnarled (bacterium)	vesicul/o	vesicle (seminal vesicle)
		vitr/o	glassy
super/o	above	vitre/o	glassy
synov/o	binding eggs; synovial	vulv/o	vulva
synovi/o	binding eggs; synovial	xanth/o	yellow
syndesm/o	binding together	xer/o	dry
tars/o	flat surface		

Suffix	Definition
-a	singular
-ac	pertaining to
-acusis	hearing condition
-ad	toward
-al	pertaining to
-algesia	pain
-algia	pain
-apheresis	removal
-ar	pertaining to
-ary	pertaining to
-asthenia	weakness
-atresia	closure; absence of a normal body opening
-capnia	carbon dioxide
-cele	hernia, swelling, protrusion
-centesis	surgical puncture
-clasia	break apart
-clasis	break apart
-clast	break apart
-crit	separate
-cusis	hearing condition
-cyte	cell
-desis	surgical fixation, fusion
-drome	run, running
-dynia	pain
-eal	pertaining to
-ectasis	expansion, dilation
-ectomy	excision
-elle	small
-emesis	vomiting
-emetic	vomiting
-emia	blood (condition of)
-gen	formation, cause, produce
-genesis	origin, cause
-genic	pertaining to formation, causing, producing
-gram	recording
-graph	instrument for recording
-graphy	recording process
-hemia	blood (condition of)
-ia	diseased state (condition of)
-ial	pertaining to
-iasis	condition of
-iatry	treatment, specialty
-ic	pertaining to
-ion	pertaining to
-ior	pertaining to
-is	pertaining to

Suffix	Definition
-ism	condition or disease
-ist	one who practices
-itis	inflammation
-lepsy	seizure
-logist	one who studies
-logy	study of
-lytic, -lysis	to loosen, dissolve
-malacia	softening
-meter	measuring instrument
-metry	measurement
-oid	resemblance to
-oma	abnormal swelling, tumor
-opia	vision
-opsy	view of
-osis	process or condition that is usually abnormal
-otomy	cutting into, excision
-ous	pertaining to
-oxia	oxygen
-paresis	paralysis (minor)
-pathy	disease
-penia	abnormal reduction in number, deficiency
-pepsia	digestion
-pexy	surgical fixation, suspension
-phagia	eating or swallowing
-phasia	speaking
-phil	loving, affinity for
-philia	loving, affinity for
-phobia	fear
-phonia	sound or voice
-phylaxis	protection
-physis	growth
-plasia	shape, formation
-plasm	something shaped
-plasty	surgical repair
-plegia	paralysis (major)
-pnea	breathing
-poiesis	formation
-practic	one who practices
-ptosis	falling downward (condition of)
-ptysis	spit out a fluid
-rrhagia	bleeding, hemorrhage
-rrhaphy	suturing
-rrhea	excessive discharge
-rrhexis	rupture
-salpinx	trumpet, fallopian tube

Suffix	Definition	Suffix	Definition
-sarcoma	malignant tumor	-stomy	surgical creation of an opening
-schisis	split, fissure	-tic	pertaining to
-sclerosis	hardening	-tocia	birth, labor
-scope	viewing instrument	-tome	cutting instrument
-scopy	process of viewing	-tomy	incision
-sis	state of	-tripsy	surgical crushing
-some	body	-trophy	nourishment, development
-spasm	sudden, involuntary muscle contraction	-um	pertaining to
-stasis	standing still	-uria	urine, urination
-stenosis	narrowing, constriction	-y	process of

[Endings in Medical Terminology]

1. **Plural endings.** The following list provides a summary of plural endings that are in common use with medical terms. Examples are provided to demonstrate how these endings are applied.

Endings Singular	Plural	Examples Singular	Plural
-a	-ae	fistula	fistulae
-ax	-aces	hemothorax	hemothoraces
-ex	-ices	cortex	cortices
-is	-es	mastoiditis	mastoidites
-ix	-ices	cicatrix	cicatrices
-ma	-mata	fibroma	fibromata
-on	-a	contusion	contusia
-um	-a	bacterium	bacteria
-us	-i	fungus	fungi
-y	-ies	episiotomy	episiotomies

2. **Adjective endings.** The list below provides a summary of suffixes that mean "pertaining to" and form an adjective (a description of a noun) when combined with a root.

Ending	Example	Definition
-ac	cardiac	pertaining to the heart
-al	endotracheal	pertaining to within the trachea
-ar	submandibular	pertaining to below the mandible
-ary	pulmonary	pertaining to a lung
-eal	esophageal	pertaining to the esophagus
-ic	leukemic	pertaining to leukemia
-ous	fibrous	pertaining to fiber
-tic	cyanotic	pertaining to cyanotic (blue)

3. **Diminutive endings.** The endings listed below provide the meaning of "small" to the word of origin.

Ending	Example	Definition
-icle	ossicle	small bone
-ole	bronchiole	small bronchus (airway)
-ula	macula	small macule (spot)
-ule	pustule	small pimple

4. **Diagnostic endings.** The endings in this list summarize the suffixes that are in common use to indicate measurements, treatments, and procedures.

Ending	Meaning	Example	Definition
-gram	record	bronchogram	recording of bronchus image
-graph	recording instrument	sonograph	ultrasound instrument
-graphy	process of recording	echocardiography	procedure of heart recording
-iatrics	treatment	pediatrics	treatment of children
-iatry	treatment	psychiatry	treatment of the mind
-logy	study of	oncology	study of cancer
-logist	one who studies	audiologist	one who studies hearing
-ist	one who specializes	optometrist	specialist in eye measurement
-meter	instrument of measure	spirometer	instrument measuring breathing
-metry	process of measuring	spirometry	process of measuring breathing
-scope	instrument for exam	endoscope	instrument for examination within
-scopy	examination	endoscopy	examination within

APPENDIX C: Clinical Abbreviations

These are the currently acceptable abbreviations, however, different health care facilities may use others as well.

Abbreviation	Meaning
@	at
ā	before
AB	abortion
ABGs	arterial blood gases
ac	before meals
ACAT	automated computerized axial tomography
Acc	accommodation
ACL	anterior cruciate ligament
ACTH	adrenocorticotropic hormone
AD	right ear, Alzheimer's disease
ad lib	as desired
ADD	attention deficit disorder
ADH	antidiuretic hormone
ADHD	attention-deficit-hyperactivity disorder
ADL	activities of daily living
AE	above elbow
AF	atrial fibrillation
AGN	acute glomerulonephritis
AHF	autihemophilic factor
AI	artificial insemination
AIDS	acquired immunodeficiency syndrome
AK	above knee
ALL	acute lymphocytic leukemia
ALS	amyotropic lateral sclerosis
ALT	alanine transaminase
am, AM	morning
AMI	acute myocardial infarction
AML	acute myelogenous leukemia
amt	amount
Angio	angiography
ANS	autonomic nervous system
ante	before
AP	anteroposterior
APAP	acetaminophen (Tylenol)
aq	aqueous (water)
ARC	AIDS-related complex
ARD	acute respiratory disease
ARDS	adult respiratory distress syndrome
ARF	acute respiratory failure, acute renal failure
ARMD	age-related macular degeneration
AROM	active range of motion
AS	aortic stenosis, arteriosclerosis, left ear
ASA	aspirin
ASCVD	arteriosclerotic cardiovascular disease
ASD	atrial septal defect
ASHD	arteriosclerotic heart disease
ASL	American Sign language
AST	aspartate transaminase
Astigm.	astigmatism
ATN	acute tubulor necrosis
AU	both ears
AuD	doctor of audiology
AV, A-V	atrioventricular
Ba	barium
BaE	barium enema
basos	basophil
BBB	bundle branch block (L for left; R for right)
BC	bone conduction
BCC	basal cell carcinoma
BDT	bone density testing
BE	barium enema, below elbow
bid	twice a day
BK	below knee
BM	bowel movement
BMR	basal metabolic rate
BMT	bone marrow transplant
BNO	bladder neck obstruction
BP	blood pressure
BPD	bipolar disorder
BPH	benign prostatic hypertrophy
bpm	beats per minute
Bronch	bronchoscopy

Abbreviation	Meaning
BS	bowel sounds
BSE	breast self-examination
BSN	bachelor of science in nursing
BUN	blood urea nitrogen
BX, bx	biopsy
c̄	with
C	100
C1, C2, etc.	first cervical vertebra, second cervical vertebra, etc.
Ca^{2+}	calcium
CA	cancer, chronological age
CABG	coronary artery bypass graft
CAD	coronary artery disease
cap(s)	capsule(s)
CAPD	continuous ambulatory peritoneal dialysis
CAT	computerized axial tomography
cath	catheterization
CBC	complete blood count
CBD	common bile duct
cc	cubic centimeter
CC	clean catch urine specimen, cardiac catheterization, chief complaint
CCC	speech-language pathologist
CCS	certified coding specialist
CCU	cardiac care unit, coronary care unit
CD4	protein on T-cell helper lymphocyte
CDH	congenital dislocation of the hip
c.gl.	correction with glasses
CGL	chronic granulocytic leukemia
chemo	chemotherapy
CHF	congestive heart failure
chol	cholesterol
Ci	curie
CIS	carcinoma in situ
Cl^-	chloride
CLL	chronic lymphocytic leukemia
CLS	clinical laboratory scientist
CLT	clinical laboratory technician
CMA	certified medical assistant
CML	chronic myelogenous leukemia
CNA	certified nurse aide
CNIM	certification in neurophysiologic intraoperative monitoring
CNS	central nervous system
CO_2	carbon dioxide
CoA	coarctation of the aorta
COLD	chronic obstructive lung disease
COPD	chronic obstructive pulmonary disease
COTA	certified occupational therapy assistant
CP	cerebral palsy, chest pain
CPD	cephalopelvic disproportion
CPK	creatine phosphokinase
CPR	cardiopulmonary resuscitation
CRF	chronic renal failure
crit	hematocrit
CRT	certified respiratory therapist
C & S	culture and sensitivity test
CS, CS-section	Cesarean section
CSD	congenital septal defect
CSF	cerebrospinal fluid
CT	computerized tomography, cytotechnologist
CTA	clear to auscultation
CTS	carpal tunnel syndrome
CUC	chronic ulcerative colitis
CV	cardiovascular
CVA	cerebrovascular accident
CVD	cerebrovascular disease
CVS	chorionic villus biopsy
Cx	cervix
CXR	chest X-ray
cyl lens	cylindrical lens
cysto	cystoscopic exam
d	day
D	diopter (lens strength)
D & C	dilation and curettage
D/C, d/c	discontinue
dB	decibel
DC	doctor of chiropractic
DDM	doctor of dental medicine

Abbreviation	Meaning
DDS	doctor of dental surgery
DEA	Drug Enforcement Agency
decub	lying down, decubitus ulcer
Derm, derm	dermatology
DI	diabetes insipidus, diagnostic imaging
diff	differential
dil	dilute
disc	discontinue
disp	dispense
DJD	degenerative joint disease
DM	diabetes mellitus
DO	doctor of osteopathy
DOB	date of birth
DOE	dyspnea on exertion
DPT	diphtheria, pertussis, tetanus; doctor of physical therapy
dr	dram
DRE	digital rectal exam
DSA	digital subtraction angiography
DSM-IV	*Diagnostic and Statistical Manual for Mental Disorders*, Fourth edition
DTR	deep tendon reflex; dietetic technician, registered
DUB	dysfunctional uterine bleeding
DVA	distance visual acuity
DVT	deep vein thrombosis
Dx	diagnosis
E. coli	*Escherichia coli*
EAU	exam under anesthesia
EBV	Epstein-Barr virus
ECC	endocervical curettage, extracorporeal circulation
ECCE	extracapsular cataract extraction
ECG	electrocardiogram
Echo	echocardiogram
ECT	electroconvulsive therapy
ED	erectile dysfunction
EDC	estimated date of confinement
EEG	electroencephalogram, electroencephalography
EENT	eyes, ears, nose, throat

Abbreviation	Meaning
EGD	esophagogastro-duodenoscopy
EKG	electrocardiogram
ELISA	enzyme-linked immunosorbent assay
elix	elixir
EM	emmetropia (normal vision)
EMB	endometrial biopsy
EMG	electromyogram
EMT-B	emergency medical technician-basic
EMT-I	emergency medical technician-intermediate
EMT-P	emergency medical technician-paramedic
emul	emulsion
Endo	endoscopy
ENT	ear, nose, throat
EOM	extraocular movement
eosins, eos	eosinophil
ER	emergency room
ERCP	endoscopic retrograde cholangiopancreatography
ERT	estrogen replacement therapy
ERV	expiratory reserve volume
ESR	erythrocyte sedimentation rate
ESRD	end-stage renal disease
e-stim	electrical stimulation
ESWL	extracorporeal shock-wave lithotripsy
et	and
ET	endotracheal
FBS	fosting blood sugar
FDA	Federal Drug Administration
Fe	iron
FEF	forced expiratory flow
FEKG	fetal electrocardiogram
FEV	forced expiratory volume
FHR	fetal heart rate
FHT	fetal heart tone
fl	fluid
FOBT	fecal occult blood test
FRC	functional residual capacity
FS	frozen section
FSH	follicle-stimulating hormone
FTND	full-term normal delivery

Abbreviation	Meaning
FVC	forced vital capacity
Fx,FX	fracture
GI	first pregnancy
Ga	gallium
GA	general anesthesia
GB	gallbladder
GC	gonorrhea
GERD	gastroesophageal reflux discase.
GH	growth hormone
GI	gastrointestinal
gm	gram
GOT	glutamic oxaloacetic transaminase
gr	grain
grav I	first pregnancy
gt	drop
gtt	drops
GTT	glucose tolerance test
GU	genitourinary
GVHD	graft vs. host disease
GYN, gyn	gynecology
H_2O	water
HA	headache
HAV	hepatitis A virus
Hb	hemoglobin
HBOT	hyperbaric oxygen therapy
HBV	hepatitis B virus
HCG, hCG	human chorionic gonadotropin
HCO_3^-	bicarbonate
HCT, Hct	hematocrit
HCV	hepatitis C virus
HD	Hodgkin's disease
HDL	high-density lipoproteins
HDN	hemolytic disease of the newborn
HEENT	head, ears, eyes, nose, throat
Hgb, HGB	hemoglobin
HIV	human immunodeficieny virus
HMD	hyaline membrane disease
HNP	herniated nucleus polposus
HPV	human papilloma virus
HRT	hormone replacement therapy
hs	hour of sleep
HSG	hysterosalpingography

Abbreviation	Meaning
HSV	*Herpes simplex* virus
HTN	hypertension
HZ	Hertz
ṫ	one
IBD	inflammatory bowel disease
IBS	irritable bowel syndrome
IC	inspiratory capacity
ICCE	intracapsular cataract cryoextraction
ICP	intracranial pressure
ICU	intensive care unit
I & D	incision and drainage
ID	intradermal
IDDM	insulin-dependent diabetes mellitus
Ig	immunoglobins (IgA, IgD, IgE, IgG, Igm)
ii	two
iii	three
IM	intramuscular
inj	injection
I & O	intake and output
IOL	intraocular lens
IOP	intraocular pressure
IPD	intermittent peritoneal dialysis
IPPB	intermittent positive pressure breathing
IRDS	infant respiratory distress syndrome
IRV	inspiratory reserve volume
IU	international unit
IUD	intrauterine device
IV	intravenous
IVC	intravenous cholangiogram
IVF	*in vitro* fertilization
IVP	intravenous pyclogram
JRA	juvenile rheumatoid arthritis
JVP	jugular venous pulse
K^+	potassium
kg	kilogram
KS	Kaposi's sarcoma
KUB	kidney, ureter, bladder
L	left, liter
L1, L2, etc.	first lumbar vertebra, second lumbar vertebra, etc.
LASIK	laser-assisted in-situ keratomileusis

Abbreviation	Meaning
LAT, lat	lateral
LAVH	laparoscopic-assisted vaginal hysterectomy
LBW	low birth weight
LDH	lactate dehydrogenase
LDL	low-density lipoproteins
LE	lower extremity
LGI	lower gastrointestinal series
LH	luteinizing hormone
liq	liquid
LL	left lateral
LLE	left lower extremity
LLL	left lower lobe
LLQ	left lower quadrant
LMP	last menstrual period
LP	lumbar puncture
LPN	licensed practical nurse
LUE	left upper extremity
LUL	left upper lobe
LUQ	left upper quadrant
LVAD	left ventricular assist device
LVH	left ventricular hypertrophy
lymphs	lymphocyte
LVN	licensed vocational nurse
mA	milliampere
MA	mental age
MAO	monoamine oxidase
mcg	microgram
mCi	millicurie
MCV	mean corpuscular volume
MD	doctor of medicine, muscular dystrophy
mEq	milliequivalent
mets	metastases
mg	milligram
MH	marital history
MI	myocardial infarction, mitral insufficiency
mL	milliliter
MLT	medical laboratory technician
mm	millimeter
MM	malignant melanoma
mm Hg	millimeters of mercury
MMPI	Minnesota Multiphasic Personality Inventory
Mono	mononucleosis
monos	monocyte

Abbreviation	Meaning
MR	mitral regurgitation
MRA	magnetic resonance angiography
MRI	magnetic resonance imaging
MS	mitral stenosis, multiple sclerosis, musculoskeletal
MSII	melanocyte-stimulating hormone
MSN	master of science in nursing
MT	medical technologist
MTX	methotrexate
MUA	manipulation under anesthesia
MV	minute volume
MVP	mitral valve prolapse
n & v	nausea and vomiting
Na^+	sodium
NB	newborn
NG	nasogastric (tube)
NGU	nongonococcal urethritis
NHL	non-Hodgkin's lymphoma
NIDDM	non-insulin-dependent diabetes mellitus
NK	natural killer cells
NMR	nuclear magnetic resonance
no sub	no substitute
noc	night
non rep	do not repeat
NP	nurse practitioner
NPDL	modular, poorly differentiated lymphocytes
NPH	neutral protamine Hagedorn (insulin)
NPO	nothing by mouth
NS	normal saline
NSAID	nonsteroidal anti-inflammatory drug
NSR	normal sinus rhythm
O_2	oxygen
OA	osteoarthritis
OB	obstetrics
OCD	obsessive-compulsive disorder
OCPs	oral contraceptive pills
OD	overdose, right eye, doctor of optometry
oint.	ointment
OM	otitis media

Abbreviation	Meaning
O & P	ova and parasites
Ophth.	ophthalmology
OR	operating room
ORIF	open reduction-internal fixation
Orth, ortho	orthopedics
OS	left eye
OT	occupational therapy
OTC	over the counter
Oto	otology
OTR	occupational therapist
OU	each eye
oz	ounce
$\bar{p}$	after
P	pulse
PI	first delivery
PA	posteroanterior, physician assistant, pernicious anemia
PAC	premature atrial contraction
PAP	Papanicolaou test, pulmonary arterial pressure
para I	first delivery
PARR	postanesthetic recovery room
PBI	protein-bound iodine
pc	after meals
PCA	patient-controlled administration
PCP	*Pneumocystis carinii* pneumonia
PCV	packed cell volume
PDA	patent ductus arteriosus
PDR	*Physician's Desk Reference*
PE tube	polyethylene tube placed in the eardrum
PEG	pneumoencephalogram, percutaneous endoscopic gastrostomy
per	with
PERRLA	pupils equal, round, react to light and accommodation
PET	positron emission tomography
PFT	pulmonary function test
pH	acidity or alkalinity of urine
PharmD	doctor of pharmacy
PID	pelvic inflammatory disease
PKU	phenylketonuria
PM, pm	evening
PMNs	polymorphonuclear neutrophil
PMP	previous menstrual period
PMS	premenstrual syndrome
PND	paroxysmal nocturnal dyspnea, postnasal drip
PNS	peripheral nervous system
PO, po	phone order, by mouth
polys	polymorphonuclear neutrophil
PORP	partial ossicular replacement prosthesis
pp	postprandial (after meals)
PPD	purified protein derivative (tuberculin test)
preop, pre-op	preoperative
prep	preparation, prepared
PRK	photo refractive keratectomy
PRL	prolactin
prn	as needed
Pro-time	prothrombin time
PROM	passive range of motion
prot	protocol
PSA	prostate specific antigen
pt	pint
PT	prothrombin time, physical therapy, physical therapist
PTA	physical therapy assistant
PTC	percutaneous transhepatic cholangiography
PTCA	percutaneous transluminal coronary angioplasty
PTII	parathyroid hormone
PUD	peptic ulcer disease
PVC	premature ventricular contraction
$\bar{q}$	every
qam	every morning
qd	once a day, every day
qh	every hour
qhs	every night
qid	four times a day
qod	every other day
qs	quantity sufficient
R	respiration, right, roentgen
Ra	radium
RA	rheumatoid arthritis
rad	radiation absorbed dose

Abbreviation	Meaning
RAI	radioactive iodine
RAIU	radioactive iodine uptake
RBC	red blood cell
RD	respiratory disease, registered dietitian
RDA	recommended daily allowance
RDH	registered dental hygienist
RDS	respiratory distress syndrome
REEGT	registered electroencephalography technologist
REM	rapid eye movement
REPT	registered evoked potential technologist
Rh-	Rh-negative
Rh+	Rh-positive
RHIA	registered health information administrator
RHIT	registered health information technician
RIA	radioimmunoassay
RL	right lateral
RLE	right lower extremity
RLL	right lower lobe
RLQ	right lower quadrant
RML	right mediolateral, right middle lobe
RN	registered nurse
ROM	range of motion
RP	retrograde pyelogram
RPh	registered pharmacist
RPR	rapid plasma reagin (test for syphilis)
RPSGT	registered polysomnographic technologist
RRT	registered radiologic technologist, registered respiratory therapist
RUE	right upper extremity
RUL	right upper lobe
RUQ	right upper quadrant
RV	reserve volume
Rx	take
$\bar{s}$	without
S1	first heart sound
S2	second heart sound
SA, S-A	sinoatrial

Abbreviation	Meaning
SAD	seasonal affective disorder
SAH	subarachnoid hemorrhage
SBFT	small bowel follow-through
SC, sc	subcutaneous
SCC	squamous cell carcinoma
SCI	spinal cord injury
SCIDS	severe combined immunodeficiency syndrome
Sed-rate	erythrocyte sedimentation rate
SEE-2	Signing Exact English
SG	skin graft, specific gravity
s.gl.	without correction or glasses
SGOT	serum glutamic oxaloacetic transaminase
SIDS	sudden infant death syndrome
Sig	label as follows/directions
SK	streptokinase
sl	under the tongue
SLE	systemic lupus erythematosus
SMAC	sequential multiple analyzer computer
SMD	senile macular degeneration
SOB	shortness of breath
sol	solution
SOM	serous otitis media
SPP	suprapubic prostatectomy
SR	erythrocyte sedimentation rate
ss	one-half
st	stage
ST	skin test, esotropia
stat, STAT	at once, immediately
STD	skin test done, sexually transmitted disease
STSG	split-thickness skin graft
subcu	subcutaneous
subq	subcutancons
supp.	suppository
suppos	suppository
susp	suspension
syr	syrup
T	tablespoon
t	teaspoon
T & A	tonsillectomy and adenoidectomy

Abbreviation	Meaning
T1, T2, etc.	first thoracic vertebra, second thoracic vertebra, etc.
T_3	triiodothyronine
T_4	thyroxine
T_7	free thyroxine index
tab	tablet
TAH-BSO	total abdominal hysterectomy-bilateral salpingo-oophorectomy
TB	tuberculosis
tbsp	tablespoon
TENS	transcutaneous electrical nerve stimulation
TFT	thyroid function test
THA	total hip arthroplasty
THR	total hip replacement
TIA	transient ischemic attack
tid	three times a day
tinc	tincture
TKA	total knee arthroplasty
TKR	total knee replacement
TLC	total lung capacity
TMJ	temporomandibular joint
TNM	tumor, nodes, metastases
TO	telephone order
top	apply topically
TORP	total ossicular replacement prosthests
tPA	tissue-type plasminogen activator
TPN	total parenteral nutrition
TPR	temperature, pulse, and respiration
tr	tincture
TSH	thyroid-stimulating hormone

Abbreviation	Meaning
tsp	teaspoon
TSS	toxic shock syndrome
TUR	transurethral resection
TURP	transurethral resection of prostate
TV	tidal volume
TX, Tx	traction, treatment
u	unit
U/A, UA	urinalysis
UC	uterine contractions, urine culture
UE	upper extremity
UGI	upper gastrointestinal, upper gastrointestinal series
ung	ointment
URI	upper respiratory infection
US	ultrasound
UTI	urinary tract infection
UV	ultraviolet
VA	visual acuity
VC	vital capacity
VCUG	voiding cystourethrography
VD	venereal disease
VF	visual field
VFib	ventricular fibrillation
VLDL	very low density lipoproteins
VO	verbal order
VS	vital signs
VSD	ventricular septal defect
VT	ventricular tachycardia
WBC	white blood cell
wt	weight
x	times
XT	exotropia

APPENDIX D: Laboratory Reference Values

HEMATOLOGY TESTS ABBREVIATIONS USED IN REPORTING LABORATORY VALUES

cm^3	cubic centimeter
cu µ	cubic microns
dL	deciliter
fL	femtoliter
g	gram
g/dL	grams per deciliter
IU	International Unit
kg	kilogram
L	liter
mol (M)	mole
mEq	milliequivalent
mg	milligram
mg/dL	milligram per deciliter
mm	millimeter
mmol	millimole
mm^3	cubic millimeter
mm Hg	millimeter of mercury
ng	nanogram
ng/dL	nanogram per deciliter
ng/mL	nanogram per milliliter
pg	picogram
U	unit
U/L	units per liter
uIU/mL	units International Unit per milliliter
µ g (mcg)	microgram

HEMATOLOGY TESTS

Normal Ranges (these values may vary between hospital laboratories)

Erythrocytes–Red blood cells (RBC)
- Females 4.2–5.4 million/mm^3
- Males 4.6–6.2 million/mm^3
- Children 4.5–5.1 million/mm^3

Hemoglobin (HGB, Hgb)
- Females 12.0–14.0 g/dL
- Males 14.0–16.0 g/dL

Hematocrit (HCT) 37.0–54 %
- Females 37–47 %
- Males 40–54 %

Leukocytes–White blood cells (WBC) 4500–11,000/mm^3

Differential
- Neutrophils 54–62 %
- Lymphocytes 20–40 %
- Monocytes 2–10 %
- Eosinophils 1–2 %
- Basophils 0–1 %

Thrombocytes–Platelets 200,000–400,000/mm^3

COAGULATION TESTS

Bleeding time 2.75–8.0 min
Prothrombin time (PT) 12–14 sec
Partial Thromboplastin Time (PTT) 30–45 sec

CHEMISTRIES

Normal Ranges

A/G ratio 0.7–2.0 g/dL
Alanine aminotransferase 5–30 U/L (ALT, SGPT)
Albumin 3.5–5.5 g/dL
Alkaline phosphatase (ALP) 20–90U/L
Anion gap 10–17 mEq/L
Aspartate aminotransferase 10–30 U/L (AST, SGOT)
Bilirubin 0.3–1.1 mg/dL
Blood urea nitrogen (BUN) 8–20 mg/dL
Calcium (Ca) 9.0–11.0 mg/dL
Chloride (Cl) 100–108 mmol/L
Cholesterol <200 mg/dL
- High density lipoprotein (HDL) >60 mg/dL
- Low density lipoprotein (LDL) <100 mg/dL

CO_2 21–32 mmol/L
Creatine phosphokinase (CPK)
- Females 30–135 U/L
- Males 55–170 U/L

Creatinine 0.9–1.5 mg/dL
Free T_4 0.8–1.8 ng/dL
Globulin 1.4–4.8 g/dL
Glucose (fasting) 70–115 mg/dL
Lactate dehydrogenase (LDH) 100–190 U/L
Phosphate (PO_4) 3.0–4.5 mg/dL

Potassium (K) 3.5–5.0 mEq/L
Prostate specific antigen 0.0–4.0 ng/mL
(PSA) Male
Sodium (Na) 136–145 mEq/L
Testosterone 241–827 ng/dL
Thyroid stimulating 0.5–6.0 ulU/mL
hormone (TSH)
Thyroxine (T_4) 4.4–9.9 μg/dL
Triglycerides <150 mg/dL
Uric acid
Females 1.5–7.0 mg/dL
Males 2.5–8.0 mg/dL

URINALYSIS

	Normal Ranges
Color	yellow to amber
Turbidity (Appearance)	Clear to slightly hazy
Specific gravity	1.003–1.030
Reaction (pH)	5.0–7.0
Odor	Faintly aromatic
Output	1–1.5 liters per day
Protein	Negative
Glucose	Negative
Ketones	Negative
Bilirubin	Negative
Blood	Negative
Urobilinogen	0.1–1.0
Nitrite	Negative
Leukocytes	Negative

NORMAL VALUES OF ARTERIAL BLOOD GASES*

pH 7.35–7.45
Pa_{O_2} 80–100 mm Hg
Pa_{CO_2} 35–45 mm Hg
HCO32 22–26 mEq/L
Base excess 22 to 12 mEq/L
O_2 saturation 95–98%

*Some normal values will vary according to the kind of test carried out in the laboratory.

MOST COMMON BLOOD CHEMISTRIES AND EXAMPLES OF DISORDERS THEY INDICATE

			Examples of Possible Diagnosis	
Test	Abbreviation	Normal Range	Results Increased	Results Decreased
Alkaline phosphate	ALP	30–115 mU/mL	Liver disease, bone disease, mononucleosis	Malnutrition, hypothyroidism, chronic nephritis
Blood urea nitrogen	BUN	8–25 mg/dL	Kidney disease, dehydration, GI bleeding	Liver failure, malnutrition
Calcium	CA	8.5–10.5 mg/dL	Hypercalcemia, bone metastases, Hodgkin's disease	Hypocalcemia, renal failure, pancreatitis
Chloride	Cl	96–11 mEq/L	Dehydration, eclampsia, anemia	Ulcerative colitis, burns, heat exhaustion
Cholesterol	CHOL	120–200 mg/dL	Atherosclerosis, nephrosis, obstructive jaundice	Malabsorption, liver disease, hyperthyroidism
Creatinine	Creat	0.4–1.5 mg/dL	Chronic nephritis, muscle disease, obstruction of urinary tract	Muscular dystrophy

			Examples of Possible Diagnosis	
Test	**Abbreviation**	**Normal Range**	**Results Increased**	**Results Decreased**
Globulin	Glob	1.0–3.5 g/dL	Brucellosis, rheumatoid arthritis, hepatic carcinoma	Severe burns
Glucose fasting blood sugar	FBS	70–110 mg/100 mL	Diabetes mellitus	Excess insulin
Two-hour postprandial	2-hr PPBS	140 mg/dL	Cushing syndrome, brain damage	Addison's disease, CA of pancreas
Lactic acid	LDH	100–225 mU/mL	Acute MI, acute leukemia, hepatic disease	
Potassium	K	3.5–5.5 mEq/L	Renal failure, acidosis, cell damage	Malabsorption, severe burn, diarrhea
Serum glutamic-oxaloacetic	SGOT	0–41 mU/mL	MI, liver disease, pancreatitis	Uncontrolled diabetes mellitus with acidosis
Serum glutamicpyruvic transaminase	SGPT	0–45 mU/mL	Active cirrhosis, pancreatitis, obstructive jaundice	
Sodium	NA	135–145 mEq/L	Diabetes insipitus, coma, Cushing syndrome	Severe diarrhea, severe nephritis, vomiting
Free thyroxine	T4	1–2.3 mg/dL	Thyroiditis, hyper-thyroidism, Graves disease	Goiter, myledema, hypothyroidism
Total bilirubin	TB	0.1–1.2 mg/dL	Liver disease, hemolytic anemia, lupus erythemia	
Triglycerides	TRIG	40–170 mg/dL	Liver disease, atherosclerosis, pancreatitis	Malnutrition
Uric acid	UA	2.2–9.0 mg/dL	Renal failure, gout, leukemia, eclampsia	

Glossary

abdominopelvic cavity *(ab dom ih noh PELL vik KAV ih tee)* Continuous cavity within the abdomen and pelvis that contains the largest organs of the gastrointestinal system.

abduction *(ahb DUK shun)* Moving a body part away from the midline of the body.

absorption *(ab SORP shun)* Process by which digested food nutrients move through villi of the small intestine into the bloodstream or substances move from the kidney tubules into the bloodstream.

accessory muscles Muscles in the neck, chest, and abdomen that can be used, if necessary, to help expand the thoracic cavity on inspiration.

acetylcholine *(ass SET ul KOE leen)* Neurotransmitter between neurons in the brain and spinal cord, also between a neuron and a voluntary skeletal muscle.

actin *(ak TIN)* The thin filament needed for muscle contraction.

action potential The change of the electrical charge of a nerve or muscle fiber when stimulated. Action Potentials are all or none.

active transport The movement of cellular material that requires energy.

adaptation The adjustment of an organism to changing environments.

adduction *(add DUK shun)* Moving a body part toward the midline of the body.

adenoid *(AD eh noid)* Lymphoid tissue in the superior part of the nasopharynx. Also known as the pharyngeal tonsils.

adenosine diphosphate (ADP) The compound that can be converted to ATP for energy storage. When ATP is broken down to ADP energy is released that can be used for cellular energy.

adenosine triphosphate (ATP) Energy storage molecule used to power muscle contraction and other cellular reactions.

adrenal *(ad REE nal)* Referring to the adrenal gland.

adrenal cortex *(ad REE nal KOR teks)* Outermost part of the adrenal gland. It produces and secretes 3 groups of hormones: mineralocorticoids (aldosterone), glucocorticoids (cortisol), and some androgens (male hormones).

adrenal medulla *(ad REE nal meh DULL lah)* Innermost part of the adrenal gland. It produces and secretes the hormones epinephrine and norepinephrine.

adventitia *(add ven TISH ah)* The outmost covering of a structure or organ.

afferent arterioles *(AFF er ent ahr TEE ree ohlz)* Small arteries traveling toward an organ.

agglutinate *(ah GLUE tin ate)* To clump.

agonist *(AG on ist)* The muscle that contracts while another muscle relaxes at the same time to cause movement.

albumin *(AL byoo men)* Most abundant plasma protein.

aldosterone *(al DOSS ter ohn)* Most abundant and biologically active of the mineralocorticoid hormones secreted by the adrenal cortex. It regulates the balance of electrolytes, keeping sodium (and water) in the blood while excreting potassium in the urine.

alimentary tract *(al ah MEN tar ee)* Alternate name for the gastrointestinal system.

alveoli *(al VEE oh lye)* Hollow spheres of cells in the lungs where oxygen and carbon dioxide are exchanged.

amblyopia *(am blee OH pee ah)* To prevent double vision, the brain ignores visual images from a misaligned eye (strabismus). Also known as lazy eye.

anabolism *(ah NAH bow lizm)* Assembly of new molecules in the body.

anastomosis *(ah NASS te MOE sis)* The suturing of one blood vessel to another.

anatomical position *(an ah TOM ih kal)* This is a standard position in which the body is standing erect, the head is up with the eyes looking forward, the arms are by the sides with the palms facing forward, and the legs are straight with the toes pointing forward.

anatomy *(ah NAH tom ee)* The study of the structures of the human body.

anemia *(ah NEE mee ah)* Any condition in which the number of erythrocytes in the blood is decreased.

anesthesia *(an ess THEE zee ah)* Condition in which sensation of any type, including touch, pressure, proprioception, or pain, has been completely lost.

aneurysm *(AN yoo rizm)* Area of dilation and weakness in the wall of an artery. This can be congenital or where arteriosclerosis has damaged the artery. With each heartbeat, the weakened artery wall balloons outward. Aneurysms can rupture without warning. A dissecting aneurysm is one that is enlarging by tunneling between the layers of artery wall.

Antagonists Something that does the opposite of the agonist.

Antebrachial The area of the forearm.

Antecubital The area in front of the elbow.

anterior *(an TEE ree or)* The front of the body.

anterior commissure *(an TEE ree or KAH mih sure)* A nerve pathway in the anterior part of the brain that allows communication between the right and left halves of the cerebrum.

antibody *(AN tee bahd ee)* Proteins secreted by B lymphocytes (Plasma cells) that attack infected cells.

antibody mediated immunity Immunity that results from a formation of antibodies in response to antigens.

antidiuretic hormone (ADH) *(AN tye dye yoo RET ik)* Hormone secreted by the posterior pituitary gland. It stimulates the kidneys to move water back into the blood to increase the volume of blood.

antigen displaying cells (ADC) Cells that engulf antigens and display them as markers.

antigens *(AN tih jenns)* Substance that causes a formation of antibodies. Cell surface markers that help the immune system identify cells.

antiseptic A substance capable of destroying microorganisms.

anus *(AYE nuss)* External opening of rectum, located between the buttocks. The external anal sphincter is under voluntary control. The perianal area is around the anus.

anvil One of the three small bones in the ear.

apex The rounded top of each lung and the gently rounded tip of the outer surface of the heart. The ventricles lie beneath the apex.

apocrine glands *(APP oh crin)* Sweat glands found in the pubic and axillary regions which open into the hair follicles.

appendicitis *(ah pen dih SIGH tiss)* Inflammation and infection of the appendix.

appendicular skeleton *(app en DIK yoo lahr SKELL eh ton)* The bones of the shoulders, arms, hips, and legs.

appendix *(ah PEN dicks)* Long, thin pouch on the exterior wall of the cecum. It does not play a role in digestion. It contains lymphatic tissue.

aqueous humor *(AY kwee uss HYOO mer)* Clear, watery fluid produced by the ciliary body. It circulates through the posterior and anterior chambers and takes nutrients and oxygen to the cornea and lens.

arachnoid mater *(ah RAK noyd MAY ter)* Web-like connective tissues that attach to the pia mater. The space under the arachnoid mater (subarachnoid space) contains cerebralspinal fluid.

Arteries Blood vessels that carry blood away from the heart.

arteriole *(ahr TEE ree ohl)* Smallest branch of an artery.

arteriosclerosis *(ar tee ree oh skleh ROH sis)* Progressive degenerative changes that produce a narrowed, hardened artery.

arthritis *(ahr THRYE tiss)* Inflammation of the joints.

articulation *(AHR tick you lay shun)* A joint where 2 bones come together and join or articulate.

artificial active immunity Vaccination. Intentional exposure to pathogens so patient makes own antibodies.

artificial passive immunity Injection of antibodies to help patient fight infection.

asthma *(AZ mah)* Sudden onset of hyperreactivity of the bronchi and bronchioles with bronchospasm (contraction of the smooth muscle). Inflammation and swelling severely narrow the lumen of the airways.

astrocyte *(ASS tre SITE)* Star-shaped cell that provides structural support for neurons, connects them to capillaries, and forms the blood-brain barrier.

ataxia *(ah TAK see ah)* Lack of coordination of the muscles during movement, particularly the gait. Caused by diseases of the brain or spinal cord, cerebral palsy, or an adverse reaction to a drug.

atelectasis *(at ee LEK tah sis)* Incomplete expansion or collapse of part or all of a lung due to mucus, tumor, or a foreign body that blocks the bronchus. The lung is said to be atelectatic. Also known as collapsed lung.

atherosclerosis *(ath er oh skleh ROH siss)* Hardening of the arteries as a result of plaque buildup in the lumen of the arteries.

atrial natriuretic peptide *(AY tree al nay tree your RET ick PEP tide)* Hormone released by the atria when blood pressure rises. Cause increased excretion of water by the kidney, thereby decreasing blood pressure.

atrioventricular node *(ay tree oh vehn TRIK yoo lahr)* Small knot of tissue located between the right atrium and right ventricle. The AV node is part of the conduction system of the heart and receives electrical impulses from the SA node.

atrioventricular valve *(ay tree oh vehn TRIK yoo lahr)* The valve situated between the atrium and the ventricle.

atrium *(atria) (AY tree um, AY tree ah)* Two upper chambers of the heart. Intra-atrial structures are located within the atria.

atrophy *(AT roh fee)* Loss of muscle bulk in one or more muscles. It can be caused by malnutrition or can occur in any part of the body that is paralyzed and the muscles receive no electrical impulse from the nerves.

auditory canal One of two canals that lead to the ear.

auricle *(AW rih kl)* The visible external ear. Also known as the pinna.

autonomic nervous system Division of the peripheral nervous system that carries nerve impulses to the heart, involuntary smooth muscles, and glands. It includes the parasympathetic nervous system (active during sleep and light activity) and the sympathetic nervous system (active during increased activity, danger, and stress).

autorhythmicity *(aw to rith MIH sih tee)* The heart's ability to generate its own stimulus.

axial skeleton *(AK see al SKELL eh ton)* The bones of the head, chest, and back.

Axillary Pertains to the area of the arm pit.

axon *(AK son)* Part of the neuron that is a single, elongated branch at the opposite end from the dendrites. It receives an electrical impulse and releases neurotransmitters into the synapse. Axons are covered by an insulating layer of myelin.

B lymphocytes *(B LIMF oh sights)* White blood cells which make antibodies to destroy specific pathogens.

bacteria Asexually reproducing cell capable of creating an infection.

basal nuclei *(BAY sal noo KLEE ie)* Clusters of cells (nuclei) deep in the diencephalon, midbrain and cerebrum which help fine tune voluntary movements.

base The bottom of each lung.

basophil *(BAY soh fill)* Least numerous of the leukocytes. It is classified as a granulocyte because granules in its cytoplasm stain dark blue to purple with basic dye. It releases histamine and heparin at the site of tissue damage.

benign *(bee NINE)* Not progressive, non malignant.

bicuspid A two leafed structure.

blood platelets Blood cells responsible for clotting. Also known as thrombocytes.

bolus *(BOW luss)* A mass of masticated food.

brachial artery Major artery that carries blood to the upper arm.

brain stem Most inferior part of the brain that joins with the spinal cord. It is composed of the midbrain, pons, and medulla oblongata.

bronchi *(BRONG kye)* Tubular air passages that branch off the trachea to the right and left and enter each lung. They carry inhaled and exhaled air to and from the lungs.

bronchioles *(BRONG kee ohlz)* Small tubular air passageways that branch off the bronchi. They carry inhaled and exhaled air to and from the alveoli.

buccal *(BUCK al)* Pertaining to cheek or mouth region.

bundle of His *(HISS)* Section of the conduction system of the heart after the AV node. It splits into the right and left bundle branches.

bursa *(BER sah)* Fluid-filled sac that decreases friction where a tendon rubs against a bone near a synovial joint.

calcium ion channels Pathways that allow calcium ions to pass thorugh.

cancellous bone *(CAN cell us)* Spongy bone found in the epiphyses of long bones. Its spaces are filled with red bone marrow that makes blood cells.

canine teeth Long, pointed teeth located between the incisors and the premolars. The canines sink deeply into food to hold it. There are 4 canines, 2 in the maxilla and 2 in the mandible. Also known as cuspids (because they have one large, pointed cusp) or eyeteeth.

capillaries *(KAP ih lair eez)* Smallest blood vessels in the body. Connecting blood vessels between arterioles and venules. The exchange of oxygen and carbon dioxide takes place in the capillaries.

capillary bed A network of capillaries.

capsid The protein covering around a virus particle.

cardiac Pertaining to the heart.

cardiopulmonary Pertaining to the heart and lungs.

cardiovascular system Body system that includes the heart, arteries, veins, and capillaries. It distributes blood throughout the body.

carina *(kuh RINE uh)* A structure with a projecting central ridge such as occurs at the bifurcation of the mainstem bronchi in the lung.

carotene *(CARE eh teen)* A yellow pigment found in plant and animal tissue. The pre-cursor of vitamin A.

carpal bones The 8 small bones of the wrist joint.

cartilage *(KAR tih lij)* Smooth, firm, but flexible connective tissue.

catabolism *(ka TAH bow lizm)* Breaking down of molecules in the body.

cataract *(KAT ah rakt)* Clouding of the lens. Protein molecules in the lens begin to clump together. Caused by aging, sun exposure, eye trauma, smoking, and some medications.

caudal *(KAWD al)* Toward the tailbone, feet, or lower part of the body.

cecum *(SEE kum)* First part of the large intestine. A short, pouchlike area. The appendix is attached to its external wall.

cell mediated immunity Destruction of pathogens by T lymphocytes. T lymphocytes directly attack infected cells, destroying them.

cell membrane Semipermeable barrier that surrounds a cell and holds in the cytoplasm. It allows water and some nutrients to enter and waste products to leave the cell.

cementum *(si MEN tum)* Continuous layer of bone-like connective tissue that covers the dentin layer of the tooth and roots below the gum line. It begins at the gum line where the enamel stops. It anchors one side of the periodontal ligaments.

central nervous system (CNS) Division of the nervous system that includes the brain and the spinal cord.

Centrioles An organelle that precedes mitosis.

Centrosomes Region of cytoplasm usually near the nucleus that contains 1-2 centrioles.

cephalic *(seh FAL ik)* Toward the head of the body.

cerebellum *(ser eh BELL um)* Small rounded section that is the most posterior part of the brain. Monitors muscle tone and position and coordinates new muscle movements.

cerebralspinal fluid *(ser eh broh SPY nal FLOO id)* The fluid cushion that protects the brain and spinal cord from shock.

cerebrum *(SER eh brum)* The largest and most visible part of the brain. Its surface contains gyri and sulci and is divided into 2 hemispheres.

cerumen *(seh ROO men)* Sticky wax that traps dirt in the external auditory canal.

ceruminous glands *(seh ROO men us)* Gland that produces the wax-like substance in the ear.

Cervical Pertaining to the region of the neck.

chemical synapse *(KEH mih cull SIH naps)* Site of communication between neurons and other excitable cells. Neurotransmitters are released from the neuron (presynaptic cell) which travel to a muscle or gland cell (the post synaptic cell), allowing communication between the two cells.

cholecystitis *(koh lee siss TYE tiss)* Acute or chronic inflammation of the gallbladder because of gallstones.

cholecystokinin (CCK) Hormone released by the duodenum when it receives food from the stomach. It causes the gallbladder to release bile and the pancreas to release its digestive enzymes.

cholelithiasis *(KOH lee lith EYE ah siss)* One or more gallstones in the gallbladder. Choledocholithiasis occurs when a gallstone becomes lodged in the common bile duct.

cholesterol Lipid-containing compound that is a component of bile (from the gallbladder), sex hormones, neurotransmitters and cell membranes.

chondrosarcoma *(KON droe sar KOE ma)* Cancer of the cartilage.

choroid *(KOH royd)* Spongy membrane of blood vessels that begins at the iris and continues around the eye. In the posterior cavity, it is the middle layer between the sclera and the retina.

Chromatin Genetic material found in the nucleus of a cell.

chronic bronchitis *(brong KYE tiss)* Chronic inflammation or infection of the bronchi. Inflammation of the bronchi is due to pollution or smoking.

chyle *(KILE)* Milk-like substance formed from digested and absorbed fats.

chyme *(KIME)* Mixed food and digestive juices in the stomach and small intestine.

cilia *(SIL ee ah)* Small hairs that flow in waves to move foreign particles away from the lungs toward the nose and the throat where they can be expelled. Also found inside the fallopian tube to propel an ovum toward the uterus.

ciliary muscles *(SILL ee air ee)* Smooth muscle that alters the lens of the eye to accommodate for near vision.

clot A thrombus or coagulated blood.

coagulation The formation of a blood clot by platelets and the clotting factors.

cochlea *(KOHK lee ah)* Structure of the inner ear that is associated with the sense of hearing. It relays information to the brain via the cochlear branch of the vestibulocochlear nerve.

collecting duct Common passageway that collects fluid from many nephrons. The final step of reabsorption takes place there and the fluid is known as urine.

colon The longest part of the large intestine. It has 4 parts: the ascending colon, the transverse colon, the descending colon, and the S-shaped sigmoid colon.

commissures *(KAH mih sures)* Transverse bands of nerve fibers; carry information from one side of the nervous system to the other.

compact bone Hard or dense bone forming the superficial layer of all bones.

complement cascade A series of chemical reactions triggered by infection that leads to the destruction of a pathogen.

conchae *(kong KA)* Shelf-like structures inside the nasal cavity.

cones Light-sensitive cells in the retina that detect colored light. There are 3 types of cones, each of which responds to either red, green, or blue light.

congestive heart failure (CHF) Inability of the heart to pump sufficient amounts of blood. Caused by chronic coronary artery disease or hypertension.

conjunctiva *(kon JUNK tih vah)* Delicate, transparent mucous membrane that covers the inside of the eyelids and the anterior surface of the eye. It produces clear, watery mucus.

conjunctivitis *(kon JUNK tih VYE tiss)* Inflamed, reddened, and swollen conjunctivae with dilated blood vessels on the sclerae. Caused by a foreign substance in the eye or an infection.

cor pulmonale *(KOR pull moh NAY lee)* Failure of the pumping ability of the right ventricle.

corium *(CORE ee um)* Layer of skin immediately under the epidermis. Also known as the true skin.

cornea Transparent layer over the anterior part of the eye. It is a continuation of the white sclera.

coronal plane *(kor ROHN al)* Also called frontal plane; an imaginary vertical plane that divides the entire body into front and back sections. The coronal plane is named for the coronal suture where the anterior and posterior skull bones meet.

corpus callosum *(KOR pus kah LOH sum)* Thick white band of nerve fibers that connects the 2 hemispheres of the cerebrum and allows them to communicate and coordinate their activities.

cortex Tissue layer of kidney just beneath the renal capsule.

corticobulbar tract *(KOR ti coe BUL bar)* Spinal cord tract that carries impulses to the brainstem from the motor cortex. Carries orders for voluntary movements.

corticospinal tract *(KOR ti coe SPY nal)* Pertains to the tract between the cerebral cortex and spinal cord. Carries orders for voluntary movements.

counter-current circulation Exchange of substances between two streams on either side of a membrane. Helps control concentration of fluids as in the nephron loop.

cramp Spasmodic muscle contraction.

cranial *(KRAY nee al)* Pertaining to the skull.

cranial nerves Twelve pairs of nerves that originate in the brain. Carry sensory nerve impulses to the brain from the nose, eyes, ears, and tongue for the senses of smell, vision, hearing, and taste. Also carry sensory nerve impulses to the brain from the skin of the face. Also carry motor nerve impulses from the brain to the muscles of the face, mouth, throat; eye, and salivary glands.

cross-sectioning Making slices of a sample for examination purposes.

crown White part of the tooth that is visible above the gum line.

crural *(CRUR al)* Pertains to the leg or thigh.

Cuspids Canine teeth.

cutaneous membranes *(cue TAY nee us)* Membranes of the skin.

cuticle Layer of dead skin that arises from the epidermis around the proximal end of the nail. It keeps microorganisms from the nail root.

cyanosis *(sigh ah NOH siss)* Bluish-gray discoloration of the skin from abnormally low levels of oxygen and abnormally high levels of carbon dioxide in the tissues.

cytokines *(SIGH tow kines)* Chemicals released by injured body tissues that summon leukocytes and cause them to move to the area.

cytoplasm *(SIGH toh plazm)* Gel-like intracellular substance. Organelles are embedded in it.

cytotoxic T cells *(sigh tow TOX ick)* Type of T lymphocyte that matures in the thymus. Cytotoxic T cells destroy all types of pathogens as well as body cells infected with viruses.

deciduous teeth *(deh SIH jew uss)* Teeth that erupt during childhood from age 6 months to 2 years. Also called the milk teeth, baby teeth, or primary teeth.

decubitus *(dee KYOO bih tus)* Lying down position; on the back.

defecation *(deh fih CAY shun)* Process by which undigested food fiber and water are removed from the body in the form of a bowel movement.

dendrite *(DEN dright)* Multiple branches at the end of a neuron that carry information to the cell body.

dendritic cells *(DEN dright ick)* One of several types of antigen displaying cells that stimulate adaptive immunity.

dentin Hard layer of tooth just beneath the enamel layer.

deoxyribonucleic acid (DNA) Sequenced pairs of nucleotides that form a double helix. A segment of DNA makes up a gene.

depolarization Changing of the permeability of the cell membrane of any excitable cell, for example cardiac muscle or a neuron, that leads to a decrease in charge across the cell membrane.

dermis (DER miss) Layer of skin under the epidermis. It is composed of collagen and elastin fibers. It contains arteries, veins, nerves, sebaceous glands, sweat glands, and hair follicles.

diagnosis *(dye ahg NOH siss)* A determination as to the cause of the patient's symptoms and signs.

diaphragm *(DYE ah fram)* Muscular sheet that divides the thoracic cavity from the abdominal cavity. Most important ventilation muscle.

diaphysis *(dye AFF ih siss)* The straight shaft of a long bone.

diastole *(dye ASS toe lee)* Resting period between contractions. It is when the heart fills with blood.

diencephalon *(dye en SEFF ah lon)* Central part of the brain that contains that thalamus and hypothalamus.

differentiation Process by which embryonic cells assume different shapes and functions in different parts of the body.

diffusion The process of movement of a substance from high concentration to low concentration.

digestion Process of mechanically and chemically breaking food down into nutrients that can be used by the body.

digital Pertaining to the fingers or toes.

disease *(dih ZEEZ)* Any change in the normal structure or function of the body.

distal *(DISS tal)* Moving from the body toward the end of a limb (arm or leg).

distal tubule Tubule of the nephron that begins at the loop of Henle. It empties into the collecting duct. Reabsorption takes place there.

dorsal *(DOR sal)* Pertaining to the posterior of the body, particularly the back.

dorsal column tract Spinal cord pathway that carries fine touch sensation from the spinal cord to the brain.

dorsal root ganglion *(DOR sal ROOT GANG lee on)* A collection of sensory neurons on the dorsal roots of the spinal cord.

duodenum *(doo ODD eh num)* First part of the small intestine. It secretes cholecystokinin, a hormone that stimulates the gallbladder and pancreas to release bile and digestive enzymes.

dura mater *(DOO ra MAY ter)* Tough, outermost layer of the meninges. The dura mater lies just under the bones of the cranium and vertebrae.

eccrine glands *(EKK rin)* Sweat glands that cover the entire skin surface.

efferent arteriole *(EFF er ent ahr TEE ree ohlz)* Small blood vessels that carry blood away from the glomeruli of the kidney.

electrolyte Chemical element that carries a positive or negative charge and conducts electricity when dissolved in a solution: Examples include sodium (Na+), potassium (K^+), chloride (Cls^-), calcium (Ca^{++}), and bicarbonate ($HCO3^-$). Electrolytes are carried in the plasma. Excess amounts in the blood are removed by the kidneys.

electromyography (EMG) *(elec troh my AH graf ee)* Diagnostic procedure to diagnose muscle disease or nerve damage. A needle electrode inserted into a muscle records electrical activity as the muscle contracts and relaxes. The electrical activity is displayed as waveforms on an oscilloscope screen and permanently recorded on paper as an electromyogram.

embolus *(EM boh luss)* Mass of undissolved matter present in the blood or lymphatic vessels that was brought there by the blood or lymph current.

emphysema *(em fih SEE mah)* Chronic pulmonary disease resulting in destruction of air spaces distal to the terminal bronchiole.

empyema *(em pye EE mah)* Localized collection of purulent material (pus) in the thoracic cavity from an infection in the lungs. Also known as pyothorax.

emulsification *(ee mull sih fih KAY shun)* Process performed by bile of breaking down large fat droplets into smaller droplets with more surface area.

enamel Glossy, thick white layer that covers the crown of the tooth. Enamel is the hardest substance in the body.

endocardium *(ehn doh KAR dee um)* Innermost layer of the heart. It covers the inside of the heart chambers and valves.

endocrine system *(EHN doh krin)* Body system that includes the testes, ovaries, pancreas, adrenal glands, thymus, thyroid gland, parathyroid glands, pituitary gland, pineal gland. It produces and releases hormones into the blood to direct the activities of other body organs.

endocytosis Ingestion of substances by a cell. Substances are taken into the cells after being surrounded by vesicles.

endolymph *(EN doe limf)* Fluid within the labyrinth of the ear.

endoplasmic reticulum Organelle that consists of a network of channels that transport materials within the cell. Also the site of protein, fat, and glycogen synthesis.

enzyme Molecules that speed up the rate of chemical reactions in cells. Enzymes are particularly important in the breakdown and synthesis of biological molecules.

eosinophils *(ee oh SIN oh fillz)* Type of leukocyte. It is classified as a granulocyte because it has granules in the cytoplasm. The nucleus has 2 lobes. Eosinophils are involved in allergic reactions and defense against parasites.

ependymal cells Specialized cells that line the walls of the ventricles and spinal canal and produce cerebrospinal fluid.

epidermis *(ep ih DER miss)* Thin, outermost layer of skin. The most superficial part of the epidermis consists of dead cells filled with keratin. The deepest part (basal layer) contains constantly dividing cells and melanocytes.

epidural space *(eh pih DURE all)* Area between the dura mater and the vertebral body.

epiglottis *(ep ih glah TISS)* Lidlike structure that seals off the larynx, so that swallowed food goes into the esophagus.

epinephrine *(EP ih NEFF rinn)* Hormone secreted by the adrenal medulla in response to stimulation by nerves of the sympathetic nervous system.

epiphyseal plate *(eh piff ih SEE al)* The growth plate.

epiphysis *(eh PIFF ih siss)* The widened ends of a long bone. Each end contains the epiphysial plate where bone growth takes place.

epithelial tissue *(ep ih THEE lee al)* Layers of cells that form the epidermis of the skin as well as the surface layer of mucous and serous membranes.

erythrocyte *(eh RITH roh sights)* A red blood cell. Erythrocytes contain hemoglobin and carry oxygen and carbon dioxide to and from the lungs and cells of the body.

erythropoiesis *(eh rith roh poy EE sis)* Formation of red blood cells.

erythropoietin *(eh RITH roh poy EH tin)* In the body, a hormone secreted by the kidneys when the number of red blood cells decreases. It stimulates the bone marrow to make more red blood cells. As a drug, erythropoietin does the same.

esophagus *(eh SOFF ah guss)* Flexible, muscular tube that moves food from the pharynx to the stomach.

etiology *(ee tee ALL oh jee)* The cause or origin of a disease.

eustachian tube *(yoo STAY she ehn)* Tube that connects the middle ear to the nasopharynx and equalizes the air pressure in the middle ear.

excretion *(ik SCREE shun)* Removal of waste matter from the body.

exocytosis Secretion. The expulsion of material from a cell using vesicles.

extension *(eks TEN shun)* Straightening a joint to increase the angle between 2 bones or 2 body parts.

extensor muscle Muscle that produces extension when it contracts.

external Near or on the outside surface of the body or an organ.

external auditory meatus *(AW dih tor ee mee AY tuss)* Opening at the entrance to the external auditory canal where sound waves enter.

external urethral sphincter *(EKS ter nal yoo REE thral SFINK ter)* One of two valves, made of circular muscle, which allows voluntary control of urination.

facilitated diffusion Also known as carrier mediated passive transport; the movement of substances into cells via carrier proteins.

femoral artery Major artery that carries blood to the upper leg.

fibrin Fiber strands that are the formed by the activation of clotting factors. Fibrin traps erythrocytes and this forms a blood clot.

fibrinogen *(fye BRINN oh jenn)* Blood clotting factor.

fibroblasts Any cell from which connective tissue is created.

fibromyalgia *(fie bro my AL je)* Pain located at specific, small trigger points along the neck, back and hips. The trigger points are very tender to the touch and feel firm. Caused by injury or trauma.

filtration Process in which water and substances in the blood are pushed through the pores of the glomerulus. The resulting fluid is known as filtrate.

fissure *(FISH er)* Deep division on the surface of the brain and spinal cord.

flaccid *(FLAH sid)* Limp or without muscle tone.

flagella hair-like processes on bacteria or protozoon that cause movement.

flexion *(FLEK shun)* Bending of a joint to decrease the angle between 2 bones or 2 body parts. Opposite of extension.

flexor muscle Muscle that produces flexion when it contracts.

flora *(FLOOR ah)* Plant life occurring in a specific environment.

follicle *(FALL ih kle)* 1. Mass of cells with a hollow center. It holds an oocyte before puberty and a maturing ovum after puberty. The follicle ruptures at the time of ovulation and becomes the corpus luteum. 2. Also a site where a hair is formed. The follicle is located in the dermis.

fornix *(FOR niks)* 1. Tract of nerves that joins all the parts of the limbic system. 2. Area of the superior part of the vagina that lies behind and around the cervix.

Fowler's position A semi-sitting position with the torso at a 45–60 degree angle.

frenulum *(FREN you lum)* Structure that attaches the lower side of the tongue to the gum.

frontal lobe Lobe of the cerebrum that predicts future events and consequences. Exerts conscious control over the skeletal muscles.

frontal plane An imaginary plane parallel with the long axis of the body that divides the body into an anterior and posterior section.

fundus *(FUN duss)* A larger part, base, or body of a hollow organ such as the dome-shaped top of the bladder, uterus above the fallopian tubes, or rounded, most superior part of the stomach.

fungi *(FUN jie)* A plant-like organism that includes mold and yeasts.

furuncle *(FOO rung kle)* A boil.

ganglion *(GANG lee on)* Mass of nervous tissue composed mostly of nerve cell bodies and lying outside the brain and spinal cord.

gastrin (GAS trin) Hormone produced by the stomach that stimulates the release of hydrocholoric acid and pepsinogen in the stomach.

gastrointestinal (GI) system Body system that includes the oral cavity, pharynx, stomach esophagus, small and large intestines, and the accessory organs of the liver, gallbladder, and pancreas. Its function is to digest food and remove undigested food from the body. Also known as the gastrointestinal tract and digestive system or tract.

gene An area on a chromosome that contains all the DNA information needed to produce 1 type of protein molecule.

genitourinary system *(gen i toe YOUR in air EE)* Combination of 2 closely related body systems: the male genitalia and the urinary system. Also known as the urogenital system.

gingival *(jin jih VAL)* Referring to the gum.

glaucoma *(glaw KOH mah)* Increased intraocular pressure (IOP) because aqueous humor cannot circulate freely. In open-angle glaucoma, the angle where the edges of the iris and cornea touch is normal and open, but the trabecular meshwork is blocked. Open-angle glaucoma is painless but destroys peripheral vision, leaving the patient with tunnel vision. In closed-angle glaucoma, the angle is too small and blocks the aqueous humor. Closed-angle glaucoma causes severe pain, blurred vision, and photophobia. Glaucoma can progress to blindness.

glia *(GLEE ah)* Non-nervous or supporting tissue found in the brain and spinal cord; made of glial cells.

glial cells *(GLEE all sells)* Cells that include astrocytes, oligodendrocytes, epenymal cells, microglia cells, schwann cells and satellite cells.

glomerular filtrate *(gla MARE you ler FILL trate)* The filtered fluid within the glomerulus.

glomerulus *(gloh MAIR yoo luss)* Network of intertwining capillaries within Bowman's capsule in the nephron. Filtration takes place in the glomerulus.

glottis *(GLOT is)* V-shaped structure of mucous membranes and vocal cords within the larynx.

glucose *(GLOO kohs)* 1. A simple sugar found in foods and also the sugar in the blood. 2. Glucose is not normally found in the urine. Its presence (glycosuria) indicates uncontrolled diabetes mellitus with excess glucose in the blood "spilling" over into the urine.

gluteal *(GLOO tee al)* Pertains to buttocks.

glycogen *(GLIE co jin)* The form that glucose (sugar) takes when it is stored in the liver and skeletal muscles.

golgi apparatus Organelle of the cell that packages cellular material for transport.

Guillian Barre syndrome A neuromuscular disease that ususally leads to ascending flaccid paralysis.

gustatory sense *(GUSS ta tore ee)* Sense of taste.

gyri *(JIE rie)* Convolutions of the cerebral hemispheres of the brain.

Hammer One of the three small bones of the ear, also known as the malleus.

helper T cell Helper T cells stimulate the production of cytotoxic T cells and B cells. Also known as a CD4 cell.

hemisphere One half of the cerebrum, either the right hemisphere or the left hemisphere. The right hemisphere deals with recognizing patterns and 3-dimensional structures (including faces) and the emotions of words. The left hemisphere deals with mathematical and logical reasoning, analysis, and interpreting sights, sounds, and sensations. The left hemisphere is active in reading, writing, and speaking.

hemoglobin *(HEE moh GLOH binn)* Substance in an erythrocyte that binds to oxygen and carbon dioxide. Its globin chains give it a round shape. When it is bound to oxygen it forms the compound oxyhemoglobin.

hemophilia *(HEE moh FILL ee ah)* Inherited genetic abnormality of a gene on the X chromosome that causes an absence or deficiency of a specific clotting factor. When injured, hemophiliac patients cannot easily form a blood clot and continue to bleed for long periods of time.

hemopoiesis *(HEME ah poy ee sus)* Formation of blood cells.

hemostasis *(HEE moh STAY siss)* The cessation of bleeding after the formation of a blood clot.

hemothorax *(HEEM oh THOH raks)* Presence of blood in the thoracic cavity, usually from trauma.

heparin Substance that inhibits coagulation of blood.

hepatic duct *(hepp ah TIC duct)* Duct that carries bile from the liver.

hernia A weakness in the muscles of the abdominal wall that allows loops of intestine to balloon outward.

hilum *(HIGH lim)* 1. Indentation on the medial side of each lung where the bronchus, pulmonary artery, pulmonary vein, and nerves enter the lung. 2. Indentation in the medial side of each kidney where the renal artery enters and renal vein and the ureter leave.

histamine *(HISS tah meen)* Released by basophils. Heparin dilates blood vessels and increases blood flow to damaged tissue. Allows protein molecules to leak out of blood vessels into the surrounding tissue. This produces redness and swelling.

homeostasis *(hoh mee oh STAY siss)* State of equilibrium of the internal environment of the body, including fluid balance, acid-base balance, temperature, metabolism, and so forth, to keep all the body systems functioning optimally.

horizontal plane Another name for the transverse plane.

hormone *(HOR mohn)* Chemical messenger of the endocrine system that is released by a gland or organ and travels through the blood.

hyperopia *(HIGH per OH pee ah)* Farsightedness. Light rays from a far object focus correctly on the retina, creating a sharp image. However, light rays from a near object come into focus posterior to the retina, creating a blurred image.

hyperpolarized The charge across the cell membrane is more negative than resting.

hypertrophy *(high PER troh fee)* Greater than normal growth.

hypodermis The fatty tissue layer below the dermis of the skin.

hypothalamus *(high poh THAL ah mus)* Endocrine gland located in the brain just below the thalamus. It produces (but does not secrete) antidiuretic hormone (ADH) and oxytocin. The hypothalamis is in the center of the brain just below the thalamus and coordinates the activities of the pons and medulla oblongata. It also controls heart rate, blood pressure, respiratory rate, body temperature, sensations of hunger and thirst, and the circadian rhythm. It also produces hormones as part of the endocrine system. In addition, the hypothalamus helps control emotions (pleasure, excitement, fear, anger, sexual arousal) and bodily responses to emotions; regulates the sex drive; contains the feeding and satiety centers; and functions as part of the "fight or flight" response of the sympathetic nervous system.

ilium *(ILL ee um)* Most superior hip bone. Bony landmarks include the iliac crest and the anterior-superior iliac spine (ASIS). Posteriorly, each ilium joins one side of the sacrum.

incisors Chisel-shaped teeth in the middle of the dental arch that cut and tear food on their incisal surface. There are 8 incisors, 4 in the maxilla and 4 in the mandible.

incus *(ING kuss)* Second bone of the middle ear. It is attached to the malleus on one end and the stapes on the other end. Also known as the anvil.

infarct *(in FARKT)* Cellular death due to lack of blood flow (perfusion).

inferior Pertaining to the lower half of the body or a position below an organ or structure.

inferior vena cava The vena cava is the largest vein in the body. The inferior vena cava receives blood from the abdomen, pelvis, and lower extremities and takes it to the heart.

inflammation *(in flah MAY shun)* Tissue reaction to injury that includes swelling and reddening due to increase blood flow to the area.

Ingestion Process of taking in material (particularly food).

inguinal region The groin.

innate immunity *(ih NATE im YOO nih tee)* Defense against pathogens that you are born with and that does not improve with experience or remember specific pathogens. The first line of defense.

inotropism An influence on the force of muscular contraction.

insula The deep lobes of the cerebral hemispheres.

intercalated discs *(in ter KUH late ed)* Structures that connect heart tissue cells to facilitate a smooth contraction.

interferon *(in ter FIR on)* Substance released by macrophages that have engulfed a virus. Interferon stimulates body cells to produce an antiviral substance that keeps a virus from entering a cell and reproducing.

interleukin *(in ter LOO kin)* Released by macrophages, it stimulates B cell and T lymphocytes and activates NK cells. It also produces the fever associated with inflammation and infection.

internal Structures deep within the body or an organ.

interneurons *(in ter NURE ons)* Neurons that facilitate communication between neurons.

iris *(EYE riss)* Colored ring of tissue whose muscles iris (colored part contract or relax to change the size of the of the eye) pupil in the center of the iris.

ischemia *(iss KEE mee ah)* Tissue injury due to a decrease in blood flow.

jejunum *(jee JOO num)* Second part of the small intestine.

joint Area where 2 bones come together.

keratin *(KAIR ah tin)* Hard protein found in the cells of the outermost part of the epidermis and in the nails.

keratinization *(KAIR ah tin eye ZAY shun)* The process of forming a horny growth such as fingernails.

kidney Organ of the urinary system that filters blood and produces urine, controlling fluid and ionic balance.

labia *(LAY bee ah)* An outer pair of vertical fleshy lips covered with pubic hair (the labia majora) and a smaller, thinner, inner pair of lips (the labia minora) that partially cover the clitoris, and urethral and vaginal openings. Part of the external female genitalia.

labyrinth *(LAB ih rinth)* Intricate communicating passage of the inner ear essential for maintaining equilibrium.

labyrinthitis *(LAB ih rinn THYE tiss)* Bacterial or viral infection of the semicircular canals of the inner ear, causing severe vertigo.

lacrimal apparatus *(LAK rim al app ah RA tuss)* Structures involved with the secretion and production of tears.

lacteal *(LACK te al)* Pertains to milk.

large intestine Organ of absorption between the small intestine and the anal opening to the outside of the body. The large intestine includes the cecum, appendix, colon, rectum, and anus. Also known as the large bowel.

laryngitis *(lar in JIGH tis)* Hoarseness or complete loss of the voice, difficulty swallowing, and cough due to swelling and inflammation of the larynx.

laryngopharynx *(lah ring goh FAR inks)* Relates to both the larynx and pharynx.

larynx *(LAR inks)* Triangular-shaped structure in the anterior neck (visible as the laryngeal prominence or Adam's apple) that contains the vocal cords and is a passageway for inhaled and exhaled air. Also known as the voice box.

lateral *(LAT er al)* Pertaining to the side of the body or the side of an organ or structure.

lens Clear, hard, disk in the internal eye. The muscles and ligaments of the ciliary body change its shape to focus light rays on the retina.

lesion *(LEE zhun)* General category for any area of visible damage on the skin, whether it is from disease or injury.

leukemia Cancer of leukocytes (white blood cells), including mature lymphocytes, immature lymphoblasts, as well as myeloblasts and myelocytes that mature into neutrophils, eosinophils, or basophils). The malignant leukocytes crowd out the production of other cells in the bone marrow. Leukemia is named according to the type of leukocyte that is the most prevalent and whether the onset of symptoms is acute or chronic. Types of leukemia include acute myelogenous leukemia (AML), chronic myelogeous leukemia (CML), acute lymphocytic leukemia (ALL), and chronic lymphocytic leukemia (CLL).

leukocytes *(LOO koh sights)* White blood cells. There are five different types of mature leukocytes: neutrophils, eosinophils, basophils, lymphocytes, and monocytes.

leukocytosis Increase in the number of white blood cells above normal.

leukopenia Abnormal decrease of white blood cells.

lingual *(LING gwal)* Pertaining to the tongue.

ligament Fibrous bands that hold 2 bone ends together in a synovial joint.

limbic system *(LIM bick)* Processes memories and controls emotions, mood, motivation, and behavior. Links the conscious to the unconscious mind. Limbic system consists of the thalamus, hypothalamus, hippocampus, amygdaloid bodies, and fornix.

lipocyte Cell in the subcutaneous layer that stores fat.

lithotripsy *(LITH oh trip see)* Medical or surgical procedure that uses sound waves to break up a kidney stone.

lobes 1. Large divisions of the lung, visible on the outer surface. 2. Large area of the hemisphere of the cerebrum. Each lobe is named for the bone of the skull that is next to it: frontal lobe, parietal lobe, temporal lobe, and occipital lobe.

local potential Change in the charge across a cell membrane that is proportional to the size of the stimulus.

lower esophageal sphincter (LES) Ringed muscle leading into the stomach.

lumbar region Two of the 9 regions of the abdominopelvic area. The right and left lumbar regions are inferior to the right and left hypochondriac regions. Also refers to the lower back, spinal cord and spinal column.

lumen Opening in the center of a large tube, for example the center of the tubes in the digestive and respiratory systems and the blood vessels.

lunula *(LOO nyoo lah)* Whitish half-moon visible under the proximal portion of the nail plate. It is the visible tip of the nail root.

lymph *(LIMF)* Fluid that flows through the lymphatic system.

lymph nodes *(LIMF nohdz)* Small, encapsulated pieces of lymphoid tissue located along the lymphatic vessels. Lymph nodes filter and destroy invading microorganisms and cancerous cells present in the lymph.

lymphatic system *(lim FAT ik)* Body system that includes lymphatic vessels, lymph nodes, lymph fluid, and lymphoid tissues (tonsils and adenoids, appendix, Peyer's patches), lymphoid organs (spleen and thymus), and the blood cells, lymphocytes and macrophages.

lymphatic fluid *(lim FAT ik FLOO id)* Clear and colorless fluid of the lymphatic system.

lymphatic vessels *(lim FAT ik)* Vessels that begin as capillaries carrying lymph, continue through lymph nodes, and empty into the right lymphatic duct and the thoracic duct.

lymphocyte activation Stimulation of lymphocytes, "waking them up" to fight a pathogen.

lymphocyte proliferation Reproduction of activated lymphocytes so there are many copies.

lysis *(LYE siss)* Destruction or breakdown.

lysosome *(LIE so soam)* Organelle that consists of a small sac with digestive enzymes in it. These destroy pathogens that invade the cell.

macrophages *(MAC reh fage ez)* Cells that take fragments of the pathogen they have eaten and present them to a B cell (lymphocyte). This stimulates the B cell to become a plasma cell and make antibodies against that specific pathogen. Macrophages also activate Helper T cells in this way. Macrophages also produce special immune response chemicals: interferon, interleukin, and tumor necrosis factor.

macroscopic anatomy *(MAK roh scop ic ah NAH tom ee)* Study of large structures of the body.

major calyx, minor calyces *(KAY licks, KAY leh seez)* Tubes in the kidney which carry urine from the nephrons to the renal pelvis.

malignant *(mah LIG nant)* Cancerous, able to spread to distant parts of the body.

malleus *(MALL ee us)* First bone of the middle ear. It is attached to the tympanic membrane on one end and to the incus on the other end. Also known as the hammer.

mast cells Connective tissue cells that are important in cellular defense and contain heparin and histamine.

mastication *(MASS tih CAY shun)* Process of chewing, during which the teeth and tongue together tear, crush, and grind food. This is part of the process of mechanical digestion.

medial *(MEE dee al)* Pertaining to the middle of the body or the middle of an organ or structure.

mediastinum *(me dee ah STY num)* Central area within the thoracic cavity. It contains the trachea, esophagus, heart, and other structures.

medulla oblongata *(meh DULL lah ob long GALL ah)* Most inferior part of the brainstem that joins to the spinal cord. It relays nerve impulses from the cerebrum to the cerebellum. It contains the respiratory center. Cranial nerves IX through XII originate there.

melanin *(MELL an in)* Dark brown or black pigment that gives color to the skin and hair.

melanocytes *(mell AN oh sights)* Cell that produces melanin.

melanoma A malignant pigmented mole or tumor.

melatonin *(MELL ah TOH ninn)* Hormone secreted by the pineal body. It maintains the 24-hour wake-sleep cycle known as the circadian rhythm.

membrane A thin soft pliable layer of tissue which can line a cavity or cover an organ or structure.

memory B cells Antibody producing cells which are produced when a pathogen is encountered the first time. Memory B cells are stored until the pathogen comes again. They are responsible for secondary response.

memory T cells Memory cells responsible for cell mediated immunity. They are produced when a pathogen is encountered the first time. Memory T cells are stored until the pathogen comes again. They are responsible for secondary response.

Meniere's disease *(MEN yerz)* Recurring and progressive disease that includes progressive deafness, ringing ears, dizziness and the feeling of fullness in the ears.

meninges *(men IN jeez)* Three separate membranes that envelope and protect the entire brain and spinal cord. The meninges include the dura mater, arachnoid, and pia mater.

meningitis *(men in JYE tiss)* Inflammation of the meninges of the brain or spinal cord by a bacterial or viral infection. Initial symptoms include fever, headache, nuchal rigidity (stiff neck) lethargy, vomiting, irritability, and photophobia.

mesentery *(MEZ in tare ee)* Membranous sheet of peritoneum that supports the jejunum and ileum.

metabolism *(me TAH bow lizm)* Process of using oxygen and glucose to produce energy for cells. Metabolism also produces byproducts like carbon dioxide and other waste products. The ongoing cycle of anabolism and catabolism.

metastasis *(meh TASS tah siss)* Process by which cancerous cells break off from a tumor and move through the blood vessels or lymphatic vessels to other sites in the body.

metric system Sytem of measurement based on the power of 10.

microglia *(mie crow GLEE ah)* Cells that move, engulf, and destroy pathogens anywhere in the central nervous system.

microscopic anatomy *(MY kroh scop ic ah NAH tom ee)* Study of structures that require the aid of magnification.

midbrain An area that connects the pons and the cerebellum with the hemispheres of the cerebrum.

midsagittal plane *(mid SAJ ih tal)* An imaginary vertical plane that divides the entire body into right and left sides and creates a midline. The midsagittal plane is named for the sagittal suture of the skull.

Mitochondria The energy organelle of the cell.

Mitral Pertains to the bicuspid or mitral valve of the heart.

mixed nerve A nerve that carries both sensory and motor information.

molars Largest tooth, located posterior to the premolar. It crushes and grinds food on its large, flat occlusal surface.

motor neurons Neuron that innervates muscle tissue.

motor system The system responsible for movement.

mucosa 1. Lining throughout the gastrointestinal system that consists of a mucous membrane that produces mucus and an underlying smooth muscle layer that contracts to move food. 2. Mucous membrane that lines the respiratory tract. It warms and humidifies incoming air. It produces mucus to trap foreign particles. 3. Mucous membrane lining the inside of the bladder. 4. Mucous membranes lining the nasal cavity that warm and moisturize the incoming air. They also produce mucus to trap foreign particles.

Mucous Pertaining to mucus.

muscle Many muscle fascicles grouped together and surrounded by fascia.

muscular dystrophy *(MUSS kyoo lahr DISS troh fee)* Genetic disease due to a mutation of the gene that makes the muscle protein dystrophin. Without dystrophin, the muscles weaken and then atrophy. Symptoms appear in early childhood as weakness first in the lower extremities and then in the upper extremities. The most common and most severe form is Duchenne's muscular dystrophy; Becker's muscular dystrophy is a milder form.

muscularis externa The outside muscular layer of an organ or tubule.

myalgia *(my AL jee ah)* Pain in one or more muscles due to injury or muscle disease. Polymyalgia is pain in several muscle groups.

myasthenia gravis *(my ass THEE nee ah)* Abnormal and rapid fatigue of the muscles, particularly evident in the muscles of the face; there is ptosis of the eyelids. Symptoms worsen during the day and can be relieved by rest. The body produces antibodies against its own acetylcholine receptors located on muscle fibers. The antibodies destroy many of the receptors. There are normal levels of acetylcholine, but too few receptors remain to produce sustained muscle contractions.

myelin *(MY eh lin)* Fatty sheath around the axon of a neuron. It acts as an insulator to keep the electrical impulse intact. Myelin around the axons of the brain and spinal cord is produced by oligodendrocytes. Myelin around axons of the cranial and spinal nerves is produced by Schwann cells. An axon with myelin is said to be myelinated.

myofibril *(my ah FIE bril)* Thin filament (actin) and thick filament (myosin) within the muscle fiber that give it its characteristic striated appearance.

myopia *(my OH pee ah)* Nearsightedness. Light rays from a near object focus correctly on the retina, creating a sharp image. However, light rays from a far object come into focus anterior to the retina, creating a blurred image.

myosin *(MY ah sin)* The thick filament needed for muscle contraction.

nares *(NAIR eez)* The paired external openings of the nasal cavity.

nasal Pertaining to the nose.

nasal cavity *(NAY zl CAV ih tee)* Hollow area inside the nose that is lined with mucosa or mucous membrane.

nasopharynx *(nay zoh FAR inks)* Uppermost portion of the throat where the posterior nares unite. The nasopharynx contains the opening for the eustachian tubes and the adenoids.

natural active immunity Antibodies developed due to exposure to a pathogen.

natural killer (NK) cell Type of lymphocyte that matures in the red marrow and is the body's first cellular defense against invading microorganisms. Without the help of antibodies or complement, an NK cell recognizes a pathogen by the antigens on its cell wall and releases chemicals that penetrate and destroy it.

natural passive immunity Immunity due to the passage of antibodies from mother to child across the placenta or in breast milk.

neck Transitional area between the root and crown where the tooth becomes narrower. The neck of the tooth is located just above and below the gum line.

necrosis *(neh KROH siss)* Gray-to-black discoloration of the skin in areas where the tissue has died.

negative feedback loop Physiological process that works against the trend. Most often brings a variable back to set point. For example, as blood pressure rises, heart rate may decrease to bring blood pressure back to "normal".

negative selection The destruction of lymphocytes which react to "self" antigens. These lymphocytes must be deleted to prevent autoimmunity.

nephron *(NEFF rahn)* Microscopic functional unit of the kidney.

nephropathy *(neff ROPP ah thee)* General word for any disease process involving the kidney. Diabetic nephropathy involves progressive damage to the glomeruli because of diabetes mellitus. The tiny arteries of the glomerulus harden (glomerulosclerosis) because of accelerated arteriosclerosis throughout the body.

nerves Bundles of individual axons.

nervous system Body system that includes the brain, cranial nerves, spinal cord, spinal nerves, and neurons. It receives signals from parts of the body and interprets them as pain, touch, temperature, body position, taste, sight, smell, and hearing. It coordinates body movement. It maintains and interprets memory and emotion.

neuroglia *(glial cells) (noo ROH glee ah)* Cells that hold neurons in place and perform specialized tasks. Includes astrocytes, ependymal cells, microglia, oligodendrocytes, satellite cells and Schwann cells.

neuromuscular Pertaining to the nervous and muscular system.

neuromuscular junction Area on a single muscle fiber where a nerve connects.

neuron *(NER on)* An individual nerve cell. The functional part of the nervous system.

neurotransmitter *(noo roh TRANS mit ter)* Chemical messenger that travels across the synapse between a neuron and another neuron, muscles fiber or gland.

neutrophils *(NOO troh fill)* A type of leukocyte that perform non-specific phagocytosis.

nodes of Ranvier Constriction of the myelin sheath on a myelinated nerve fiber that facilitates nodal transmission of the impulse.

norepinephrine *(NOR ep ih NEFF rinn)* 1. Neurotransmitter for the sympathetic nervous system. It goes between neurons and an involuntary muscle, organ, or gland. Controls the flight or fight response. 2. Hormone secreted by the adrenal medulla in response to stimulation by nerves of the sympathetic nervous system.

nucleolus Round, central region within the nucleus. It makes ribosomes.

occipital lobe *(ok SIP eh tal)* Lobe of the cerebrum that receives sensory information from the eyes. Contains the visual cortex for the sense of sight.

oligodendrocytes *(AH li go DEN droe site)* Neuroglial cells which produce myelin in the CNS.

ophthalmologist *(off thal MALL oh jee)* A doctor who specializes in the eyes.

Oral Pertaining to the mouth.

orbit Bony socket in the skull that surrounds all but the anterior part of the eyeball.

Organ A part of the body comprised of tissues, that has a specialized function.

organelles Small structures in the cytoplasm that have various specialized functions. Organelles include mitochondria, ribosomes, the endoplasmic reticulum, the Golgi apparatus, and lysosomes.

oropharynx *(oh roh FAR inks)* Middle portion of the throat just behind the oral cavity. It begins at the level of the soft palate and ends at the epiglottis.

Osmosis The passage of the solvent through a semi-permeable membrane to equalize concentrations.

osmotic pressure The pressure which develops when there are two solutions of varying concentrations that are separated by a semi-permeable membrane.

osseous tissue *(AH see us)* Bone, a type of connective tissue.

ossicles *(AH sih kel)* Three tiny bones in the middle ear that function in the process of hearing: malleus, incus, and stapes.

ossification *(AH siff ih cay shun)* Process by which cartilaginous tissue is changed into bone from infancy through puberty. Also known as osteogenesis.

osteoarthritis *(OSS tee oh ahr THRYE tiss)* Chronic inflammatory disease of the joints, particularly the large weightbearing joints of the knees and hips, although it often occurs in the joints that move repeatedly like the shoulders, neck, and hands.

osteoblasts Osteocytes that form new bone.

osteoclasts Osteocytes that break down old or damaged areas of bone.

osteocytes *(OSS tee oh site)* Bone cells. There are two types of osteocytes: osteoclasts and osteoblasts.

osteomalacia *(OSS tee oh mah LAY she ah)* Abnormal softening of the bones due to a deficiency of vitamin D. Chondromalacia is abnormal softening of the cartilage, specifically of the patella.

osteoporosis *(OSS tee oh por OS sis)* Condition of increased bone porosity that weakens the bones, usually seen in the elderly.

otitis media *(oh TYE tiss MEH dee ah)* Acute or chronic bacterial infection of the middle ear.

oval window Opening in the temporal bone between the middle ear and the vestibule of the inner ear. The opening is covered by the end of the stapes.

oxytocin *(AHK see TOH sin)* Hormone secreted by the posterior pituitary gland. It stimulates the uterus to contract and begin labor. It stimulates the "let-down reflex" to get milk flowing for breastfeeding.

pacemaker Cells cells or group of cells that automatically generate electrical impulses.

palate *(PAHL aht)* Roof of the mouth

palatine tonsils *(PAL ah tighn TAHN sill)* Lymphoid tissue on either side of the throat where the soft palate arches downward in the oropharynx.

pancreas *(PAN kree ass)* A digestive and endocrine organ located in the abdominal cavity that produces digestive enzymes (amylase, lipase, protease, peptidase) and releases them into the duodenum. It also contains the islets of Langerhans (alpha, beta, and delta cells) that produce and secrete the hormones glucagon, insulin, and somatostatin.

pancreatitis *(PAN kree ah TYE tiss)* Inflammation or infection of the pancreas.

paralysis Temporary or permanent loss of muscle function.

parasympathetic nervous system Division of the autonomic nervous system that uses the neurotransmitter acetlycholine and carries nerve impulses to the heart, involuntary smooth muscles, and glands while the body is at rest.

parathyroid glands *(PAIR ah THIGH royd)* Endocrine glands, 4 of them, on the posterior lobes of the thyroid gland. They produce and secrete parathyroid hormone.

parietal lobe *(pah RYE eh tal)* Lobe of the cerebrum that receives sensory information about temperature, touch, pressure, vibration, and pain from the skin and internal organs.

parietal pleura *(pah RYE eh tal PLOO rah)* One of the 2 layers of the pleura. It lines the thoracic cavity.

parotid salivary gland *(pah RAH tid SAHL ih vair ee gland)* Gland that secretes saliva that helps to lubricate food so that it is easier to chew and swallow.

passive transport The general term for the transportation of cellular material without the use of energy.

Patellar Pertaining to the knee cap.

pathogen *(PATH oh jenn)* Microorganism that causes a disease. Pathogens include bacteria, viruses, protozoa, and other microorganisms, as well as plant cells like fungi or yeast.

pathology *(path ALL oh jee)* The study of disease.

Pedal Pertaining to the foot or feet.

pepsin Digestive enzyme produced by the stomach that breaks down food protein into smaller protein molecules.

perforin Chemical secreted by cytotoxic T cells which makes holes in the cell membranes of pathogens or infected cells, killing them.

perfusion Blood flow to a particular region.

perilymph *(per ih LIMF)* Pale lymph fluid found the labyrinth of the inner ear.

periodontal *(perr ee oh DAHN til)* Literally means "around the teeth" and may refer to the area of the gum.

periosteum *(pair ee OSS tee um)* Thick, fibrous membrane that goes around and covers the outside of a bone.

Peripheral Referring to "away from center" or the extremities.

peripheral nervous system (PNS) Division of the nervous system that includes the cranial nerves and the spinal nerves.

peripheral vascular disease (PVD) Any disease of the arteries of the extremities.

peristalsis *(pair ih STALL siss)* Contractions of the smooth muscle of the gastrointestinal tract that propel food through it. Can also be the process of smooth muscle contractions that propel urine through the ureter.

peritubular capillaries *(per ee TUBE you ler)* Capillaries surrounding the renal tubules.

pH A test of how acidic or alkaline the a substance is.

phagocytosis *(fag oh sigh TOH siss)* The process by which a phagocyte destroys a foreign cell or cellular debris; a type of endocytosis.

pharyngitis *(far in JIGH tis)* Bacterial or viral infection of the throat. When the bacteria group A beta-hemolytic streptococcus causes the infection, it is known as strep throat.

pharynx *(FAR inks)* The throat; contains the passageways for food and for inhaled and exhaled air.

physiology *(fiz ee ALL oh jee)* The study of the function of the body's structures.

pia mater *(PEE ah MAY ter)* Thin, delicate innermost layer of the meninges that covers the surface of the brain and spinal cord. It contains many small blood vessels.

pineal gland *(pih NEE al)* Endocrine gland in the brain that lies posterior to the pituitary gland. It secretes the hormone melatonin.

pinna *(PINN ah)* The auricle of the exterior ear that collects sound waves.

Pinocytosis Process in which a cell absorbs fluid material.

pituitary gland *(pih TOO ih tair ee)* Endocrine gland in the brain that is connected by a stalk of tissue to the hypothalamus. Also known as the hypophysis. It is known as the master gland of the body. It consists of the anterior and the posterior pituitary gland.

plantar Referring to sole of the foot.

plasma *(PLAZ mah)* Clear, straw-colored fluid portion of the blood that carries blood cells and contains dissolved substances like proteins, glucose, minerals, electrolytes, clotting factors, complement proteins, hormones, bilirubin, urea, and creatinine.

plasma proteins *(PLAZ mah)* Protein molecules in the plasma. The most important one is albumin.

pleural cavities *(PLOO ral)* The space between the parietal and visceral layers of the pleura.

pleural effusion *(PLOO ral eh FYOO zhun)* Accumulation of fluid within the pleural space due to inflammation or infection of the pleura and lungs.

plexus *(PLECK sus)* A network of nerves or vessels.

plicae circulares One of the transverse folds in the small intestine.

pneumothorax *(NOO moh THOH raks)* Large volume of air that forms in the pleural space and progressively separates the 2 pleural membranes.

polycythemia *(pall ee sigh THEE mee ah)* Increased number of erythrocytes due to uncontrolled production by the red marrow. The cause is unknown. The viscosity of the blood increases; it becomes viscous (thick), and the total blood volume is increased.

pons Area of the brainstem that relays nerve impulses from the body to the cerebellum and back to the body. Area where nerve tracts cross from one side of the body to the opposite side of the cerebrum. Cranial nerves V through VIII originate there.

positive feedback Vicious cycle. During positive feedback, physiological processes send body chemistry or other attributes further and further away from equilibrium (set point). The trend will continue until something breaks the cycle.

positive selection During lymphocyte development, only those lymphocytes which can actually react to antigens will survive.

postcentral gyrus Ridge on the surface of the cerebrum posterior to the central sulcus in each hemisphere. The postcentral gyrus contains the primary somatic sensory area for your sense of touch.

posterior The back of the body.

precentral gyrus Ridge on the surface of the cerebrum anterior to the central sulcus in each hemisphere. The postcentral gyrus contains the primary motor cortex for voluntary movements.

presbyopia *(PRESS bee OH pee ah)* Loss of flexibility of the lens with blurry near vision and loss of accommodation.

prognosis *(prog NOH siss)* The predicted outcome of a disease.

prolactin *(proh LAK tinn)* Hormone secreted by the anterior pituitary gland. It stimulates milk glands of the breasts to develop during puberty and to produce milk during pregnancy.

prone position Lying with the anterior section of the body down.

prothrombin *(pro THROM bin)* Blood clotting factor that is activated just before the thrombus is formed.

Protozoa Unicellular organisms.

proximal *(PROK sim al)* Referring to "near" a reference point.

proximal tubule The part of the renal tubule closest to the glomerulus. Many substances are secreted or absorbed in this part of the renal tubule.

pulmonary artery Artery that carries blood from the heart to the lungs. The pulmonary artery is the only artery in the body that carries blood that has low levels of oxygen.

pupil *(PYOO pill)* Round opening in the iris that allows light rays to enter the internal eye.

pustule *(PUS tyool)* A small elevation of skin filled with lymph or pus.

pyloric sphincter *(pye LOR ik SFINK ter)* Muscular ring that keeps food in the stomach from entering the duodenum.

pylorus *(pye LOR uss)* Narrowing canal of the stomach just before it joins the duodenum. It contains the pyloric sphincter.

rapid eye movement (REM) The dream stage of sleep.

reabsorption Process by which water and substances in the filtrate move out of the renal tubule and into the blood in a nearby capillary.

rectum Final part of the large intestine. It is a short, straight segment that lies between the sigmoid colon and the outside of the body.

reflex Involuntary muscle reaction that is controlled by the spinal cord. In response to pain, the spinal cord immediately sends a command to the muscles of the body to move. All of this takes place without conscious thought or processing by the brain. The entire circuit is also known as a reflex arc.

refractory period Short period of time when the myocardium is resting and unresponsive to electrical impulses.

regulatory T cells Type of T cell that shuts down decreases immune response.

renal artery *(REE nal AHR ter ee)* Major artery that carries blood to the kidney.

renal corpuscle *(REE nal KOR puss el)* The filtration apparatus of the kidney, consists of the glomerulus and the glomerular capsule.

renal nephron Fundamental functional unit of the kidney, consists of the renal corpuscle and renal tubule.

renal pelvis *(REE nal PELL vis)* Funnel-shaped part of the kidney that collects urine.

renal vein Major blood vessels that carries blood away from the kidneys.

renin-angiotensin-aldosterone *(REE nen—an gee oh TEN sen—al DOSS ter ohn)* A complex hormone system that regulates blood volume and blood pressure. The system is triggered when blood flow to the kidney decreases.

repolarization The opposite of depolarization.

respiration *(ress pih RAY shun)* The process of gas exchange at the lungs or tissue sites. Oxygen and carbon dioxide are exchanged in the alveoli during external respiration. Oxygen and carbon dioxide are exchanged at the cellular level during internal respiration.

retina *(RETT in ah)* Membrane lining the posterior cavity. It contains rods and cones. Landmarks include the optic disk and macula.

Rh factor A blood group discovered on the surface of erythrocytes of Rhesus monkeys and found to a variable degree in humans. Can be Rh-negative or Rh-positive.

rhinoplasty *(RYE noh plass tee)* Surgical procedure that uses plastic surgery to change the size or shape of the nose.

ribonucleic acid (RNA) Molecule contained in ribosomes and necessary for making proteins.

ribosome Granular organelle located throughout the cytoplasm and on the endoplasmic reticulum. Ribosomes contain RNA and proteins and are the site of protein synthesis.

rigor mortis *(RIG er MORE tiss)* A stiffness that occurs in dead bodies as a result of retained calcium and decreased ATP.

rods Light-sensitive cells in the retina. They detect black and white and function in daytime and nighttime vision.

root Part of the tooth that is hidden below the gum line. The premolars have 1 or more roots. The molars have multiple roots.

rotation Spin a body part on its axis.

rugae *(ROO guy)* 1. Deep folds in the gastric mucosa. 2. Folds in the mucosa of the bladder that disappear as the bladder fills with urine.

sarcomeres *(SAR ca meres)* Portion of striated muscle fibril that lies between the two adjacent dark lines.

satellite cells Neuroglia cells that enclose the cell bodies of neurons in the spinal ganglia.

Schwann cell *(SHWAN sells)* Cell that forms the myelin sheaths around axons of the cranial and spinal nerves.

sclera *(SKLAIR ah)* White, tough, fibrous connective tissue that forms the outer layer around most of the eye. Also known as the white of the eye.

sebaceous glands *(see BAY shuss)* An exocrine gland of the skin that secretes sebum. Sebaceous glands are located in the dermis. Their ducts join with a hair and sebum coats the hair shaft as it moves toward the surface of the skin. Also known as oil glands.

sebum *(SEE bum)* Oily substance secreted by sebaceous glands.

secondary response Increased immune response mediated by memory cells when meeting a pathogen which it recognizes.

secretion *(sih CREE shun)* The movement of a chemical out of a cell or gland.

segmentation Division into similar parts.

self vs. non-self recognition The ability of the immune system to distinguish between the body's cells and cells that do not belong in the body.

semicircular canals Three canals in the inner ear that are oriented in different planes (horizontally, vertically, obliquely) that help the body keep its balance. It relays information to the brain via the vestibular branch of the vestibulocochlear nerve.

septum *(SEHP tum)* 1. Wall of cartilage and bone that divides the nasal cavity into right and left sides. 2. Partitioning wall that divides the right atrium from the left atrium (interatrial septum) and the right ventricle from the left ventricle (interventricular septum).

serosa *(seh ROSE ah)* A serous membrane.

serous membrane *(SEER us)* double layered membrane lining a serous cavity. The parietal layer lines the wall of the cavity and the visceral layer covers the organs in the cavity. There is a potential, fluid-filled cavity between the layers.

sinoatrial node *(sigh noh AY tree al)* Pacemaker of the heart. Small knot of tissue located in the posterior wall of the right atrium in a shallow channel near the entrance of the superior vena cava. The SA node dictates the heart rate at 70–80 beats per minute when the body is at rest. It generates the electrical impulse for the entire conduction system of the heart.

sinus Hollow cavity within a bone of the cranium.

skeletal muscle *(SKELL eh tal)* One of 3 types of muscles in the body, but the only muscle that is under voluntary, conscious control. Under the microscope, skeletal muscle has a striated appearance.

smooth muscle One of three types of body muscles that is involuntarily controlled and found in the lining of the airways, blood vessels and uterus.

somatic nervous system *(so MAT ick)* Division of the peripheral nervous system that uses the neurotransmitter acetylcholine and carries nerve impulses to the voluntary skeletal muscles.

spasm involuntary contraction of a muscle.

sphincter *(SFING ter)* Muscular ring around a tube; a valve.

spinal cavity *(SPY nal)* A continuation of the cranial cavity as it travels down the midline of the back. The spinal cavity lies within and is protected by the bones (vertebrae) of the spinal column. The spinal cavity contains the spinal cord, the spinal nerves, and spinal fluid.

spinal cord Part of the central nervous system. Continuous with the medulla oblongata of the brain and extends down the back in the spinal cavity. Ends at L2 and separates into individual nerves (cauda equina).

spinal nerves Thirty-one pairs of nerves. Each pair comes out from the spinal cord between 2 vertebrae. An individual spinal nerve consists of dorsal nerve roots and ventral nerve roots.

spinal roots Axon bundles attached to each spinal cord segment. The dorsal roots are sensory and the ventral roots are motor. The dorsal and ventral roots join to form the spinal nerves.

spinocerebellar tract *(SPY no ser eh BELL ar)* Sensory pathway from the spinal cord to the cerebellum.

spinothalamic tract *(SPY no THAL ah mic)* Sensory pathway from the spinal cord to the thalamus and eventually the primary somatic sensory cortex. Contains pain and crude touch information.

spleen Lymphoid organ located in the abdominal cavity behind the stomach. The spleen destroys old erythrocytes, breaking their hemoglobin into heme and globins. It also acts as a storage area for whole blood. Its white pulp is lymphoid tissue that contains B and T lymphocytes.

Spores A protective barrier to allow for future reproduction in a hostile environment.

sprain Overstretching or tearing of a ligament.

squamous cells *(SKWAY muss sells)* A flat, scaly epithelial cell.

stapes *(STAY peez)* Third bone of the middle ear. It is attached to the incus on one end and the oval window on the other end. Also known as the stirrup.

Sternal Pertaining to the sternum.

sternum *(STER num)* Vertical bone of the anterior thorax to which the clavicle and ribs are attached. Also known as the breast bone.

steroids Ringed lipids that function as extremely powerful hormones.

strain Overstretching of a muscle, often due to physical overexertion. This causes inflammation, pain, swelling, and bruising as the capillaries in the muscle tear. There can be small tears in the muscle itself. Also known as a pulled muscle.

stratified *(STRAT ih fied)* Having more than one layer.

stratum basale The stem cell layer of the epidermis.

stratum corneum *(STRAY tum core NEE um)* The outer most horny layer of the epidermis.

striated muscle *(STRY ate ed)* Skeletal muscle

subarachnoid space *(SUB ah RACK noyd)* Space beneath the arachnoid layer of the meninges. It is filled with cerebrospinal fluid.

subcutaneous fascia *(sub cue TAY nee us FAY she ah)* Connective tissue layer beneath the skin.

subdural space *(sub DOO ral)* The space between the arachnoid and dura matter.

sublingual salivary glands *(sub LIN gwill SAHL ih vair ee glands)* Smallest of salivary glands found between the tongue and the mandible, one on each side.

submandibular salivary glands (sub MAN dih bue lar SAHL ih vair ee glands) Salivary gland beneath the mandible or jaw.

submucosa Layer of connective tissue under a mucous membrane.

sulcus *(SULL cuss)* One of many shallow grooves between the gyri in the cerebrum and cerebellum. Plural: sulci.

superior Pertaining to the upper half of the body or a position above an organ or structure.

superior vena cava Largest vein that drains venous blood from the upper portions of the body.

supine position *(sue PINE)* Position of lying on the posterior part of the body. Also known as the dorsal supine position.

surfactant *(sir FAC tent)* Protein-fat compound that creates surface tension and keeps the walls of the alveolus from collapsing inward with each inhalation.

sympathetic nervous system Division of the autonomic nervous system that uses the neurotransmitter norepinephrine and carries nerve impulses to the heart, involuntary muscles, and glands during times of increased activity, danger, or stress.

synapse *(SIH naps)* Space between the axon of one neuron and the dendrites of the next neuron.

syndrome *(SIN drohm)* A set of symptoms and signs associated with and characteristic of one particular disease.

Synergistic A cooperating action of certain muscles.

synovial fluids *(sin OH vee al)* Clear lubricating fluid that is secreted by the synovial membrane.

synovial membrane *(sin OH vee al)* The membrane lining a capsule of the joint.

systems An organized grouping of related structures or parts that perform specific functions.

systole *(SISS toh lee)* Combined contractions of the atria and the ventricles.

T lymphocytes *(T LIMF oh sights)* White blood cells involved in adaptive immunity. There are four types of T lymphocytes: Helper T cells, Cytotoxic T cells, Memory T cells and Regulatory T cells.

tactile corpuscles *(TAK tle KOR puss els)* Elongated bodies found in nerve ends that act as receptors for slight pressure or touch.

taste buds Sensory end organs that provide us with a sense of taste.

temporal lobe Lobe in the cerebrum that receives sensory information from the auditory cortex for hearing and the olfactory cortex for smelling.

tendonitis Inflammation of any tendon from injury or overuse.

tendon Cordlike white band of non-elastic fibrous connective tissue that attaches a muscle to a bone.

testes *(TESS teez)* Small, egg-shaped glands in the scrotum. Also known as the testicles. They contain interstitial cells that secrete testosterone. They also contain the seminiferous tubules that produce spermatozoa.

tetanus *(TETT ah nuss)* An acute infectious disease caused by a bacterium that can lead to severe spasms of voluntary muscles.

thalamus *(THAL ah mus)* Relay station in the brain that receives sensory nerve impulses from the optic nerves and sends them to the visual centers in the occipital lobes of the brain.

thoracic cage *(tho RASS ik)* The portion of the skeleton to include the ribs, sternum and thoracic vertebrae that house and protect the lungs, heart and great vessels.

thoracic cavity *(thoh RASS ik KAV ih tee)* Hollow space within the thorax that is filled with the lungs and structures in the mediastinum.

thoracic duct *(thoh RASS ik)* The main lymph duct of the body.

thrombin *(THROM bin)* An enzyme that reacts with fibrinogen , converting it to fibrin which forms a clot.

thrombocyte *(THROM boh sights)* Cell fragment that is flat and does not have a nucleus. It is active in the blood clotting process. Thrombocytes are also known as blood platelets.

thrombocytopenia *(THROM boh sigh TOH PEE nee ah)* Deficiency in the number of thrombocytes. This can be due to exposure to radiation or toxic chemicals or drugs that damage the stem cells in the bone marrow.

thrombus *(THROM buss)* A blood clot.

thymus *(THIGH muss)* Lymphoid organ in the thoracic cavity. As an endocrine gland, it releases hormones known as thymosins. The thymosins cause lymphoblasts in the thymus to mature into T lymphocytes.

thyroid gland *(THIGH royd)* Endocrine gland in the neck that produces and secretes the hormones T3, T4, and calcitonin. Its 2 lobes and narrow connecting bridge (isthmus) give it a shield-like shape.

tinnitus *(tinn EYE tuss)* Sounds (buzzing, ringing, hissing, or roaring) that are heard constantly or intermittently in one or both ears, even in a quiet environment.

tissues Collection of similar cells that form a particular function,

tongue Large muscle that fills the oral cavity and assists with eating and talking. It contains taste buds and receptors for the sense of taste.

tonus *(TONE us)* A partial steady contraction of a muscle; firmness.

trabecula *(tra BECK you la)* A fibrous cord of connective tissues that acts as a supporting fiber.

trachea *(TRAY kee ah)* Rigid tubular air pipe between the larynx and the bronchi that is a passageway for inhaled and exhaled air.

transitional *(tran ZISH ion al)* Moving from one state to another.

transverse plane *(tranz VERS)* Plane that divides the body into top and bottom sections, superior and inferior.

tricuspid Pertains to having three cusps or points as in the tricuspid valve of the right heart.

tuberculosis (TB) *(too ber kew LOH sis)* Lung infection caused by the bacterium mycobacterium tuberculosis and spread by air-borne droplets expelled by coughing.

tubular reabsorption Movement of substances out of the renal tubule and back into the blood. The substances will be retained in the body.

tubular secretion Movement of substances from the blood into the renal tubule. These substances will leave the body in the urine.

tumor necrosis factor (TNF) *(neh KROH siss)* Released by macrophages, it destroys endotoxins produced by certain bacteria. It also destroys cancer cells.

tunica externa *(TOO nik ah ex TERN ah)* The outer layer of an artery.

tunica interna *(TOO nik ah in TERN ah)* The inner lining of an artery.

tunica media *(TOO nik ah mee DEE ah)* The middle muscular layer of an artery.

turbinates Three long projections (superior, middle, inferior) of the ethmoid bone that jut into the nasal cavity: superior, middle, and inferior. They break up the stream of air as it enters the nose. Also known as the nasal conchae.

tympanic membrane *(tihm PAN ik)* Membrane that divides the external ear from the middle ear. Also known as the eardrum.

universal donor A person who has the type O blood that can be transfused to any individual of the ABO blood groups.

universal recipient A person who has type AB blood who can receive blood from the ABO blood groups.

upper respiratory infection (URI) Bacterial or viral infection of the nose that can spread to the throat and ears. The nose is a part of the respiratory system as well as the ENT system. Also known as a common cold or head cold.

ureter *(yoo REE ter)* Tube that connects the pelvis of the kidney to the bladder.

urethra *(yoo REE thrah)* Tube that connects the bladder to the outside of the body.

urinary bladder Holding receptacle for urine before it is expelled (voided) from the body.

vagus nerve Cranial nerve X. Sensation and movement of the throat. Sensory and motor for thoracic and abdominal organs.

vasculature Network of blood vessels in a particular organ.

vasoconstriction *(vaz oh kon STRIK shun)* Constriction of the smooth muscle in the artery wall causes the artery to become smaller in diameter.

vasodilation *(vaz oh DYE lay shun)* Relaxation of the smooth muscle in the artery wall causes the artery to become larger in diameter.

vein Blood vessel that carries oxygen-poor blood as well as carbon dioxide and waste products of cellular metabolism away from the cells and back to the heart. Veins have one-way valves that keep blood from flowing backwards, away from the heart. The exception is the pulmonary vein, which carries oxygenated blood from the lungs to the heart.

ventilation *(ven tih LAY shun)* The bulk movement of gas into and out of the lungs.

ventral Pertaining to the anterior of the body particularly the abdomen.

ventricles *(VEN trik lz)* 1. Two lower chambers of the heart. Intraventricular structures are located in the ventricles. 2. Four hollow chambers within the brain that contain cerebrospinal fluid. The 2 lateral ventricles are within the right and left hemispheres of the cerebrum. The third ventricle is small and connects the lateral ventricles to the fourth ventricle, which is at the level of the pons and medulla oblongata.

venules *(VEHN yules)* Smallest branch of a vein.

vertebrae *(VER teh bray)* One of 33 irregularly shaped bony segments of the spinal column.

vertigo Sensation of being off balance when the body is not moving. Caused by upper respiratory infection, middle or inner ear infection, head trauma, or degenerative changes of the semicircular canals.

vesicle *(VESS ih kle)* A small bladder or blister; a membrane bound storage sac inside a cell.

vestibule chamber *(VESS tih byool)* A small cavity or space at the beginning of a canal.

Vestibulocochlear nerve *(VESS tih byool KOHK lee are)* The eighth cranial nerve responsible for hearing and balance. Sometimes called the acoustic nerve.

villi *(VILL eye)* Microscopic projections of the mucosa within the lumen of the small intestine.

Virus A parasitic microorganism that depends on other cells for its metabolic and reproductive needs.

visceral *(VISS er al)* Pertaining to organs.

visceral pleura *(VISS er al PLOO rah)* One of the 2 membranes of the pleura. It covers the surface of the lung.

vital signs Medical procedure during a physical examination in which the temperature, pulse, and respirations (TPR), as well as the blood pressure, are measured.

vitreous humor *(VITT ree uss HYOO mer)* Clear, gel-like substance that fills the posterior cavity of the eye.

vocal cords Connective tissue bands in the larynx that vibrate and produce sounds for speaking and singing.

white blood cells (WBCs) Leukocytes; responsible for the immune response.

z lines Lines visible on the surface of skeletal muscle that mark the ends of each sarcomere.

Index